Clinical Atlas of Cardiac and Aortic CT and MRI

Patricia M. Carrascosa · Carlos M. Capuñay
Alejandro Deviggiano
Gastón A. Rodríguez-Granillo
Editors

Clinical Atlas of Cardiac and Aortic CT and MRI

Springer

Editors
Patricia M. Carrascosa
Department of Cardiovascular Imaging
Associate Professor of Radiology
Buenos Aires University
Diagnostico Maipú
Buenos Aires
Buenos Aires
Argentina

Alejandro Deviggiano
Department of Cardiovascular Imaging
Diagnostico Maipú
Buenos Aires
Buenos Aires
Argentina

Carlos M. Capuñay
Department of Cardiovascular Imaging
Diagnostico Maipú
Buenos Aires
Buenos Aires
Argentina

Gastón A. Rodríguez-Granillo
Department of Cardiovascular Imaging
Department of Research
Diagnostico Maipú
Buenos Aires
Buenos Aires
Argentina

ISBN 978-3-030-03681-2 ISBN 978-3-030-03682-9 (eBook)
https://doi.org/10.1007/978-3-030-03682-9

Library of Congress Control Number: 2019930252

Illustrations by Daniel Cirigliano: Diagnostico Maipu, Departmento de Investigacion. Av. Maipú 1668, Vicente López B1602ABQ, Buenos Aires, Argentina

This Springer imprint is published by the registered company Springer Nature Switzerland AG
The registered company address is: Gewerbestrasse 11, 6330 Cham, Switzerland

Foreword

It is just about 20 years ago when the concept of "Advanced Cardiac Imaging" emerged, adding multi-slice cardiac CT and contrast-enhanced cardiac MRI to the curriculum of trainees in the sub-specialty of cardiovascular medicine and rapidly becoming a subspecialty of interest for cardiologists and radiologists. It was about that time when I met Patricia Carrascosa, a radiologist with an unmatched energy level, who over the years has proven excellence as a clinician and as a clinical investigator. Among her many strengths, Dr. Carrascosa has shown a vision to move clinical research beyond any limits but focusing on unmet clinical needs, discovered through her collaboration with local and international leaders from both the radiology and cardiology worlds. I have been fortunate to have the opportunity of participating with her in many projects, and I am a witness of her creativity and perseverance, both essential qualities for a leader. Most of the authors and editors of this book have been our colleagues and have also emerged as leaders in the field, coming together now to produce a comprehensive compendium of images accompanied by a summary of the essential technical and clinical information that should be relevant to the practice of advanced cardiac imaging.

This Atlas should be equally useful to those who are involved in the interpretation of cardiovascular imaging studies, regardless of their technical area of expertise, as well as to clinicians who often wonder what the most appropriate method to establish a diagnosis is. Each chapter has been carefully crafted to cover all clinical aspects of cardiovascular imaging succinctly and comprehensively at the same time. High-quality images are accompanied by clear diagrams and tables that will be useful to readers and consultants.

"*Now, here, you see, it takes all the running you can do, to keep in the same place. If you want to get somewhere else, you must run at least twice as fast as that!*" – written by Lewis Carroll in *Through the Looking-Glass* defines Carrascosa as the Alice in the Wonderland of Imaging. Congratulations to her and her colleagues in another great accomplishment.

Mario J. Garcia
Division of Cardiology, Medicine and Radiology
Montefiore-Einstein Center for Heart and Vascular Care
New York, NY
USA

Contents

Contributors

Fernando Abramzon, MD Cardiovascular Imaging, Department of Radiology, Hospital de Trauma y Emergencias "Dr. Federico Abete", University of Buenos Aires, Buenos Aires, Argentina

Maria Jose Bosaleh, MD Department of Pediatrics, Pediatric Cardiology Section, Department of Radiology, Section of CT and MR, Hospital Nacional Alejandro Posadas, Buenos Aires, Argentina

Carlos M. Capuñay, MD Departments of CT, MR, and Research, Department of Cardiovascular Imaging, Diagnostico Maipu, Buenos Aires, Argentina

Jimena B. Carpio, MD Department of CT and MR, Diagnóstico Maipú, Buenos Aires, Argentina

Patricia M. Carrascosa, MD, PhD, FACC, FSCCT Departments of CT, MR, and Research, Department of Cardiovascular Imaging, Diagnostico Maipu, Buenos Aires, Argentina

University of Buenos Aires, Buenos Aires, Argentina

Latin American Committee of the Society of Cardiovascular Computed Tomography, Buenos Aires, Argentina

Alejandro H. de la Vega, MD Cardiovascular Imaging, CT and MR of Clinica de Imagenes and Fundación Médica de Río Negro y Neuquén, Cipolletti, Argentina

Macarena C. De Zan, MD Cardiovascular CT and MR, CEMIC and Fundación Centro Diagnostico Nuclear, Buenos Aires, Argentina

Alejandro Deviggiano, MD Department of Cardiovascular Imaging, Diagnostico Maipu, Buenos Aires, Argentina

Cardiac CT and MRI Council of the Argentinian Society of Cardiology, Buenos Aires, Argentina

Mariano L. Falconi, MD Universidad del Salvador, Buenos Aires, Argentina

Cardiology Specialist Career, Instituto Universitario Hospital Italiano, Buenos Aires, Argentina

Cardiovascular Imaging Unit, Cardiology Division, Hospital Italiano of Buenos Aires, Buenos Aires, Argentina

Andrea Maria Giovannini Bercht, MD Cardiovascular Magnetic Resonance and Computed Tomography Department, Heart Institute (InCor), University of Sao Paulo Medical School, Sao Paulo, Brazil

Ezequiel Levy Yeyati, MD Cardiovascular Imaging, Department of Radiology, Hospital Municipal de Merlo "Eva Perón", University of Buenos Aires, Buenos Aires, Argentina

Cesar Nomura, MD Cardiovascular Magnetic Resonance and Computed Tomography Department, Heart Institute (InCor), University of Sao Paulo Medical School, Sao Paulo, Brazil

Diego Pérez de Arenaza, MD Cardiovascular Imaging Section, Department of Cardiology, Hospital Italiano de Buenos Aires, Buenos Aires, Argentina

Pablo Pollono, MD Department of Cardiovascular Imaging, Hospital del Cruce, Florencio Varela, Buenos Aires, Argentina

Gastón A. Rodríguez-Granillo, MD, PhD, FACC Department of Cardiovascular Imaging, Department of Research, Diagnostico Maipu, Buenos Aires, Argentina

National Council of Scientific and Technical Investigations (CONICET), Buenos Aires, Argentina

Natalia Aldana Sepulveda, MD Clinical Radiology Universidad CES, Medellín, Colombia

Clinical Radiology Universidad Pontificia Bolivariana, Medellín, Colombia

CEDIMED, Body and Cardiovascular Imaging sections, Medellín, Colombia

Juan Wolcan, MD Department of Cardiovascular Imaging, Hospital del Cruce, Florencio Varela, Buenos Aires, Argentina

Alejandro Zuluaga Santamaría, MD, FSCMR Clinical Radiology Universidad CES, Medellín, Colombia

Clinical Radiology Universidad Pontificia Bolivariana, Medellín, Colombia

Radiology Residence Universidad Pontificia Bolivariana, Medellín, Colombia

CEDIMED, Body and Cardio-vascular Imaging sections, Medellín, Colombia

Cardiac Anatomy and Coronary Artery Anomalies

1

Patricia M. Carrascosa and Carlos M. Capuñay

Normal Anatomy of the Coronary Arteries

The left main coronary artery (LMCA) normally originates from the left coronary sinus of Valsalva, giving rise to the left anterior descending (LAD) artery and the left circumflex (LCx) artery (Fig. 1.1). In 7–8% of patients it gives a third branch, known as the ramus intermedius. Major branches of LAD are the septal and diagonal arteries, whereas the LCx branches are the obtuse marginal (lateral) branches. In cases of left dominance, the LCx gives the posterior descending artery (PDA) and posterolateral branch.

The right coronary artery (RCA) normally arises from the right coronary sinus (Fig. 1.1). Branches include the conus artery (50–60% of cases) and acute marginal branches. In 85% of cases, there is right dominance, giving rise to PDA and posterolateral branch (Fig. 1.2).

Coronary artery segmentation, adapted from the standard American Heart Association (AHA) classification, has been proposed to facilitate description and reporting of findings on coronary CT angiography (Fig. 1.2).

Based on the myocardial 17-segment model proposed by the AHA, the arterial blood flow distribution can be assigned to the most frequent corresponding coronary artery territory (Fig. 1.3).

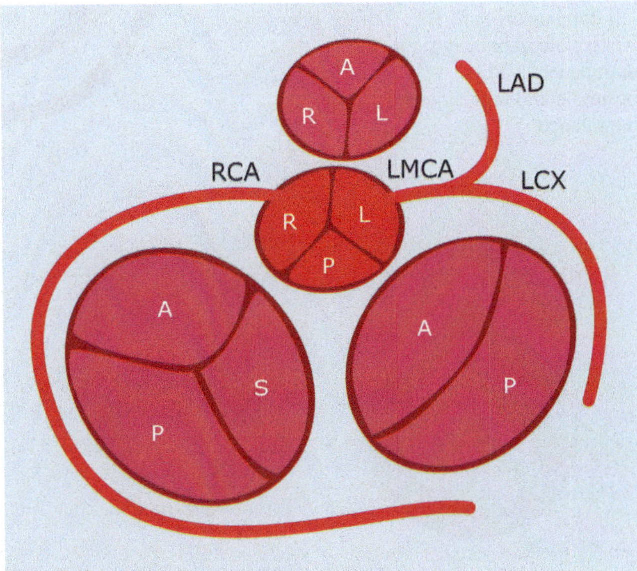

Fig. 1.1 Normal relationship between the coronary arteries and cardiac valves. The pulmonary artery is the most anterior structure and its valve has three cusps (anterior, A; left, L; and right, R). The aortic valve has three cusps (left, L; right, R; and the noncoronary posterior cusp, P). The LMCA arises from the left coronary sinus of Valsalva and the right coronary artery (RCA) from the right sinus. The posterior coronary cusp does not originate any vessel. The left anterior descending artery (LAD) has a course through the anterior interventricular septum and the left circumflex (LCX) courses through the left atrioventricular sulcus, related to the mitral valve (with two cusps/leaflets, anterior, A; and posterior, P). The RCA has a course through the right atrioventricular sulcus, related to the tricuspid valve (with three cusps, anterior, A; septal, S; and posterior, P)

P. M. Carrascosa (✉)
Departments of CT, MR, and Research, Department of Cardiovascular Imaging, Diagnostico Maipu, Buenos Aires, Argentina

University of Buenos Aires, Buenos Aires, Argentina

Latin American Committee of the Society of Cardiovascular Computed Tomography, Buenos Aires, Argentina
e-mail: patriciacarrascosa@diagnosticomaipu.com.ar

C. M. Capuñay
Departments of CT, MR, and Research, Department of Cardiovascular Imaging, Diagnostico Maipu, Buenos Aires, Argentina

P. M. Carrascosa et al. (eds.), *Clinical Atlas of Cardiac and Aortic CT and MRI*, https://doi.org/10.1007/978-3-030-03682-9_1

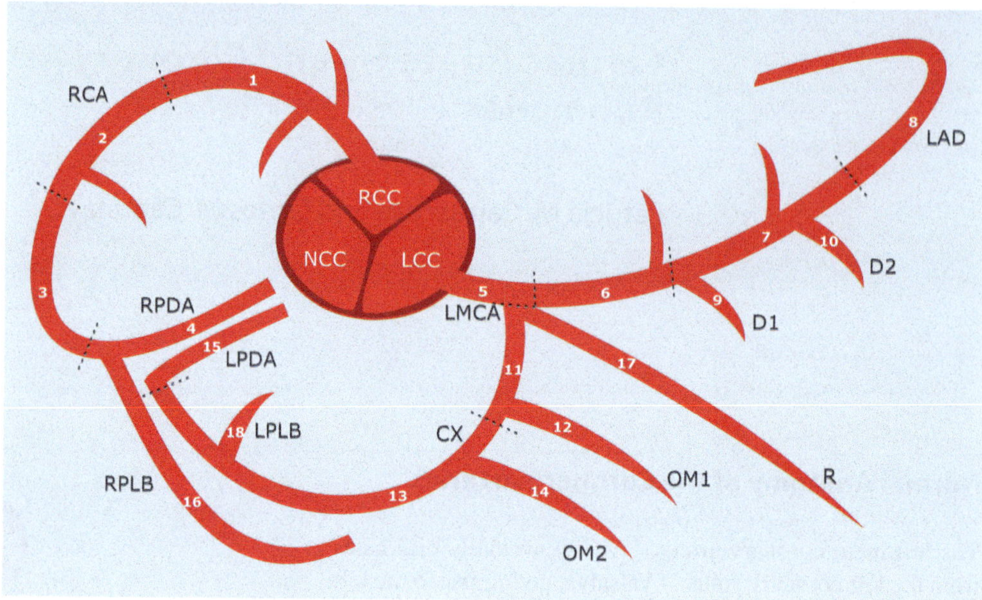

Fig. 1.2 Coronary artery segmentation diagram proposed by the Society of Cardiovascular Computed Tomography based on the standard American Heart Association classification. LMCA left main coronary artery, D diagonal branch, LAD left anterior descending artery, R ramus intermedius, OM obtuse marginal, CX left circumflex artery, RCA right coronary artery, R-PDA posterior descending artery, right dominance, L-PDA posterior descending artery, left dominance, R-PLB posterolateral branch, right dominance, L-PLB posterolateral branch, left dominance

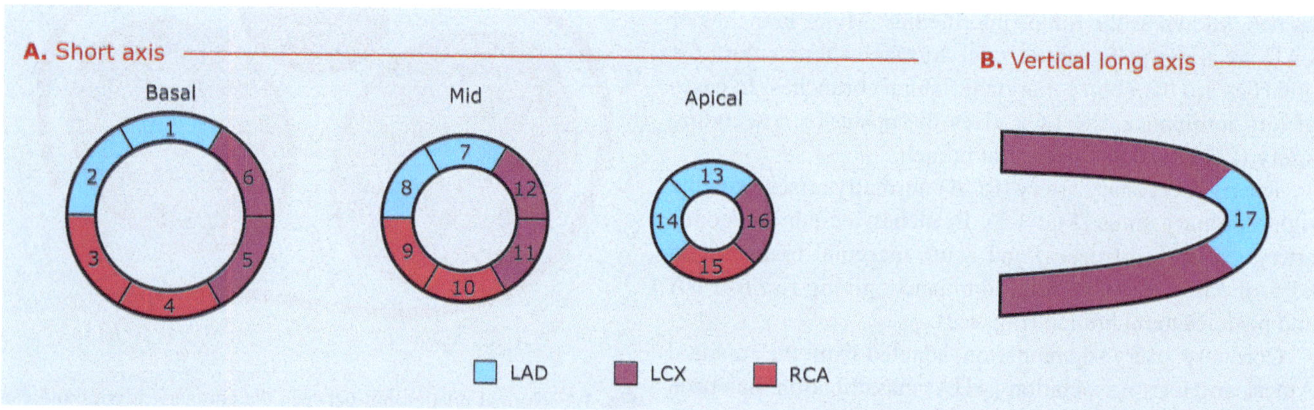

Fig. 1.3 (**a**) Left ventricular 17-segment myocardial model as proposed by the American Heart Association, with corresponding coronary artery territories. 1, Basal anterior; 2, basal anteroseptal; 3, basal inferoseptal; 4, basal inferior; 5, basal inferolateral; 6, basal anterolateral; 7, mid anterior; 8, mid-anteroseptal; 9, mid-inferoseptal; 10, mid-inferior; 11, mid-inferolateral; 12, mid-anterolateral; 13, apical anterior; 14, apical septal; 15, apical inferior; 16, apical lateral; 17, apex. LAD left anterior descending artery, RCA right coronary artery, LCx left circumflex artery (**b**) Left ventricular segmentation

Coronary Artery Anomalies

Isolated coronary artery anomalies are rare, with an incidence of 0.5–1% of the general population. Most of them are asymptomatic and without clinical relevance. Nevertheless, they can have hemodynamic significance according to their origin and proximal course.

Cross-sectional noninvasive imaging modalities such as cardiac magnetic resonance (MR) and especially computed tomography coronary angiography (CTCA) provide accurate two-dimensional and three-dimensional images, enabling the visualization of coronary artery anatomy and the relationship of the vessels to adjacent structures.

Coronary artery anomalies can be classified into anomalies of origin and course, anomalies of intrinsic anatomy, and anomalies of termination. Also, they can be classified according to the hemodynamic significance: either nonsignificant or significant coronary anomalies, including in the last group an anomalous origin of the RCA or LMCA from the pulmo-

Table 1.1 Coronary artery anomalies classification

Anomalies of origination and course
Absent left main trunk (split origination of LAD and LCx)
Anomalous location of coronary ostium within the aortic root or near proper aortic sinus High Low Commissural
Anomalous location of coronary ostium outside normal coronary aortic sinuses Posterior "noncoronary" aortic sinus Ascending aorta Left ventricle – Right ventricle Pulmonary artery Aortic arch Innominate artery Descending thoracic aorta
Anomalous location of coronary ostium at improper sinus RCA that arises from left anterior sinus, with anomalous course Retroaortic Between aorta and pulmonary artery (inter-arterial) Intraseptal (transeptal) Anterior to pulmonary outflow Posteroanterior interventricular groove (wraparound) LAD that arises from right anterior sinus, with anomalous course Between aorta and pulmonary artery (inter-arterial) Intraseptal (transeptal) Anterior to pulmonary outflow Posteroanterior interventricular groove (wraparound) LCx that arises from right anterior sinus, with anomalous course Retroaortic LMCA that arises from right anterior sinus, with anomalous course Retroaortic Between aorta and pulmonary artery (inter-arterial) Intraseptal (transeptal) Anterior to pulmonary outflow
Single coronary artery
Anomalies of intrinsic coronary arterial anatomy
Congenital ostial stenosis or atresia
Coronary ectasia or aneurysm
Absent coronary artery
Coronary hypoplasia
Intramural coronary artery (myocardial bridging)
Subendocardial coronary course
Coronary crossing
Split RCA
Split LAD
Anomalies of termination
Coronary artery fistula

LMCA left main coronary artery, *RCA* right coronary artery, *LCx* circumflex artery, *LAD* left anterior descending artery

nary artery, an anomalous course of the RCA or LMCA between the aorta and the pulmonary artery, congenital coronary artery fistula, and complete myocardial bridging (Table 1.1; Fig. 1.4). Finally, it is important to discriminate major coronary anomalies (anomalous origin of a coronary artery from the opposite sinus with inter-arterial course between the aorta and pulmonary artery), related to a higher risk of sudden cardiac death.

Normal Cardiac Anatomy

In order to understand cardiac anatomy and the relationship between structures, it is important to have a clear picture through conventional axial views of the chest from the supra-aortic trunks to the coronary sinus/inferior vena cava (Fig. 1.5). The relevance of understanding these images is of outmost importance for the assessment of complex cases such as patients with congenital heart disease.

Nomenclature of short, horizontal long (four-chamber), and vertical long (two-chamber) axes has been recommended for the cardiac planes generated by cross-sectional or tomographic imaging methods such as CT and MR. These planes must be oriented at 90° angles relative to each other.

Relationship between cardiac chambers, evaluation of the myocardium, assessment of cardiac valves and ventricular function, and determination of the area of any cardiac structure (valves, chambers) can be assessed based on these cardiac planes.

Three short-axis slices of the basal, mid-cavity, and apical region of the left ventricle are selected for regional analysis of left ventricular systolic function or myocardial perfusion, while the true apex (segment AHA-17) must be assessed on the vertical long axis and horizontal or four-chamber views.

The three-chamber view optimizes the evaluation of the left ventricular outflow tract, aortic valve and root, and the ascending aorta.

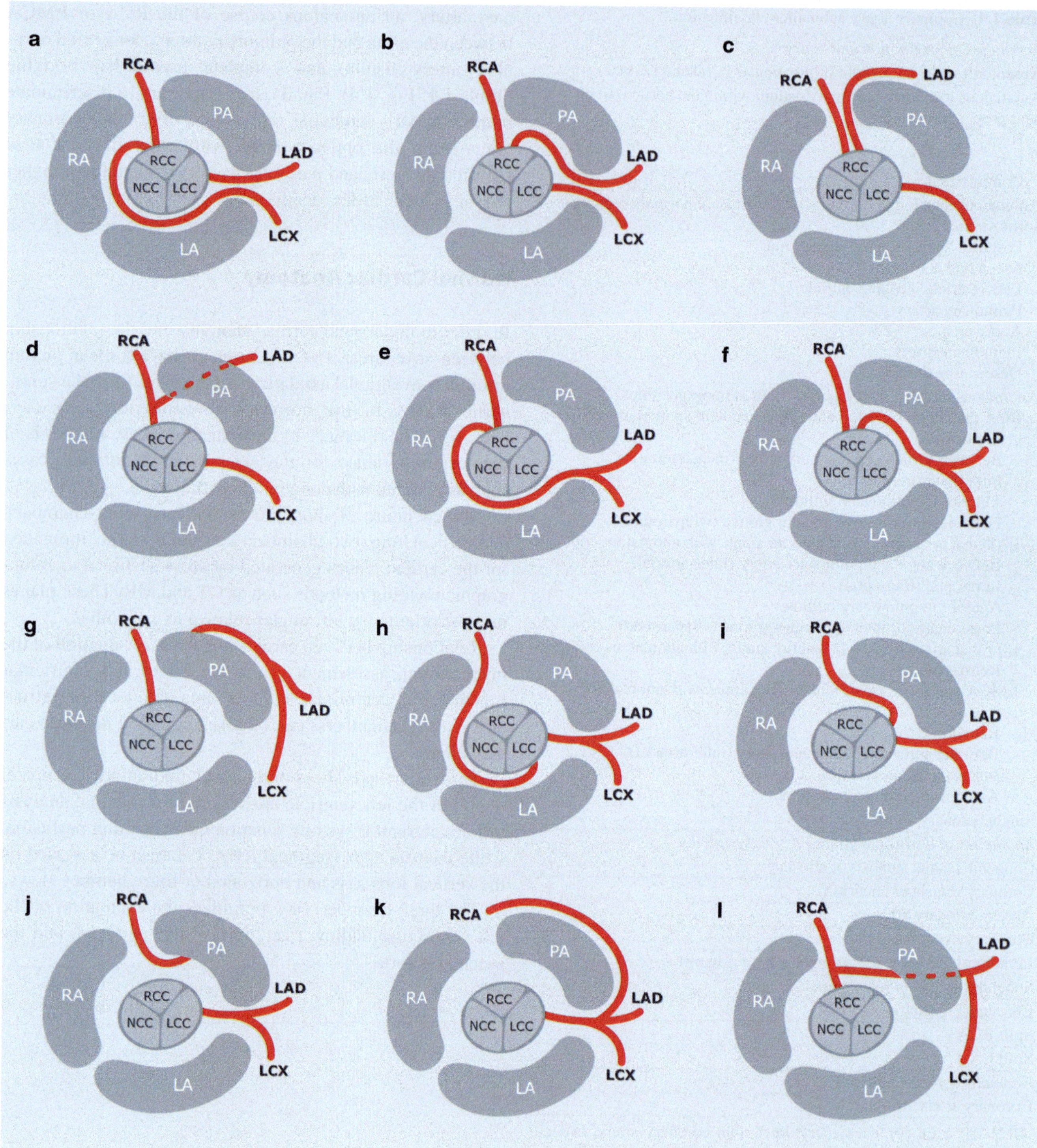

Fig. 1.4 Most common coronary artery anomalies. (**a**) LCx arising from the right coronary sinus, with retroaortic course. (**b**) LAD arising from the right coronary sinus, with inter-arterial course between the aorta and the pulmonary artery (PA). (**c**) LAD arising from the right coronary sinus, with pre-pulmonary course. (**d**) LAD arising from the right coronary artery, with transeptal/sub-pulmonary course. (**e**) LMCA arising from the right coronary sinus, with retroaortic course between the aorta and the left atrium (LA). (**f**) LMCA arising from the right coronary sinus, with inter-arterial course (between aorta and pulmonary artery) (**g**) LMCA arising from the pulmonary trunk (ALCAPA) (**h**) RCA arising from the left coronary sinus, with retroaortic course. (**i**) RCA arising from the left coronary sinus, with inter-arterial course (between aorta and pulmonary artery). (**j**) RCA arising from the pulmonary trunk. (**k**) Single coronary artery arising from the left coronary sinus with RCA course anterior to RV pulmonary trunk. (**l**) LMCA arising from the RCA, with transseptal/sub-pulmonary course

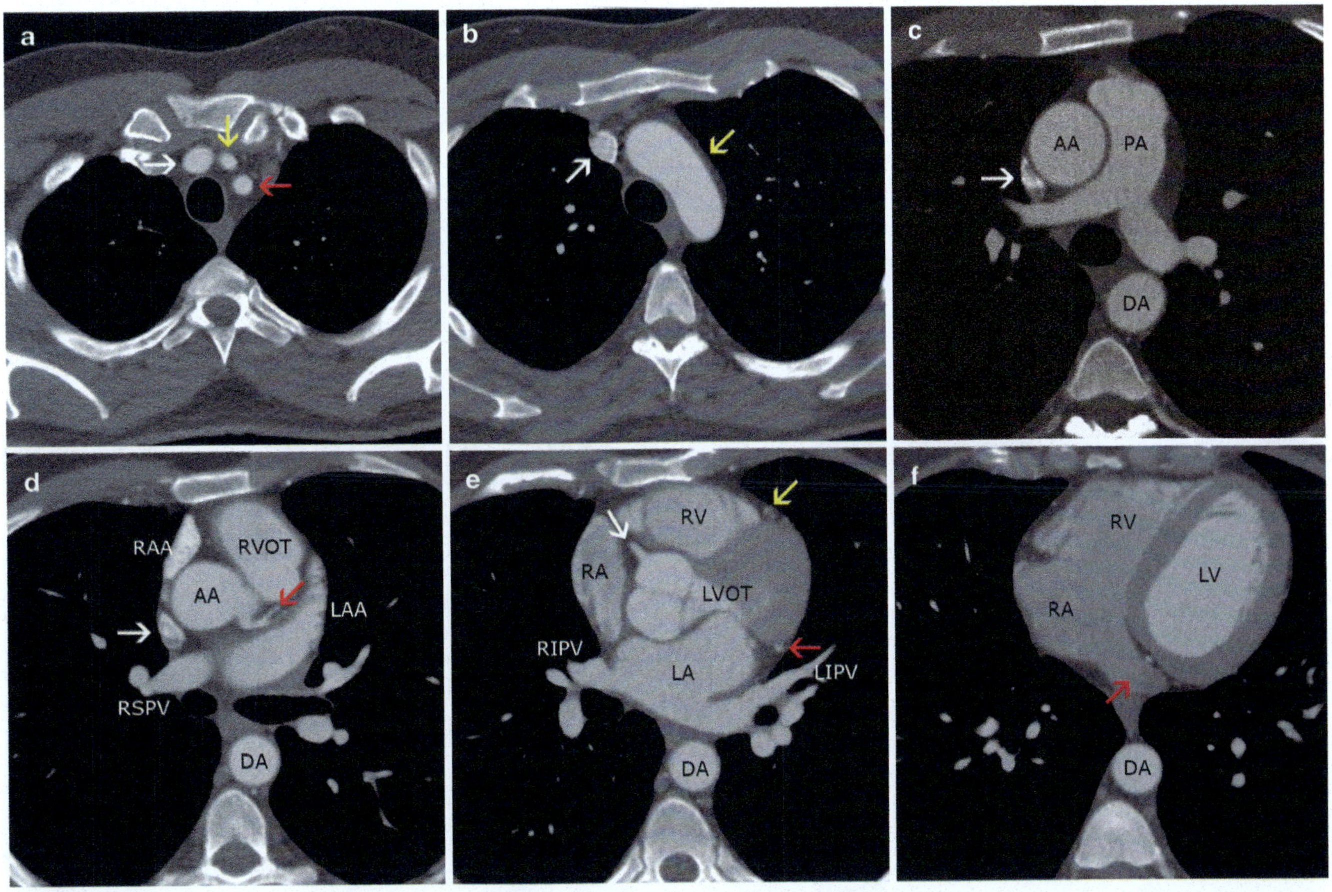

Fig. 1.5 Computed tomography angiography axial views from the supraaortic trunks to the coronary sinus. Panel (**a**): axial view at the supraaortic trunks (white arrow, innominate trunk; yellow arrow, left common carotid; red arrow, left subclavian artery). Panel (**b**): axial view at the aortic arch (yellow arrow) level, also showing the superior vena cava (SVC, white arrow). Panel (**c**): axial view at the ascending aorta (AA) level, also showing the pulmonary artery (PA), the descending aorta (DA), and the SVC (white arrow). Panel (**d**): axial view at the aortic root level (AA), showing the right ventricular outflow tract (RVOT), the right atrial appendage (RAA), the left atrial appendage (LAA), the right superior pulmonary vein (RSPV), the SVC (white arrow), and the left coronary artery (red arrow). Panel (**e**): slightly lower axial view showing the origin of the right coronary artery (white arrow), the left anterior descending artery (yellow arrow), the left circumflex (red arrow), the right ventricle (RV), the left ventricular outflow tract (LVOT), the right atrium (RA), the left atrium (LA), the right inferior pulmonary vein (RIPV), and the left inferior pulmonary vein (LIPV). Panel (**f**): a lower axial view shows the coronary sinus (red arrow) draining to the RA, the left ventricle (LV), and the RV

Further Reading

Angelini P. Coronary artery anomalies: an entity in search of an identity. Circulation. 2007;115(10):1296–305.

Angelini P, Villason S, Chan A, et al. Normal and anomalous coronary arteries in humans. In: Angelini P, Fairchild VD, editors. Coronary artery anomalies: a comprehensive approach. Philadelphia: Lippincott Williams & Wilkins; 1999. p. 27–150.

Cerqueira MD, Weissman NJ, Dilsizian V, Jacobs AK, Kaul S, Laskey WK, et al. Standardized myocardial segmentation and nomenclature for tomographic imaging of the heart: a statement for healthcare professionals from the Cardiac Imaging Committee of the Council on Clinical Cardiology of the American Heart Association. Circulation. 2002;105:539–42.

Heermann P, Heindel W, Schülke C. Coronary artery anomalies: diagnosis and classification based on cardiac CT and MRI (CMR) - from ALCAPA to anomalies of termination. Rofo. 2017;189:29–38.

Lee S, Uppu SC, Lytrivi ID, Sanz J, Weigand J, Geiger MK, et al. Utility of multimodality imaging in the morphologic characterization of anomalous aortic origin of a coronary artery. World J Pediatr Congenit Heart Surg. 2016;7:308–17.

Leipsic J, Abbara S, Achenbach S, Cury R, Earls JP, Mancini GJ, et al. SCCT guidelines for the interpretation and reporting of coronary CT angiography: a report of the Society of Cardiovascular Computed Tomography Guidelines Committee. J Cardiovasc Comput Tomogr. 2014;8:342–58.

Case 1

Normal Coronary Arteries

Clinical History

- Forty-six-year-old female.
- Patient with low pretest probability of coronary artery disease (CAD) with equivocal stress test findings.
- Medical history indicates controlled hypertension and a history of hyperlipidemia.
- The patient was referred to computed tomography coronary angiography (CTCA) to rule out CAD.

Images

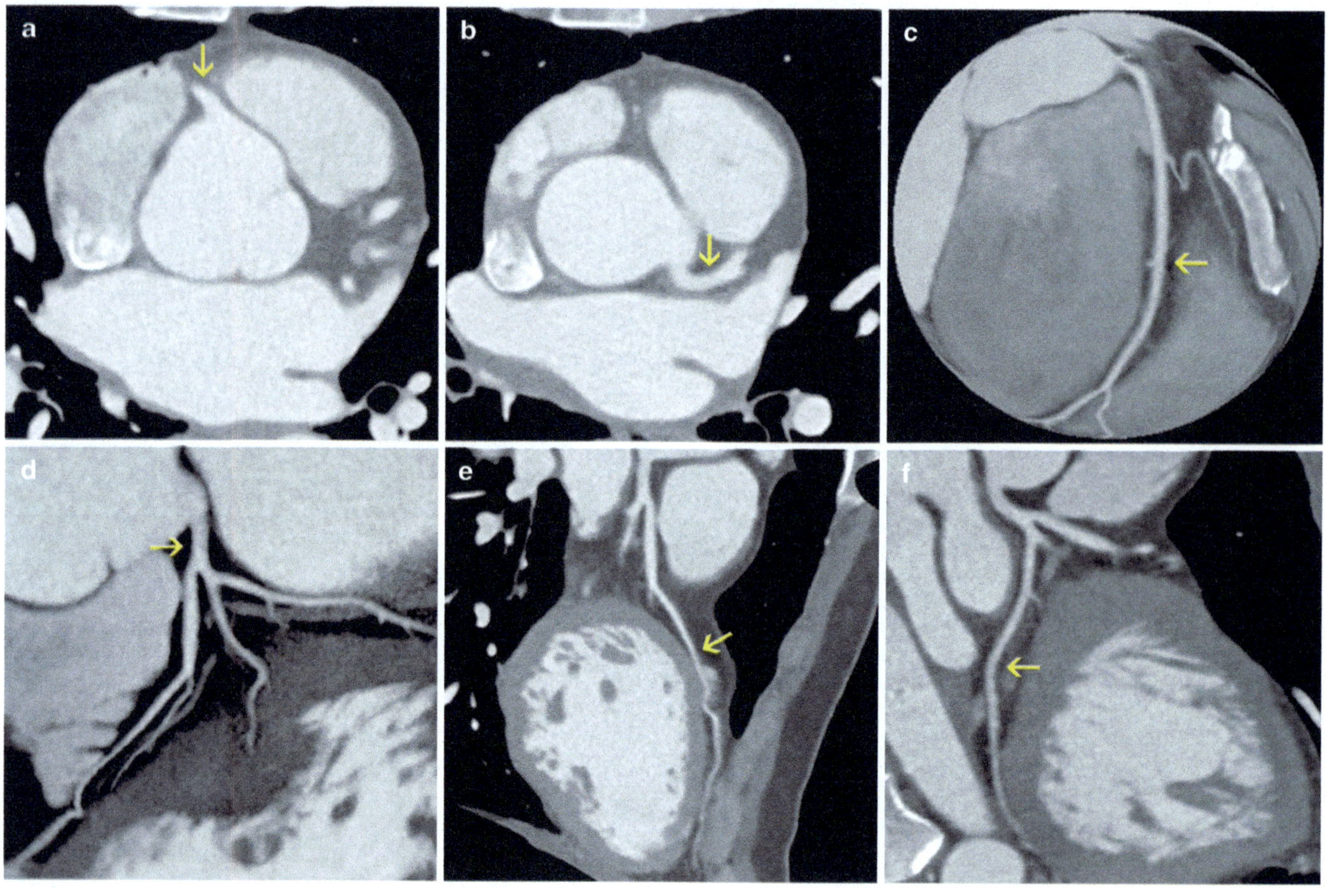

Findings and Interpretation

- CTCA was performed demonstrating normal coronary arteries.
- Axial CT image (panel A) shows normal origin of the right coronary artery (RCA) from the right anterior coronary sinus (arrow). Axial CT image (panel B) shows normal origin of the left main coronary artery (LMCA) from the left anterior coronary sinus (arrow). Curved multiplanar reconstructions show a normal RCA (panel C), a normal LMCA and its two branches (panel D), a normal left anterior descending coronary artery (panel E), and a normal left circumflex artery (panel F).
- CTCA can assess the presence, as well as the extent, of coronary artery stenosis.
- A normal CTCA has a high negative predictive value (98–100%) for excluding CAD.
- In patients with a low to intermediate probability of CAD who are unable to exercise or with inconclusive functional test results, current guidelines recommend the use of CTCA.

Further Reading

Sheikh M, Ben-Nakhi A, Shukkur AM, Sinan T, Al-Rashdan I. Accuracy of 64-multidetector-row computed tomography in the diagnosis of coronary artery disease. Med Princ Pract. 2009;18:323–8.

Stein PD, Beemath A, Kayali F, Skaf E, Sanchez J, Olson RE. Multidetector computed tomography for the diagnosis of coronary artery disease: a systematic review. Am J Med. 2006;119:203–16.

Thomas DM, Branch KR, Cury RC. PROMISE of coronary CT angiography: precise and accurate diagnosis and prognosis in coronary artery disease. South Med J. 2016;109:242–7.

Case 2

Normal Coronary Arteries

Clinical History

- Fifty-six-year-old female.
- Patient presents a prolonged episode of chest pain associated to shortness of breath. The electrocardiogram showed negative T waves in the anterior leads, and cardiac markers are nonconclusive.
- The patient has intermediate pretest probability of coronary artery disease (CAD).
- Medical history indicates controlled hypertension.
- The patient was referred to computed tomography coronary angiography (CTCA) to rule out CAD.

Images

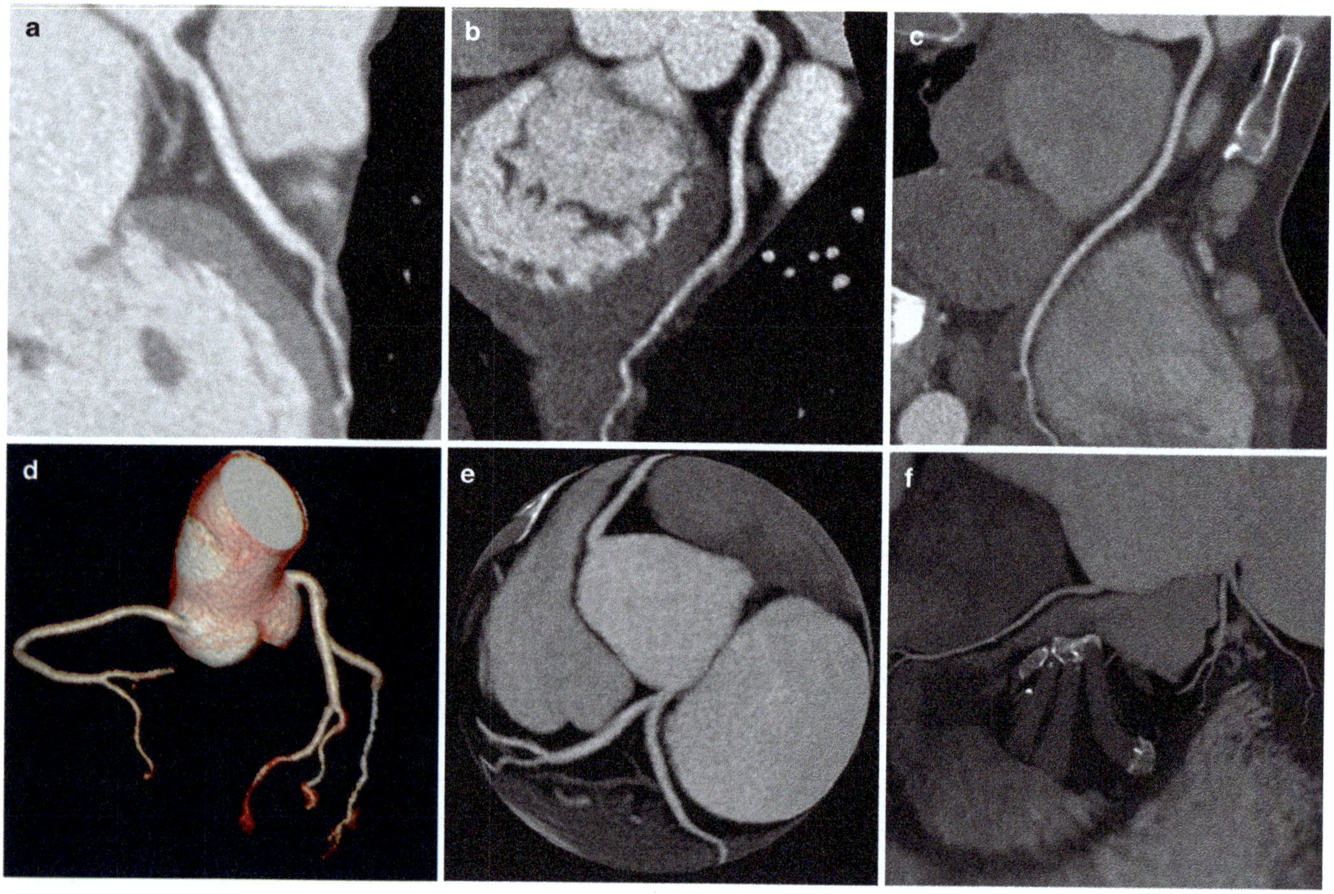

Findings and Interpretation

- CTCA was performed demonstrating normal coronary arteries.
- Curved multiplanar reconstructions show a normal left main coronary artery (LMCA) and left anterior descending coronary artery (LAD, panel A), normal left circumflex artery (LCX, panel B), and normal right coronary artery (RCA, panel C).
- Volume rendering reconstruction of the coronary tree (panel D), 3D-globe maximum intensity projection (MIP) image (panel E), and 2D-MIP image (panel F) demonstrate the absence of coronary artery disease (CAD).
- Cardiovascular disease remains a leading cause of morbidity and mortality worldwide. CAD requires accurate and timely diagnosis, being a challenge according to each patient characteristics and the clinical setting.
- CTCA is a noninvasive, expeditious, and in some instances more cost-effective alternative diagnostic test to rule out CAD in the appropriate clinical scenario.
- A normal CTCA has a high negative predictive value (98–100%) for excluding CAD. The 2010 Cardiac CT Appropriateness Criteria considered appropriate the use of cardiac CT in low- to intermediate-risk patients with acute chest pain and nondiagnostic ECG and serum biomarkers.

Further Reading

Stein PD, Beemath A, Kayali F, Skaf E, Sanchez J, Olson RE. Multidetector computed tomography for the diagnosis of coronary artery disease: a systematic review. Am J Med. 2006;119:203–16.

Taylor AJ, Cerqueira M, Hodgson JM, Mark D, Min J, O'Gara P, Rubin GD. ACCF/SCCT/ACR/AHA/ASE/ASNC/NASCI/SCAI/SCMR 2010 appropriate use criteria for cardiac computed tomography. J Cardiovasc Comput Tomogr. 2010;4:407.e1–33.

Thomas DM, Branch KR, Cury RC. PROMISE of coronary CT angiography: precise and accurate diagnosis and prognosis in coronary artery disease. South Med J. 2016;109:242–7.

Case 3

Complete Myocardial Bridging

Clinical History

- Fifty-four-year-old male.
- He had a recent hospitalization for atrial fibrillation with rapid ventricular response.
- Stress echocardiography did not show evidence of myocardial ischemia.
- A computed tomography coronary angiography (CTCA) was indicated.

Images

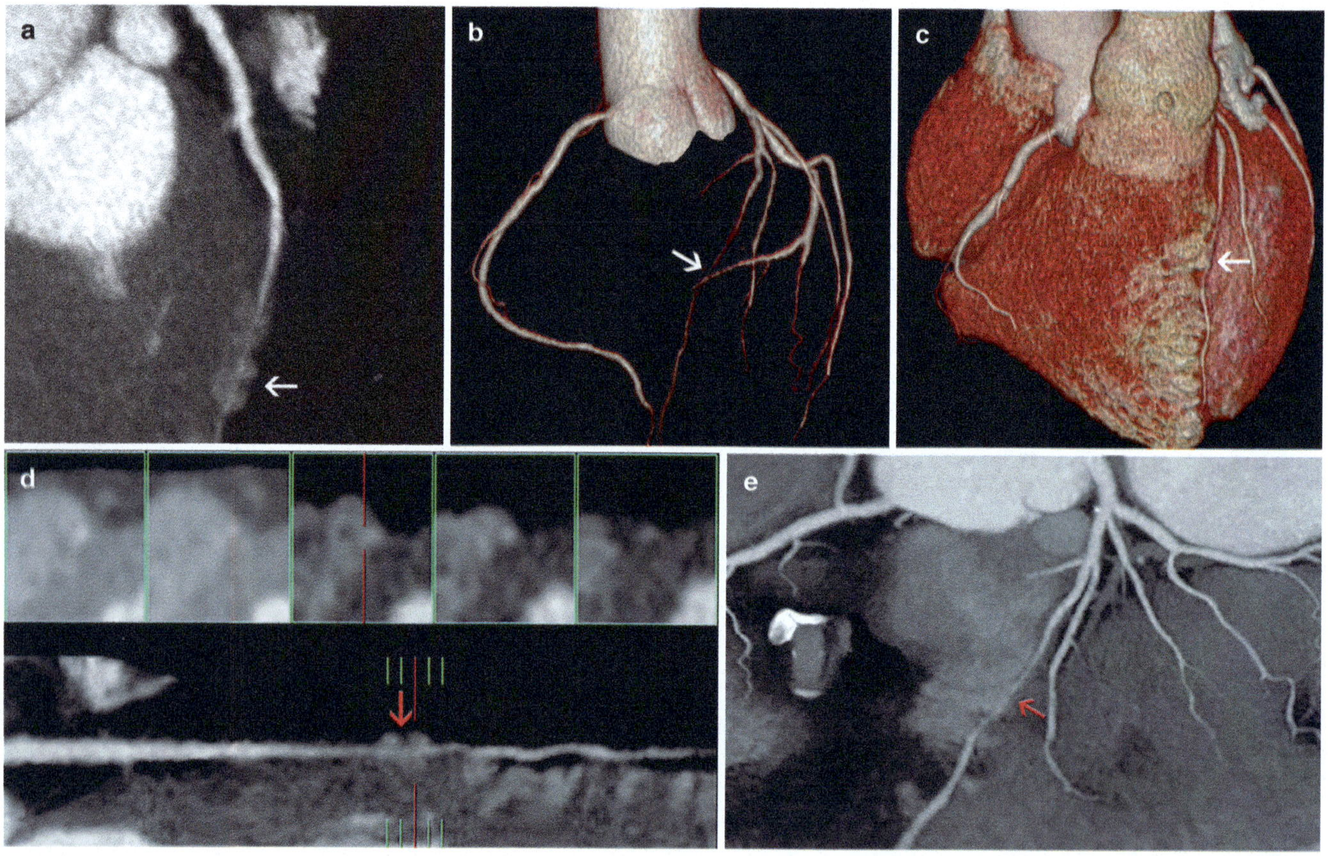

Findings and Interpretation

- Curved multiplanar reconstruction (MPR) of the left anterior descending coronary artery (LAD, panel A). There is a complete myocardial bridging of the mid LAD (arrow) where the artery takes an intramyocardial course in the right ventricle. A severe reduction in the artery diameter is observed at that level. Distally, the LAD artery emerges with normal diameter and extends to the apex (panels C and E).
- Volume rendering images of the coronary tree (panel B) and of the hole heart (panel C), respectively, showing the mid LAD myocardial bridging. The diameter reduction is clearly identified (arrow).
- Extended MPR of the LAD artery with orthogonal views in the upper part of the image (panel D). The red line shows the narrowest portion of the myocardial bridging (arrow).
- Two-dimensional maximum intensity projection of the coronary tree (panel E). Myocardial bridging of the mid LAD artery is shown (arrow).
- Myocardial bridging is a common finding in CTCA. In most cases these are incidental findings not associated with any symptoms. Only in few cases they can produce chest pain (systolic compression) and even perfusion defects (diastolic compression). The vessel most frequently involved is the LAD artery.

Further Reading

Lee MD, Chen CH. Myocardial bridging: An up-to-date review. J Invasive Cardiol 2015;27:521–8.

Case 4

Anomalous Left Circumflex Artery

Clinical History

- Fifty-four-year-old male.
- He presented at the emergency department with acute chest pain.
- He had normal ECG and cardiac enzyme levels.
- A computed tomography coronary angiography (CTCA) was then indicated.

Images

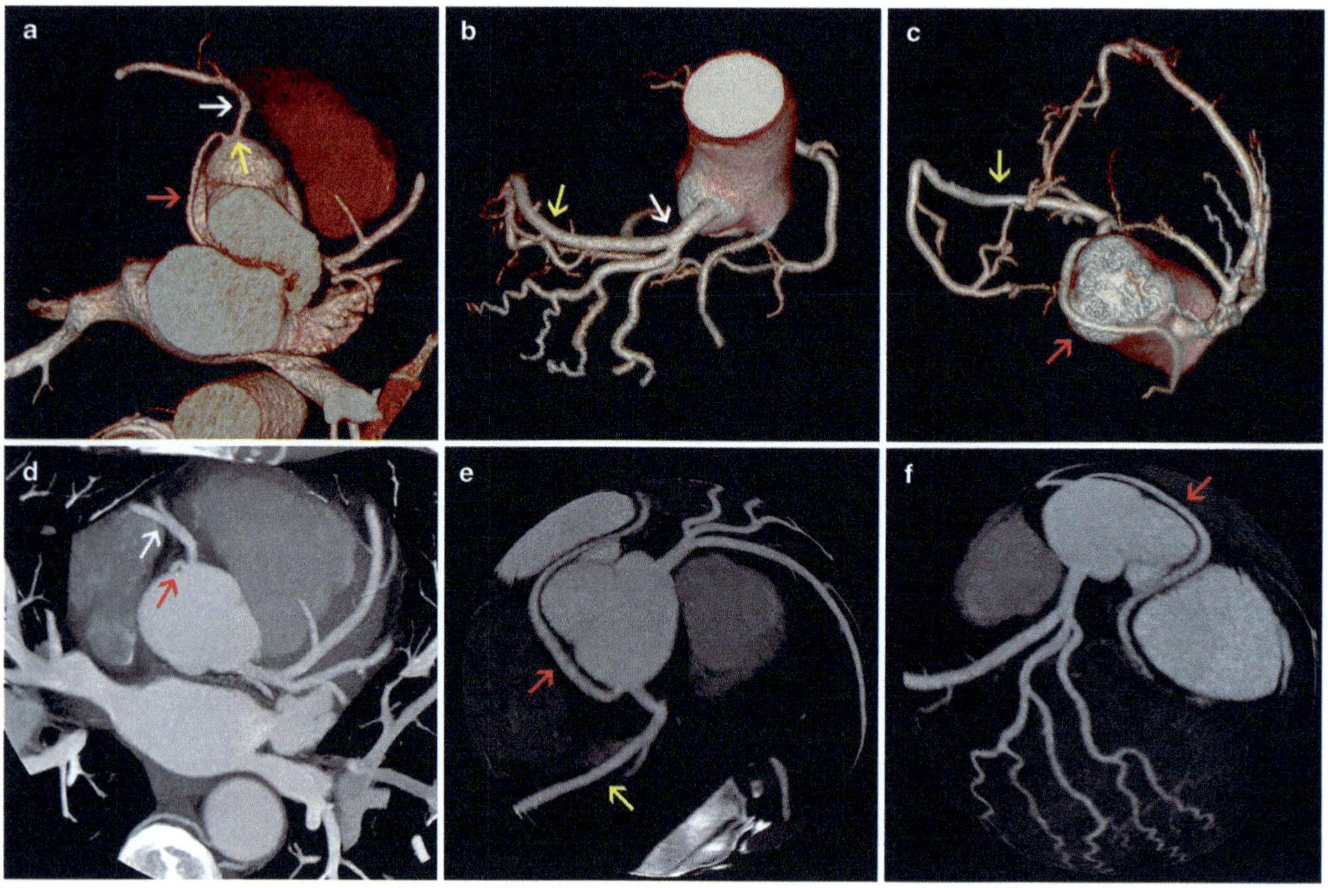

Findings and Interpretation

- Volume rendering image in an axial view (panel A). From the right coronary sinus (yellow arrow) originate the right coronary artery (RCA) (white arrow) and the left circumflex (LCX) artery (red arrow). The anomalous LCX artery has a retroaortic course surrounding the lateral aortic root wall, going backwards between the posterior portion of the aortic root and the left atrium.
- Volume rendering image of the coronary tree in a sagittal view (panel B). The left coronary artery (white arrow) originates exclusively the left anterior descending (LAD) artery (yellow arrow).
- Volume rendering image of the coronary tree in an axial view (panel C). The LCX artery is clearly displayed from its anomalous origin to the distal portion (red arrow).
- Axial maximum intensity projection (MIP, panel D). The anomalous origin of the LCX artery from the right coronary sinus is shown (red arrow), whereas the RCA has a normal origin (white arrow).
- Two-dimensional MIP globe views (panels E and F). The LCX artery is shown at different angles.
- In most series of patients, anomalous LCX artery is the most frequent of the coronary anomalies of origin. It is considered a benign variant, and it can arise from a common trunk with the RCA, directly from the RCA, or with an independent origin.

Further Reading

Erol C, Seker M. Coronary artery anomalies: the prevalence of origination, course, and termination anomalies of coronary arteries detected by 64-detector computed tomography coronary angiography. J Comput Assist Tomogr. 2011;35:618–24.

Rodríguez-Granillo GA, Rosales MA, Pugliese F, Fernandez-Pereira C, Rodríguez AE. Prevalence and characteristics of major and minor coronary artery anomalies in an adult population assessed by computed tomography coronary angiography. EuroIntervention. 2009;4(5):641–7.

Case 5

Anomalous Right Coronary Artery

Clinical History

- Fifty-one-year-old male.
- Former smoker. He presented a rest, oppressive chest pain radiated to jaw that lasted 1 h and solved spontaneously. The ECG was normal.
- The case was interpreted as low-risk unstable angina.
- Echocardiogram showed normal global and regional left ventricular wall motion.
- Stress echocardiogram identified inconclusive postero-basal ischemia.
- A computed tomography coronary angiography (CTCA) was indicated to evaluate coronary anatomy.

Images

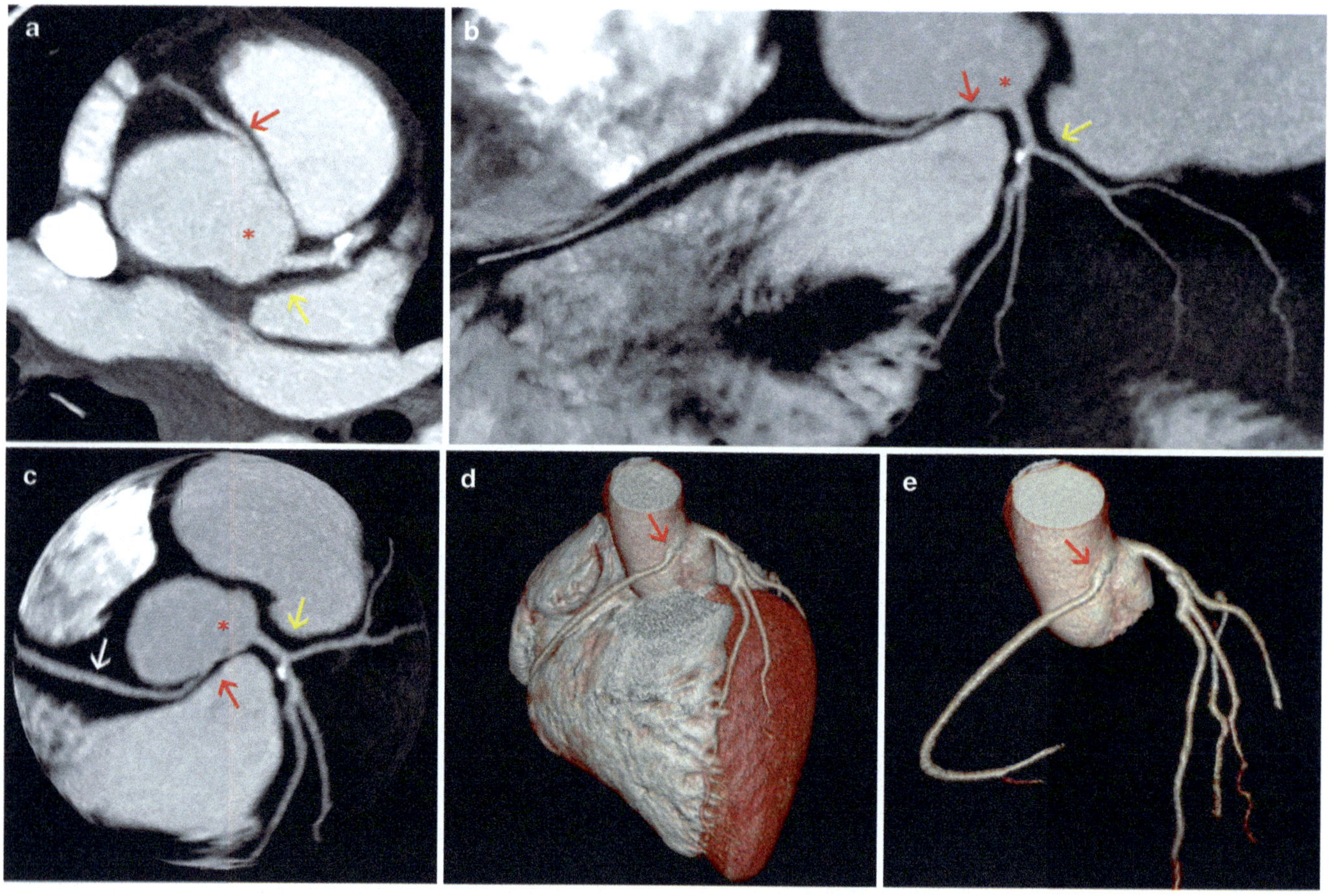

Findings and Interpretation

- Axial CT image at the coronary sinus level (panel A). The left coronary sinus (red asterisk) originates the left main coronary artery (LMCA, yellow arrow). The right coronary artery (RCA, red arrow) is originating at the sinotubular junction, in the intersection between the left and right coronary sinus. The proximal RCA has an acute take-off angle, passing through the aortic root and the pulmonary trunk, leading to moderate compression at that level. This is clearly shown using a two-dimensional maximum intensity projection of the coronary tree (panel B) and in a globe display (panel C). In the mid portion, the RCA diameter is restored (white arrow in panel C).
- Volume rendering image of the whole heart (panel D). RCA origin at the left aspect of the sinotubular junction and crosses to the right side. A diameter reduction is observed (red arrow). Volume rendering image of the coronary tree (panel E) shows similar findings.
- Coronary artery variants can be classified into two groups: benign or malignant. Benign variants are those that are not associated with symptoms or risks such as absence of LMCA, anomalous origin of the left circumflex artery, and myocardial bridging among the most frequent. In the second group, the RCA arising from the left sinus, the LMCA arising from the right coronary sinus, and the LMCA arising from the pulmonary artery are the most relevant. This group is considered malignant as they can be associated with chest pain, myocardial ischemia, or even cardiac death.
- Among the cases of the second group, the RCA arising from the left side portends a better prognosis. However in certain cases, it can be compressed between the aortic root and the pulmonary trunk. CTCA is an excellent modality to detect and classify coronary artery variants.

Further Reading

Zeitjian V, Moazez C, Saririan M, August DL, Roy R. Manifestation of non-ST elevation myocardial infarction due to hyperthyroidism in an anomalous right coronary artery. Int J Gen Med. 2017;10:409–13.

Case 6

Single Coronary Artery

Clinical History

- Thirty-four-year-old male.
- Family history of coronary artery disease.
- He was hospitalized for a non-transmural infarct. An invasive coronary angiography was performed, showing no significant lesions. A coronary anomaly was suspected.
- A computed tomography coronary angiography (CTCA) was indicated to evaluate coronary anatomy.

Images

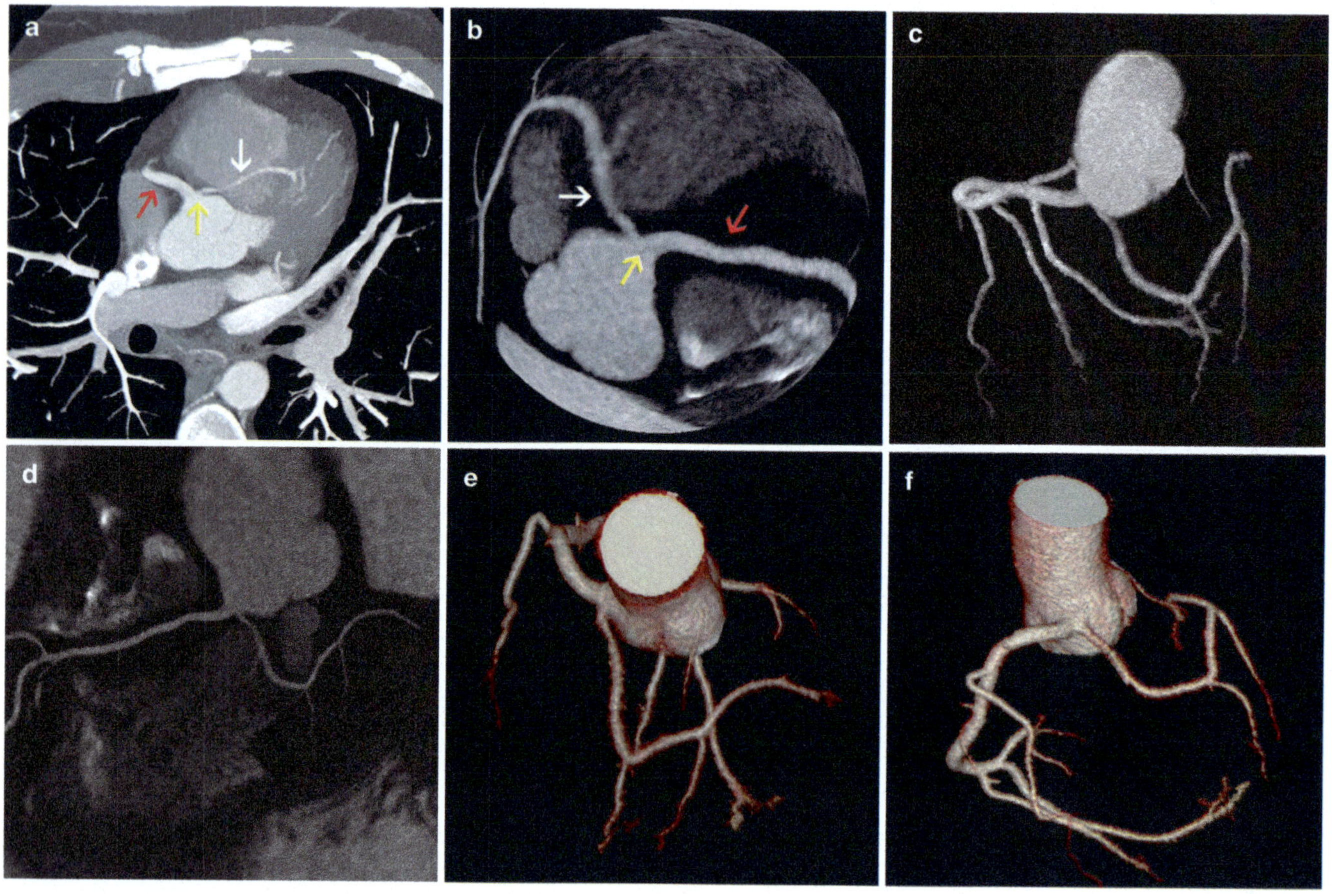

Findings and Interpretation

- Axial view with thick maximum intensity projection (MIP, panel A) showing a single coronary artery arising from the right coronary sinus (yellow arrow). The right coronary artery (red arrow) and the left main coronary artery (white arrow) originate from a common trunk.
- Two-dimensional MIP globe views (panel B), three-dimensional MIP of the coronary tree (panel C), two-dimensional MIP (panel D), and volume rendering (panels E and F) views showing similar findings.
- Single coronary artery arising from the right coronary sinus is one of the malignant coronary artery anomalies. It is rare and it can be associated with chest pain, myocardial ischemia, or even cardiac death.
- CTCA can clearly detect the different coronary variants and determine their origin and course.

Further Reading

Rubinshtein R, Flugelman MY, Jubran A, Shiran A, Jaffe R. Varying clinical presentations of anomalous origin of the left main coronary artery from the right coronary sinus with an interarterial course in adults. Int J Cardiol. 2017;248:149–51.

Case 7

Anomalous Left Coronary Artery from the Pulmonary Artery (ALCAPA)

Clinical History

- Thirty-nine-year-old female.
- No cardiovascular risk factors.
- Presented with heart failure symptoms. Echocardiogram identified abnormal flow at the pulmonary trunk.
- She was suspected of having an ALCAPA. For that reason a computed tomography coronary angiography (CTCA) was requested.

Images

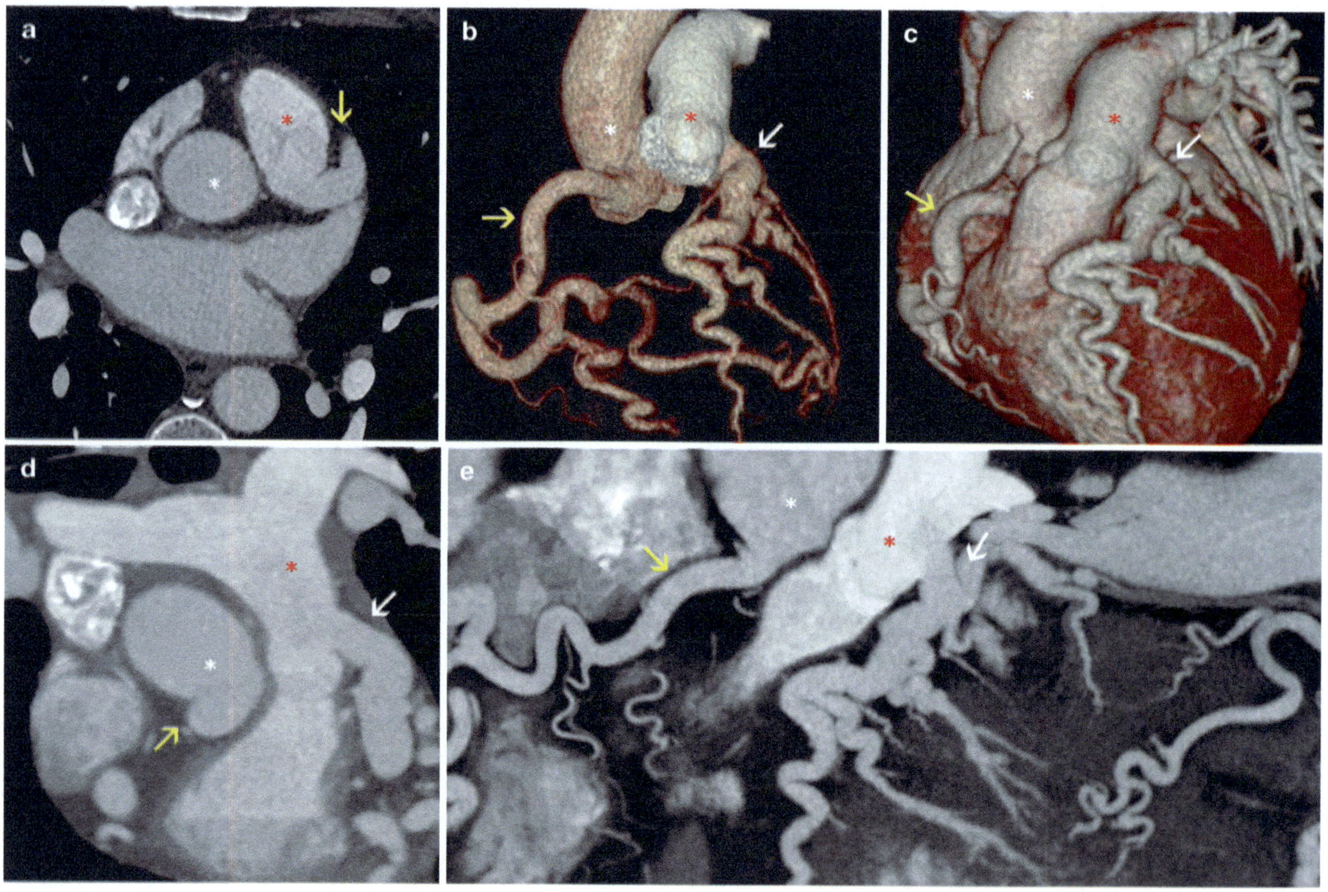

Findings and Interpretation

- Axial CT image at the pulmonary trunk level (panel A). The left main coronary artery (LMCA, arrow), markedly dilated, originates from the trunk of the pulmonary artery (red asterisk).
- Volume rendering image of the coronary tree (panel B). The aorta (white asterisk) originates the right coronary artery (RCA) (yellow arrow), while the pulmonary trunk (red asterisk) originates the LMCA (white arrow). Whole heart volume rendering (panel C) shows dilatation of both coronary arteries.
- Maximum intensity projection (MIP) reconstruction (panel D). The aorta (white asterisk) originates the RCA, while the pulmonary artery (red asterisk) originates the LMCA (white arrow).
- Two-dimensional MIP display of the complete coronary tree (panel E) showing the same findings.
- Anomalous origin of the left coronary artery arising from the pulmonary artery (ALCAPA or Bland-White-Garland syndrome) is a rare but serious congenital coronary artery anomaly, with a poor prognosis without surgical repair. There are two types of ALCAPA syndrome: infant type and adult type. Infant type has worse prognosis as it does not develop collaterals. Patients in general die before the first year of life. On the other hand, the adult type reveals giant and tortuous coronary arteries with many collaterals between the left and right coronary system with better prognosis, similar to the presented case.

Further Reading

Patrianakos AP, Hatzidakis A, Marketou M, Parthenakis FI. Adult-type ALCAPA syndrome: a rare coronary artery anomaly. Echocardiography. 2018;35:1056–9.

Ischemic Cardiomyopathy

2

Gastón A. Rodríguez-Granillo, Patricia M. Carrascosa, and Alejandro H. de la Vega

Background

The advent of cardiac computed tomography (CT) and cardiac magnetic resonance (CMR) has had a major impact in the shifting paradigms of the evaluation of coronary artery disease (CAD), originally defined straightforward by binary antagonic concepts such as the presence or absence of obstructive disease and the presence or absence of myocardial ischemia. These noninvasive imaging techniques, particularly cardiac CT, can provide a comprehensive pathophysiological assessment rather than a merely anatomical approach, including subclinical assessment and enhanced risk stratification (coronary artery calcium score), plaque characterization (including identification of high-risk features), detailed anatomical information aimed at improving guidance of percutaneous coronary interventions, stent and graft evaluation, and physiological assessment using either stress myocardial perfusion or by extracting functional information from anatomical data, and computational fluid dynamics (fractional flow reserve). Consequently, computed tomography coronary angiography (CTCA) is possibly the noninvasive technique with the highest likelihood to provide a one-stop-shop tool, potentially addressing the anatomy, spatial distribution, burden, and physiological assessment in a single session. Furthermore, CTCA can identify patients previously considered as low risk such as those with nonobstructive but extensive CAD, recently shown to pose a similar risk of events than those with obstructive but non-extensive disease, and also patients at very low risk of events (those with absence of plaques/calcifications). On the other hand, the role of CMR in the evaluation of CAD is more related to the functional assessment (stress myocardial perfusion) and to the accurate phenotyping of the presence, characteristics, mechanisms, extension, and complications of myocardial infarction.

Anatomical Assessment: Key Concepts

Coronary Artery Calcium Score (CACS)

Technical Aspects Non-contrast-enhanced CT scan, low radiation dose (≤1 mSv), axial scan, 2.5–3 mm thickness. Agatston classification score is established for each calcified area and is based on a weighted density (Hounsfield units) score given to the highest density, multiplied by the calcified area (computing as calcifications plaques with a density >130 Hounsfield units within a ≥3 pixel area).

Prognosis CACS has been extensively validated as an independent predictor of major adverse cardiac events and total mortality in asymptomatic patients, providing a significant incremental value over traditional risk factors and functional studies.

G. A. Rodríguez-Granillo (✉)
Department of Cardiovascular Imaging, Department of Research, Diagnostico Maipu, Buenos Aires, Argentina

National Council of Scientific and Technical Investigations (CONICET), Buenos Aires, Argentina

P. M. Carrascosa
Departments of CT, MR, and Research, Department of Cardiovascular Imaging, Diagnostico Maipu, Buenos Aires, Argentina

University of Buenos Aires, Buenos Aires, Argentina

Latin American Committee of the Society of Cardiovascular Computed Tomography, Buenos Aires, Argentina

A. H. de la Vega
Cardiovascular Imaging, CT and MR of Clinica de Imagenes and Fundación Médica de Río Negro y Neuquén, Cipolletti, Argentina

P. M. Carrascosa et al. (eds.), *Clinical Atlas of Cardiac and Aortic CT and MRI*, https://doi.org/10.1007/978-3-030-03682-9_2

Classification (Agatston Classification)

CACS 0	Absence of coronary artery calcifications. Very low risk of major cardiovascular events (~0.10% annual risk), providing a ≥5-year safety window (non-vulnerable patient)
CACS 1–10	Minimal coronary calcifications. Low risk of events but higher than patients CACS 0
CACS 11–99	Mild-moderate coronary calcifications. Mild-moderate risk of events. Very low (<2%) prevalence of abnormal functional tests
CACS 100–399	Moderate coronary calcifications. Incremented risk of events. Asymptomatic patients with CACS 100–399 might benefit from further risk stratification with CTCA. Threshold above which patients might benefit from primary prevention strategies (aspirin and statins) independent of coronary risk factors (RF)
CACS 400–999	Extensive coronary artery calcification. High risk of events (>2% annual risk), independent of RF and functional tests
CACS ≥1000	Very extensive coronary artery calcification. Very high risk of events, independent of RF and functional tests
CACS >75th percentile	Extensive coronary artery calcification. High risk of events, independent of RF and functional tests

Plaque Characterization with CT Coronary Angiography (CTCA)

Technical Aspects CTCA can be acquired using prospective or retrospective ECG gating. The former requires a low (<65 bpm) and stable heart rate and leads to large reductions in radiation doses. Low tube voltage (100 kV or even 80 kV in very small subjects) and iterative reconstruction algorithms allow further reductions in radiation dose. Retrospective ECG-gated acquisitions are chosen among patients with higher or irregular heart rates and obese patients. In this case, tube modulation techniques (full X-ray tube output only in a pre-established cardiac phase) can reduce significantly the radiation dose.

Prognosis A normal CTCA has a very high negative predictive value for the prediction of events (~0.20% annual risk), with ≥5-year warranty period (non-vulnerable patient). The presence of any plaque (particularly if proximal) is related to a higher risk of events. The presence of high-risk characteristics (particularly positive remodeling and low-attenuation plaque) entails a higher risk of events, although with a low positive predictive value.

A schematic representation of key CTCA plaque phenotype features, both of *de novo* lesions and stented vessels, including the detection of in-stent restenosis, is displayed in Fig. 2.1.

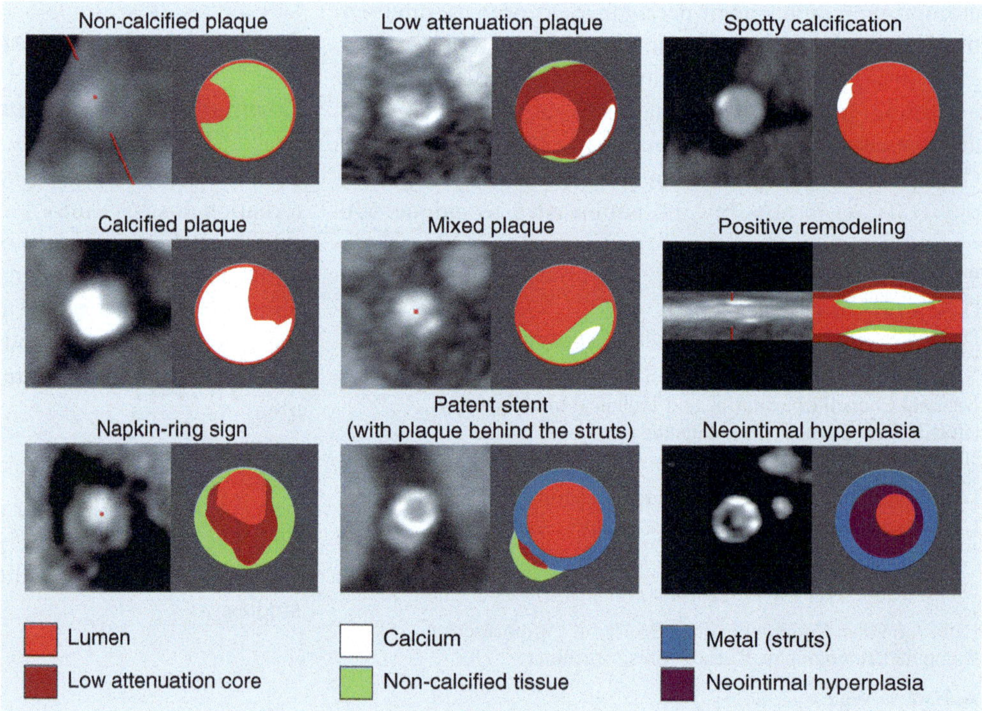

Fig. 2.1 Schematic representation of key CTCA plaque phenotype features, both of *de novo* lesions and stented vessels

High-Risk Features

The three main CTCA features related to high-risk plaques are positive remodeling, low-attenuation plaque, and napkin-ring sign.

Low-attenuation plaque	Generally defined as plaques with attenuation <30 Hounsfield units
Positive remodeling	Lesion with vessel area >10% larger than a proximal normal reference site (remodeling index> 1.1)
Napkin-ring sign	Low-attenuation core surrounded by a rim-like area of higher attenuation (but less than 130 HU)
Spotty calcification	<3 mm length calcifications comprising <90° of the vessel circumference

Other Key Concepts

Segment involvement score (SIS)	Total number of coronary artery segments involved irrespective of the degree of stenosis (SIS >5 indicates a large atherosclerotic plaque burden). Patients with extensive (SIS>5) but nonobstructive disease are at similar risk of events than those with obstructive but not extensive disease
CAD-RADS 0	No plaque or stenosis
CAD-RADS 1	1–24% stenosis
CAD-RADS 2	25–49% stenosis
CAD-RADS 3	50–69% stenosis
CAD-RADS 4A	70–99% stenosis
CAD-RADS 4B	Left main >50% stenosis or 3-vessel obstructive disease >70%
CAD-RADS 5	Total occlusion
CAD-RADS modifiers	N (non-diagnostic); S (stent); G (graft); V (vulnerable features)

Physiological Assessment: Key Concepts

Using stress-rest myocardial perfusion imaging (or dobutamine stress for wall motion abnormalities in some institutions) and late-enhancement imaging, cardiac CT and CMR enable the assessment of the presence of ischemia (defined as reversible myocardial perfusion defects, with lack of late contrast enhancement), myocardial infarcts (defined as fixed myocardial perfusion defects, coincident with late contrast enhancement), and residual perinecrotic ischemia (defined as partially reversible perfusion defects, with late contrast enhancement involving a smaller extension of irreversible damage). These pathophysiological findings are summarized in Fig. 2.2.

Stress CT Myocardial Perfusion

CTCA has a relatively low specificity in patients with intermediate to high likelihood of CAD, predominantly in those with diffusely calcified coronary vessels. Besides, there is a weak correlation between the degree of luminal stenosis of lesions detected by CTCA and the presence of ischemia. Furthermore, recent studies suggest that coronary revascularization improves the outcome only among patients with moderate to severe ischemia. CT myocardial perfusion imaging (CTP) under pharmacological stress has been extensively validated for the evaluation of the hemodynamic significance of coronary lesions.

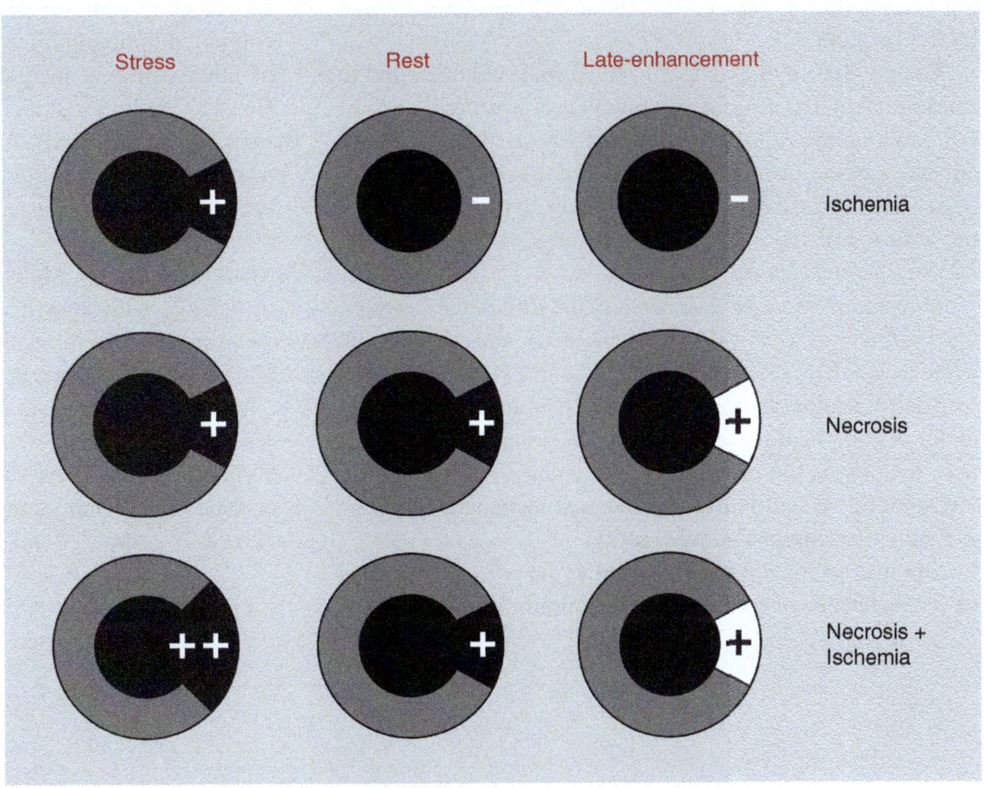

Fig. 2.2 Schematic representation of myocardial ischemia (reversible perfusion defect, with lack of late contrast enhancement), myocardial infarct (fixed myocardial perfusion defect, coincident with late contrast enhancement), and residual perinecrotic ischemia (partially reversible perfusion defect, with late contrast enhancement involving a smaller extension)

FFR-CT

Computational fluid dynamics applied to standard CTCA images is a novel method that allows prediction of blood flow and pressure in coronary arteries and calculation of lesion-specific fractional flow reserve (FFR-CT). However, it usually requires complex and/or remote evaluation and demands very high image quality. An FFR-CT <0.80 defines the presence of lesion-specific ischemia.

Cardiac Magnetic Resonance (CMR)

Patients with ischemic cardiomyopathy can be evaluated with CMR, allowing estimation of ventricular morphology (wall thickness and mechanical complications of myocardial infarction) and systolic function without the acoustic window restrictions of echocardiography, myocardial perfusion, and discrimination between myocardial edema (T2-weighted images) and necrosis (late gadolinium enhancement, LGE).

Stress CMR Myocardial Perfusion and Infarct Imaging

CMR allows the evaluation of myocardial perfusion by means of a validated non-ionizing radiation technique. Stress imaging using CMR can be induced using different pharmacological strategies including vasodilators (adenosine, dipyridamole, regadenoson) or dobutamine. Since gadolinium and iodine have similar contrast kinetics, CT can be an alternative to CMR among patients with contraindications, providing comparable assessment including myocardial CTP and infarct imaging.

The presence and extent of LGE (from subendocardial to transmural in ischemic cardiomyopathy) are predictors of left ventricular systolic dysfunction, heart failure, major adverse cardiac events, and death. The likelihood of functional recovery after revascularization is inversely related to the transmural extent of wall thickness with LGE (0%; <25%; 25–49%; 50–75%; >75%).

Myocardial salvage is defined as the difference between myocardium at risk (T2-weighted area) and myocardial necrosis (LGE).

Microvascular obstruction/no reflow, an independent predictor of complications after myocardial infarction, is identified in CMR as the presence of hypointense regions within the infarct core and is usually assessed in images obtained 2–5 min after contrast administration.

Lipomatous metaplasia is defined as the presence of areas of fat replacement within the myocardium, more prevalent among >1-year-old (and predominantly anterior wall) infarcts.

Conclusions

Overall, cardiac CT can provide a comprehensive pathophysiological assessment of patients with CAD, from improved risk stratification of asymptomatic patients, to plaque characterization and detailed anatomical information in patients with suspected and established CAD, to physiological assessment. Therefore, CTCA might become a noninvasive one-stop-shop tool, potentially addressing the anatomy, spatial distribution, burden, and physiological assessment during a single session. Alternatively, the role of CMR in the evaluation of patients with suspected or established CAD is more related to the functional evaluation (stress-rest imaging) and to the characterization of myocardial infarction in terms of presence, patterns, mechanisms, extension, and complications.

Further Reading

Foley JR, Plein S, Greenwood JP. Assessment of stable coronary artery disease by cardiovascular magnetic resonance imaging: Current and emerging techniques. World J Cardiol. 2017;9(2):92–108.

Goncalves P de A, Rodriguez-Granillo GA, Spitzer E, et al. Functional evaluation of coronary disease by CT angiography. JACC Cardiovasc Imaging. 2015;8(11):1322–35.

Rodriguez-Granillo GA, Carrascosa P, Bruining N, et al. Defining the non-vulnerable and vulnerable patients with computed tomography coronary angiography: evaluation of atherosclerotic plaque burden and composition. Eur Heart J Cardiovasc Imaging. 2016;17(5):481–91.

Shaw LJ, Giambrone AE, Blaha MJ, et al. Long-term prognosis after coronary artery calcification testing in asymptomatic patients: a cohort study. Ann Int Med. 2015;163(1):14–21.

Vincenti G, Masci PG, Monney P, et al. Stress perfusion CMR in patients with known and suspected CAD: prognostic value and optimal ischemic threshold for revascularization. JACC Cardiovasc Imaging. 2017;10(5):526–37.

Xie JX, Cury RC, Leipsic J. The coronary artery disease–reporting and data system (CAD-RADS) prognostic and clinical implications associated with standardized coronary computed tomography angiography reporting. J Am Coll Cardiol. 2018;11:78–89.

Case 8

Subclinical Atherosclerosis: Coronary Artery Calcium Scoring (CACS)

Clinical History

- Fifty-eight-year-old male.
- Coronary risk factors: hypertension; family history of coronary artery disease.
- Asymptomatic.
- Referred for CACS to refine risk stratification.

Images

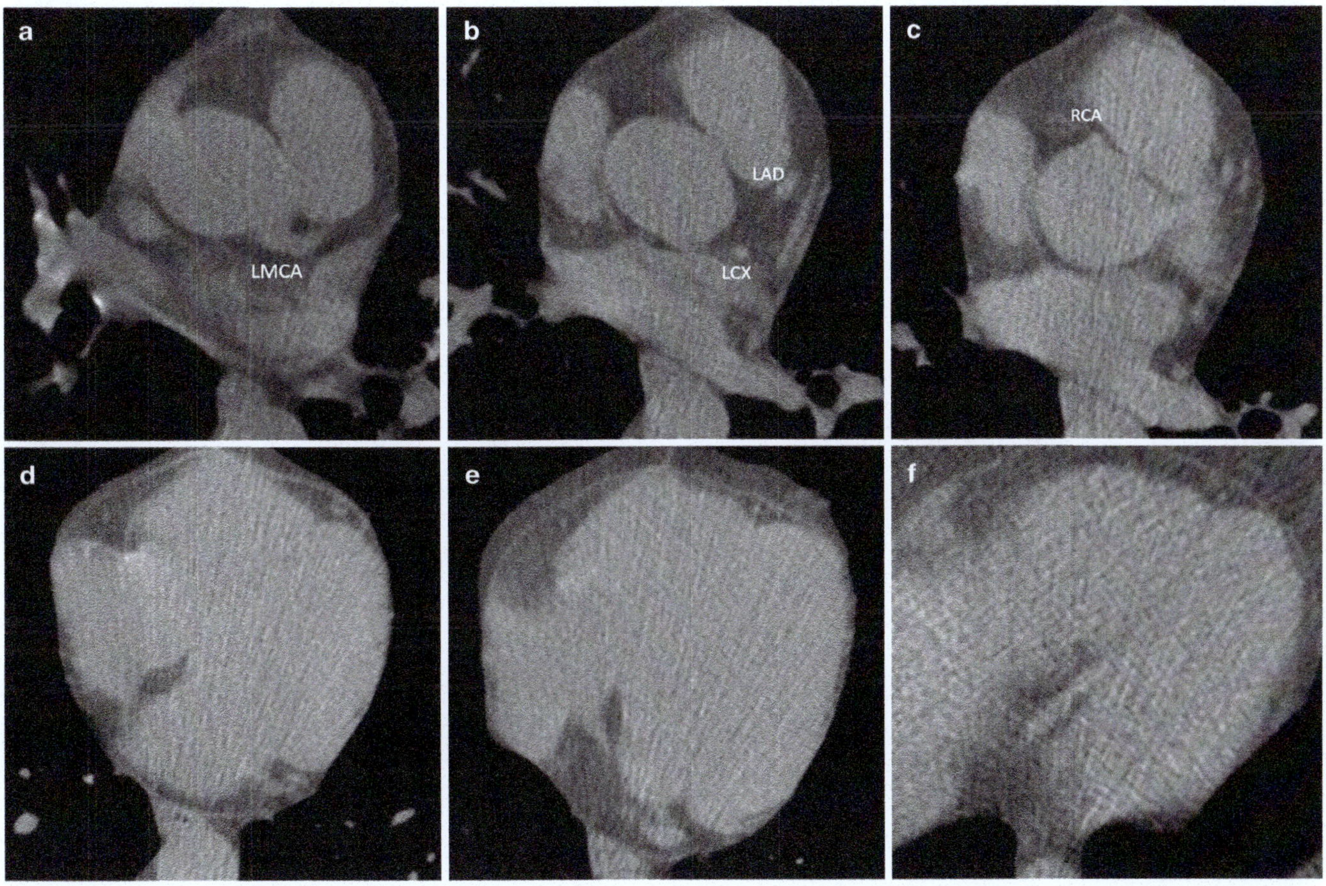

Findings and Interpretation

- Axial views of the heart from cranial to caudal (panels A–F).
- Absence of coronary calcifications (CACS 0). LMCA, left main coronary artery; LAD, left anterior descending artery; LCX, left circumflex artery; RCA, right coronary artery.
- Risk of cardiovascular events is refined, from intermediate risk to low risk of cardiovascular events.
- Asymptomatic patients with CACS 0, independent of Framingham risk score, are at very low risk of events (0.10% per year), with a safety window of at least 5 years.
- Patients with CACS 0 do not benefit from aspirin for primary prevention.
- The benefit of statins among patients with abnormal lipid profile but CACS 0, if any, is marginal.

Further Reading

Martin SS, Blaha MJ, Blankstein R, et al. Dyslipidemia, coronary artery calcium, and incident atherosclerotic cardiovascular disease: implications for statin therapy from the multi-ethnic study of atherosclerosis. Circulation 2014;129:77–86.

Miedema M, Duprez DA, Misialek JR, et al. Use of coronary artery calcium testing to guide aspirin utilization for primary prevention: estimates from the multi-ethnic study of atherosclerosis. Circ Cardiovasc Qual Outcomes. 2014;7:453–60.

Nasir K, Rubin J, Blaha MJ, et al. Interplay of coronary artery calcification and traditional risk factors for the prediction of all-cause mortality in asymptomatic individuals. Circ Cardiovasc Imaging. 2012;5:467–73.

Shaw LJ, Giambrone AE, Blaha MJ, et al. Long-term prognosis after coronary artery calcification testing in asymptomatic patients: a cohort study. Ann Int Med. 2015;163:14–21.

Case 9

Subclinical Atherosclerosis: Coronary Artery Calcium Scoring (CACS)

Clinical History

- Seventy-year-old female.
- Coronary risk factors: hypercholesterolemia.
- Asymptomatic; intolerance to statins.
- Referred for CACS in order to evaluate the possibility to withdraw statin use.

Images

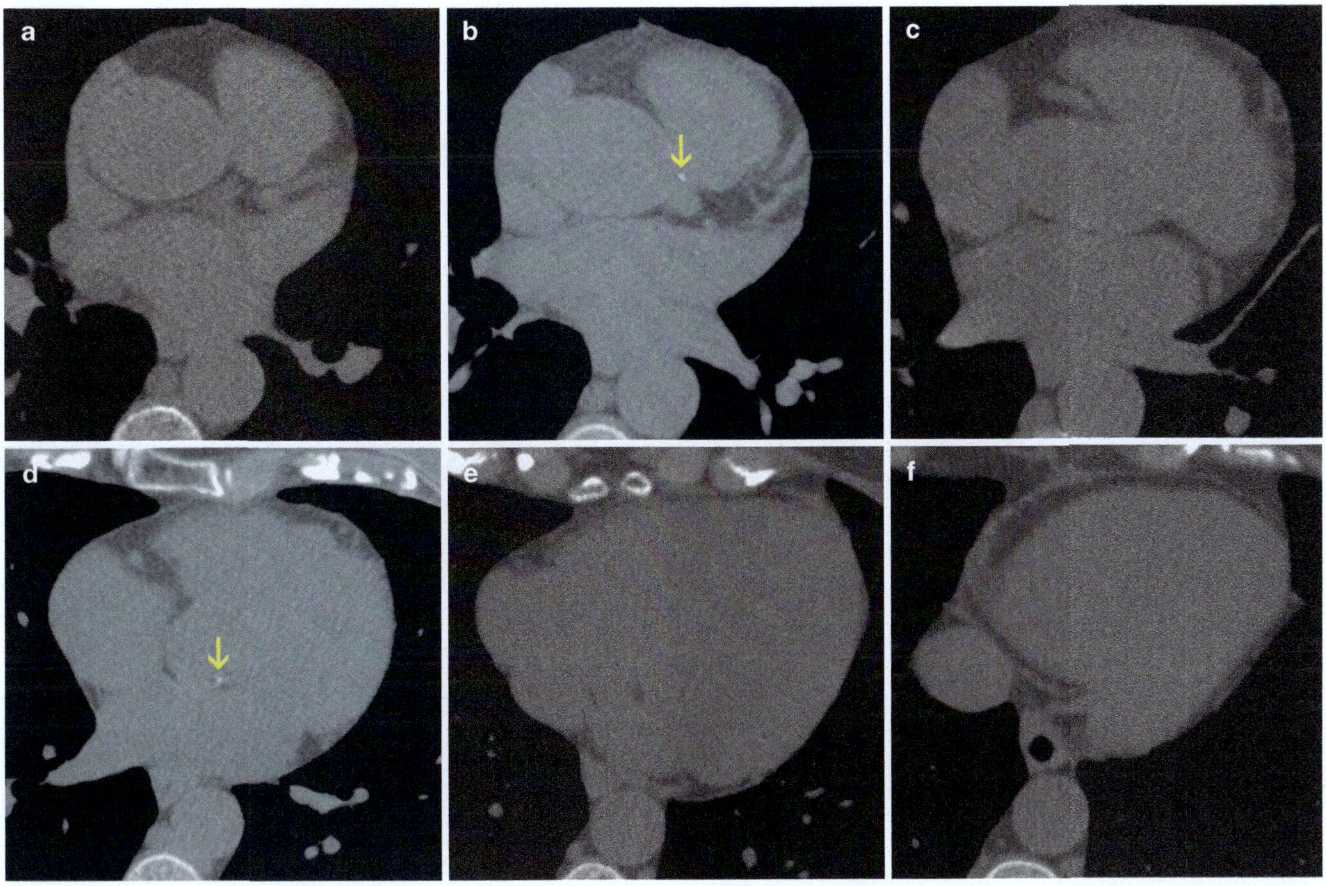

Findings and Interpretation

- Axial views from cranial to caudal (panels A–F).
- Absence of coronary artery calcifications. Note that the minimal calcifications observed (arrows) involve only the aortic root and aortic valve.
- Risk of major adverse cardiovascular events among patients with CACS 0 is very low (0.10% per year), independent of risk factors.
- The benefit of statins among patients with abnormal lipid profile but CACS 0, if any, is marginal.

Further Reading

Martin SS, Blaha MJ, Blankstein R, et al. Dyslipidemia, coronary artery calcium, and incident atherosclerotic cardiovascular disease: implications for statin therapy from the multi-ethnic study of atherosclerosis. Circulation 2014;129:77–86.

Nasir K, Rubin J, Blaha MJ, et al. Interplay of coronary artery calcification and traditional risk factors for the prediction of all-cause mortality in asymptomatic individuals. Circ Cardiovasc Imaging. 2012;5:467–73.

Shaw LJ, Giambrone AE, Blaha MJ, et al. Long-term prognosis after coronary artery calcification testing in asymptomatic patients: a cohort study. Ann Int Med. 2015;163:14–21.

Case 10

Subclinical Atherosclerosis: Coronary Artery Calcium Scoring (CACS)

Clinical History

- Sixty-eight-year-old male.
- Coronary risk factors: diabetes, hypercholesterolemia, hypertension.
- Non-anginal chest pain.
- Functional test (stress echo) without evidence of ischemia.
- Referred for CACS to refine risk stratification.

Images

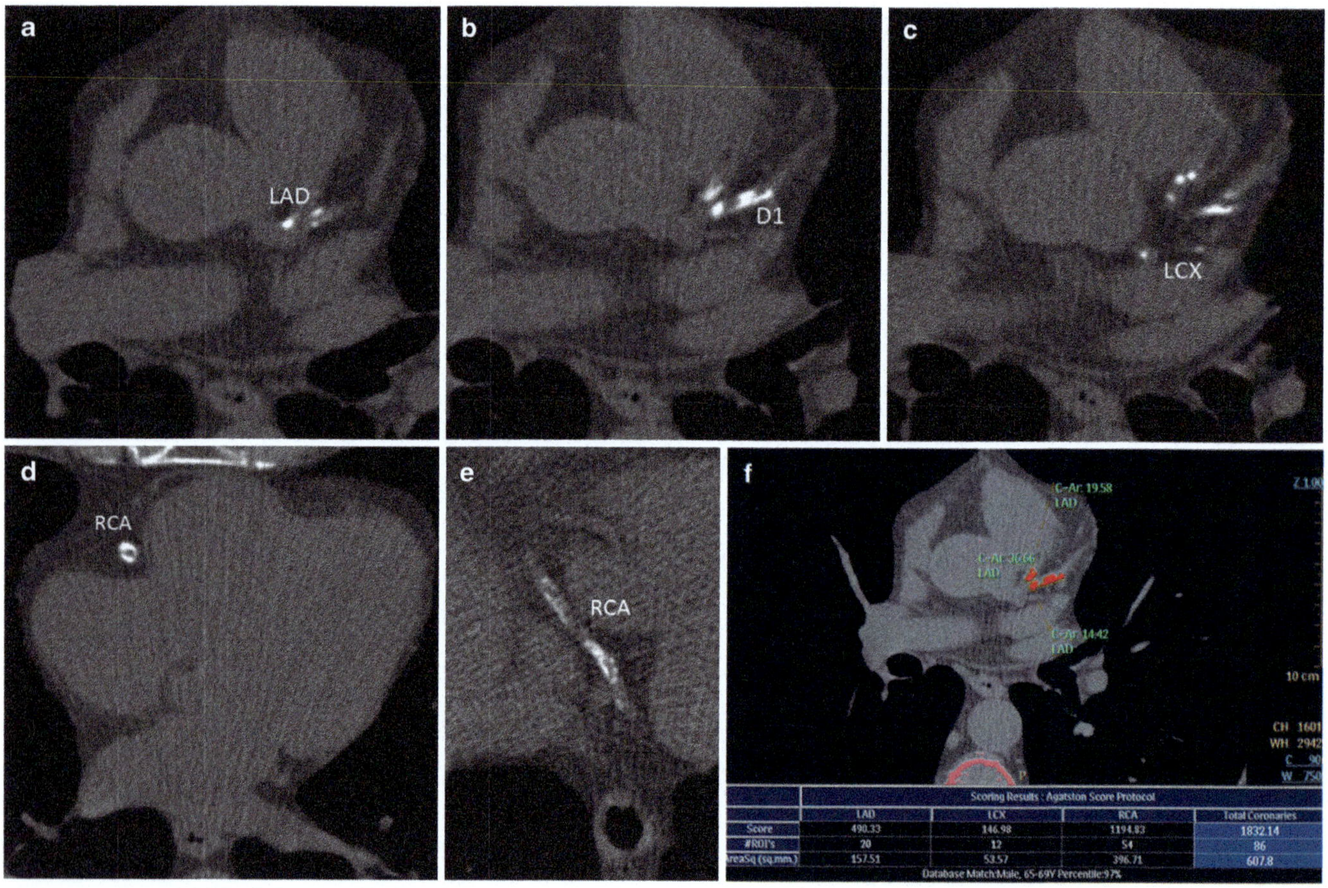

Findings and Interpretation

- Axial views from cranial to caudal (panels A–E) and CACS display (panel F). LAD, left anterior descending artery; LCX, left circumflex artery; RCA, right coronary artery; D1, diagonal branch.
- Extensive coronary calcification (CACS 1832, in panel F) involving multiple coronary segments. Total CACS and CACS discriminated by coronary artery are displayed. CACS in this patient was at 97th age- and sex-matched percentile (lower right panel).
- The three main and secondary branches are involved. Note the different calcification patterns (diffuse at the D1 and distal RCA, concentric at the mid RCA, and spotty at the ostial LAD and LCX).
- This patient is at very high risk of cardiovascular events and has a high likelihood of obstructive coronary artery disease.
- Symptomatic patients with CACS> 400 are at high risk of events (>2% per year), independent of risk factors and functional tests. Particularly, patients with CACS>1000 have significantly higher risk of major adverse events even in the presence of normal stress-rest myocardial perfusion imaging.
- Conversely, among stable symptomatic patients with low to intermediate pretest likelihood of coronary artery disease, a CACS 0 can safely exclude flow-limiting coronary disease.

Further Reading

Engbers EM, Timmer JR, Ottervanger JP, et al. Prognostic value of coronary artery calcium scoring in addition to single-photon emission computed tomographic myocardial perfusion imaging in symptomatic patients. Circ Cardiovasc Imaging. 2016;9(5). pii: e003966.

Mouden M, Timmer JR, Reiffers S, et al. Coronary artery calcium scoring to exclude flow-limiting coronary artery disease in symptomatic stable patients at low or intermediate risk. Radiology. 2013;269:77–83.

Nicoll R, Wiklund U, Zhao Y, et al. The coronary calcium score is a more accurate predictor of significant coronary stenosis than conventional risk factors in symptomatic patients: Euro-CCAD study. Int J Cardiol. 2016;207:13–9.

Case 11

Subclinical Atherosclerosis: Computed Tomography Coronary Angiography (CTCA)

Clinical History

- Thirty-five-year-old male.
- Coronary risk factors: hypercholesterolemia.
- Asymptomatic. He regularly performs strenuous physical activity.
- Abnormal findings in a routine exercise ECG treadmill test (asymptomatic ST depression).
- Referred for CTCA to rule out coronary anomalies or coronary artery disease.

Images

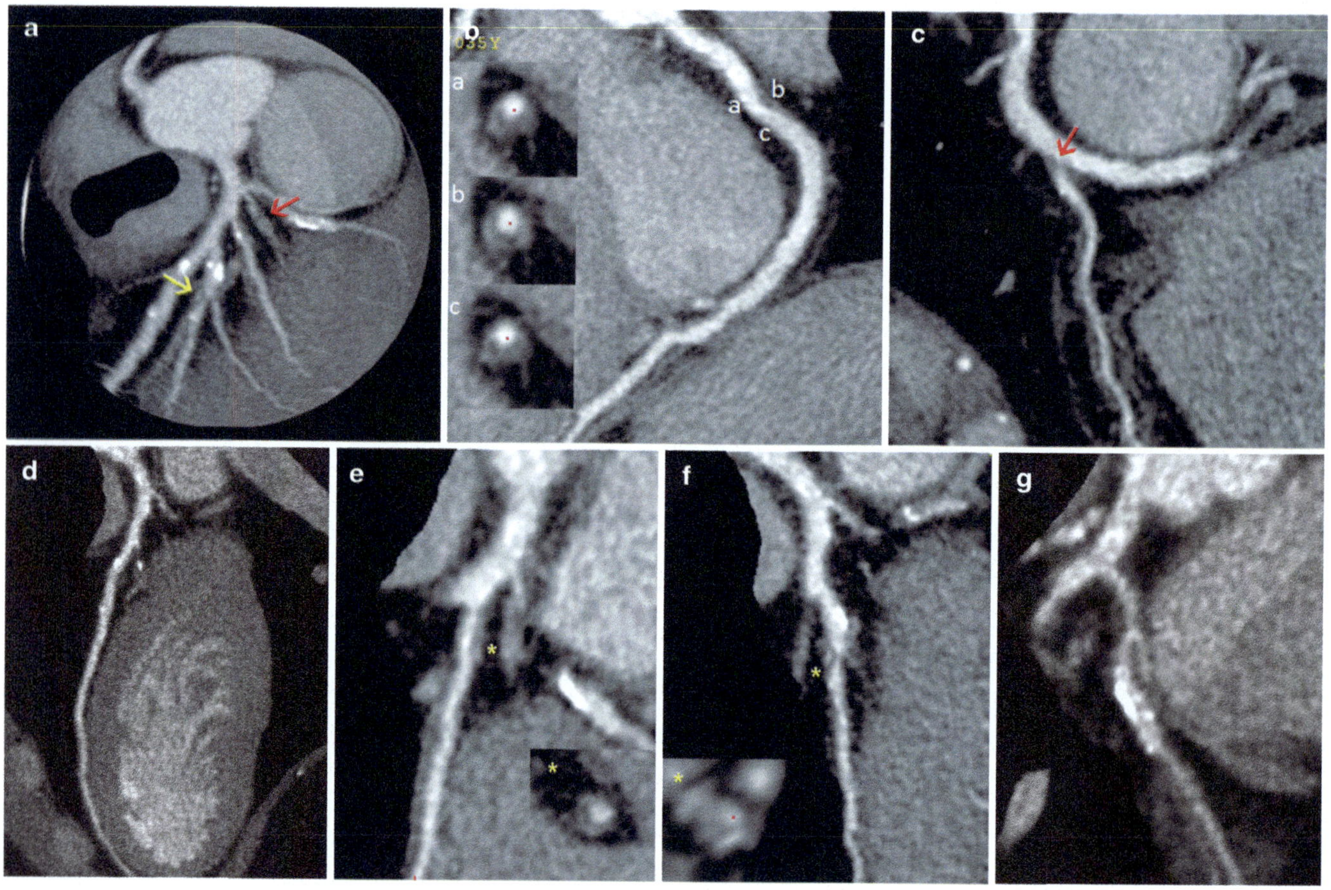

Findings and Interpretation

- Extensive coronary atherosclerosis, involving multiple segments (segment involvement score, SIS >5) and secondary branches.
- Two-dimensional maximum intensity projection (MIP) globe reconstruction (panel A) showing multiple focal lesions. Obstructive lesions involve the second diagonal branch (yellow arrow) and intermediate branch (red arrow).
- The right coronary artery (panel B) has a focal, eccentric, nonsignificant lesion (a–c) at the mid segment, with positive remodeling, low attenuation (−15 Hounsfield units), and napkin-ring sign (see orthogonal views at the left).
- The acute marginal branch (panel C) has an obstructive ostial lesion (arrow).
- The left anterior descending artery (panel D) has mild lesions.
- The first diagonal branch (panel E) has a moderate ostial lesion (*) with positive remodeling, low-attenuation core, and napkin-ring sign.
- The second diagonal branch, as seen in panel A, has a severe focal lesion (asterisk) with high-risk characteristics (panel F).
- The left circumflex artery (panel G) has moderate proximal disease.

- This patient is at very high risk of events, although the benefit of invasive management might be challenged given the lack of symptoms and the anatomy (only secondary branches with obstructive disease).
- This comprises a vulnerable patient from a lesion (multiple characteristics of plaque vulnerability) and patient [obstructive, extensive (SIS>5), and proximal disease] point of view.

Further Reading

Bittencourt MS, Hulten E, Ghoshhajra B, et al. Prognostic value of nonobstructive and obstructive coronary artery disease detected by coronary computed tomography angiography to identify cardiovascular events. Circ Cardiovasc Imaging. 2014;7:282–91.

Hadamitzky M, Taubert S, Deseive S, et al. Prognostic value of coronary computed tomography angiography during 5 years of follow-up in patients with suspected coronary artery disease. Eur Heart J. 2013;34:3277–85.

Maddox TM, Stanislawski MA, Grunwald G, et al. Nonobstructive coronary artery disease and risk of myocardial infarction. JAMA. 2014;312:1754–63.

Naoum C, Berman DS, Ahmadi A, et al. Predictive value of age- and sex-specific nomograms of global plaque burden on coronary computed tomography angiography for major cardiac events. Circ Cardiovasc Imaging. 2017;10. pii: e004896.

Case 12

Subclinical Atherosclerosis: Computed Tomography Coronary Angiography (CTCA)

Clinical History

- Fifty-eight-year-old female.
- Coronary risk factors: hypertension, smoking.
- She has symptomatic severe aortic stenosis (bicuspid valve).
- Referred for preoperative CTCA in order to rule out coronary artery disease.

Images

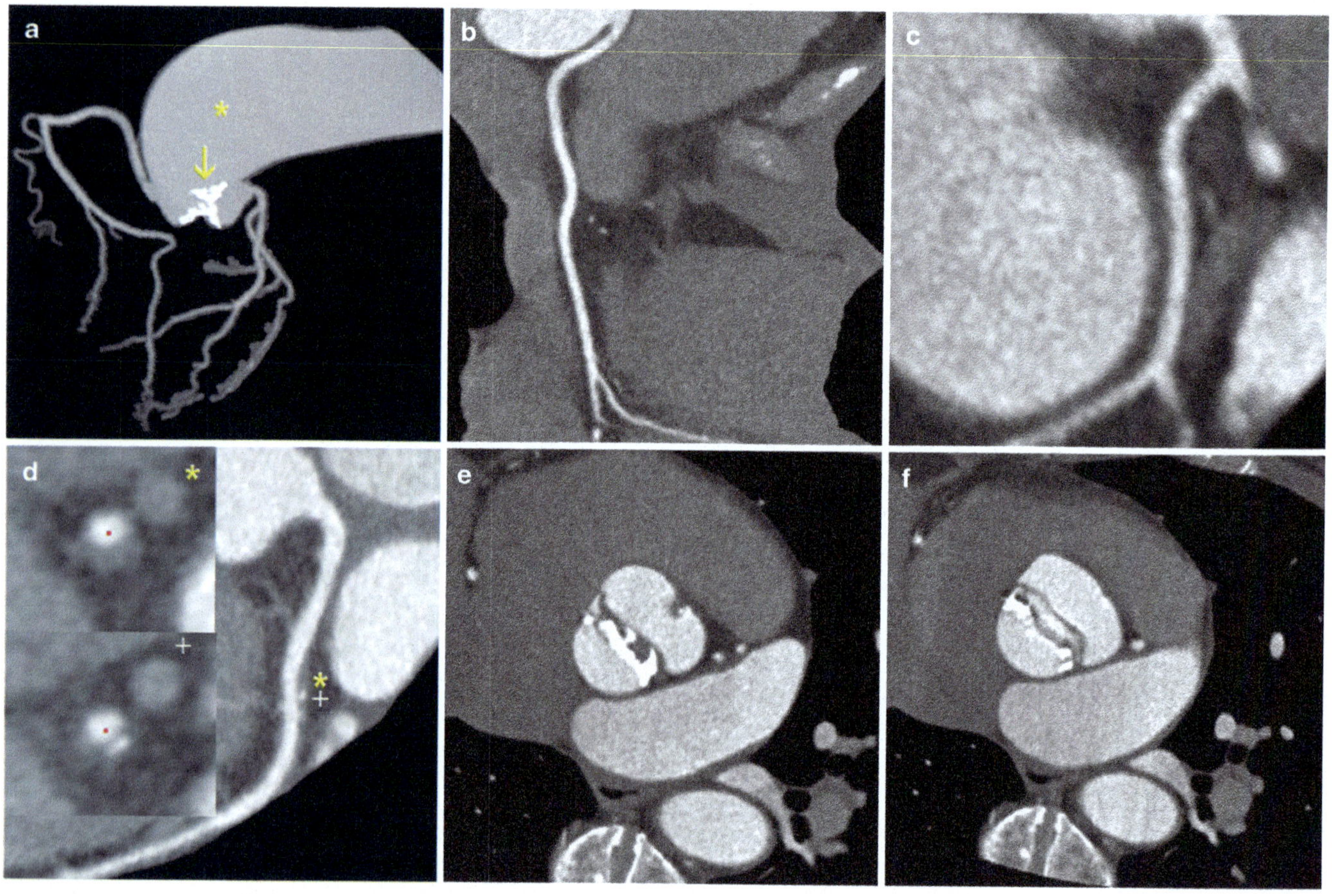

Findings and Interpretation

- Absence of obstructive coronary disease. Panel A shows a 3D maximum intensity reconstruction of the coronary tree, with absence of coronary calcifications, aortic dilatation (52 mm, *), and aortic valve calcification (arrow).
- The right coronary artery (panel B), with no evidence of atherosclerosis, has an acute angulation of the proximal segment related to the presence of aortic dilatation, without luminal narrowing.
- The left circumflex artery (panel C) has no evidence of atherosclerosis.
- The left anterior descending artery (panel D) has a nonobstructive mixed plaque (* and †), with evidence of positive remodeling. Note the relatively large plaque (orthogonal views on the left, red dot indicates the luminal center), with preserved lumen due to the positive (expansive) remodeling.
- Bicuspid aortic valve is clearly depicted (panels E and F in mid-diastolic and systolic views, respectively), with moderate calcification of the free edges of the cusps. Note the presence of raphe at 2 o'clock.
- Though nonobstructive (CAD-RADS 1 V), the presence of any plaque confers a significantly higher risk of hard

events compared to normal coronaries. Moreover, positive remodeling (defined as vessel size 10% larger than the proximal disease-free reference segment) is an independent predictor of high-risk plaques and adverse events.

- This patient might possibly benefit from statins.

Further Reading

Lin FY, Shaw LJ, Dunning AM, et al. Mortality risk in symptomatic patients with nonobstructive coronary artery disease: a prospective 2-center study of 2583 patients undergoing 64-detector row coronary computed tomographic angiography. J Am Coll Cardiol. 2011;58:510–9.

Min JK, Dunning A, Lin FY, et al. Age- and sex-related differences in all-cause mortality risk based on coronary computed tomography angiography findings results from the International Multicenter CONFIRM (Coronary CT Angiography Evaluation for Clinical Outcomes: an International Multicenter Registry) of 23,854 patients without known coronary artery disease. J Am Coll Cardiol. 2011;58:849–60.

Motoyama S, Ito H, Sarai M, et al. Plaque characterization by coronary computed tomography angiography and the likelihood of acute coronary events in mid-term follow-up. J Am Coll Cardiol. 2015;66:337–46.

Nakazato R, Otake H, Konishi A, et al. Atherosclerotic plaque characterization by CT angiography for identification of high-risk coronary artery lesions: a comparison to optical coherence tomography. Eur Heart J Cardiovasc Imaging. 2015;16:373–9.

Case 13

Subclinical Atherosclerosis: Computed Tomography Coronary Angiography (CTCA)

Clinical History

- Seventy-two-year-old male.
- Coronary risk factors: hypertension, hypercholesterolemia, former smoking, peripheral arterial disease.
- He is asymptomatic. Single photon emission computed tomography (dipyridamole) with inferior ischemia.
- Referred for CTCA to confirm findings and evaluate anatomy.

Images

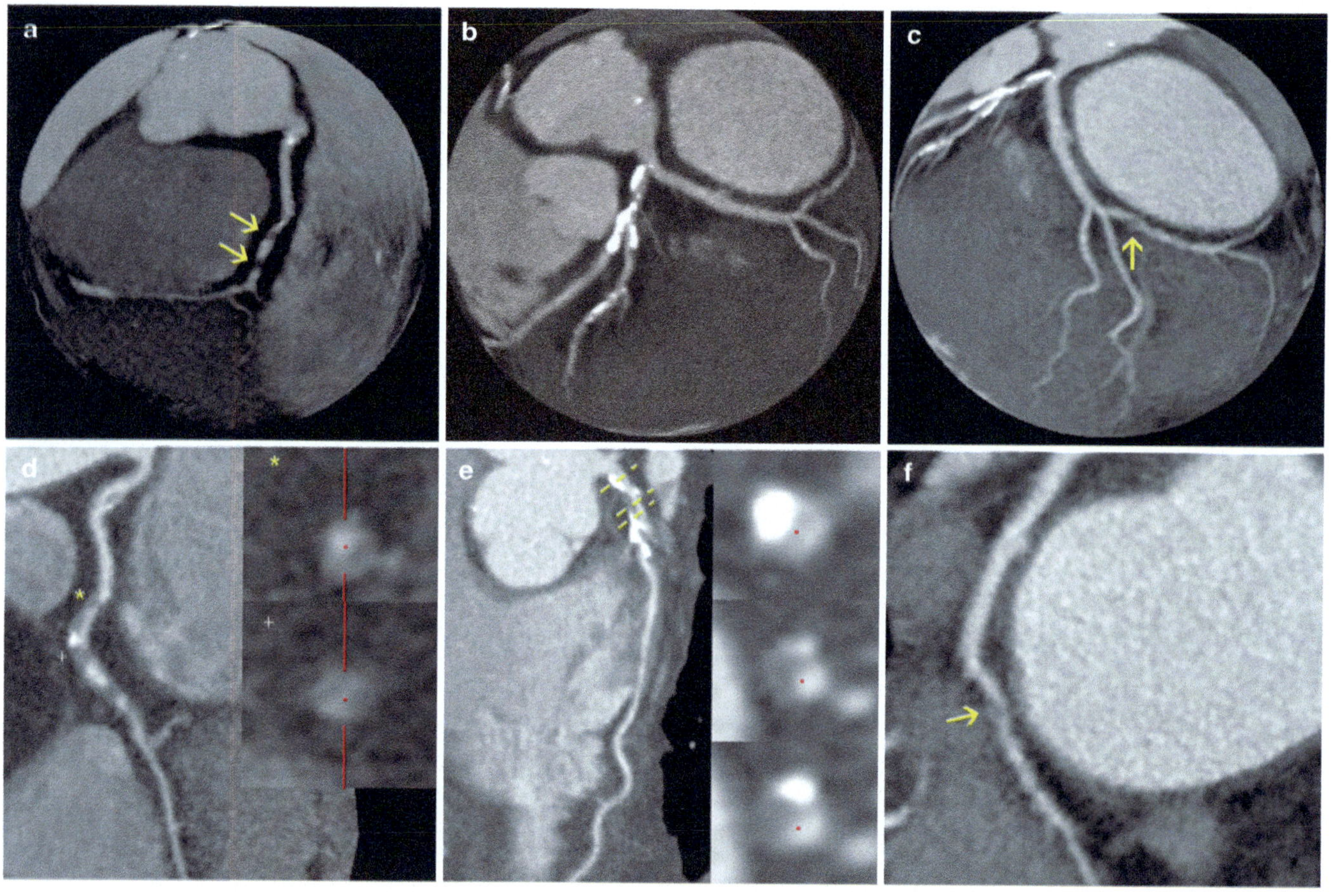

Findings and Interpretation

- Multiple vessel disease (obstructive).
- Two-dimensional maximum intensity projection (MIP) globe views (panels A–C) and multiplanar reconstructions (panels D–F).
- The right coronary artery (RCA) has two focal total occlusions (arrows in panel A). In the multiplanar reconstruction (panel D), a severe lesion with napkin-ring sign (*) is observed immediately proximal from a focal and hazy (possibly thrombotic) total occlusion (†). Note that the vessel wall boundaries are hazy and poorly defined (†), suggesting thrombotic content and perivascular adipose tissue inflammation.
- The left anterior descending artery (panel E) has moderate proximal stenosis. Note that within a few millimeter distance, three different plaque phenotypes are observed: calcified plaque (above), vulnerable (napkin-ring) plaque (mid), and mixed (below) plaques.
- The left circumflex artery (panels C and F) has a severe non-calcified distal lesion (arrow).
- This patient is at very high risk of events and warrants invasive management. He has obstructive (CAD-RADS 5 V), extensive (SIS>5), and proximal disease. Furthermore, he has multiple vulnerable lesions including a seemingly fresh total occlusion.

Further Reading

Bittencourt MS, Hulten E, Ghoshhajra B, et al. Prognostic value of nonobstructive and obstructive coronary artery disease detected by coronary computed tomography angiography to identify cardiovascular events. Circ Cardiovasc Imaging. 2014;7:282–91.

Hadamitzky M, Taubert S, Deseive S, et al. Prognostic value of coronary computed tomography angiography during 5 years of follow-up in patients with suspected coronary artery disease. Eur Heart J. 2013;34:3277–85.

Maddox TM, Stanislawski MA, Grunwald G, et al. Nonobstructive coronary artery disease and risk of myocardial infarction. JAMA. 2014;312:1754–63.

Naoum C, Berman DS, Ahmadi A, et al. Predictive value of age- and sex-specific nomograms of global plaque burden on coronary computed tomography angiography for major cardiac events. Circ Cardiovasc Imaging. 2017;10. pii: e004896.

Ohyama K, Matsumoto Y, Takanami K, et al. Coronary adventitial and perivascular adipose tissue inflammation in patients with vasospastic angina. J Am Coll Cardiol. 2018;71:414–25.

Case 14

Obstructive De Novo Lesions: Computed Tomography Coronary Angiography (CTCA)

Clinical History

- Fifty-five-year-old male.
- Coronary risk factors: former smoking.
- Ten days ago he was admitted in the emergency department with typical anginal complaints.
- ECG and enzyme levels were normal.
- He underwent a stress myocardial perfusion (single photon emission computed tomography), which was sufficient (12 METS) and did not show perfusion defects.
- Referred for CTCA to rule out coronary artery disease.

Images

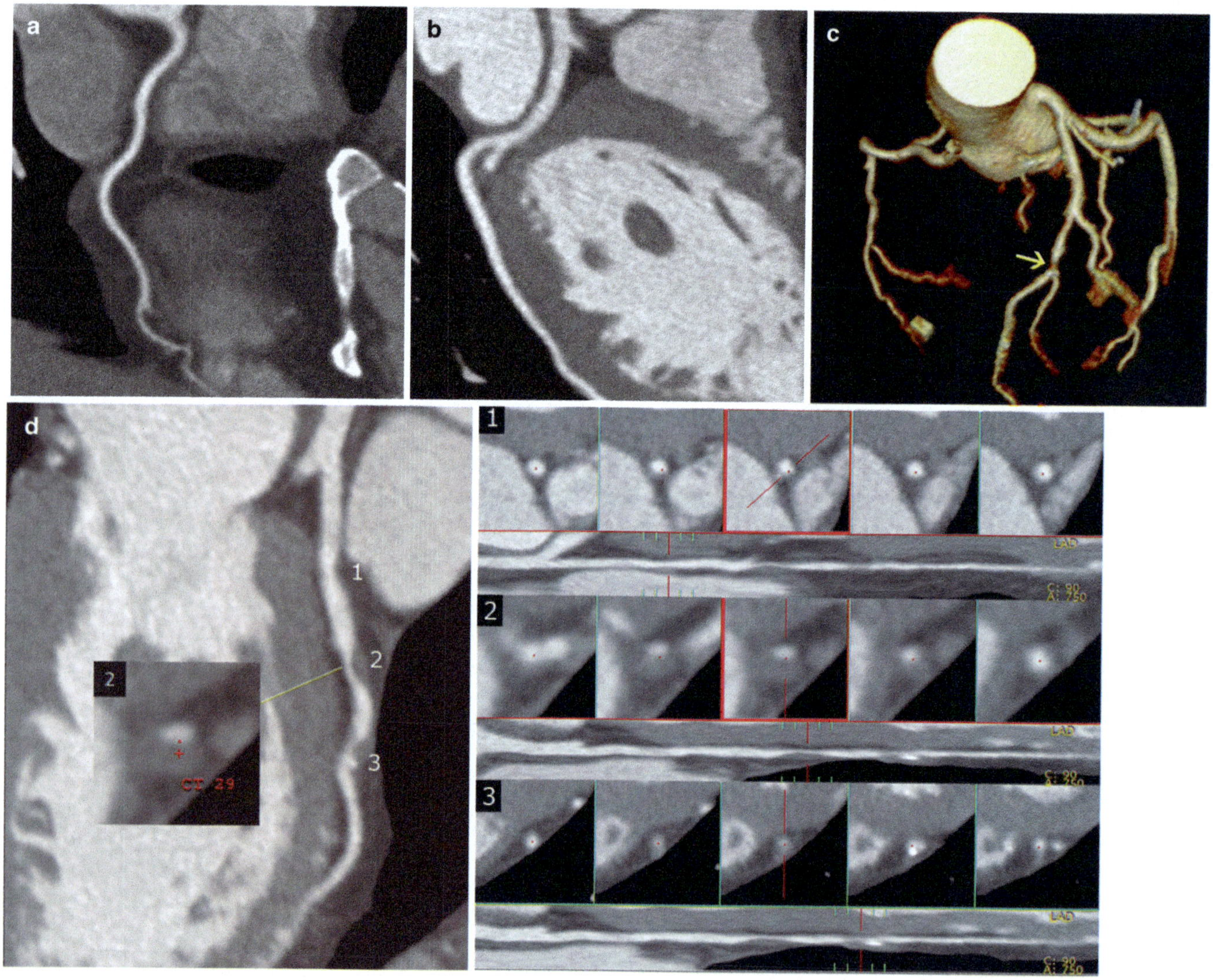

Findings and Interpretation

- Obstructive, non-extensive coronary atherosclerosis.
- The right coronary artery (panel A) and the left circumflex artery (panel B), dominant, have no evidence of disease.
- The left anterior descending (LAD) artery has a severe lesion at the mid portion (arrow in panel C, in three-dimensional volume rendering of the coronary tree).
- The multiplanar reconstruction of the LAD (panel D) shows a mild non-calcified lesion at the proximal segment

(1); confirms the severe mid lesion (2) which is focal, eccentric, with positive remodeling and a low-attenuation core (29 Hounsfield units); and demonstrates a second severe, mixed, lesion at the distal segment (3).

- This is an example of discordant findings (positive symptoms, negative functional tests, positive anatomy).
- The management in these patients remains controversial, although probably would benefit from revascularization.

Further Reading

Gray AJ, Roobottom C, Smith JE, Goodacre S, Oatey K, O'Brien R, et al. The RAPID-CTCA trial (Rapid Assessment of Potential Ischaemic Heart Disease with CTCA) – a multicentre parallel-group randomised trial to compare early computerised tomography coronary angiography versus standard care in patients presenting with suspected or confirmed acute coronary syndrome: study protocol for a randomised controlled trial. Trials. 2016;17:579.

Rodriguez-Granillo GA, Campisi R, Carrascosa P. Noninvasive cardiac imaging in patients with known and suspected coronary artery disease: what is in it for the interventional cardiologist? Curr Cardiol Rep. 2016;18:3.

Winchester DE, Jois P, Kraft SM, Wymer DC, Hill JA. Immediate computed tomography coronary angiography versus delayed outpatient stress testing for detecting coronary artery disease in emergency department patients with chest pain. Int J Cardiovasc Imaging. 2012;28:667–74.

Case 15

Obstructive De Novo Lesions: Computed Tomography Coronary Angiography (CTCA)

Clinical History

- Sixty-year-old female.
- Coronary risk factors: hypercholesterolemia, hypertension, former smoking, family history of coronary disease.
- Typical chest pain of variable functional class.
- Three years ago, she underwent invasive coronary angiography, which was normal (without angiographical evidence of lesions).
- She further underwent PET/CT with ^{13}N-amonia and cold-pressor test for the evaluation of coronary flow reserve and endothelial function, yielding endothelium-dependent microvascular dysfunction (anginal complaints, ST depression, and abnormal response to cold-pressor test).
- Given the persisting symptoms despite full medical therapy, the patient was referred for CTCA to evaluate coronary anatomy.

Images

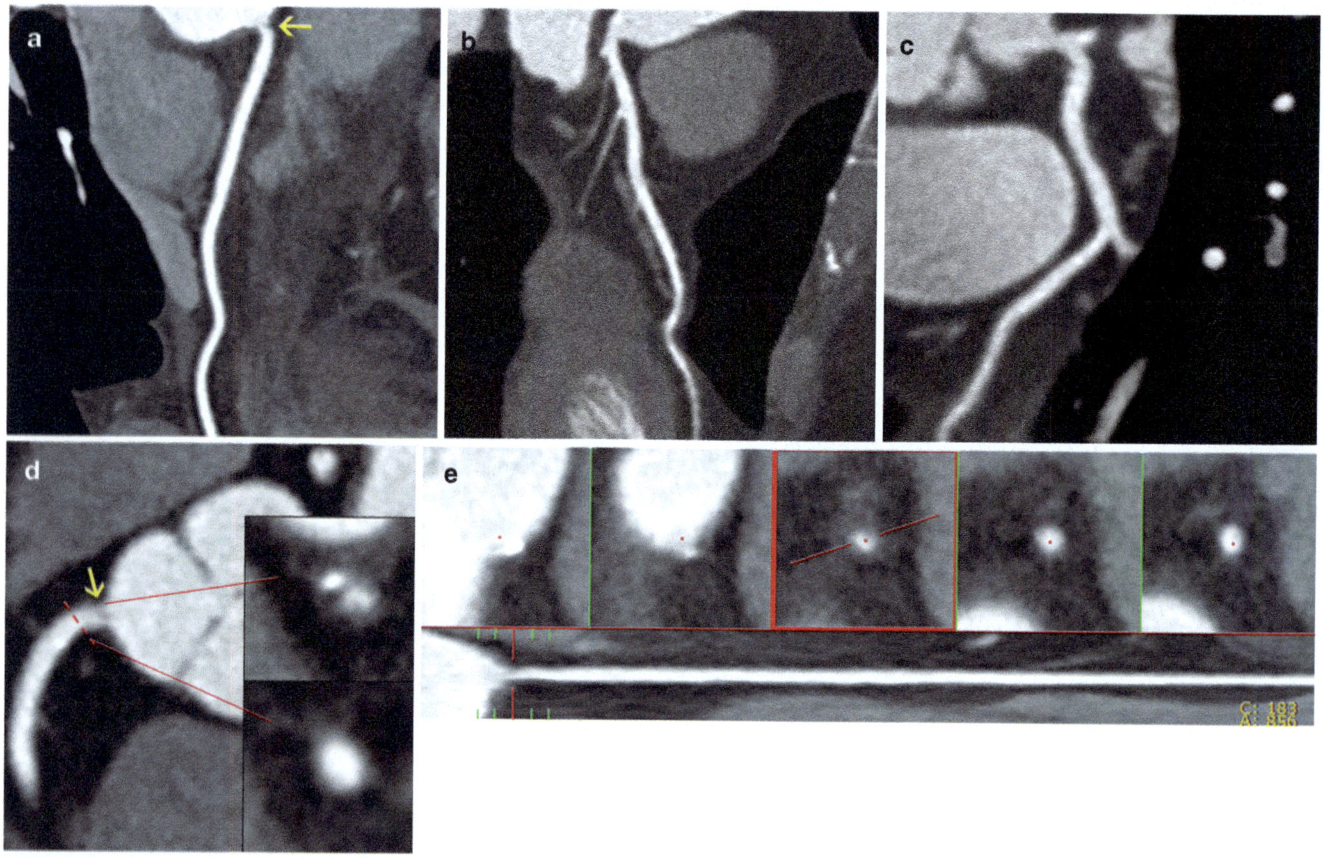

Findings and Interpretation

- Moderate ostial stenosis.
- The right coronary artery (panels A, D, and E), dominant, has a moderate ostial, predominantly non-calcified eccentric lesion (arrow), with low-attenuation core and a linear low-density intraluminal image suggestive of focal dissection.
- The left anterior descending artery (panel B) and the left circumflex artery (panel C) have no evidence of atherosclerosis.
- The presence of persisting symptoms warrants percutaneous coronary intervention (PCI). Nonetheless, this is controversial since PCI of patients with spontaneous coronary dissection presenting as acute coronary syndromes has been associated with a higher incidence of mortality compared with conservative management.

Further Reading

Afzal A, Sarmast S, Choi JW, McCullough PA, Schussler JM. Spontaneous coronary artery dissection: a review of pathogenesis, presentations, treatment, and outcomes. Rev Cardiovasc Med. 2017;18:29–36.

Mahmoud AN, Taduru SS, Mentias A, et al. Trends of incidence, clinical presentation, and in-hospital mortality among women with acute myocardial infarction with or without spontaneous coronary artery dissection: a population-based analysis. J Am Coll Cardiol Intv. 2018;11:80–90.

Case 16

Obstructive De Novo Lesions: Computed Tomography Coronary Angiography (CTCA)

Clinical History

- Seventy-three-year-old male.
- Coronary risk factors: hypercholesterolemia.
- Asymptomatic.
- In a routine stress-rest single photon emission computed tomography with optimal exertion and absence of symptoms, a 4 mm ST-segment depression in the anterolateral leads (V3 to V6) was detected, with normal myocardial perfusion.
- Such discordant findings promoted the referral to CTCA to rule out coronary artery disease.

Images

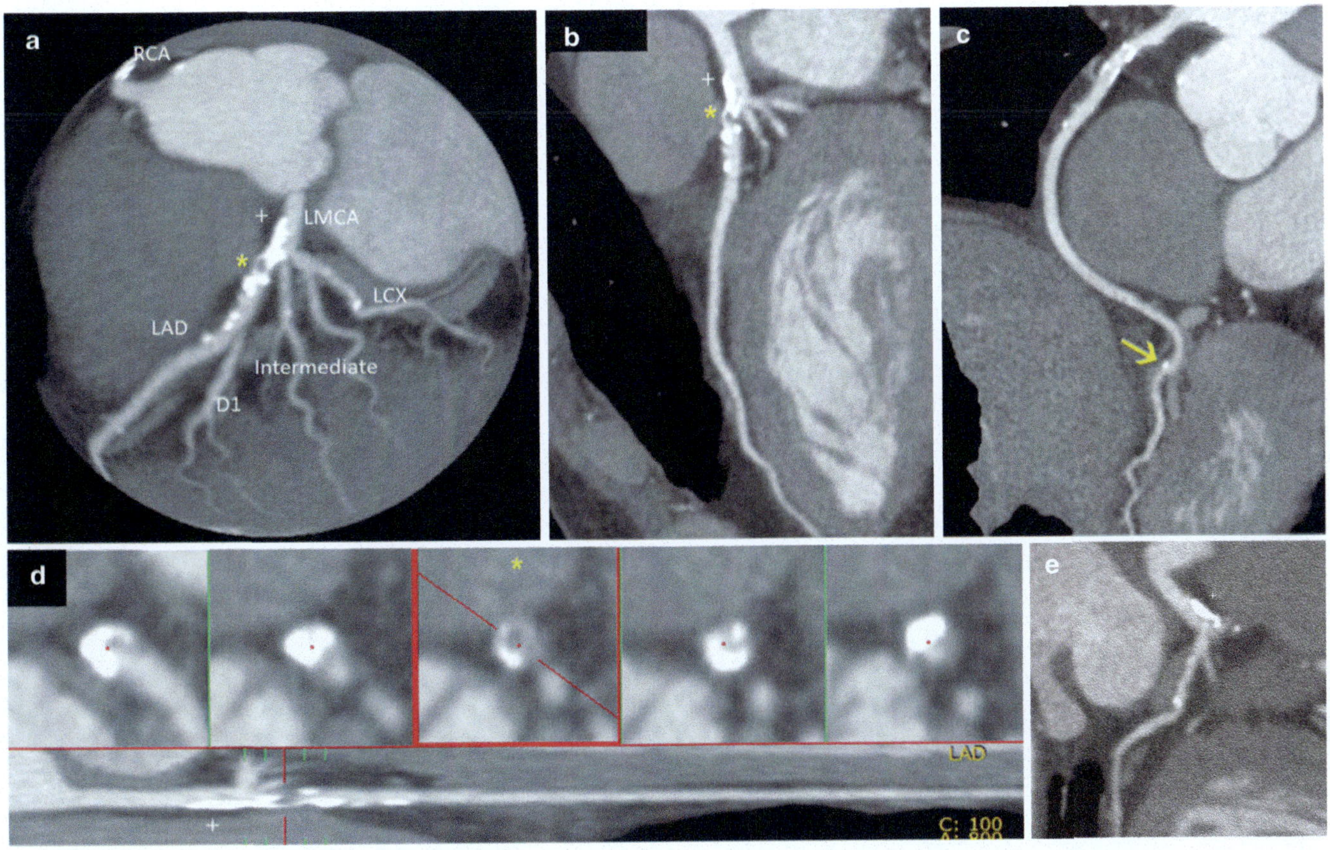

Findings and Interpretation

- Obstructive coronary atherosclerosis.
- Two-dimensional maximum intensity projection (MIP) globe reconstruction (panel A) shows calcification of the left main (LMCA), left anterior descending (LAD), and right coronary (RCA) arteries and minimal spotty calcifications of the left circumflex (LCX) and intermediate and diagonal (D1) branches.
- The LMCA has an eccentric distal nonobstructive plaque (†, in panel B).
- The LAD (panels B and D) has a focal severe proximal mix lesion (*). Mild calcifications are detected in the mid LAD, D1, and intermediate branch.
- The RCA (panel C), dominant, has a mild calcified lesion at the proximal segment and minimal calcifications at the mid RCA and posterior descending artery (arrow).
- The LCX (panel E) is small and has minimal calcifications.
- This is an example of discordant findings (negative symptoms, positive ECG/negative perfusion, and positive anatomy).
- This patient is at high risk of events given the anatomy (proximal LAD), although management in this case remains controversial (asymptomatic, with absence of perfusion defects). Before planning revascularization, an alternative stress-imaging strategy (with CMR, CT, or echo) might possibly be useful.

Further Reading

Iqbal MB, Ilsley C, De Robertis F, et al. Comparison of outcomes of coronary artery bypass grafting using internal mammary graft versus percutaneous coronary intervention for isolated proximal left anterior descending narrowing. Am J Cardiol. 2017;119:719–26.

Rodriguez-Granillo GA, Campisi R, Carrascosa P. Noninvasive cardiac imaging in patients with known and suspected coronary artery disease: what is in it for the interventional cardiologist? Curr Cardiol Rep. 2016;18:3.

Roguin A, Camenzind E, Kerner A, et al. Long-term outcomes of stenting the proximal left anterior descending artery in the PROTECT trial. JACC Cardiovasc Interv. 2017;10:548–56.

Case 17

Obstructive De Novo Lesions and Coronary Stents: Computed Tomography Coronary Angiography (CTCA)

Clinical History

- Forty-three-year-old male.
- Coronary risk factors: hypercholesterolemia, former smoking.
- He has a previous history of deep venous thrombosis.
- One month ago, he had a non-ST-segment elevation acute myocardial infarction and underwent percutaneous coronary intervention with stenting of the left circumflex (LCX) artery.
- The left anterior descending (LAD) artery had a chronic total occlusion (CTO), with collateral circulation.
- Stress-rest single photon emission computed tomography revealed perinecrotic residual ischemia in the anterior wall, suggesting viable myocardium.
- Referred for CTCA as guidance for recanalization attempt.

Images

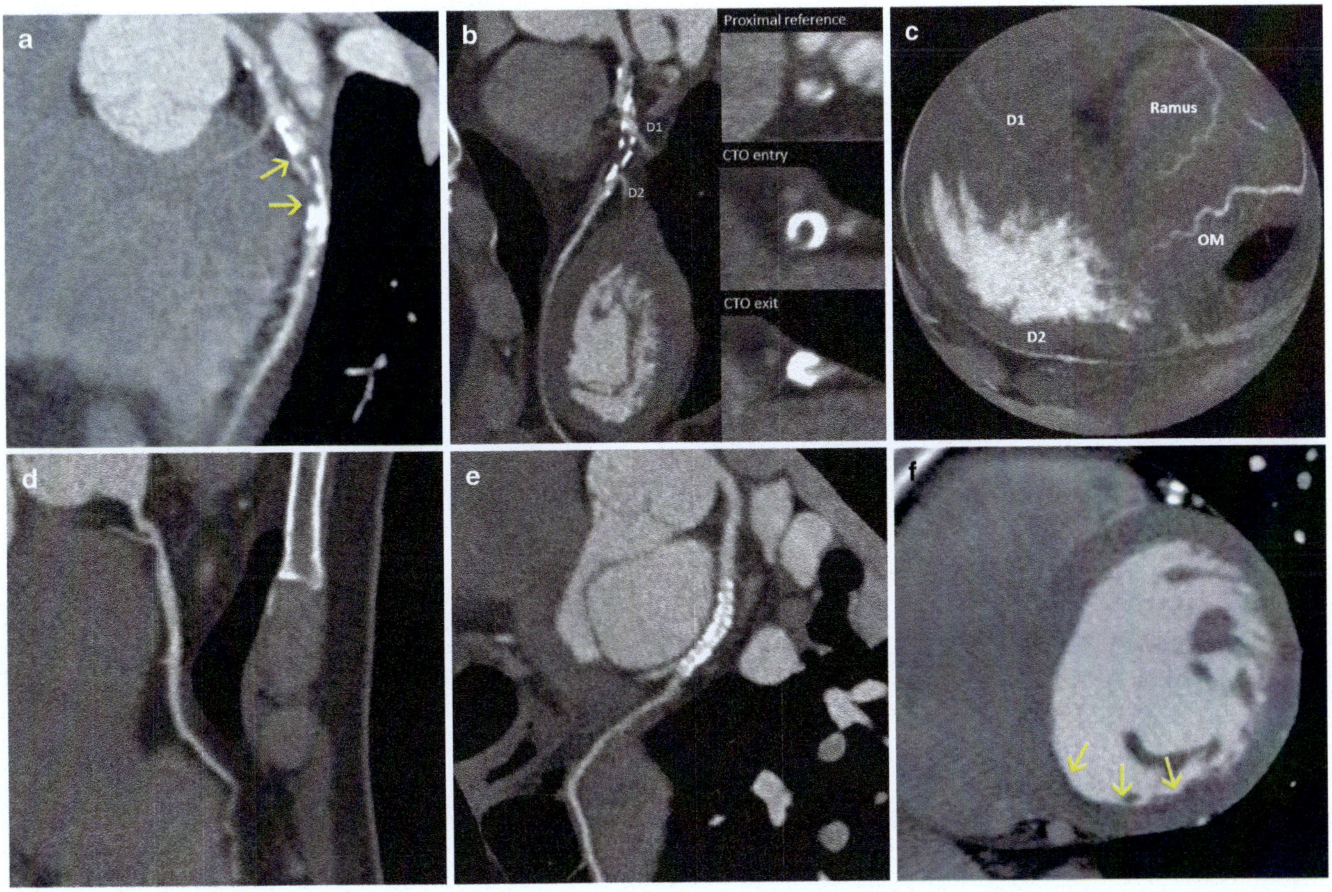

Findings and Interpretation

- Chronic total occlusion.
- The mid LAD (panels A and B) is totally occluded (arrows), with a short total occlusion between the first and second diagonal branches (D1 and D2).
- The CTO entrance has moderate eccentric calcification, with non-calcified low-attenuation core, whereas the exit has heavy concentric calcification (panel B, orthogonal views).
- There is no vessel tortuosity or angulation, and the distal coronary bed has no evidence of disease, with collateral circulation from the ramus intermedius (ramus) and obtuse marginal (OM) branches (two-dimensional MIP globe view, panel C).
- The right coronary artery (panel D), not dominant, has no evidence of disease.
- The LCX (panel E) has a patent stent at the mid segment, without evidence of neointimal hyperplasia.
- Subendocardial resting perfusion defect is present at the inferior septal wall (arrows, in panel F).
- The patient underwent PCI with successful recanalization that required rotational atherectomy.

Further Reading

García-García HM, Brugaletta S, van Mieghem CA, et al. CRosser As First choice for crossing Totally occluded coronary arteries (CRAFT Registry): focus on conventional angiography and computed tomography angiography predictors of success. EuroIntervention. 2011;7:480–6.

Mehran R, Claessen BE, Godino C, et al. Long-term outcome of percutaneous coronary intervention for chronic total occlusions. JACC Cardiovasc Interv. 2011;4:952–61.

Rodríguez-Granillo GA, Rosales MA, Llauradó C, et al. Guidance of percutaneous coronary interventions by multidetector row computed tomography coronary angiography. EuroIntervention. 2011;6:773–8.

Sudhakar G, MD. Long-term follow-up of elective chronic total coronary occlusion angioplasty: analysis from the U.K. Central Cardiac Audit Database. JACC Cardiovasc Interv. 2014;64:235–43.

Case 18

Obstructive De Novo Lesions: Computed Tomography Coronary Angiography (CTCA)

Clinical History

- Forty-eight-year-old female.
- Coronary risk factors: hypertension, hypercholesterolemia, smoking.
- Typical anginal complaints.
- Referred for CTCA to rule out coronary artery disease.

Images

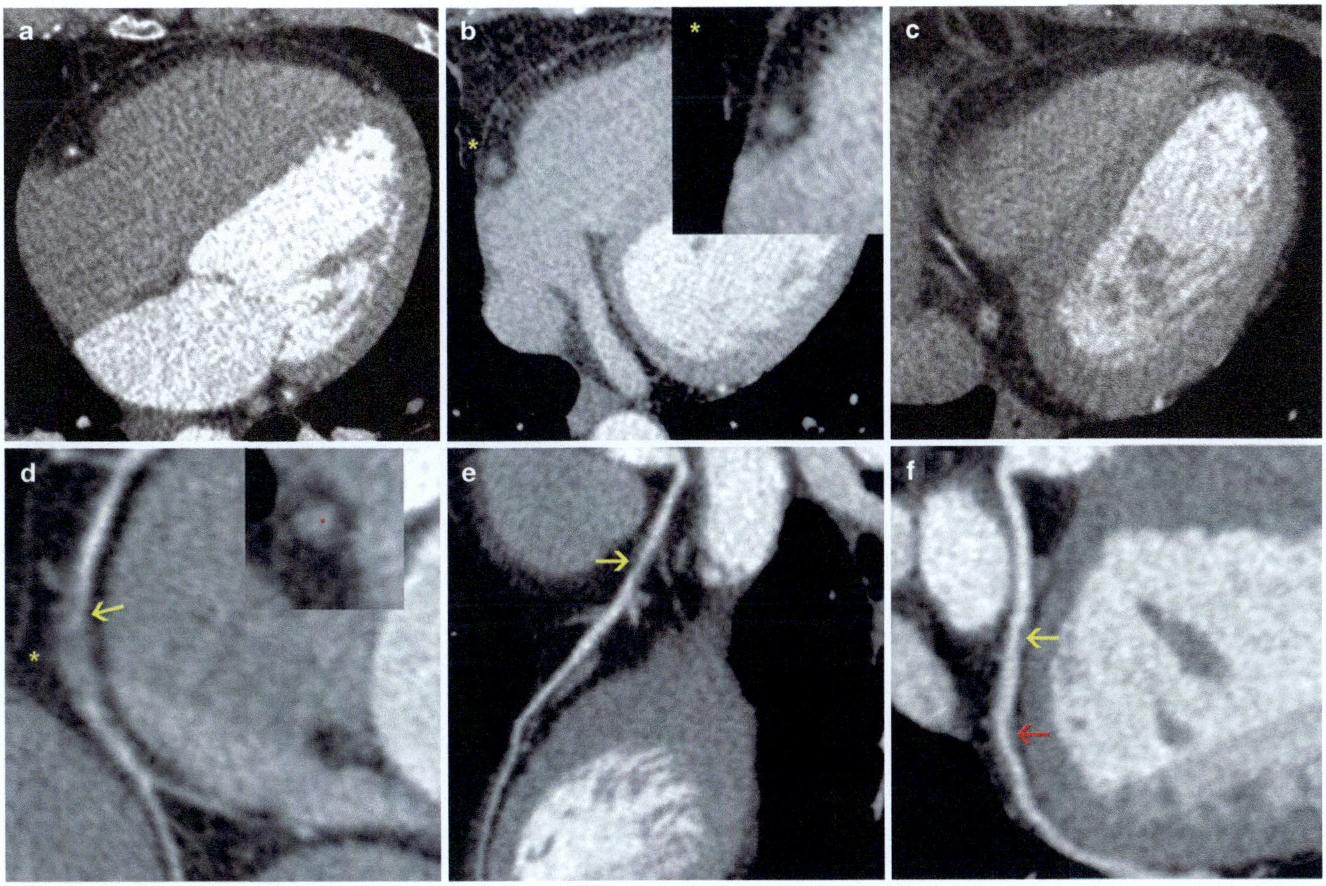

Findings and Interpretation

- Fresh total occlusion.
- Axial views of the proximal (panel A), mid (panel B), and distal (panel C) segments of the right coronary artery (RCA). The RCA, dominant, has an occlusive non-calcified lesion at the mid segment (*, in panel B). The absence of luminal contrast is clearly depicted in the axial views. Also, the vessel wall boundaries are hazy and poorly defined (*, in panels B and D). This is typically observed in acute lesions and might suggest thrombotic content with perivascular adipose tissue inflammation.
- In addition, immediately proximal, a significant non-calcified lesion with positive remodeling and napkin-ring sign is present (arrow in panel D).
- The left anterior descending artery (panel E) has a focal moderate non-calcified lesion at the mid segment (arrow).
- The left circumflex artery (panel F) has mild (yellow arrow) and moderate (red arrow) non-calcified lesions.
- This patient warrants prompt revascularization, and CTCA findings might be useful for percutaneous coronary intervention guidance.

Further Reading

Ohyama K, Matsumoto Y, Takanami K, et al. Coronary adventitial and perivascular adipose tissue inflammation in patients with vasospastic angina. J Am Coll Cardiol. 2018;71:414–25.

Rodríguez-Granillo GA, Rosales MA, Llauradó C, et al. Guidance of percutaneous coronary interventions by multidetector row computed tomography coronary angiography. EuroIntervention. 2011;6:773–8.

Case 19

Obstructive De Novo Lesions: Computed Tomography Coronary Angiography (CTCA)

Clinical History

- Sixty-two-year-old male.
- Coronary risk factors: none.
- Asymptomatic.
- A stress myocardial perfusion test (single photon emission computed tomography) identified anterior wall ischemia.
- Referred for CTCA to rule out coronary artery disease.

Images

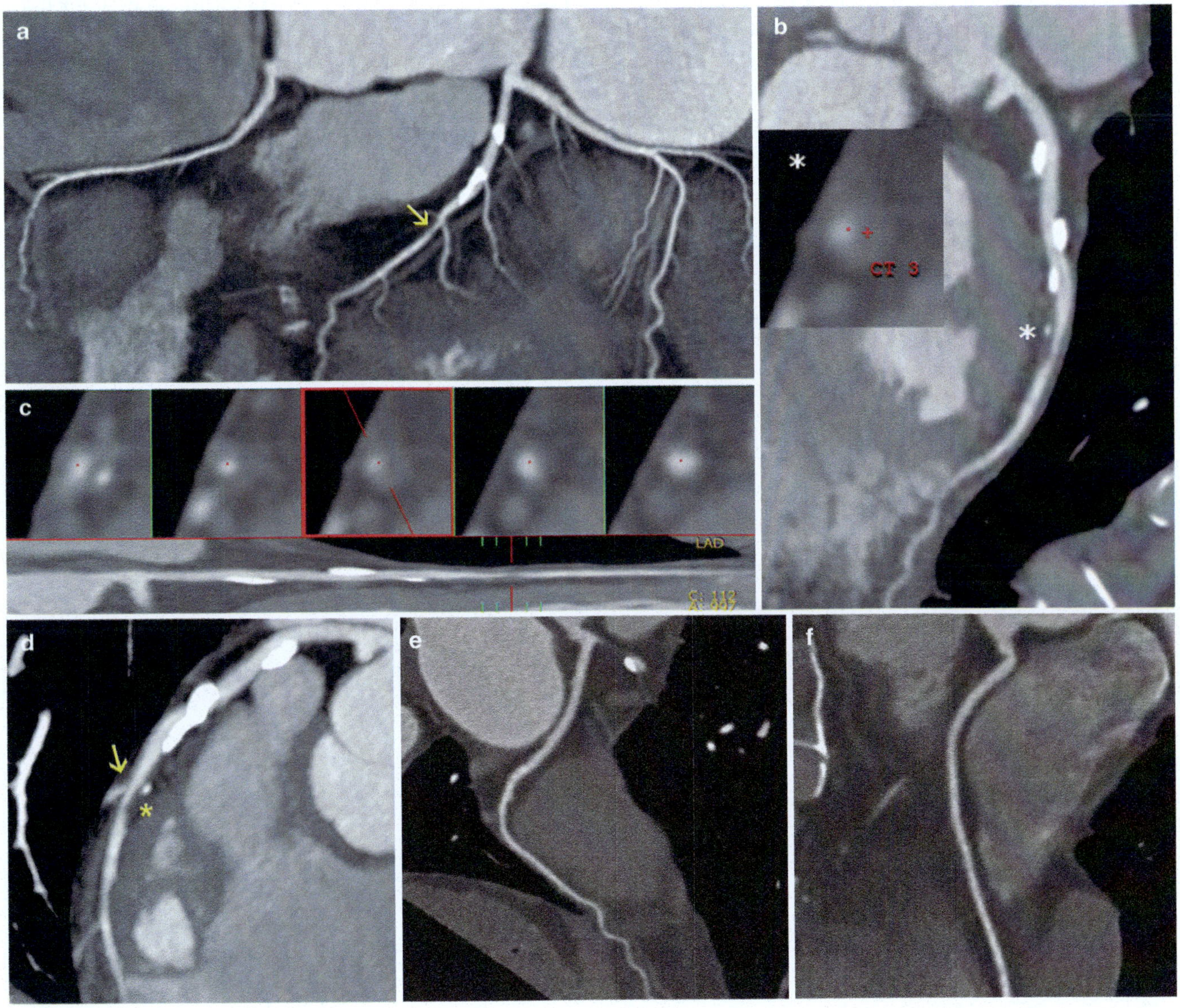

Findings and Interpretation

- Obstructive, non-extensive coronary atherosclerosis.
- Two-dimensional maximum intensity projection (MIP) reconstruction (panel A) showing calcification of the left anterior descending (LAD) artery, with a severe distal lesion (arrow).
- The LAD (panels B, C, and D) has nonsignificant calcified plaques at the proximal and mid segments and a severe (focal, eccentric, predominantly non-calcified) lesion at the mid to distal segment (*) with low-attenuation

core (3 Hounsfield units), positive remodeling, and napkin-ring sign.

- Using a thick-slab MIP (panel D), severe involvement of the ostium of the third diagonal branch (arrow) is detected (Medina classification 0, 1, 1).
- The left circumflex artery (panel E) and right coronary artery (panel F) have no evidence of disease.
- According to the extension of the ischemic burden, this patient might benefit from percutaneous revascularization.
- The Medina classification divides bifurcation lesions in three segments (proximal segment of the main branch, distal segment of the main branch, and side branch ostium; and any segment with plaque is classified as 1, whereas the absence of plaque is classified as 0).

Further Reading

Carrascosa PM, Capuñay CM, Garcia-Merletti P, Carrascosa J, Garcia MF. Characterization of coronary atherosclerotic plaques by multidetector computed tomography. Am J Cardiol. 2006;97:598–602.

Kesarwani M, Nakanishi R, Choi TY, Shavelle DM, Budoff MJ. Evaluation of plaque morphology by 64-slice coronary computed tomographic angiography compared to intravascular ultrasound in nonocclusive segments of coronary arteries. Acad Radiol. 2017;24:968–74.

Papadopoulou SL, Girasis C, Gijsen FJ, et al. A CT-based Medina classification in coronary bifurcations: does the lumen assessment provide sufficient information? Catheter Cardiovasc Interv. 2014;84:445–52.

Case 20

Obstructive De Novo Lesions: Computed Tomography Coronary Angiography (CTCA)

Clinical History

- Sixty-seven-year-old male.
- Coronary risk factors: hypertension, hypercholesterolemia, former smoking, family history.
- Atypical chest pain.
- Discordant stress-rest single photon emission computed tomography findings (2 mm ST-segment depression V2–V6; absence of myocardial perfusion defects).
- Referred for CTCA to define coronary anatomy.

Images

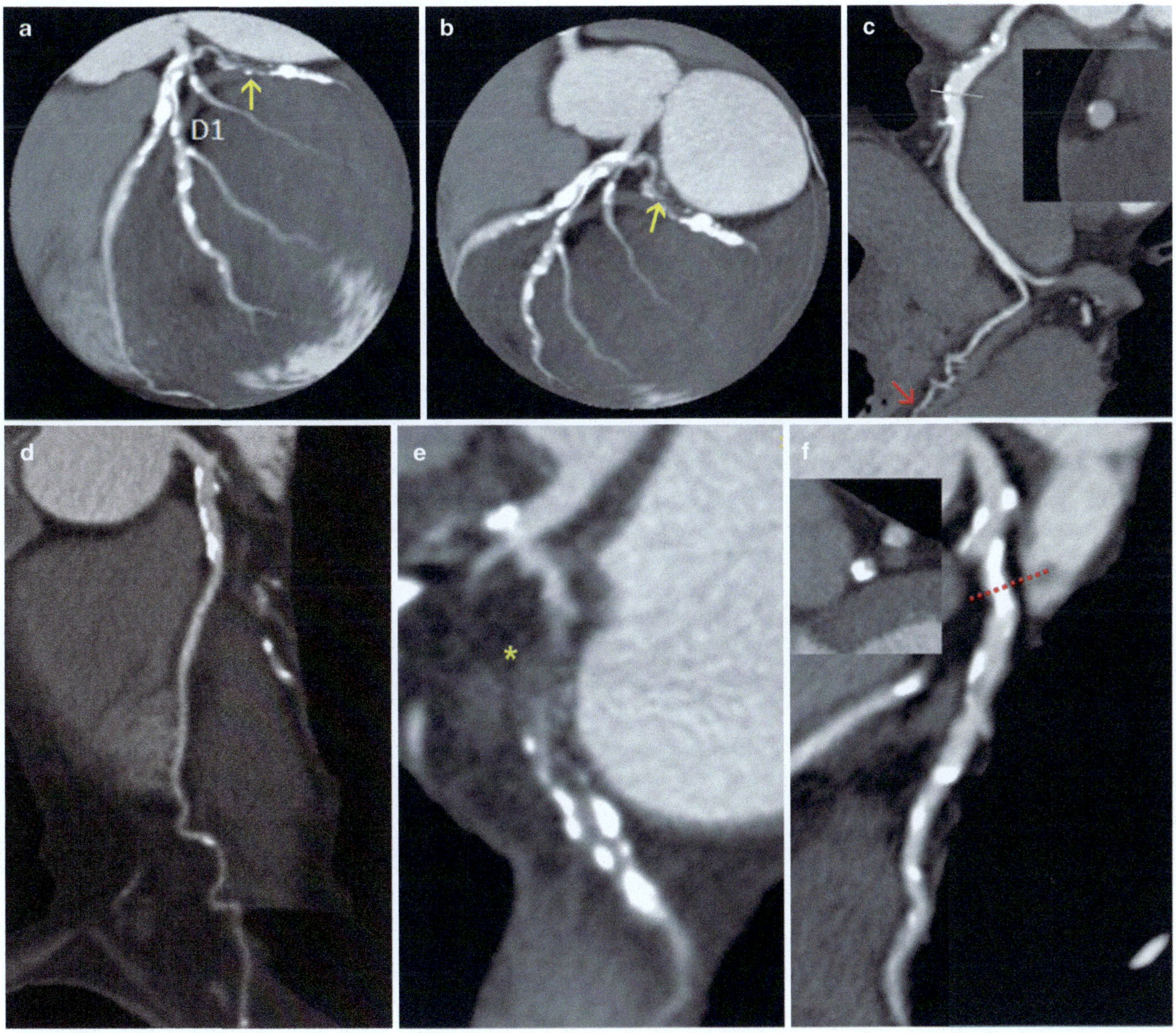

Findings and Interpretation

- Chronic total occlusion (CTO).
- Two-dimensional maximum intensity projection (MIP) globe views (panels A and B) show diffuse calcification of the first diagonal branch (D1) and a proximal total occlusion of the left circumflex artery (arrow). The occlusion site has a very large vessel size (seemingly coronary ectasia).

- There is no calcification at the occlusion entry (*, in panel E), but heavy calcification is present at the occlusion exit point. Collateral circulation (red arrow in panel C) is provided by a very large right coronary artery (RCA), and a side branch emerges at the entry site.
- The RCA (panel C), dominant, has mild calcifications. Note that the mid segment has segmental dilatation (coronary ectasia) with mild calcification.
- The left anterior descending artery (panel D) has mild calcified proximal and distal lesions.
- There is a large and bifurcated D1 (panel F) with diffuse ostial calcification that impairs the ability to accurately define the extent of luminal stenosis (possibly at least moderate).
- The likelihood of successful recanalization of the CTO in this patient is low, and the risk/benefit ratio seems unfavorable. Furthermore, the need for recanalization is dubious given the small territory involved and the presence of collateral circulation.
- On the other hand, given the complex diagonal branch anatomy, this patient might possibly be better managed with intensive medical therapy.
- CTCA has been validated as a helpful imaging tool for the characterization of CTO and provides accurate information regarding key features related to a decreased likelihood of successful percutaneous recanalization: blunt morphology of the entry point, severe calcification, tortuosity >45° proximal or within the occluded segment, and occlusion length >20 mm.

Further Reading

García-García HM, Brugaletta S, van Mieghem CA, et al. CRosser As First choice for crossing Totally occluded coronary arteries (CRAFT Registry): focus on conventional angiography and computed tomography angiography predictors of success. EuroIntervention. 2011;7:480–6.

Li Y, Xu N, Zhang J, et al. Procedural success of CTO recanalization: comparison of the J-CTO score determined by coronary CT angiography to invasive angiography. J Cardiovasc Comput Tomogr. 2015;9:578–84.

Mehran R, Claessen BE, Godino C, et al. Long-term outcome of percutaneous coronary intervention for chronic total occlusions. JACC Cardiovasc Interv. 2011;4:952–61.

Rodríguez-Granillo GA, Rosales MA, Llauradó C, et al. Guidance of percutaneous coronary interventions by multidetector row computed tomography coronary angiography. EuroIntervention. 2011;6:773–8.

Sudhakar G, MD. Long-term follow-up of elective chronic total coronary occlusion angioplasty: analysis from the U.K. Central Cardiac Audit Database. JACC Cardiovasc Interv. 2014; 64:235–43.

Sugaya T, Oyama-Manabe N, Yamaguchi T, et al. Visualization of collateral channels with coronary computed tomography angiography for the retrograde approach in percutaneous coronary intervention for chronic total occlusion. J Cardiovasc Comput Tomogr. 2016;10:128–34.

Case 21

Obstructive De Novo Lesions: Computed Tomography Coronary Angiography (CTCA)

Clinical History

- Sixty-eight-year-old male.
- Coronary risk factors: hypertension, hypercholesterolemia, diabetes, former smoking.
- Asymptomatic.
- Stress echo with inferior and posterior septal ischemia (two segments).
- Referred for CTCA to define coronary anatomy.

Images

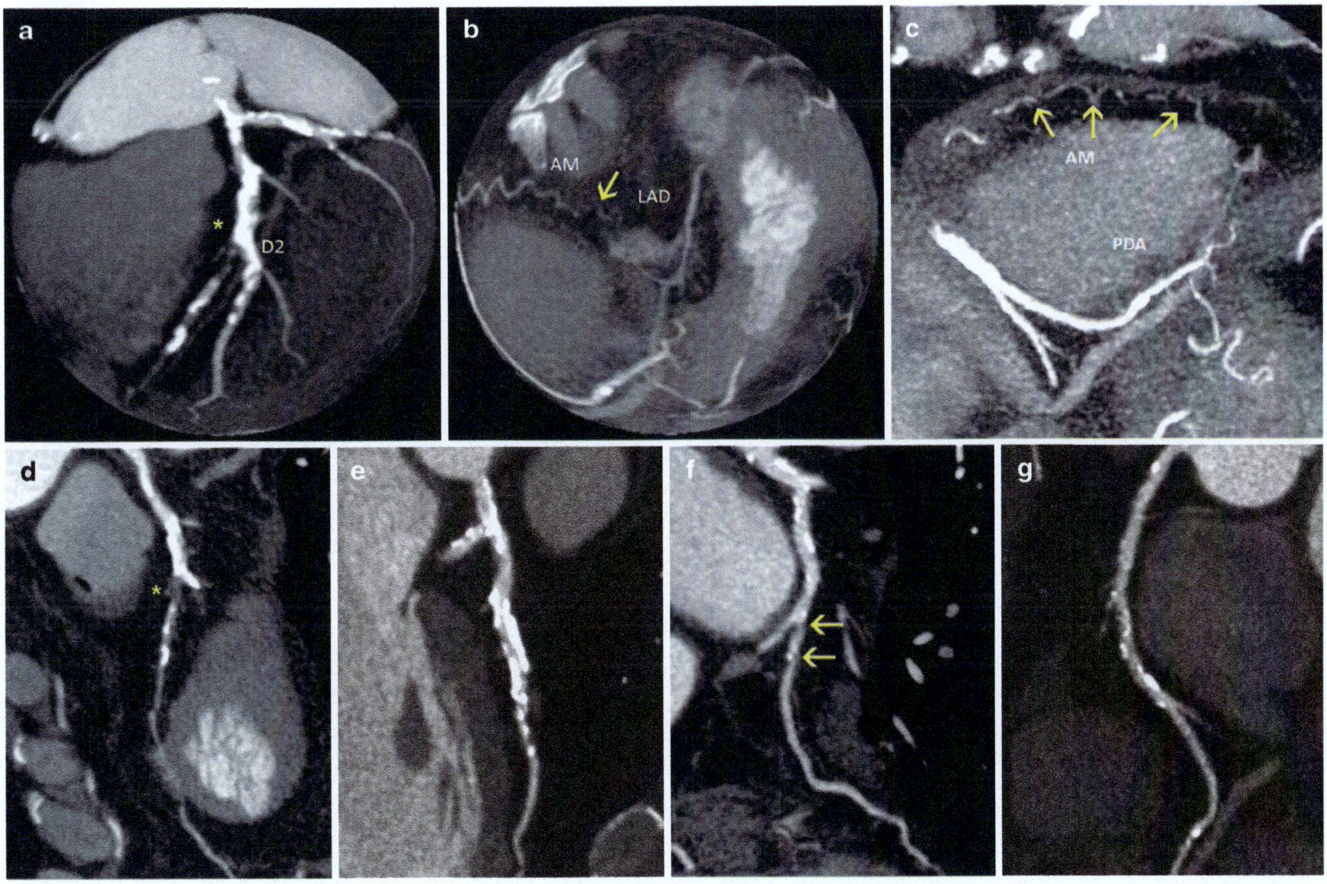

Findings and Interpretation

- Chronic total occlusion (CTO).
- The left coronary system is diffusely diseased (panel A), and the mid left anterior descending (LAD) artery has a CTO (*). The entry site (*) has both severe calcification and emergence of a large diagonal branch (D2), which is also heavily calcified (panels A and E).
- The distal coronary bed of the LAD has extensive collateral circulation from the acute marginal (AM) branch (arrows in panels B and C). This is particularly evident using thick maximum intensity projections (panel C).
- The obtuse marginal branch (panel F) has two severe tandem mixed lesions (arrows).
- The right coronary artery (panel G), dominant, has multiple mild calcified lesions.
- Given the heavy calcification at the entry site and the proximal side branch exit, this patient has a low likelihood of successful percutaneous recanalization of the LAD. However, the obtuse marginal lesion might warrant revascularization.

Further Reading

García-García HM, Brugaletta S, van Mieghem CA, et al. CRosser As First choice for crossing Totally occluded coronary arteries (CRAFT Registry): focus on conventional angiography and computed tomography angiography predictors of success. EuroIntervention. 2011;7:480–6.

Li Y, Xu N, Zhang J, et al. Procedural success of CTO recanalization: Comparison of the J-CTO score determined by coronary CT angiography to invasive angiography. J Cardiovasc Comput Tomogr. 2015;9:578–84.

Case 22

Obstructive De Novo Lesions: Computed Tomography Coronary Angiography (CTCA)

Clinical History

- Fifty-one-year-old male.
- Coronary risk factors: hypertension, former smoking, obesity.
- Eight months ago, he underwent primary angioplasty for an ST-elevation acute myocardial infarction, with stent implantation to the left circumflex (LCX) artery.
- Currently asymptomatic. Single photon emission computed tomography with a fixed inferior/lateral defect and no evidence of ischemia.
- Referred for CTCA to evaluate coronary anatomy.

Images

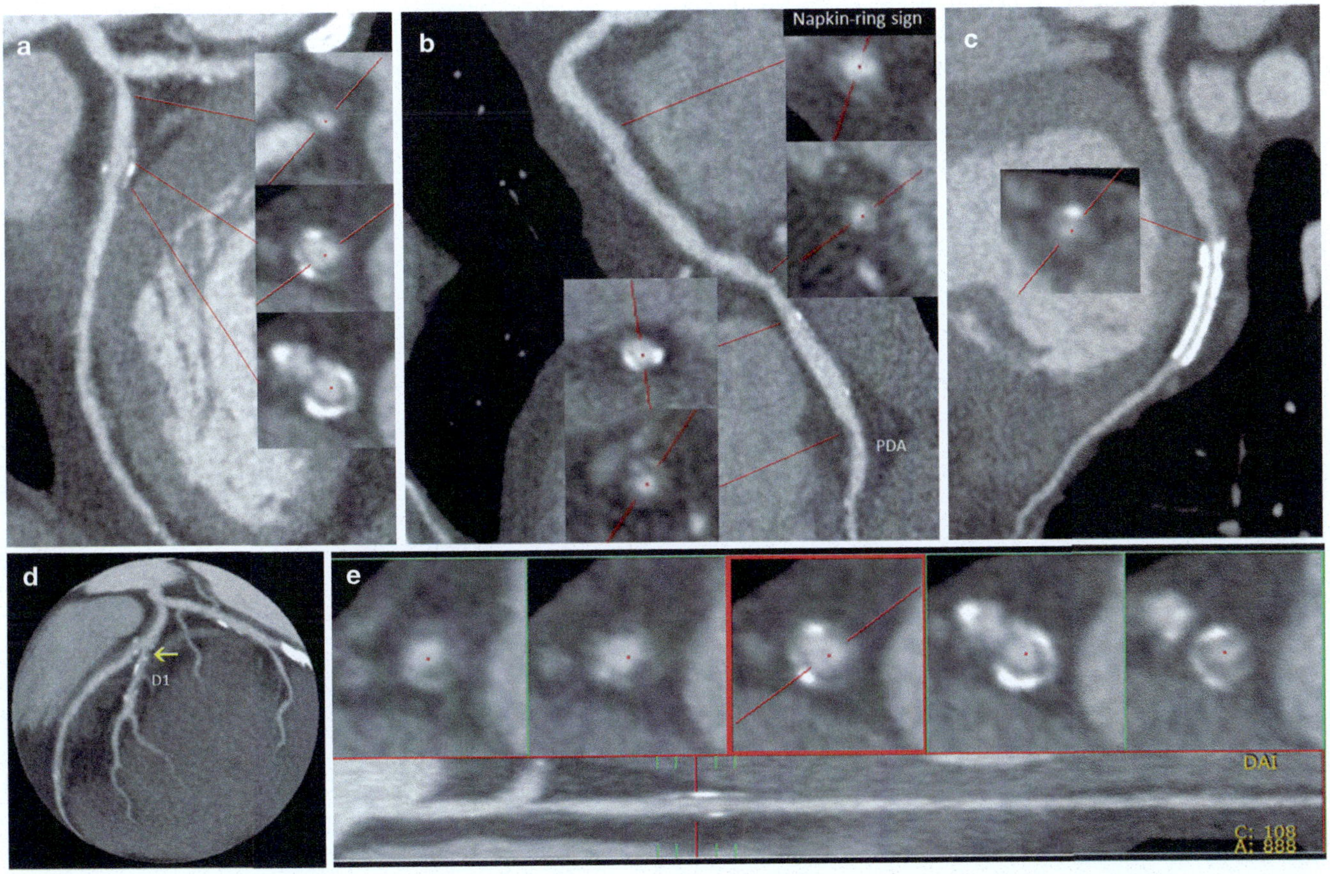

Findings and Interpretation

- Extensive coronary atherosclerosis, obstructive lesions, and high-risk plaque characteristics.
- The left anterior descending (LAD) artery is diffusely diseased in the proximal and mid segments, involving moderate ostial and proximal segment stenoses (panels A and E). The ostial lesion is eccentric and non-calcified, whereas the proximal lesion (orthogonal views in panel E) is concentric and mixed with low-attenuation core and marked positive remodeling (coronary ectasia).
- There is a large first diagonal branch (D1, in panel D), bifurcated, with a severe, mixed, ostial (arrow) lesion (Medina classification 1, 1, 1).
- The right coronary artery (panel B), dominant, is diffusely diseased and with segmental dilatation (coronary ectasia). An eccentric mild lesion with "napkin-ring" sign is present at the proximal segment (orthogonal view). A concentric significant non-calcified lesion is observed at the mid segment (orthogonal view). The posterior descending artery has a moderate, concentric, mixed lesion.
- The stent in the LCX artery (panel C) is patent and has no evidence of neointimal hyperplasia. However, a severe, concentric, mixed lesion (in-segment restenosis) is identified immediately proximal.
- This patient is at very high risk of events. He has extensive coronary atherosclerosis and multiple moderate ste-

noses, obstructive disease, and several plaques with high-risk characteristics.

- Therapeutical approach of in this patient might be controversial. The lack of symptoms and absence of ischemia might safely lead to a conservative management. However, among both stable patients and patients with previous acute coronary syndromes, more than half of events occur among patients with normal stress tests.

Further Reading

Hoffmann U, Ferencik M, Udelson JE, et al. Prognostic value of noninvasive cardiovascular testing in patients with stable chest pain: insights from the PROMISE trial (Prospective Multicenter Imaging Study for Evaluation of Chest Pain). Circulation. 2017;135:2320–32.

Nakazato R, Otake H, Konishi A, et al. Atherosclerotic plaque characterization by CT angiography for identification of high-risk coronary artery lesions: a comparison to optical coherence tomography. Eur Heart J Cardiovasc Imaging. 2015;16:373–9.

Stone GW, Maehara A, Lansky AJ, et al. A prospective natural-history study of coronary atherosclerosis. N Engl J Med. 2011;364:226–35.

Case 23

Coronary Stents: Computed Tomography Coronary Angiography (CTCA)

Clinical History

- Seventy-year-old male.
- Coronary risk factors: hypertension, smoking.
- He has a history of previous myocardial infarction (4 years ago), with primary angioplasty and stenting of the left anterior descending (LAD) artery.
- He is currently asymptomatic but only performs minimal efforts.
- Referred for CTCA to evaluate coronary anatomy.

Images

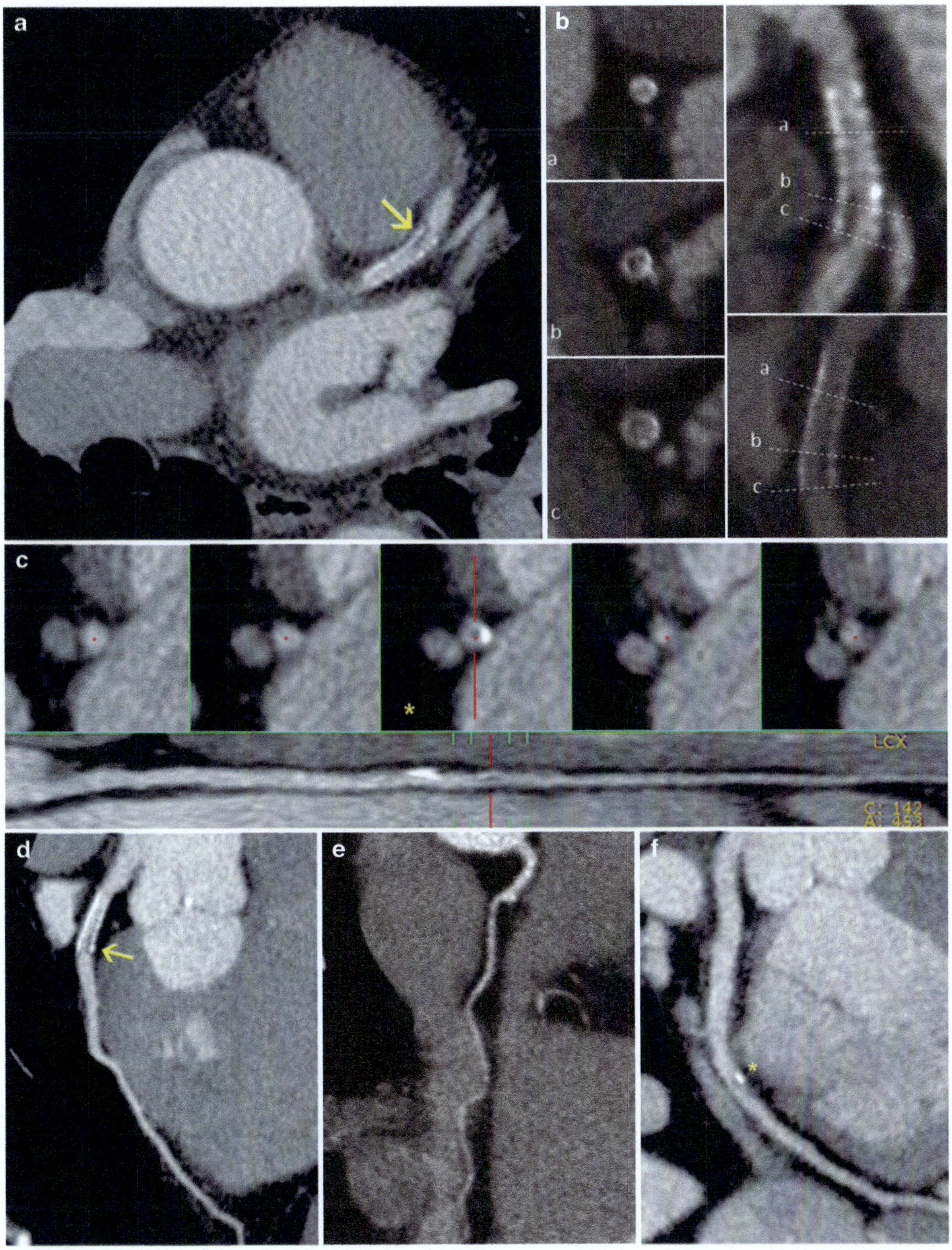

Findings and Interpretation

- In-stent restenosis.
- The proximal LAD has a patent stent, with in-stent restenosis (arrow) of the distal portion. This can be clearly observed using an axial view (panel A), as well as in multiplanar and orthogonal views (panels B and D, respectively).
- The right coronary artery (panel E), small and not dominant, has no evidence of disease.
- The mid left circumflex artery (LCX, panels C and F) has a severe focal mixed lesion (*), with a low-attenuation core.
- This patient underwent invasive coronary angiography with stenting of the proximal LAD and mid LCX arteries.
- CTCA has a good diagnostic accuracy for the evaluation of coronary stents and the detection of in-stent restenosis, particularly in the evaluation of stents ≥3 mm. Aside from the requirements of optimal quality acquisitions including low and stable heart rate and high intraluminal opacification, the ability of CTCA to assess stent patency also depends on strut thickness and material (stainless steel, chromium cobalt, tantalum, nitinol, bioabsorbable scaffolds) and cell type (open or closed struts).

Further Reading

Dai T, Wang JR, Hu PF. Diagnostic performance of computed tomography angiography in the detection of coronary artery in-stent restenosis: evidence from an updated meta-analysis. Eur Radiol. 2018;28:1373–82.

Eisentopf J, Achenbach S, Ulzheimer S, et al. Low-dose dual-source CT angiography with iterative reconstruction for coronary artery stent evaluation. JACC Cardiovasc Imaging. 2013;6:458–65.

Case 24

Coronary Artery Bypass Surgery: Computed Tomography Coronary Angiography (CTCA)

Clinical History

- Seventy-year-old male.
- Coronary risk factors: hypercholesterolemia, hypertension, diabetes, former smoker.
- He has a history of previous coronary artery bypass surgery in 1995. Three years ago he underwent percutaneous coronary intervention of the left internal mammary artery and of the left anterior descending (LAD) artery.
- He has persistent anginal symptoms despite optimal medical treatment.
- Referred for CTCA to evaluate coronary anatomy.

Images

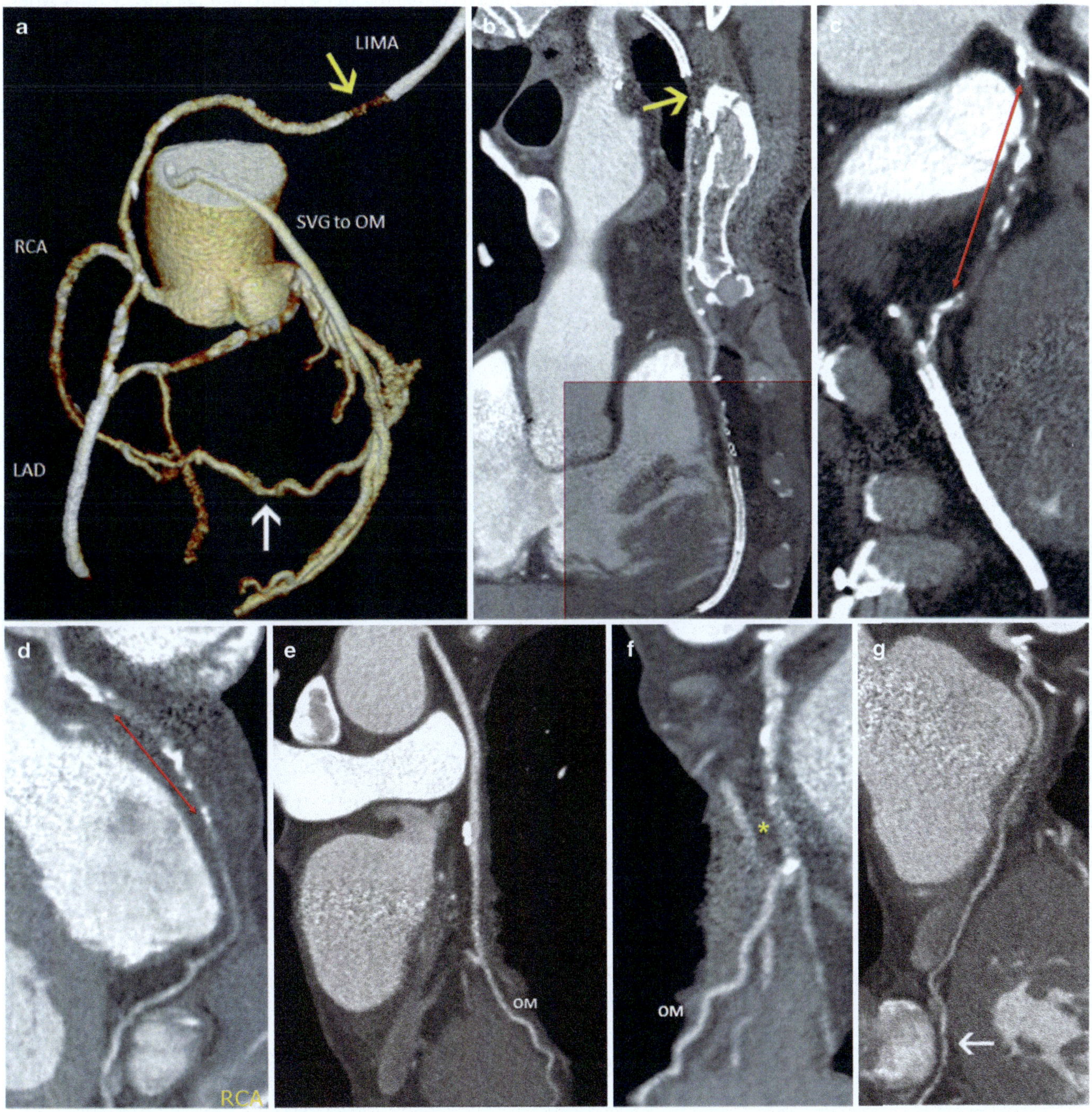

Findings and Interpretation

- Occluded left internal mammary artery (LIMA).
- The LIMA has a total occlusion immediately after an ostial stent (arrow in panels A and B).
- The LAD artery has an ostial long chronic total occlusion (bidirectional line), with moderate calcification at the entry site (panel C).
- The distal runoff of the LAD artery has two patent stents, without evidence of significant neointimal hyperplasia (panels B and C). The left main coronary artery has a mild calcified lesion.
- The right coronary artery (RCA, panel D), dominant, has a long chronic total occlusion (bidirectional line) at the proximal segment, with heavy entry calcification.
- The distal RCA has preserved opacification, derived from collateral circulation (white arrows in panels A and G) from the atrioventricular branch of the left circumflex (LCX) artery.
- The saphenous vein graft (SVG, panel E) to the obtuse marginal branch (OM) is patent and has no evidence of disease, with normal distal runoff.
- The LCX artery has a total occlusion of the mid segment (*, in panel F).
- In symptomatic patients with previous surgical revascularization, CTCA can be the first diagnostic approach and allows avoidance of unnecessary stress tests, unless invasive coronary angiography is preferred.

Further Reading

Levisman JM, Budoff MJ, Karlsberg RP. Long-term coronary artery graft patency as evaluated by 64-slice coronary computed tomographic angiography. Coron Artery Dis. 2011;22:521–5.

Li Y, Xu N, Zhang J, et al. Procedural success of CTO recanalization: comparison of the J-CTO score determined by coronary CT angiography to invasive angiography. J Cardiovasc Comput Tomogr. 2015;9:578–84.

Case 25

Coronary Artery Bypass Surgery: Computed Tomography Coronary Angiography (CTCA)

Clinical History

- Seventy-four-year-old male.
- Coronary risk factors: hypertension, diabetes.
- He has a history of previous coronary artery bypass surgery in 1983 and underwent multiple percutaneous revascularizations since 2009.
- He is currently being studied for syncope and has a single photon emission computed tomography dipyridamole myocardial perfusion examination with mild perinecrotic anterior wall ischemia.
- Referred for CTCA to evaluate coronary anatomy.

Images

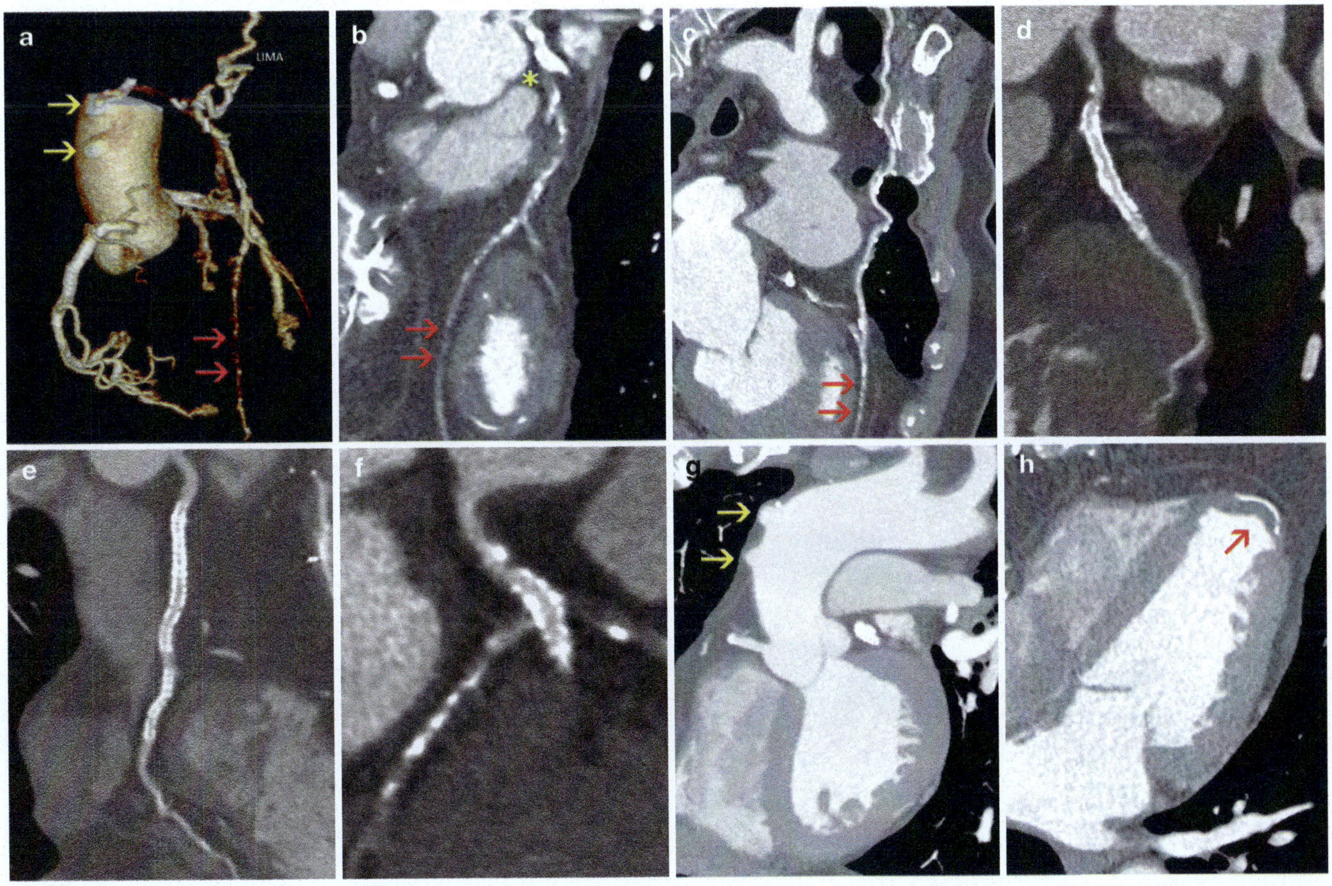

Findings and Interpretation

- Occluded coronary artery bypass grafts (CABG).
- There are two aortic grafts with ostial total occlusions (yellow arrows in panels A and G).
- The left internal mammary artery (LIMA) is patent and has no significant lesions (panels A and C). However, there is poor opacification of the distal left anterior descending (LAD) artery, with severe underlying disease (red arrows in panels A–C).
- The LAD artery has an ostial chronic total occlusion, with heavy calcification at the entry site (*, in panel B).
- The left main coronary artery has a long patent stent that extends to the intermediate branch (panel D).
- The right coronary artery (panel E), dominant, has multiple patent stents, with no evidence of neointimal hyperplasia.
- The left circumflex artery (panel F) is small and has a total occlusion with diffuse disease.
- The left ventricular four-chamber view (panel H) clearly depicts an apical mural ventricular thrombus (arrow), with myocardial wall thinning and calcification.
- CTCA has a very high diagnostic accuracy for the evaluation of CABG since coronary grafts (1) are gen-

erally larger than native vessels, (2) have less motion artifacts than native vessels, and (3) atherosclerotic disease within grafts is usually non-calcified. However, careful interpretation must be undertaken due to the metal artifacts associated with vascular clips. Furthermore, occasionally, suboptimal contrast opacification of distal runoffs impairs the ability to rule out distal stenosis.

Further Reading

Levisman JM, Budoff MJ, Karlsberg RP. Long-term coronary artery graft patency as evaluated by 64-slice coronary computed tomographic angiography. Coron Artery Dis. 2011;22:521–5.

Weustink AC, Nieman K, Pugliese F, et al. Diagnostic accuracy of computed tomography angiography in patients after bypass grafting: comparison with invasive coronary angiography. JACC Cardiovasc Imaging. 2009;2:816–24.

Case 26

Coronary Artery Bypass Surgery: Computed Tomography Coronary Angiography (CTCA)

Clinical History

- Seventy-year-old female.
- Coronary risk factors: hypertension, hypercholesterolemia.
- She has a history of previous myocardial infarction and coronary artery bypass surgery 15 months ago.
- Referred for CTCA to evaluate coronary anatomy due to atypical chest pain.

Images

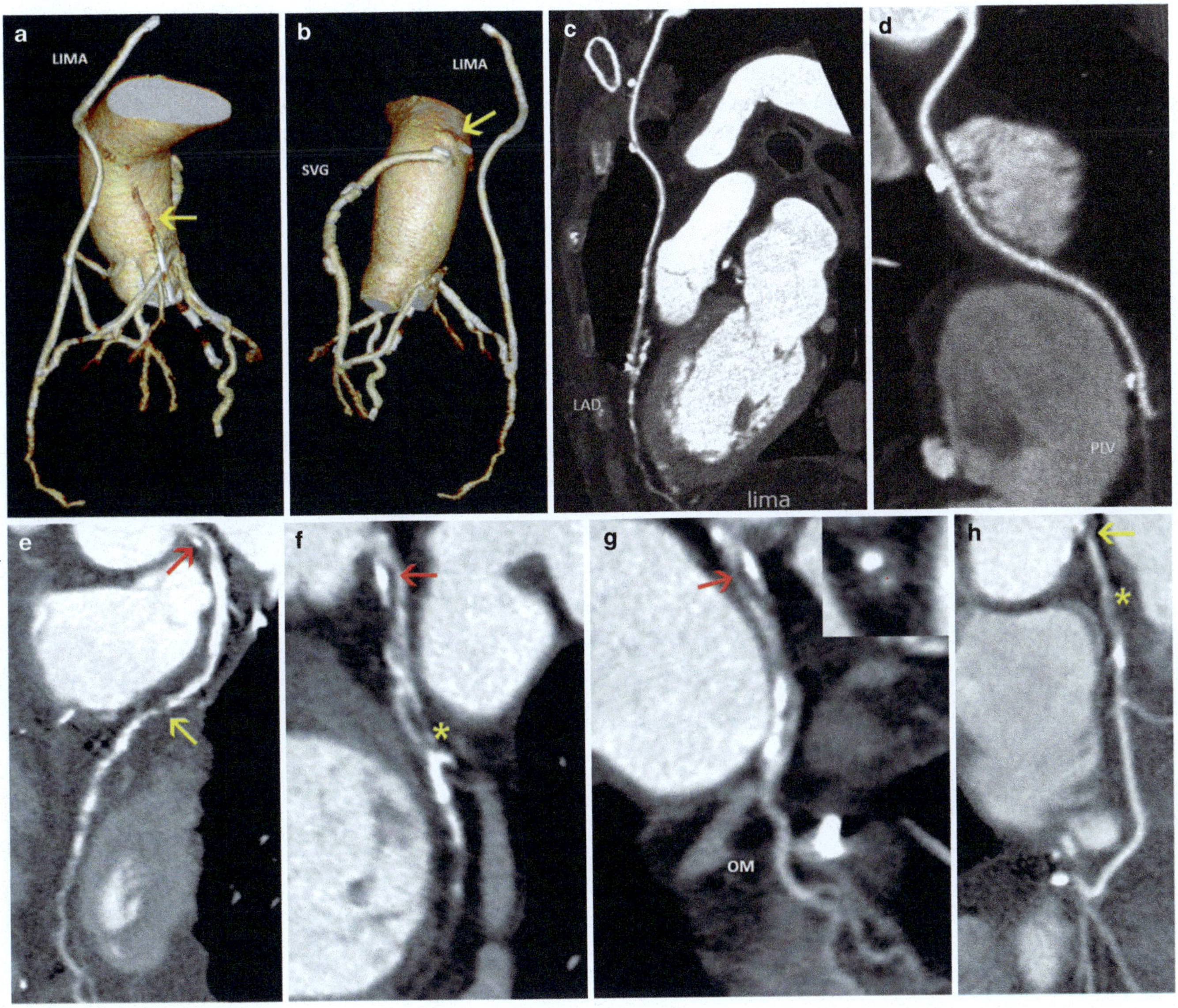

Findings and Interpretation

- Occluded coronary artery bypass graft (CABG) with small runoff vessels.
- The left internal mammary artery (LIMA) is patent and has no significant lesions (panels A–C).
- The saphenous vein graft (SVG) to the posterior left ventricular branch (PLV) of the right coronary artery (RCA) is patent and has no evidence of disease (panels B and D). The PLV is very small and has threadlike opacification.

- At the posterior wall of the ascending aorta (panel B), an occluded SVG to the obtuse marginal branch (OM) is observed [yellow arrows in panels A and B and panel G (obtuse marginal)].
- The left main coronary artery has a severe mixed lesion with positive remodeling and low-attenuation plaque (red arrows in panels E–G).
- The left anterior descending (LAD) artery has diffuse proximal calcification and a severe stenosis at the mid segment (yellow arrow in E). The distal LAD artery is irregular, with mild to moderate stenosis.
- The left circumflex artery (panel F) is diffusely diseased and has a total occlusion of the mid portion (*).
- The RCA, dominant, has a severe ostial lesion (yellow arrow, in H) and has a total occlusion (*) of the proximal/mid portion.
- In this patient with very complex anatomy, CTCA provided excellent visualization of vessels as well as of the coronary grafts, aiding clinical decision-making.

Further Reading

Levisman JM, Budoff MJ, Karlsberg RP. Long-term coronary artery graft patency as evaluated by 64-slice coronary computed tomographic angiography. Coron Artery Dis. 2011;22:521–5.

Weustink AC, Nieman K, Pugliese F, et al. Diagnostic accuracy of computed tomography angiography in patients after bypass grafting: comparison with invasive coronary angiography. JACC Cardiovasc Imaging. 2009;2:816–24.

Case 27

Coronary Artery Bypass Surgery: Computed Tomography Coronary Angiography (CTCA)

Clinical History

- Sixty-five-year-old male.
- Coronary risk factors: hypercholesterolemia.
- He has a history of previous coronary artery bypass surgery in 2002.
- He is currently asymptomatic.
- Single photon emission computed tomography myocardial perfusion revealed mild apical inferior ischemia.
- Referred for CTCA to evaluate coronary anatomy.

Images

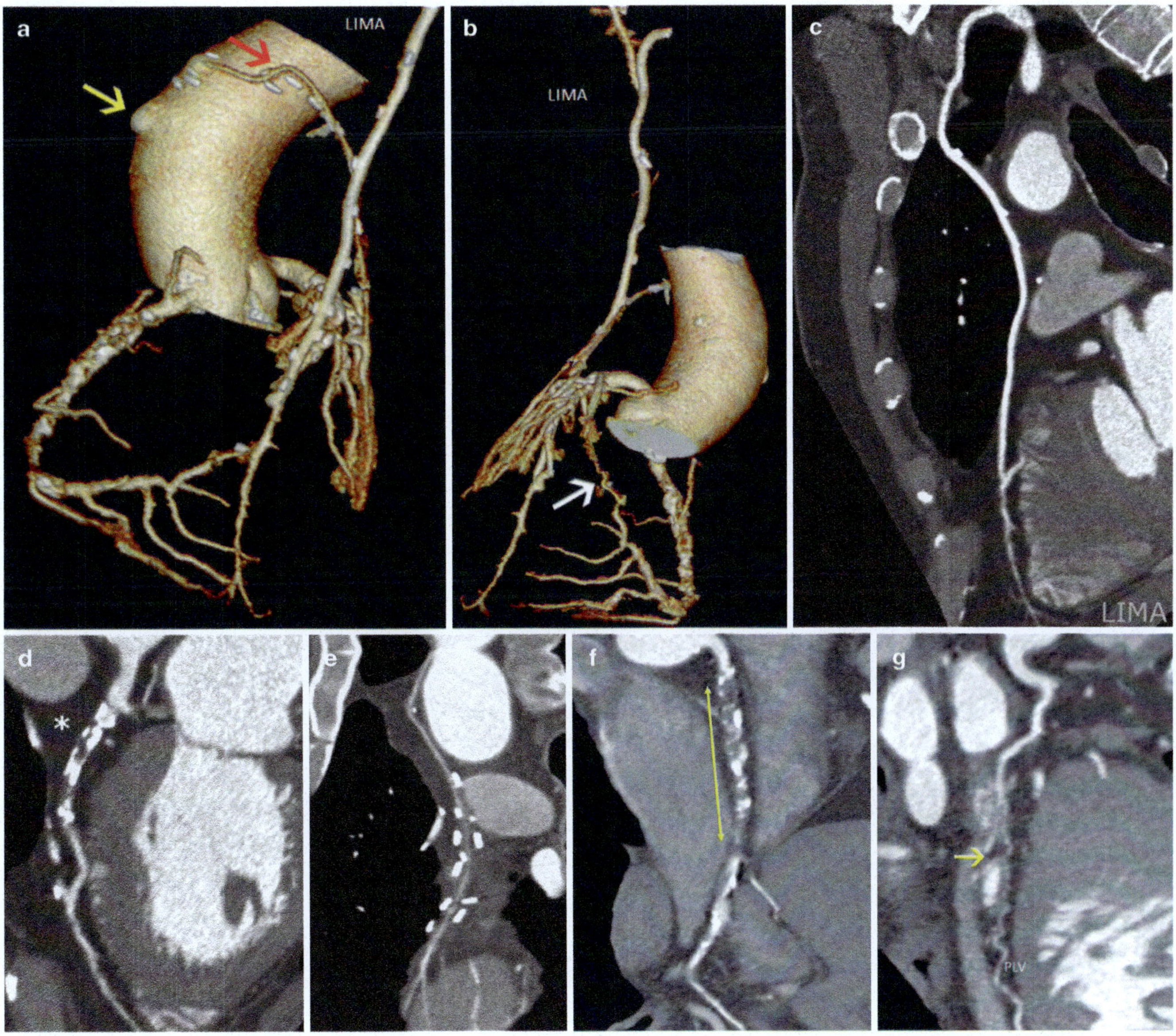

Findings and Interpretation

- Occluded coronary artery bypass graft (CABG) with collateral circulation.
- There is an occluded saphenous vein graft (yellow arrow in panel A) at the ostium.
- The small radial graft to a diagonal branch is patent (red arrow in panels A and E).
- The left internal mammary artery (LIMA) is patent and has no significant lesions (panels A–C). The distal runoff

of the anterior descending (LAD) artery has no significant lesions (panels C–D).

- The LAD artery has a proximal chronic total occlusion (*, in panel D), with heavy calcification at the entry site. The left main coronary artery has no evidence of disease.
- The right coronary artery (RCA, panel F), dominant, has a long chronic total occlusion (*) at the proximal segment, with mild entry calcification.
- The distal RCA has good opacification, derived from visible collateral circulation from the left circumflex artery to the posterior left ventricular (PLV) branch (arrow, in panel G).
- CTCA provides good visualization of collaterals in chronic total occlusions that can be used to guide retrograde recanalization with percutaneous coronary intervention.

Further Reading

Li Y, Xu N, Zhang J, et al. Procedural success of CTO recanalization: Comparison of the J-CTO score determined by coronary CT angiography to invasive angiography. J Cardiovasc Comput Tomogr. 2015;9:578–84.

Sugaya T, Oyama-Manabe N, Yamaguchi T, et al. Visualization of collateral channels with coronary computed tomography angiography for the retrograde approach in percutaneous coronary intervention for chronic total occlusion. J Cardiovasc Comput Tomogr. 2016;10:128–34.

Case 28

Physiological Assessment: Stress Myocardial Perfusion by Computed Tomography (CT)

Clinical History

- Seventy-five-year old female.
- Cardiovascular risk factors: hypertension, dyslipidemia, diabetes.
- Presents typical angina functional class II–III.
- Positive stress-rest myocardial perfusion single photon emission computed tomography (SPECT), with severe ischemia in the apical and inferior wall at low exercise workload.
- Patient refused to perform an invasive coronary angiography.
- A dual-energy CT coronary angiography (CTCA) with stress-rest static CT perfusion assessment was then performed.

Images

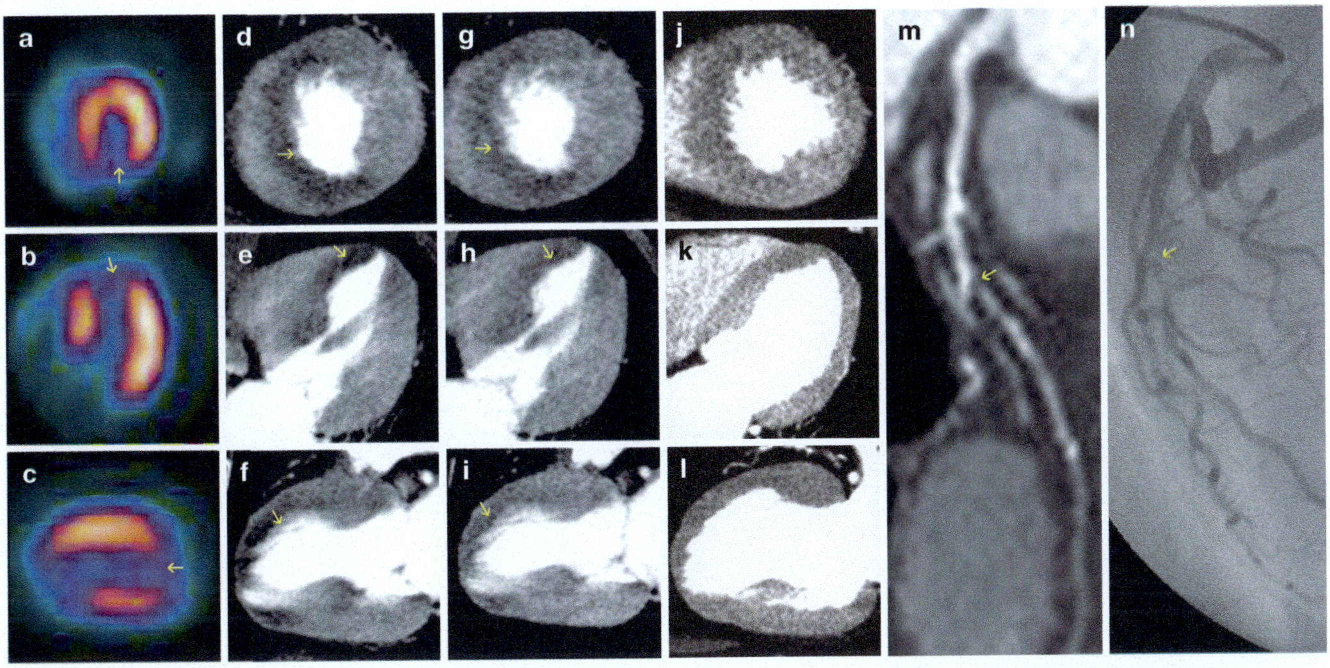

Findings and Interpretation

- Static CT perfusion using conventional (single-energy) CT scanners has some limitations for the evaluation of myocardial perfusion in relation to the polychromatic nature of X-rays. Some imaging artifacts on these scanners can mimic perfusion defects in certain myocardial segments such as posterobasal segments (AHA 5) and apical segments (AHA 13, 14, 16). They are known as beam-hardening artifacts (BHA).
- Dual-energy CT helps in cancelling this artifact and reduces false-positive rates.
- Dual-energy CT uses two different tube potentials simultaneously at low (80kvp) and high (140kvp) levels. There are different options to scan in dual-energy CT, using single-source or dual-source CT scanners, in all cases applying the same physical principle.
- After the CT scan is carried out, images can be analyzed in a range of energies from 40 keV to 140–200 keV. Intermediate levels above 80 keV cancel the hypoattenuation if it is due to a BHA, but if the hypoattenuation is a true myocardial perfusion defect, it will persist in all energy levels.
- Stress SPECT in short-axis (panel A), four-chamber (panel B), and two-chamber (panel C) views. A myocardial perfusion defect is detected in the apical, anterior and inferior, and anteroseptal walls (arrows).
- Stress CT images in short-axis (panel D), four-chamber (panel E), and two-chamber (panel F) views at 45 keV. A severe myocardial hypoperfusion is observed in the septal wall from the apex to the base (arrow).
- Stress CT imaging at 85 keV using the same views (panels G–I), with similar findings (arrow).
- Rest CT imaging using the same views (panels J–L) showing normalization of myocardial perfusion.
- Curved multiplanar reconstruction (panel M) and invasive coronary angiographic images (panel N) demonstrate

severe disease at the mid portion of the left anterior descending artery (arrows).

- Severe reversible perfusion defects in the apical, anterior, and septal walls from base to apex and in apical inferior segments are observed at all energy levels (low, medium, and high levels). These findings confirm a true myocardial perfusion defect at the monochromatic range of dual-energy CT. The normalization of defects during stress is a hallmark of myocardial ischemia. Coronary stenosis is detected in the same coronary territory.

Further Reading

Carrascosa PM, Cury RC, Deviggiano A et al. Comparison of myocardial perfusion evaluation with single versus dual-energy CT and effect of beam-hardening artifacts. Acad Radiol. 2015;22:591–9.

Rodriguez-Granillo GA, Carrascosa P, Cipriano S et al. Beam hardening artifact reduction using dual energy computed tomography: implications for myocardial perfusion studies. Cardiovasc Diagn Ther. 2015;5:79–85.

Case 29

Physiological Assessment: Stress Myocardial Perfusion by Computed Tomography (CT)

Clinical History

- Sixty-six-year old male.
- Cardiovascular risk factors: smoking, dyslipidemia.
- History of percutaneous coronary intervention in 1995 due to unstable angina. Under full medical treatment with dual antiplatelet therapy, statins, ACE inhibitors, and beta-blockers.
- CT coronary angiography (CCTA) with assessment of stress-rest myocardial perfusion and late-enhancement evaluation was performed.

Images

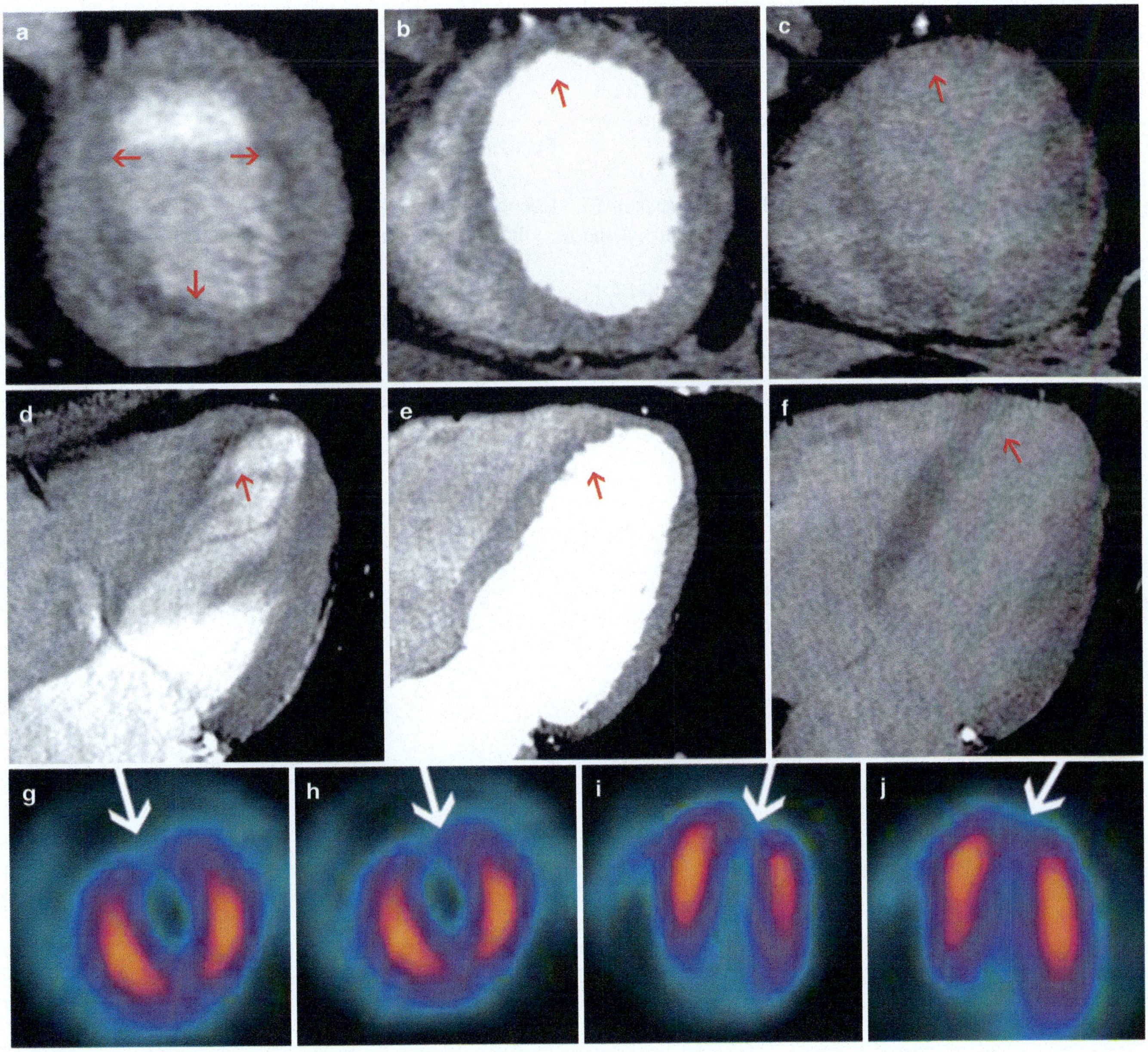

Findings and Interpretation

- Vasodilator stress myocardial perfusion images were acquired 2 min after administration of dipyridamole (0.56 mg/kg). Rest images were acquired after administration of aminophylline (1–2 mg/kg).
- Stress myocardial CT perfusion. In an apical short-axis view (panel A), a subendocardial myocardial perfusion defect is detected (red arrows).
- Rest CT images in the same short-axis view (panel B) demonstrate only mildly decreased myocardial perfusion in the anteroseptal wall, with normal myocardial perfusion of the other segments.
- Short-axis late-enhancement CT image (panel C) obtained 7 min after the administration of contrast shows focal subendocardial delayed hyperenhancement compatible with myocardial necrosis.
- Stress four-chamber CT image (panel D) illustrates a subendocardial myocardial perfusion defect in the anteroseptal wall (arrow), whereas in rest image (panel E), only mild hypoperfusion persists (arrow).
- Late-enhancement four-chamber CT image (panel F) demonstrates mild laminar hyperenhancement in the anteroseptal wall (arrow).
- Single photon emission computed tomography (SPECT) myocardial perfusion exam shows on stress images (panels G and I) a severe myocardial perfusion defect in the anteroseptal wall (white arrow and inferior wall), with mild improvement during rest (panels H and J).
- The presence of a myocardial perfusion defect during stress that disappears or decreases in rest is compatible with ischemia, whereas a fixed myocardial perfusion defect is compatible with necrosis. Also, late-enhancement imaging is valuable as only necrotic myocardial segments are observed with delayed hyperenhancement, whereas ischemic but viable myocardial segments show normal density.
- Late-enhancement CT scan is performed between 5 and 7 min after the rest scan. It does not require any additional contrast and uses low radiation dose. Stress-rest CT with late enhancement is a good imaging modality to evaluate myocardial perinecrotic ischemia, with improved spatial resolution compared to SPECT.

Further Reading

Cheng W, Zeng M, Arellano C, et al. Detection of myocardial perfusion abnormalities: standard dual-source coronary computed tomography angiography versus rest/stress technetium-99 m single-photo emission CT. Br J Radiol. 2010;83:652–60.

Case 30

Physiological Assessment: Stress Myocardial Perfusion by Computed Tomography (CT)

Clinical History

- Sixty-five-year old male.
- Cardiovascular risk factors: hypertension, former smoking.
- Five months ago he had an ST-elevation acute myocardial infarction and was treated with fibrinolysis, with positive reperfusion criteria.
- Under full medical treatment including dual antiplatelet therapy, statin, ACE inhibitors, calcium channel blockers, nitrates, and trimetazidine.
- He had persisting chest pain in functional class II–III.
- A CT coronary angiography (CTCA) with assessment of stress myocardial perfusion was required.

Images

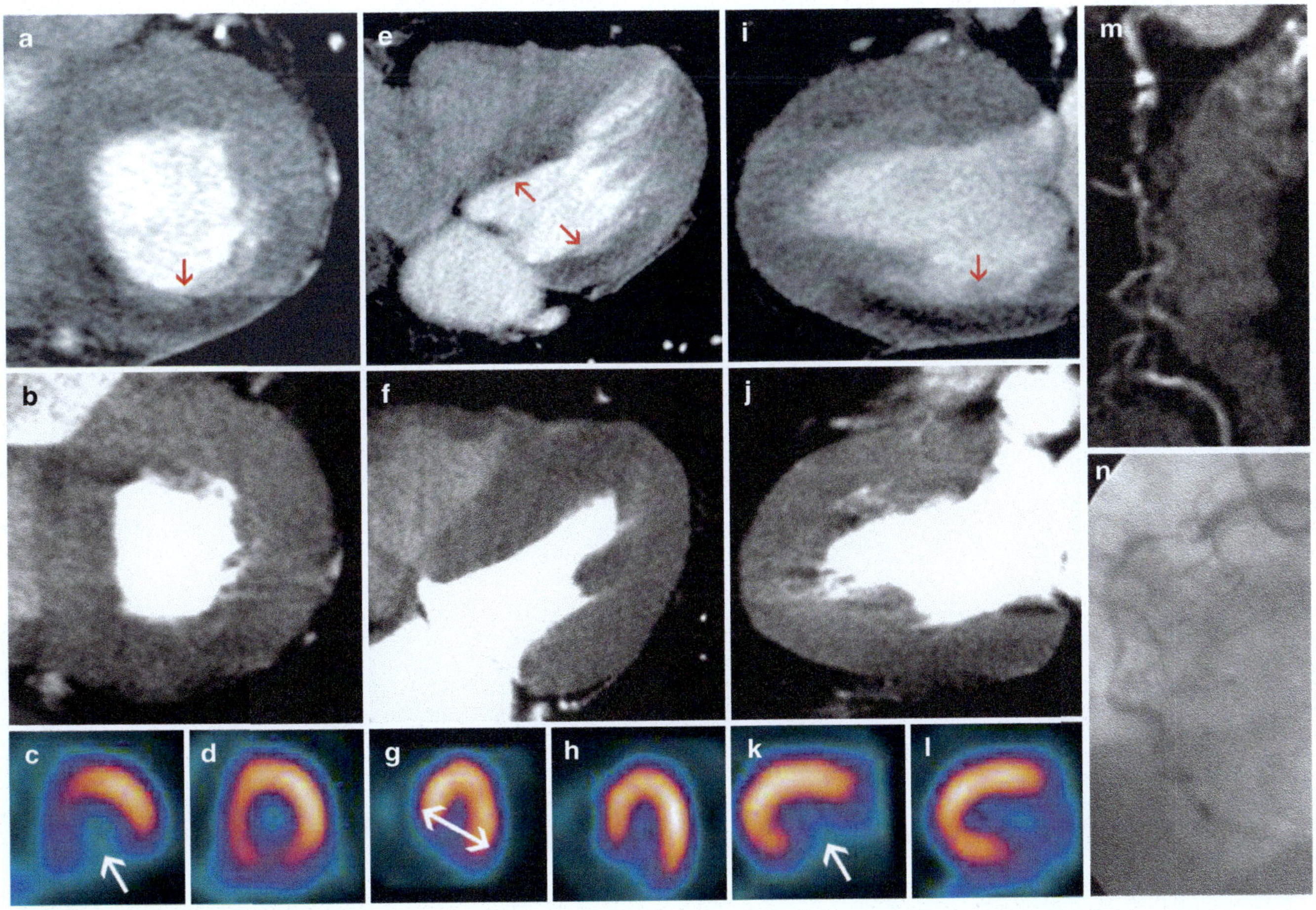

Findings and Interpretation

- Vasodilator stress myocardial perfusion images were acquired 2 min after administration of dipyridamole (0.56 mg/kg). Rest images were acquired after administration of aminophylline (1–2 mg/kg).
- Stress myocardial perfusion CT in a basal short-axis view (panel A). A severe perfusion defect is detected in the inferior wall (arrow).
- Rest images in the same short-axis view (panel B) show significant improvement in myocardial perfusion, with mild persisting defect.
- Stress (panel C) and rest (panel D) single photon emission computed tomography (SPECT) images in basal short axis demonstrate the same findings (arrow).
- Stress CT perfusion in four-chamber view (panel E). Severe perfusion defect involving basal segments including septal and lateral walls (arrows), with normal myocardial perfusion during rest (panel F).
- Stress (panel G) and rest (panel H) SPECT four-chamber views show similar findings (arrows).
- Stress CT perfusion in two-chamber view (panel I). Severe perfusion defect involving inferior basal wall

(arrow), with a mild persisting myocardial perfusion defect at rest (panel J).

- Stress (panel K) and rest (panel L) SPECT two-chamber views show similar findings.
- CTCA (panel M): subtotal occlusion of right coronary artery, with similar findings at invasive angiography (panel N).
- This case shows a good correlation between stress-rest SPECT and CT for the identification of inferior wall perinecrotic ischemia, coincident with severe disease of the right coronary artery.

Further Reading

Chen MY, Rochitte CE, Arbab-Zadeh A, et al. Prognostic value of combined CT angiography and myocardial perfusion imaging versus invasive coronary angiography and nuclear stress perfusion imaging in the prediction of major adverse cardiovascular events: the CORE320 Multicenter Study. Radiology. 2017;284:55–65.

Cury RC, Kitt TM, Feaheny K, Blankstein R, et al. A randomized, multicenter, multivendor study of myocardial perfusion imaging with regadenoson CT perfusion vs single photon emission CT. J Cardiovasc Comput Tomogr. 2015;9:103–12.

Case 31

Physiological Assessment: Stress Myocardial Perfusion by Computed Tomography (CT)

Clinical History

- Sixty-nine-year-old female.
- Cardiovascular risk factors: hypertension, dyslipidemia.
- Baseline medical treatment: statins, beta-blockers, and ACE inhibitors.
- Typical exertional angina functional class II–III.
- A CT coronary angiography (CTCA) with stress-rest static (first-pass) CT perfusion assessment was performed.

Images

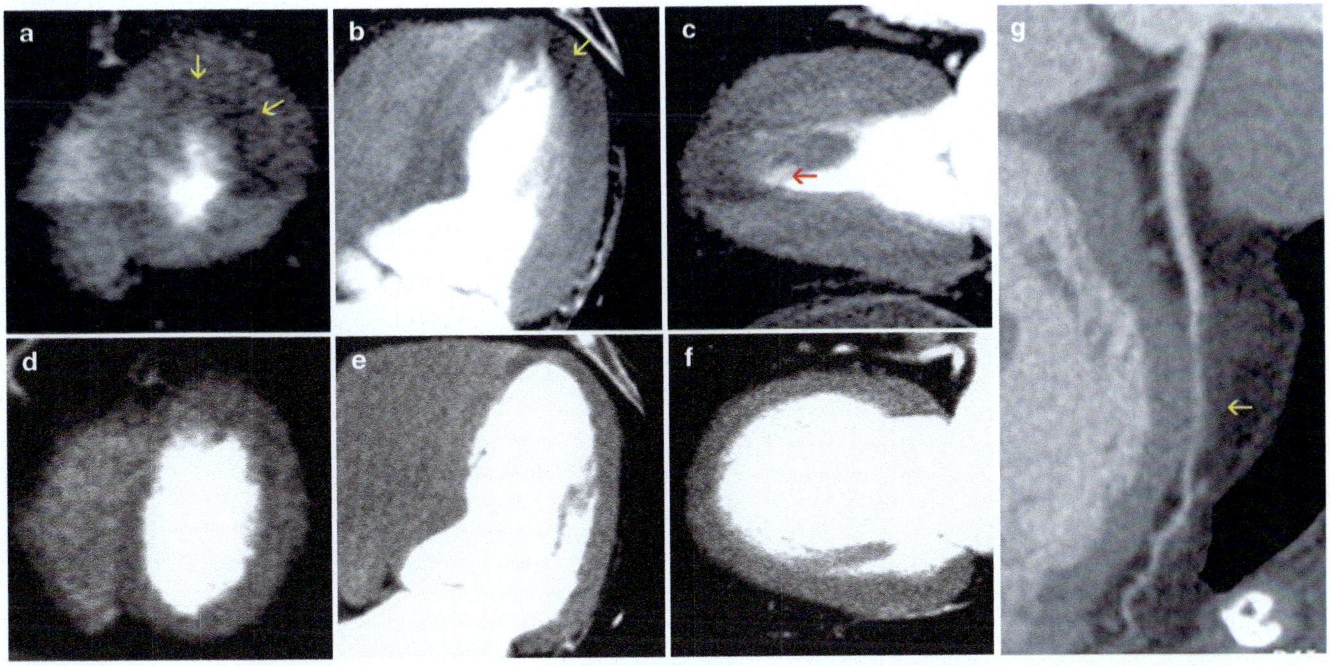

Findings and Interpretation

- Vasodilator stress myocardial perfusion images were acquired 2 min after administration of dipyridamole (0.56 mg/kg). Rest images were acquired after administration of aminophylline (1–2 mg/kg).
- Stress short-axis view in apical plane (panel A). There is a severe subendocardial myocardial perfusion defect in the anterior and anterolateral wall (arrows).
- Stress four-chamber view (panel B) shows the same perfusion defect (arrow).
- Decreased myocardial perfusion of the apex is observed (arrow) in the stress two-chamber view (panel C).
- Rest short-axis, four-chamber, and two-chamber views (panels D–F) showing normal perfusion of all myocardial segments.
- CTCA (panel G) demonstrates myocardial bridging in the mid portion of the left anterior descending (LAD) artery (arrow) that reduces the artery diameter at that level.
- The stress-induced myocardial perfusion defect displayed in all planes that disappears completely in rest is compatible with myocardial ischemia.
- The presence of myocardial bridging in the mid LAD artery, with diastolic luminal narrowing, seems to be responsible for the myocardial perfusion defect in that territory.
- Myocardial bridging is a common finding in CTCA studies. The majority of them are incomplete (when the artery is only covered by fat) or complete (when the artery is introduced into the myocardium), and usually none of them is associated with vascular compression.
- However, in certain situations of complete bridging, the artery can be compressed during systole or in systole and diastole. In the first scenario, the patient can present chest pain, and in the second scenario (systole and diastole), perfusion abnormalities can be observed.

- CT perfusion can help in the detection of the presence and significance of myocardial bridging. In cases where there is a suspected myocardial bridge with functional relevance, rest CT should be performed in retrospective modality with tube current modulation to evaluate the behavior of the bridge during the cardiac phases with the least possible radiation dose. Stress phase will help in evaluating the functional relevance.

Further Reading

Karfis I, Dresios C, Kotsalou I, Voyatzis M, Antoniadis D, Dimakopoulos N. Myocardial bridge: an unusual cause of asymptomatic ST-elevation during treadmill stress test causing functional ischaemia. Hell J Nucl Med. 2012;15:147–9.

Ker WDS, Neves DG, Damas ASAA, Mesquita CT, Nacif MS. Myocardial bridge and angiotomography of the coronary arteries: perfusion under pharmacological stress. Arq Bras Cardiol. 2017;108:572–5.

Case 32

Physiological Assessment: Stress Myocardial Perfusion by Computed Tomography (CT)

Clinical History

- Seventy-nine-year old male.
- Cardiovascular risk factors: hypertension and dyslipidemia.
- History of previous myocardial infarction.
- Currently he presented with angina pectoris functional class II under treatment with nitrates, beta-blockers, statins, and aspirin. He also receives amiodarone.
- Myocardial perfusion imaging with single photon emission computed tomography (SPECT) demonstrated a reversible perfusion defect of the lateral and inferolateral wall, compatible with myocardial ischemia.
- A CT coronary angiography (CTCA) with assessment of stress-rest myocardial perfusion was requested to evaluate coronary anatomy.

Images

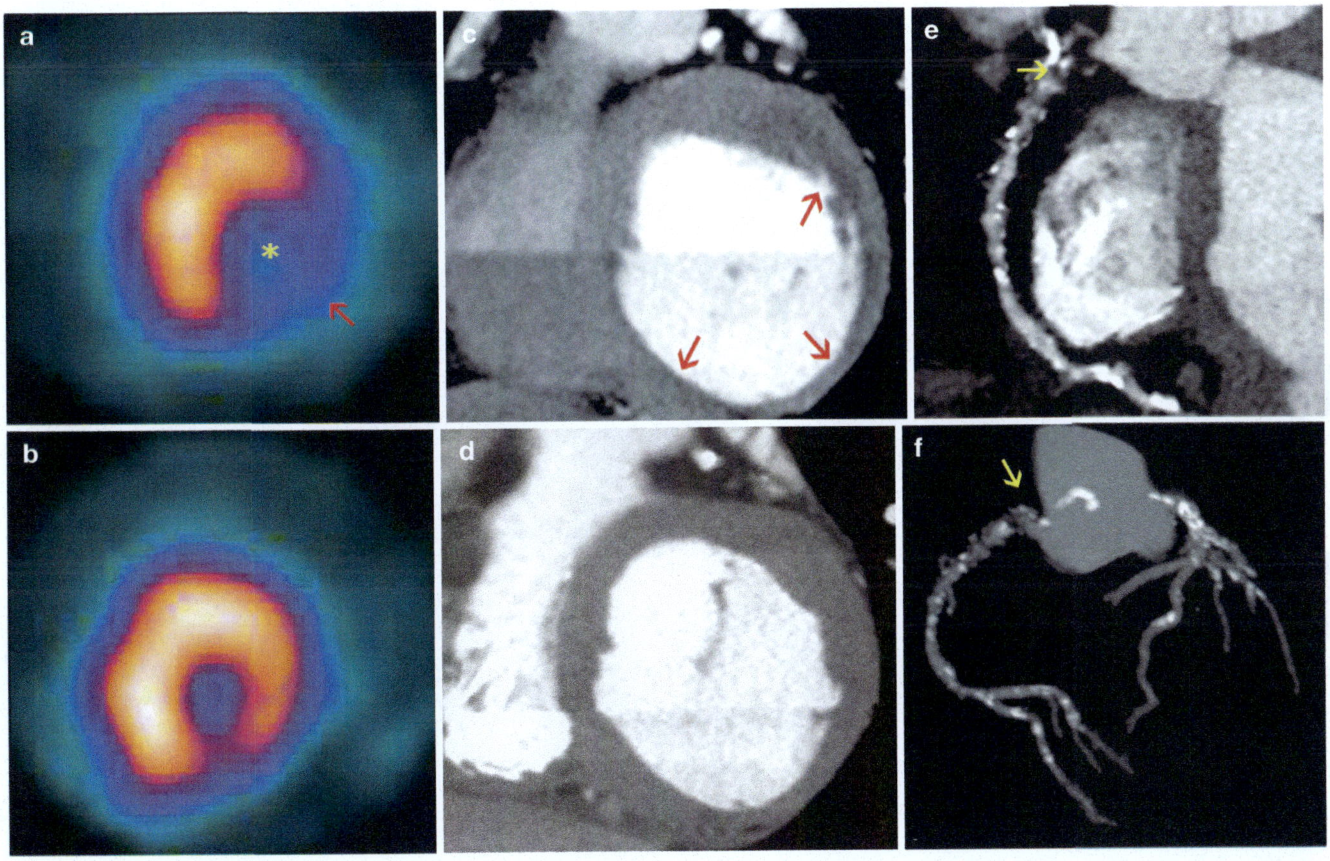

Findings and Interpretation

- Stress SPECT in a short-axis mid-ventricular plane (panel A). A severe perfusion defect is observed in the lateral and inferolateral walls (red arrow). The left ventricular cavity is dilated (asterisk).
- Rest SPECT in the same short-axis view (panel B) showing normal myocardial perfusion.
- Myocardial perfusion imaging with CT. Stress short-axis view (panel C) shows similar results than SPECT, with subendocardial lateral, inferolateral, and inferior myocardial perfusion defects (red arrows).
- At rest, CT myocardial perfusion is normal (panel D), without perfusion defects.
- Curved multiplanar reconstruction of the right coronary artery (RCA, panel E) showing diffuse atherosclerosis and proximal total occlusion (arrow).
- Three-dimensional maximum intensity projection (panel F) image shows diffuse calcification of the coronary tree, with total occlusion of the proximal RCA.
- This case demonstrates a good correlation between stress-rest SPECT and CT for the identification of dilated ischemic cardiomyopathy. Severe reversible perfusion defects

are detected by both methods in the lateral and inferior walls, compatible with ischemia within RCA territory.

Further Reading

Carrascosa PM, Deviggiano A, Capunay C, et al. Incremental value of myocardial perfusion over coronary angiography by spectral computed tomography in patients with intermediate to high likelihood of coronary artery disease. Eur J Radiol. 2015;84:637–42.

Song I, Yi JG, Park JH, Kim MY, Shin JK, Ko SM. Diagnostic performance of static single-scan stress perfusion cardiac computed tomography in detecting hemodynamically significant coronary artery stenosis: a comparison with combined invasive coronary angiography and cardiovascular magnetic resonance-myocardial perfusion imaging. Acta Radiol. 2018;59:1184–93.

Case 33

Physiological Assessment: Stress Myocardial Perfusion by Computed Tomography (CT)

Clinical History

- Fifty-six-year old male.
- Cardiovascular risk factors: smoking.
- History of coronary artery disease (CAD).
- He presents with angina with variable functional class.
- An invasive angiogram showed an occluded mid left anterior descending coronary artery, requiring percutaneous coronary intervention with stent deployment.
- Six months later he started with new-onset angina.
- A CT coronary angiography (CTCA) with stress-rest static (first-pass) CT perfusion assessment was performed.

Images

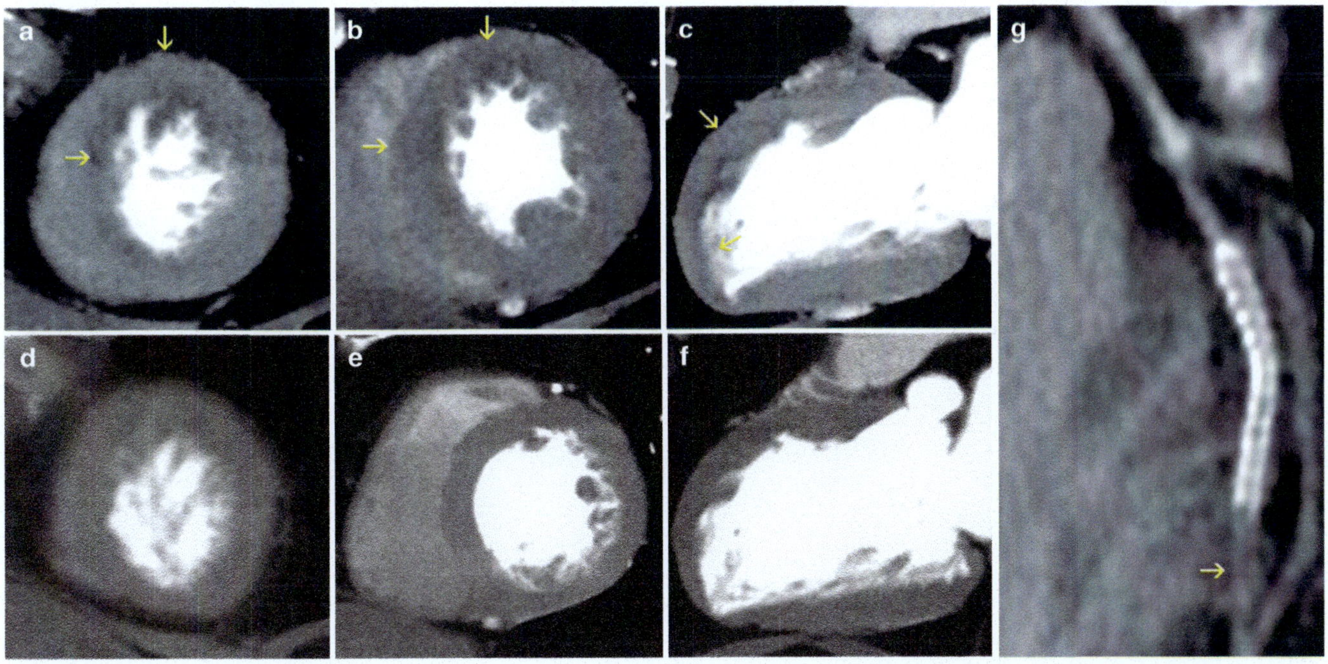

Findings and Interpretation

- Vasodilator stress myocardial perfusion images were acquired 2 min after administration of dipyridamole (0.56 mg/kg). Rest images were acquired after administration of aminophylline (1–2 mg/kg).
- Stress short-axis views in apical (panel A) and mid-ventricular (panel B) planes. There is a severe subendocardial perfusion defect in the anterior and anteroseptal walls (arrows).
- Stress vertical long-axis view (panel C) showing a subendocardial perfusion defect in the apical and anterior walls (arrow).
- Rest short-axis views in apical (panel D) and mid-ventricular (panel E) planes, showing normalization of myocardial perfusion of aforementioned segments.
- Rest vertical long-axis (panel F) image showing resolution of the perfusion defect.
- Curved multiplanar reconstruction of the left anterior descending (LAD) artery with a stent in the mid segment. There is a distal occlusion of the artery after the stent (panel G, arrow).
- Myocardial CT perfusion can also be used to evaluate stent patency. In this case ischemic defects are present in the anterior, anteroseptal walls in the apical and mid-ventricular planes. There is a distal total occlusion of the LAD artery after the stent coincident with the coronary territory identified in the perfusion evaluation.
- Stress-rest static myocardial CT perfusion is a good technique to assess the functional relevance of a coronary stenosis. It requires to perform at least two CT scans, one with pharmacologic stress using dipyridamole at a dose of 0.56 mg-kg or adenosine (in this case an infusion pump is required) and a second rest CT scan. Patient's coronary artery disease pretest probability and calcium score help in deciding which is the best phase to start with. In cases

with high pretest probability or calcium score ≥400 is recommended to start with stress CT scan to prioritize ischemia. Any perfusion defect in stress that disappears in rest corresponds to an ischemia, whereas if the myocardial perfusion defect persists in stress and rest, this corresponds to necrosis. Myocardial perfusion defects have to be correlated with coronary anatomy to determine anatomo-functional correlation.

- In cases of severe calcifications or coronary stents, CT perfusion helps in assessing the functional relevance of a coronary stenosis, as it has been shown in this case.

Further Reading

Carrascosa P, Capunay C. Myocardial CT perfusion imaging for ischemia detection. Cardiovasc Diagn Ther. 2017;7:112–28.

Case 34

Stress Myocardial Perfusion with Cardiac Magnetic Resonance (CMR)

Clinical History

- Fifty-nine-year-old male.
- Coronary risk factors: hypercholesterolemia, hypertension, sedentary lifestyle, former smoker.
- Medication: beta-blocker, angiotensin II receptor antagonist.
- Symptoms: dyspnea and chest pain at mild physical exertion.
- Routine ECG test on treadmill stopped due to muscle exhaustion, (inconclusive functional test).
- Referred for stress-rest CMR to rule out myocardial ischemia.

Images

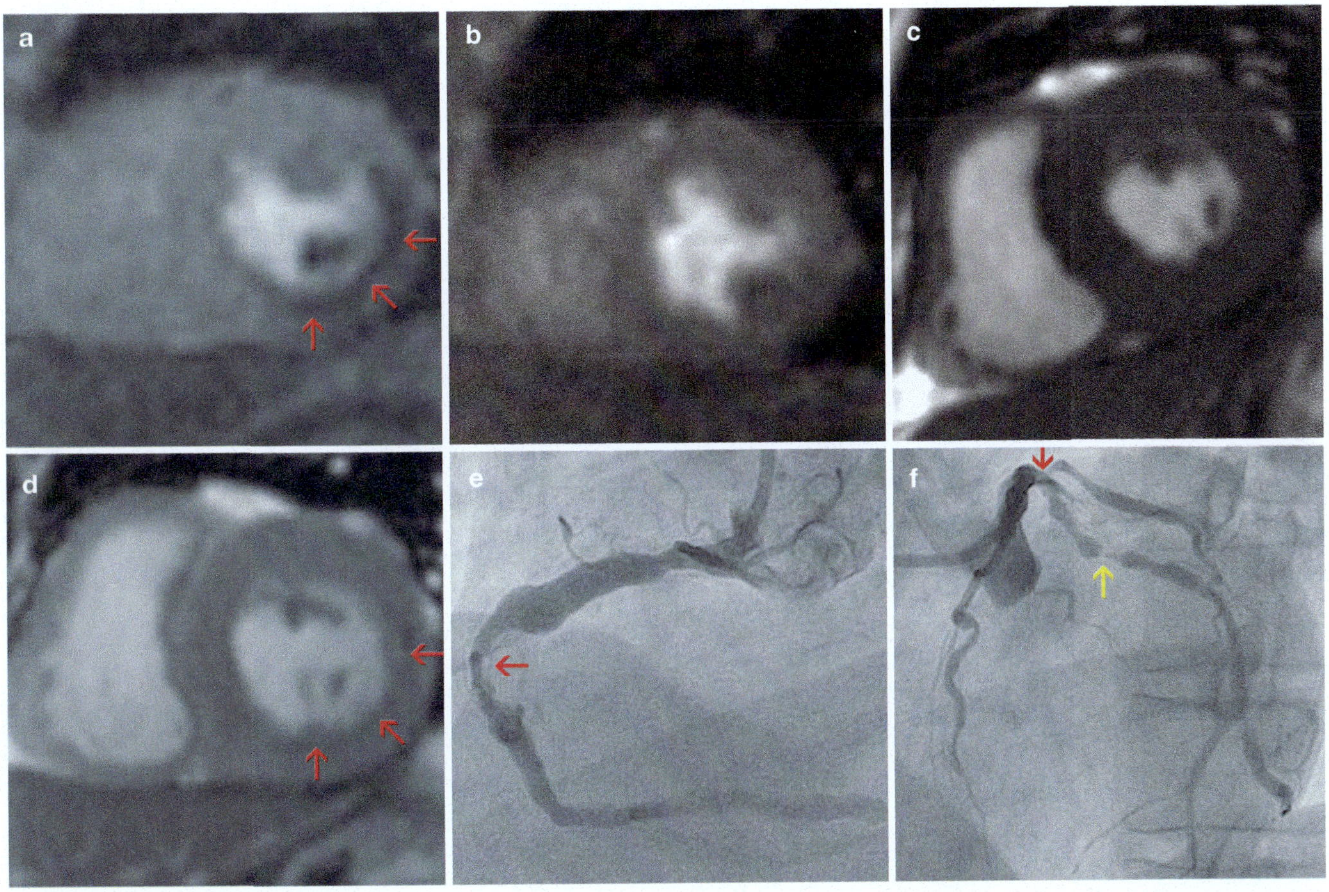

Findings and Interpretation

- High-dose dipyridamole (0.84 mg/kg in 6 min) stress perfusion CMR showed a perfusion deficit of the inferolateral wall from the base to apical segments during stress (arrows in panel A). Perfusion images acquired at rest were normal (panel B) demonstrating the reversible character of the perfusion anomaly.
- Mid-ventricular cine systolic short-axis view showed normal regional myocardial contractility during rest (panel C) and abnormal stress wall motion response in hypoperfused segments corresponding to hypokinetic wall during the stress phase induced by vasodilatation (arrows in panel D).
- In this case it is possible to affirm that there is depletion of the coronary flow reserve of the right coronary artery and left circumflex territories and depletion of contractile reserve corresponding to ischemia.
- Subsequent invasive coronary angiography showed significant stenosis at the mid segment of the right coronary artery (panel E) and severe stenosis of the proximal segment of the left circumflex coronary artery (yellow arrow in panel F). The first marginal branch of the circumflex artery shows moderate ostial stenosis (red arrow in panel F).
- The left main coronary artery and left anterior descending artery were confirmed to be free of significant stenosis.

- One of the most interesting aspects of dipyridamole stress CMR is that it allows the evaluation of different stages of the ischemic cascade. In this regard, inducible perfusion defects with normal contractile function during stress reflect less-severe perfusion defects.

Further Reading

Pingitore A, Lombardi M, Scattini B, De Marchi D, Aquaro GD, Positano V, et al. Head to head comparison between perfusion and function during accelerated high-dose dipyridamole magnetic resonance stress for the detection of coronary artery disease. Am J Cardiol. 2008;101:8–14.

Pontone G, Andreini D, Bertella E, Loguercio M, Guglielmo M, Baggiano A, et al. Prognostic value of dipyridamole stress cardiac magnetic resonance in patients with known or suspected coronary artery disease: a mid-term follow-up study. Eur Radiol. 2016;26:2155–65.

Case 35

Stress Myocardial Perfusion with Cardiac Magnetic Resonance (CMR)

Clinical History

- Fifty-two-year-old male.
- Coronary risk factors: diabetes mellitus type 2.
- Medication: oral hypoglycemic agents.
- Symptoms: effort dyspnea.
- Treadmill ECG test stopped prematurely due to muscle exhaustion (inconclusive).
- Echocardiogram: non-dilated cavities, with normal systolic and valve function.
- Referred for stress-rest CMR to rule out myocardial ischemia.

Images

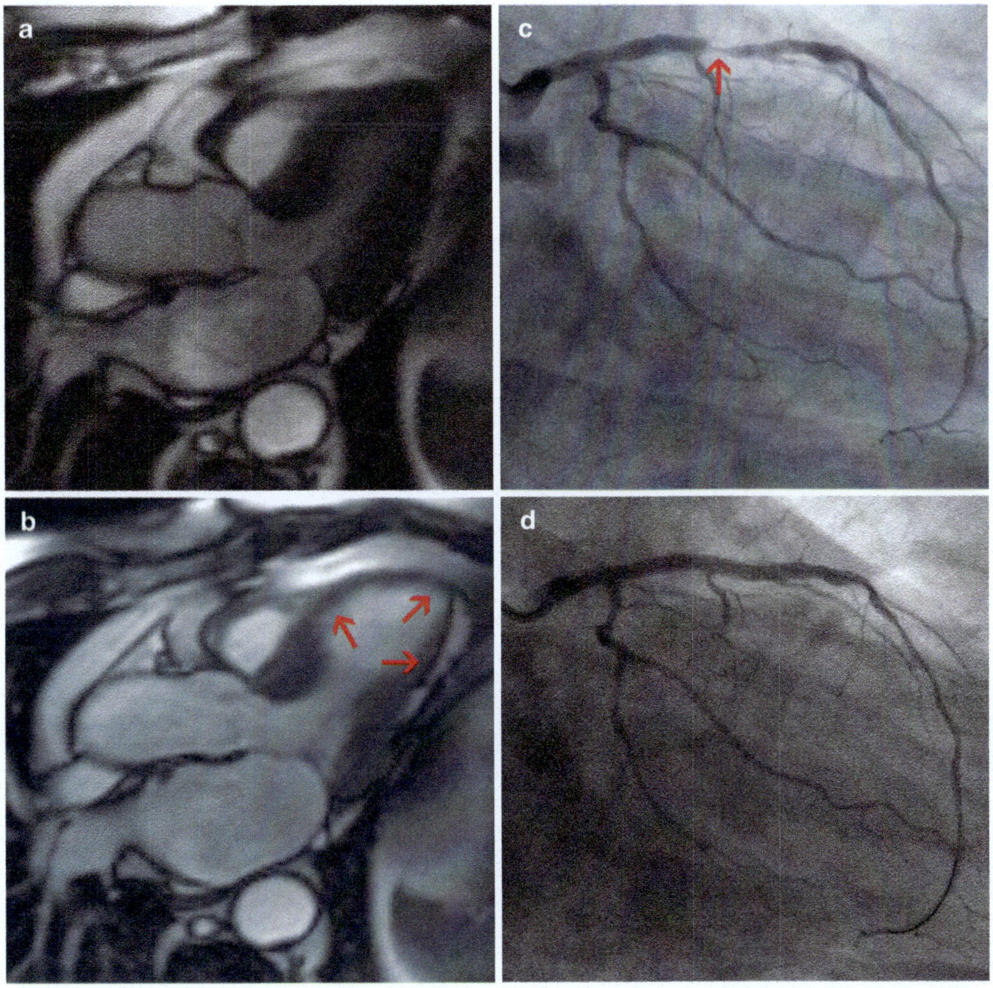

Findings and Interpretation

- Cine imaging using a left ventricular outflow tract view showed normal regional myocardial contractility at rest (panel A) and abnormal wall motion response (hypokinesia) in the anteroseptal mid to apex and infero-apical segment during the stress phase (panel B). This indicates systolic dysfunction due to ischemia, as a result of depletion of the contractile reserve in the left anterior descending artery territory.
- Invasive coronary angiography (arrow in panel C) shows severe stenosis of the mid left anterior descending artery after the origin of the first septal branch, with abnormal coronary flow (TIMI II).
- Percutaneous coronary intervention with stent placement (3.5 × 18 mm) was performed to restore blood flow to the left anterior descending coronary artery (panel D).

Further Reading

de Jong MC, Genders TS, van Geuns RJ, Moelker A, Hunink MG. Diagnostic performance of stress myocardial perfusion imaging for coronary artery disease: a systematic review and meta-analysis. Eur Radiol. 2012;22:1881–95.

Hamon M, Fau G, Née G, Ehtisham J, Morello R, Hamon M. Meta-analysis of the diagnostic performance of stress perfusion cardiovascular magnetic resonance for detection of coronary artery disease. J Cardiovasc Magn Reson. 2010;12:29.

Jahnke C, Nagel E, Gebker R, Kokocinski T, et al. Prognostic value of cardiac Magnetic Resonance stress Test. Circulation. 2007;115:1769–76.

Case 36

Stress Myocardial Perfusion with Cardiac Magnetic Resonance (CMR)

Clinical History

- Sixty-six-year-old male.
- Coronary risk factors: hypercholesterolemia, hypertension, current smoking.
- Medication: beta-blocker, angiotensin II receptor antagonist.
- Symptoms: palpitations associated with malaise.
- Echocardiogram: concentric hypertrophy of the left ventricle, with preserved systolic function.
- SPECT: fixed perfusion defect of mid-anterior, septal, and apical anterior segments without evidence of myocardial ischemia.
- Referred for stress CMR to rule out myocardial ischemia and to explore the extension of myocardial infarction.

Images

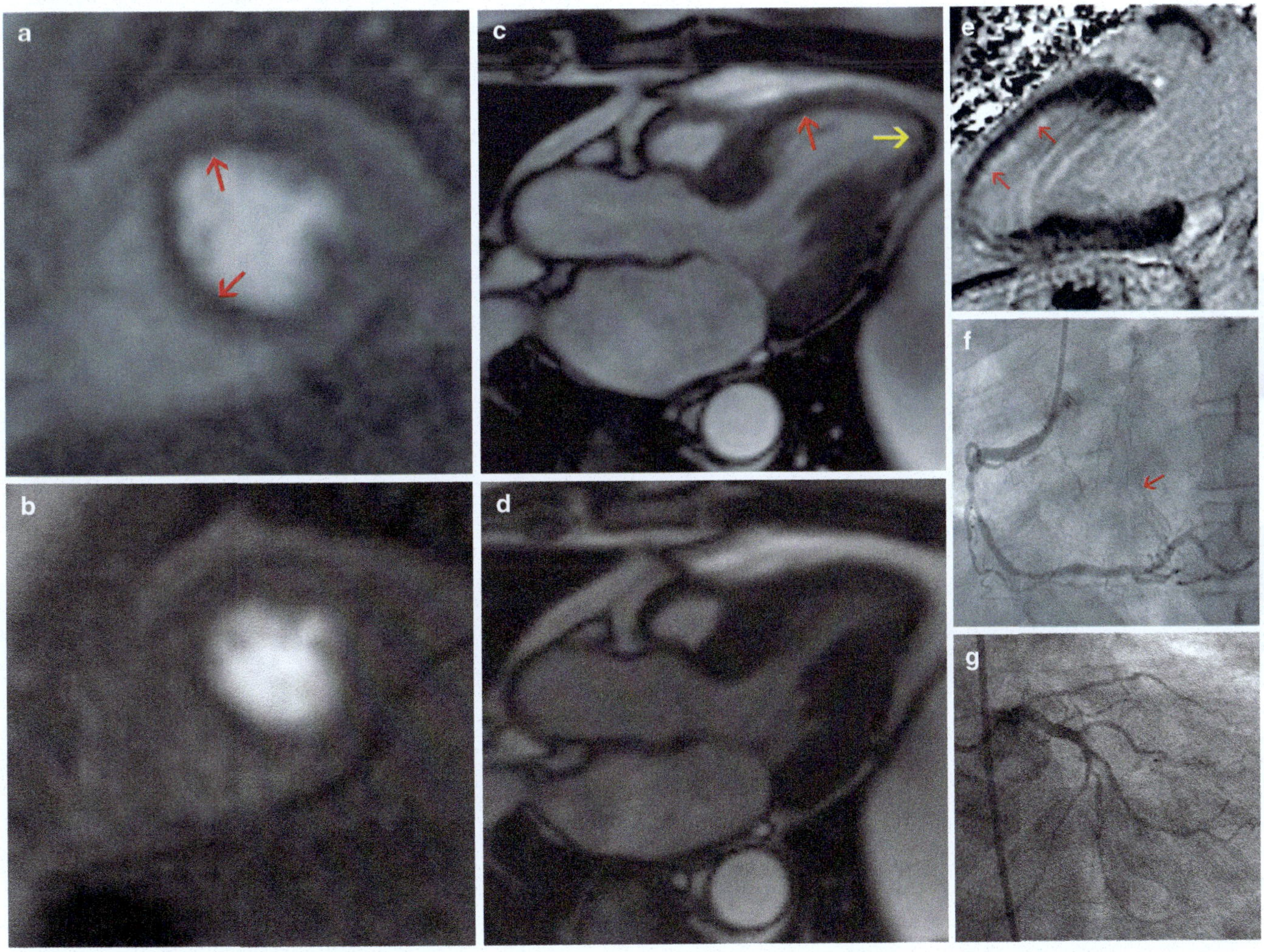

Findings and Interpretation

- High-dose dipyridamole (0.84 mg/kg in 6 min) stress perfusion images show a perfusion deficit at the anterior and anteroseptal mid-ventricular segments and anterior apical segment (panel A). Rest perfusion images were normal, demonstrating the reversible perfusion anomaly (panel B).
- The impairment of the systolic function was illustrated using left ventricular outflow tract cine view, where compared to rest (panel D), stress images (panel C) showed progression from hypokinetic to akinetic motion of the anteroseptal mid-apical segments. Dyskinetic wall motion of the apex is also observed (yellow arrow).
- The late-enhancement (phase-sensitive inversion recovery, PSIR) sequence images in vertical long axis showed a subendocardial anterior mid and apical late gadolinium enhancement (panel E), a typical ischemic-necrotic pattern.

- Coronary angiography of the right coronary artery showed moderate stenosis of the mid and distal segments, as well as the opacification of the left anterior descending artery through collateral circulation through septal branches (arrow in panel F).
- The left coronary artery catheterization showed occlusion of the left anterior descending coronary artery at the origin (panel G).
- In this way it is possible to comprehensively evaluate coronary disease, to determine the presence and extent of infarction in the territory of the anterior descending coronary artery, and to determine the existence of viable myocardium (late gadolinium enhancement comprising less than 50% of the myocardial wall thickness) and the presence of perinecrotic residual ischemia.
- The patient underwent successful coronary artery bypass surgery, with resolution of symptoms and excellent post-surgical outcome.

Further Reading

Pontone G, Andreini D, Bertella E, Loguercio M, Guglielmo M, Baggiano A, et al. Prognostic value of dipyridamole stress cardiac magnetic resonance in patients with known or suspected coronary artery disease: a mid-term follow-up study. Eur Radiol. 2016;26:2155–65.

Saeed M, Lund G, Wendland MF, Bremerich J, Weinmann H, Higgins CB. Magnetic resonance characterization of the peri-infarction zone of reperfused myocardial infarction with necrosis-specific and extracellular nonspecific contrast media. Circulation. 2001;103:871–6.

Case 37

Infarct Imaging

Clinical History

- Seventy-three-year-old male.
- He has symptomatic coronary artery disease.
- He underwent invasive coronary angiography, demonstrating severe stenosis of the mid left anterior descending (LAD) artery and distal occlusion, severe stenosis of the posterior ventricular branch (left circumflex artery), and sub-occluded (99%) distal right coronary artery (RCA).
- Referred for delayed-enhancement cardiac magnetic resonance (DE-CMR) to assess the extent and patterns of myocardial necrosis.

Images

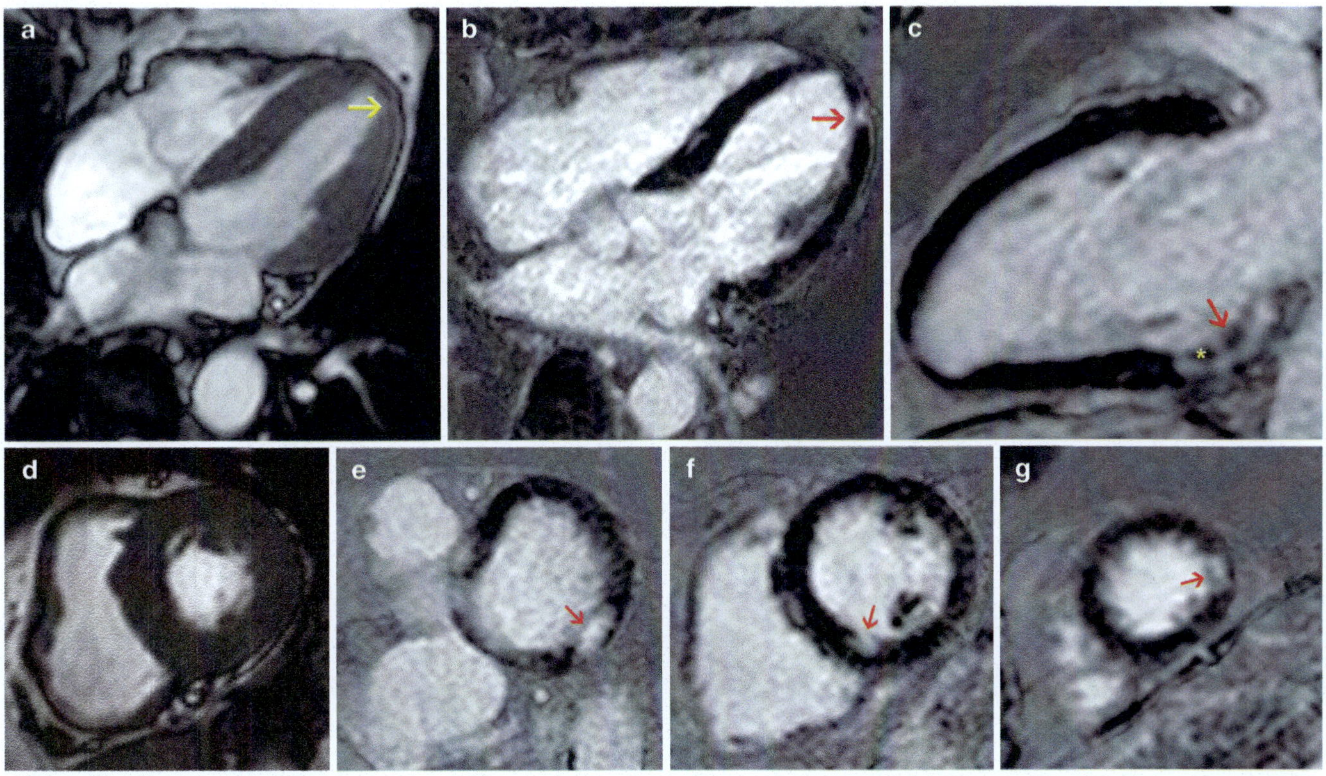

Findings and Interpretation

- Non-dilated left ventricle (end-diastolic volume 59 ml/m^2), with preserved left ventricular ejection fraction (53%).
- Systolic cine images at four-chamber (panel A) and short-axis (panel D) views demonstrate a preserved global systolic function, with a very small akinetic area at the lateral apical segment (arrow in panel A).
- Inversion-recovery images (four-chamber, panel B; two-chamber, panel C; and short-axis views, panels E–G) demonstrate small areas of late gadolinium enhancement (LGE) (red arrows). Note the different extensions of LGE, including subendocardial (panel F) and transmural (panel E), and areas of microvascular obstruction/no reflow (* in panel C).
- Microvascular obstruction, an independent predictor of final infarct size, ventricular dysfunction, and major adverse cardiac events, is not only associated to revascularization and ischemic-reperfusion damage. Indeed, it is commonly observed in patients with non-reperfused ST-elevation myocardial infarction (STEMI) and can even be detected among patients with non-STEMI.

Further Reading

Guerra E, Hadamitzky M, Ndrepepa G, et al. Microvascular obstruction in patients with non-ST-elevation myocardial infarction: a contrast-enhanced cardiac magnetic resonance study. Int J Cardiovasc Imaging. 2014;30:1087–95.

Hadamitzky M, Langhans B, Hausleiter J, et al. Prognostic value of late gadolinium enhancement in cardiovascular magnetic resonance imaging after acute ST-elevation myocardial infarction in comparison with single-photon emission tomography using Tc99m-Sestamibi. Eur Heart J Cardiovasc Imaging. 2014;15:216–25.

Hamirani YS, Wong A, Kramer CM, et al. Effect of microvascular obstruction and intramyocardial hemorrhage by CMR on LV remodeling and outcomes after myocardial infarction: a systematic review and meta-analysis. JACC Cardiovasc Imaging. 2014;7:940–52.

Khan JN, Razvi N, Nazir SA, et al. Prevalence and extent of infarct and microvascular obstruction following different reperfusion therapies in ST-elevation myocardial infarction. J Cardiovasc Magn Reson. 2014;16:38.

Case 38

Infarct Imaging

Clinical History

- Fifty-nine-year-old male.
- Coronary risk factors: diabetes, hypertension, hypercholesterolemia, smoking.
- He had a history of previous myocardial infarction and coronary artery bypass surgery.
- Referred for delayed-enhancement cardiac magnetic resonance (DE-CMR) for the evaluation of the extent and pattern of myocardial necrosis.

Images

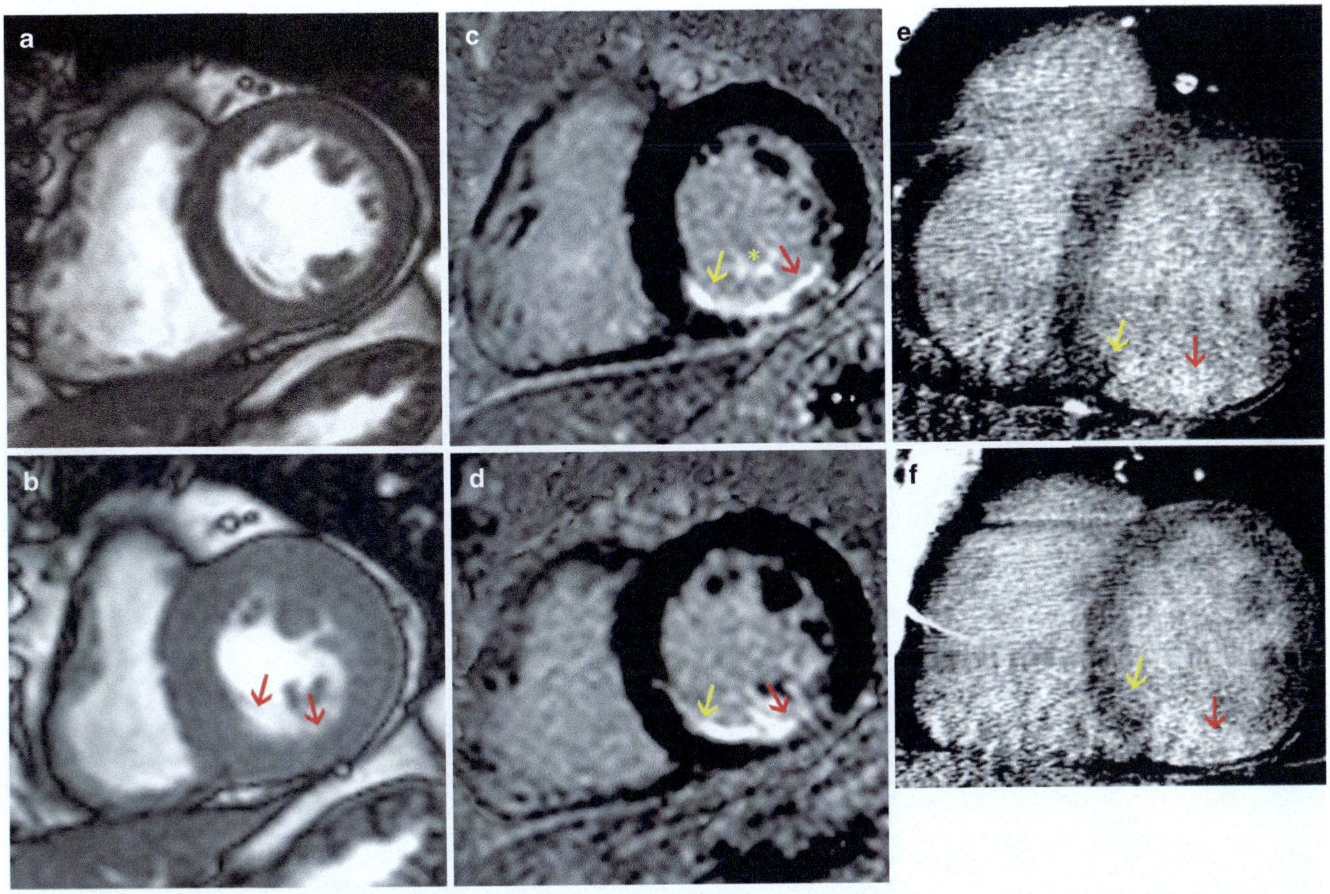

Findings and Interpretation

- The left ventricle had normal dimensions (end-diastolic volume 66 ml/m^2), with an ejection fraction of 53%.
- Cine short-axis images (diastolic, panel A; systolic, panel B) showed inferior wall motion abnormalities (arrows in panel B).
- Short-axis inversion-recovery images (basal, panel C; mid-ventricular, panel D) demonstrated areas of subendocardial (yellow arrows) and transmural (red arrows) necrosis. Also, note the presence of late gadolinium enhancement (LGE) of the posterior papillary muscle (*, in panel C).
- Delayed-enhancement computed tomography (DE-CT) images, acquired using a dual-energy CT scanner 7 min after iodine injection, identified the same findings (panels E and F), with less ability to discriminate between subendocardial and transmural necrosis extension.
- Among patients non-suitable for CMR (obesity, claustrophobia, severe renal dysfunction, cardiac implants), DE-CT provides an alternative for the assessment of myocardial necrosis.

Further Reading

Rodriguez-Granillo GA. Delayed enhancement cardiac computed tomography for the assessment of myocardial infarction: from bench to bedside. Cardiovasc Diagn Ther. 2017;7:159–70.

Case 39

Infarct Imaging

Clinical History

- Forty-six-year-old male.
- Coronary risk factors: hypertension, smoking.
- Two months ago he was admitted in the intensive care unit with an ST-elevation acute myocardial infarction and underwent primary angioplasty (thrombectomy plus stenting) of the proximal right coronary artery (RCA). The left anterior descending artery was also totally occluded but remained untreated in the index procedure based on ECG and echocardiographic findings suggesting that the RCA was the culprit lesion.
- Referred for delayed-enhancement cardiac magnetic resonance (DE-CMR) to establish the extent and patterns of myocardial necrosis.

Images

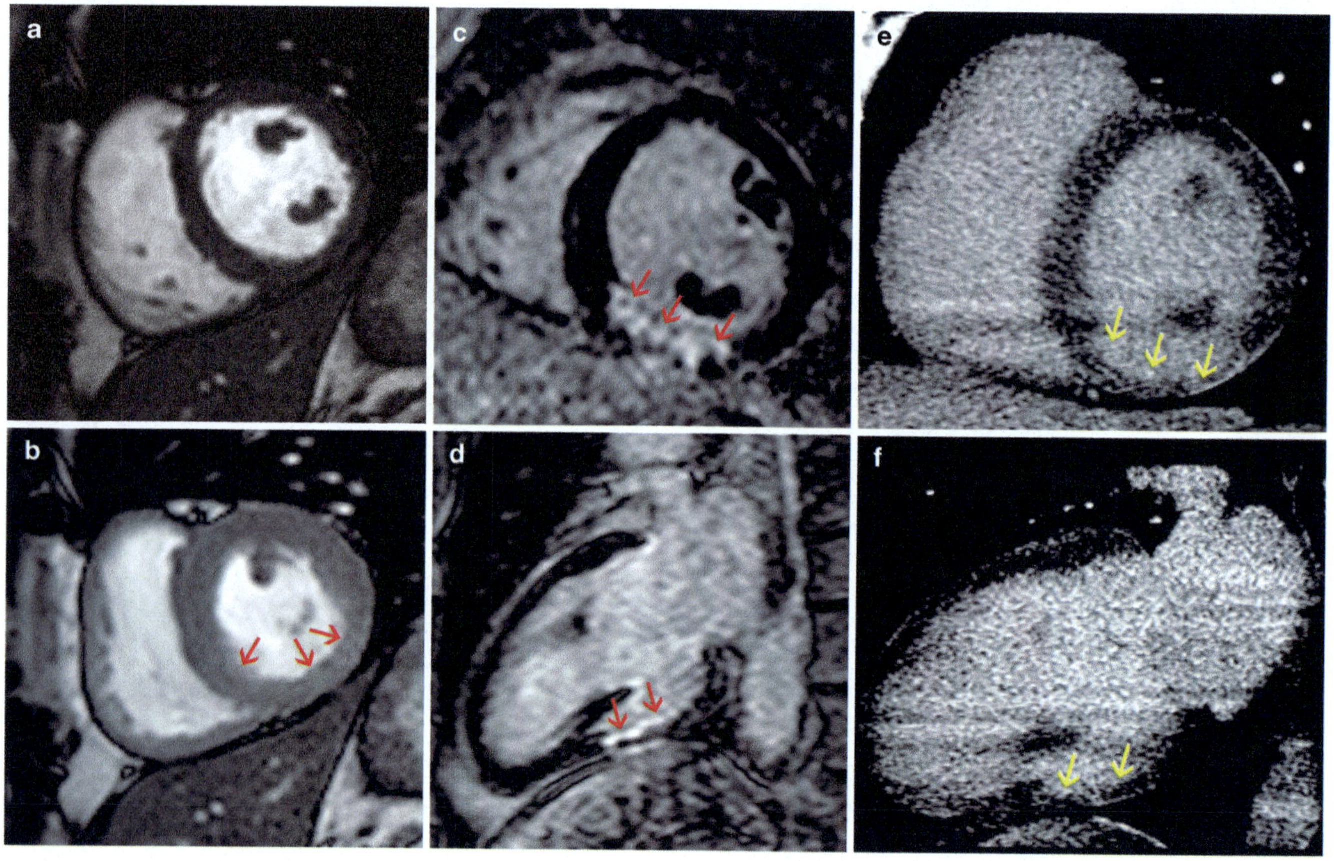

Findings and Interpretation

- The left ventricle had normal dimensions (end-diastolic volume 75 ml/m^2), with mild systolic dysfunction (left ventricular ejection fraction 45%).
- Cine short-axis images (diastolic, panel A; systolic, panel B) demonstrated akinetic basal inferior left ventricular wall (red arrows, in panel B).
- Inversion-recovery images (short-axis, panel C; two-chamber, panel D) showed a small predominantly transmural (50–75% of the myocardial wall thickness) late gadolinium enhancement (LGE) in the basal inferior wall (red arrows in panels C and D).
- Delayed-enhancement (DE) computed tomography (CT) images acquired using a dual-energy CT scanner 7 min after iodine injection demonstrated similar findings (yellow arrows in panels E and F).
- Note that the anterior wall had absence of necrosis.

Further Reading

Rodriguez-Granillo GA, Campisi R, Deviggiano A, de Munain MNL, Zan M, Capunay C, Carrascosa P. Detection of myocardial infarction using delayed enhancement dual-energy CT in stable patients. AJR Am J Roentgenol. 2017;209:1023–32.

Case 40

Infarct Imaging

Clinical History

- Sixty-six-year-old male.
- Coronary risk factors: hypercholesterolemia, smoking.
- Two months ago he was admitted in the intensive care unit with symptoms of an evolved anterior lateral myocardial infarction (interscapular pain, elevated cardiac enzymes, and negative T waves in DI, AvL, V4–V6), with conservative management.
- Referred for delayed-enhancement cardiac magnetic resonance (DE-CMR) for the evaluation of myocardial function and to establish the extent and patterns of myocardial necrosis.

Images

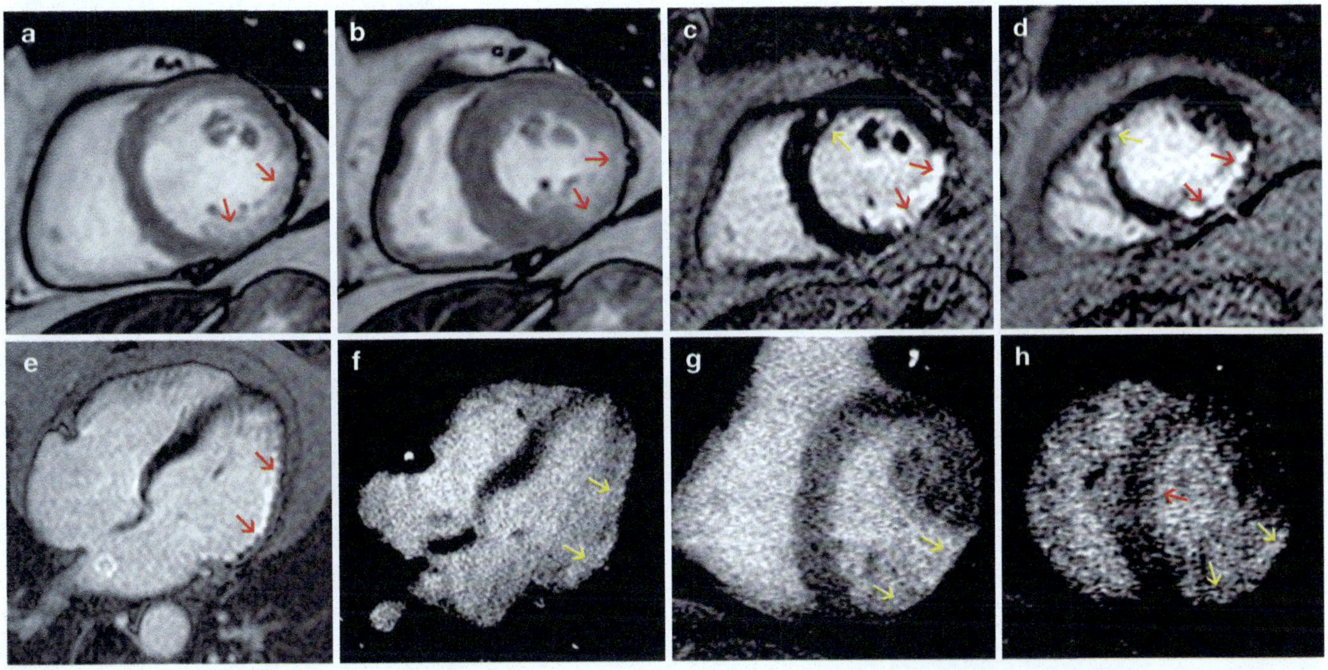

Findings and Interpretation

- The left ventricle had normal dimensions (end-diastolic volume 65 ml/m^2), with an ejection fraction of 53%.
- Cine short-axis images (diastolic, panel A; systolic, panel B) acquired in this case after administration of gadolinium demonstrated akinetic inferior lateral left ventricular wall (red arrows, in panel B). Note the increased regional myocardial signal intensity (arrows in panels A and B), reflecting residual myocardial edema.
- Inversion-recovery images (mid-ventricular, panel C; mid/apical, D; four-chamber, panel E). Predominantly transmural late gadolinium enhancement (LGE) in the left circumflex territory (red arrows, in panels C–E) and minimal subendocardial anteroseptal wall LGE (yellow arrows in panels C and D).
- Delayed-enhancement (DE) computed tomography (CT) images acquired using a dual-energy CT scanner 7 min after iodine injection demonstrated similar findings (panels F–H), although the small subendocardial septal necrosis is less clearly depicted compared to DE-CMR (panel D, yellow arrow, vs. panel H, red arrow).
- Despite the similar contrast kinetics of gadolinium and iodine, leading to comparable DE imaging in terms of infarct detection on a per patient basis, DE-CMR achieves significantly higher contrast-to-noise ratio and thus a better discrimination between necrosis and remote normal myocardium. In part, this is related to the ability of CMR to null the normal myocardium signal using specific inversion times.

Further Reading

Rodriguez-Granillo GA, Campisi R, Deviggiano A, et al. Detection of myocardial infarction using delayed enhancement dual-energy CT in stable patients. AJR Am J Roentgenol. 2017;209:1023–32.

Case 41

Infarct Imaging

Clinical History

- Forty-seven-year-old male.
- Coronary risk factors: hypertension, hypercholesterolemia, former smoking.
- He has history of previous myocardial infarction 3 years ago, with no revascularization attempt.
- Referred for delayed-enhancement cardiac magnetic resonance (DE-CMR) to assess the extent and patterns of myocardial necrosis.

Images

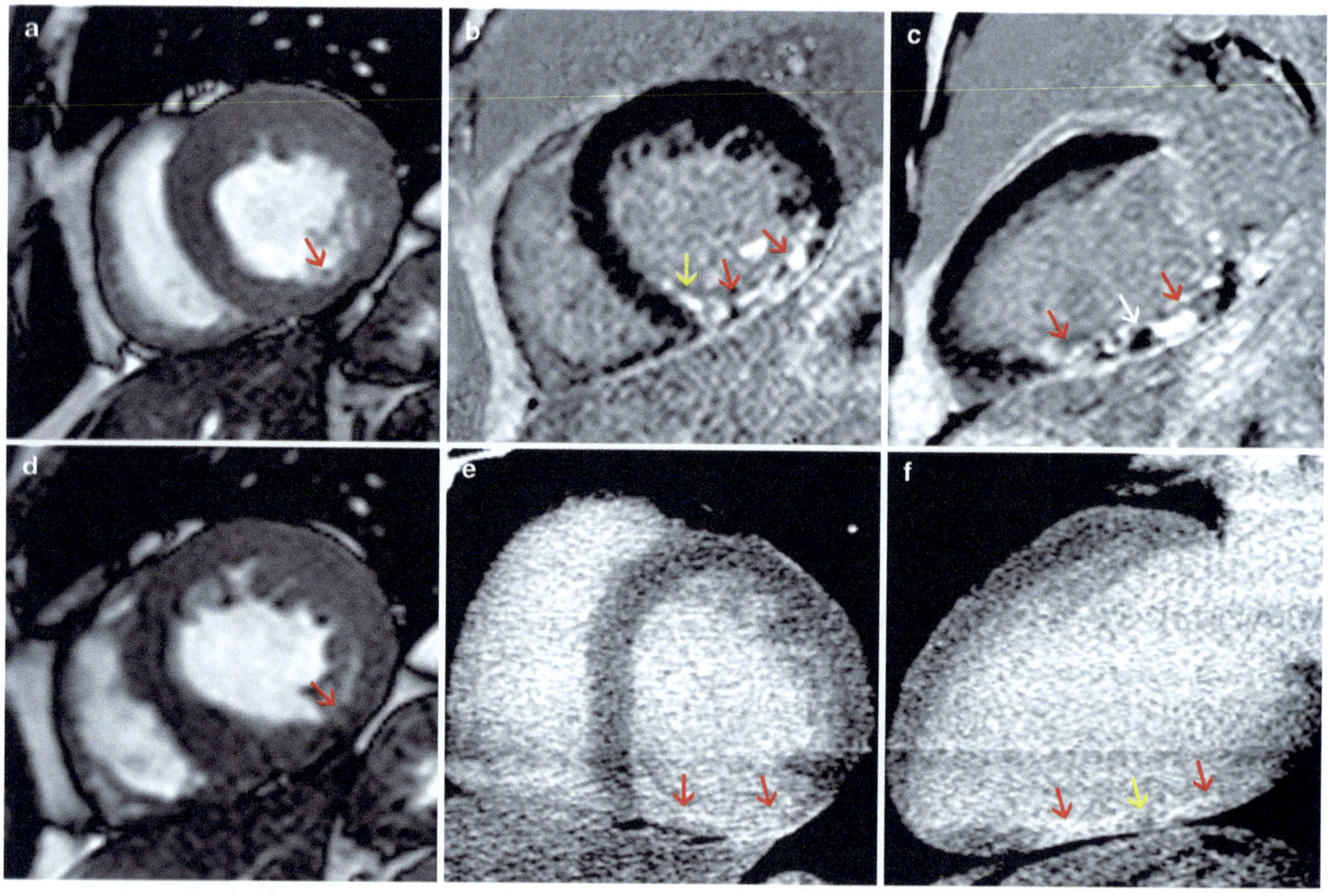

Findings and Interpretation

- He has a very mild dilatation of the left ventricle (end-diastolic dimensions: diameter 60 mm; volume 87 ml/m^2), with a left ventricular ejection fraction of 43%.
- Cine short-axis views (diastolic, panel A; systolic, panel D) demonstrate akinetic inferior lateral wall, with mild myocardial wall thinning (red arrows).
- Inversion-recovery images (short-axis, panel B; two-chamber, panel C) demonstrate a predominantly transmural myocardial infarction (red arrows) and small areas of subendocardial necrosis (yellow arrow) and microvascular obstruction/no reflow (white arrow).
- Delayed-enhancement computed tomography (DE-CT) images (panels E and F) acquired using dual-energy CT scanner 7 min after iodine administration demonstrated similar findings (arrows).
- Gadolinium- and iodinated-based contrast agents share similar kinetics. Accordingly, these techniques have a comparable ability to evaluate myocardial infarcts at both first-pass perfusion and DE imaging. DE-CT imaging offers an excellent alternative to DE-CMR in patients with acute myocardial infarction, in whom the extracellular volume (ECV) expansion is mostly related to membrane disruption. In turn, DE-CT imaging in patients with stable previous myocardial infarction (in whom the ECV increase is more associated with myocardial fibrosis) demands amendments in the acquisition parameters, including low voltage (80–100 kV), soft filters, thick reconstructions, or, if available, dual-energy CT acquisitions.

Further Reading

Chang S, Han K, Youn JC, et al. Utility of dual-energy CT-based monochromatic imaging in the assessment of myocardial delayed enhancement in patients with cardiomyopathy. Radiology. 2018;287:442–51.

Rodriguez-Granillo GA. Delayed enhancement cardiac computed tomography for the assessment of myocardial infarction: from bench to bedside. Cardiovasc Diagn Ther. 2017;7:159–70.

Case 42

Infarct Imaging

Clinical History

- Forty-six-year-old male.
- He has a history of previous myocardial infarction 6 years ago, without previous revascularization or thrombolysis attempts.
- He has frequent complex premature ventricular contractions.
- Referred for delayed-enhancement cardiac magnetic resonance (DE-CMR) to assess the extent of myocardial necrosis.

Images

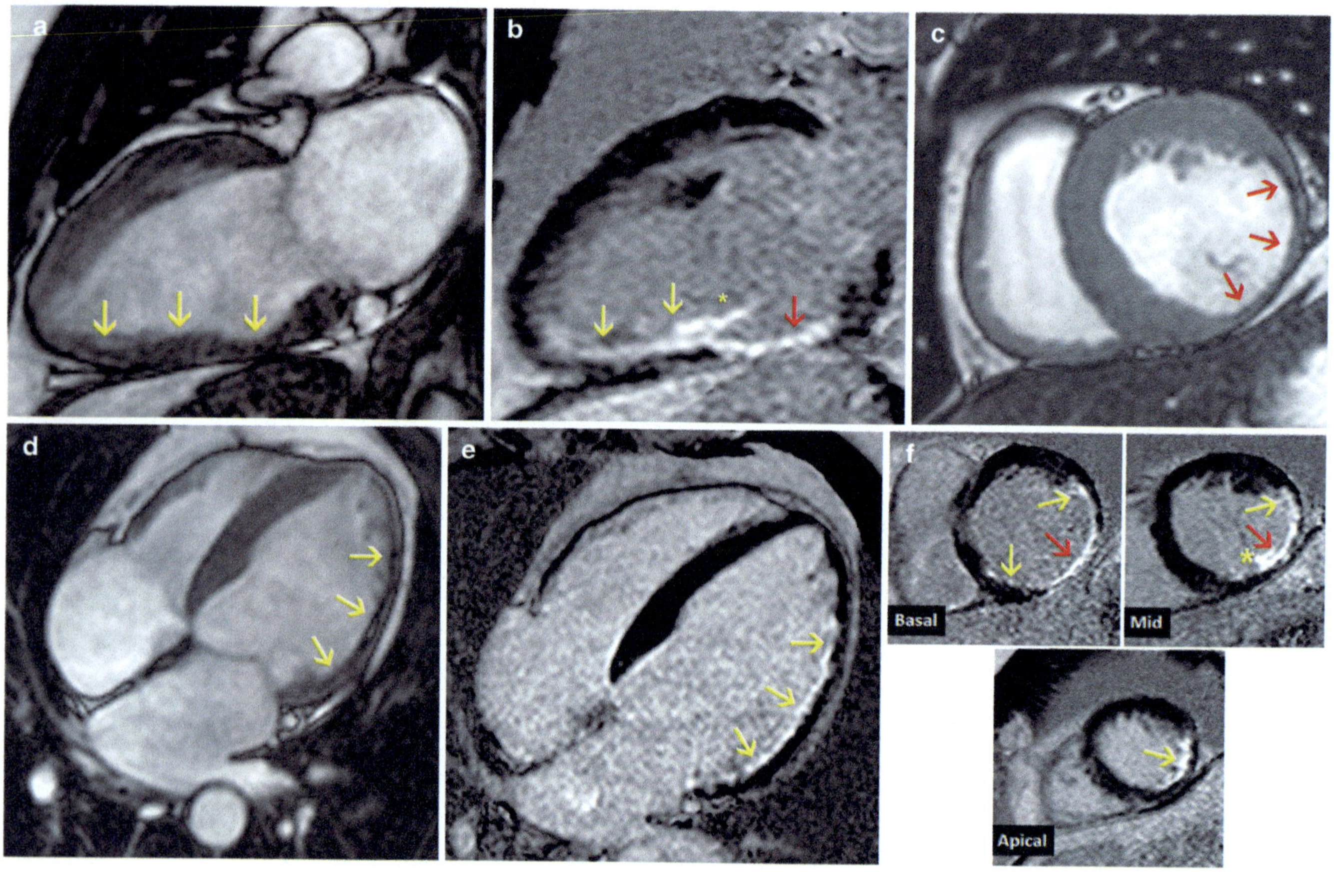

Findings and Interpretation

- Dilated left ventricle (end-diastolic volume 114 ml/m^2) with a left ventricular ejection fraction of 32%.
- Systolic cine images in two-chamber (panel A) and four-chamber (panel D) views demonstrate akinetic inferior and lateral walls (yellow arrows). Systolic basal cine short-axis view shows inferolateral dyskinesia, with marked wall thinning (red arrows, in panel C).
- Inversion-recovery delayed-enhancement images (panels B, E, and F) demonstrate late gadolinium enhancement (LGE) of the aforementioned segments (yellow arrows).

  These images depict the differences in the transmural extension of LGE (yellow arrows, subendocardial; red arrows, transmural).
- Note the presence of involvement (with LGE) of the posterior papillary muscle (* in panels B and F).
- Since LGE is predominantly subendocardial (<50% of wall thickness), coronary revascularization of the inferior wall might potentially lead to some functional recovery regardless of the presence of myocardial wall thinning.

Further Reading

Romero J, Xue X, Gonzalez W, et al. CMR imaging assessing viability in patients with chronic ventricular dysfunction due to coronary artery disease: a meta-analysis of prospective trials, J Am Coll Cardiol Img. 2012;5: 494–508.

Shah DJ, Kim HW, James O, et al. Prevalence of Regional Myocardial Thinning and Relationship. With Myocardial Scarring in Patients With Coronary Artery Disease. JAMA. 2013; 309: 909–18.

Case 43

Infarct Imaging

Clinical History

- Seventy-two-year-old male.
- He has a history of previous myocardial infarction and previous percutaneous coronary angioplasty.
- Referred for delayed-enhancement cardiac magnetic resonance (DE-CMR) to assess the extent of myocardial necrosis.

Images

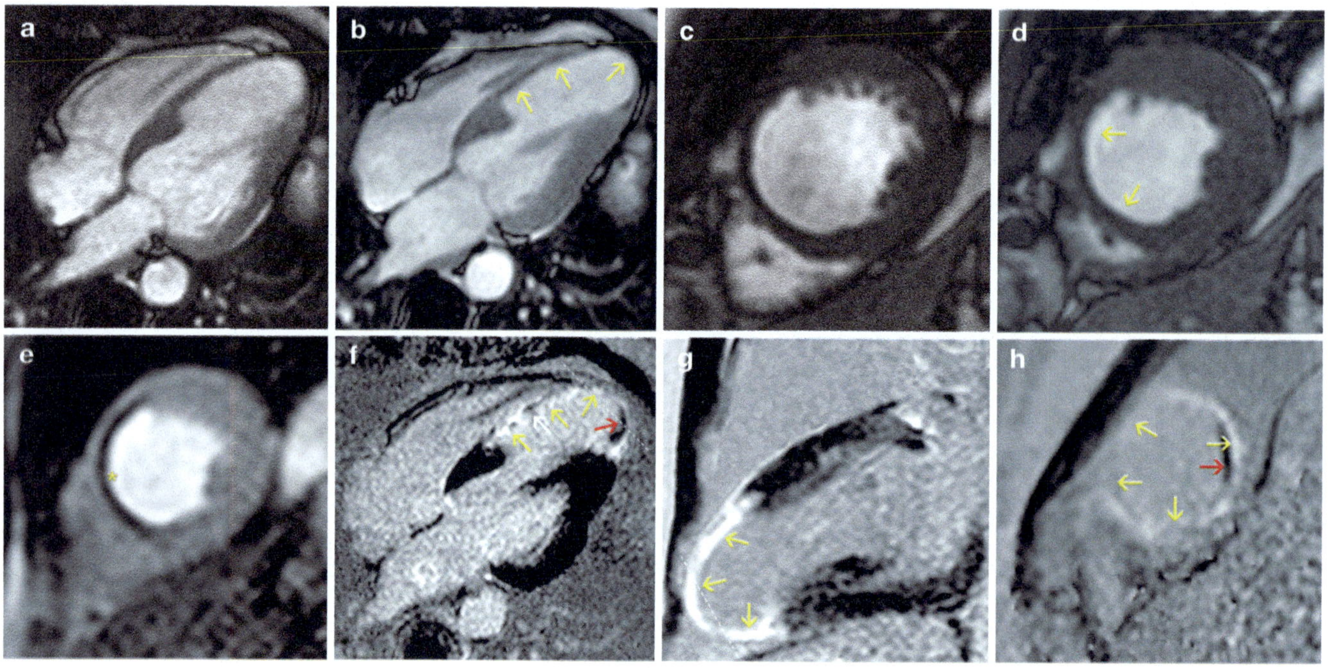

Findings and Interpretation

- Dilated left ventricle (end-diastolic volume 117 ml/m^2), with a left ventricular ejection fraction of 33%.
- Cine images at four-chamber (panel A, diastolic; panel B, systolic) and short-axis (panel C, diastolic; panel D, systolic) views demonstrate akinetic anterior septal and apical walls, with underlying myocardial wall thinning (yellow arrows in B and D).
- First-pass myocardial perfusion images (panel E) show a transmural perfusion defect of the septal wall (*).
- Inversion-recovery images (four-chamber, panel F; two-chamber, panel G; and apical short-axis, panel H) demonstrate late gadolinium enhancement (LGE) of the aforementioned segments (yellow arrows), with areas of microvascular obstruction (white arrow in panel F).
- At the apex, a laminar inferior lateral mural thrombus is observed (red arrow in panels F and H).
- Since LGE of the septal and apical walls has a transmural pattern (100% of wall thickness), this represents nonviable myocardium, and coronary revascularization of the left anterior descending artery will not lead to functional recovery.

Further Reading

Romero J, Xue X, Gonzalez W, et al. CMR imaging assessing viability in patients with chronic ventricular dysfunction due to coronary artery disease: a meta-analysis of prospective trials. J Am Coll Cardiol Img. 2012;5:494–508.

Sha D et al. Prevalence of regional myocardial thinning and relationship. With myocardial scarring in patients with coronary artery disease. JAMA. 2013; 309: 909–18.

Case 44

Complications of Myocardial Infarction

Clinical History

- Sixty-six-year-old male.
- He has history of previous myocardial infarction and surgical revascularization.
- Currently with worsening heart failure symptoms.
- Referred for delayed-enhancement cardiac magnetic resonance (DE-CMR) to evaluate the extent of myocardial viability.

Images

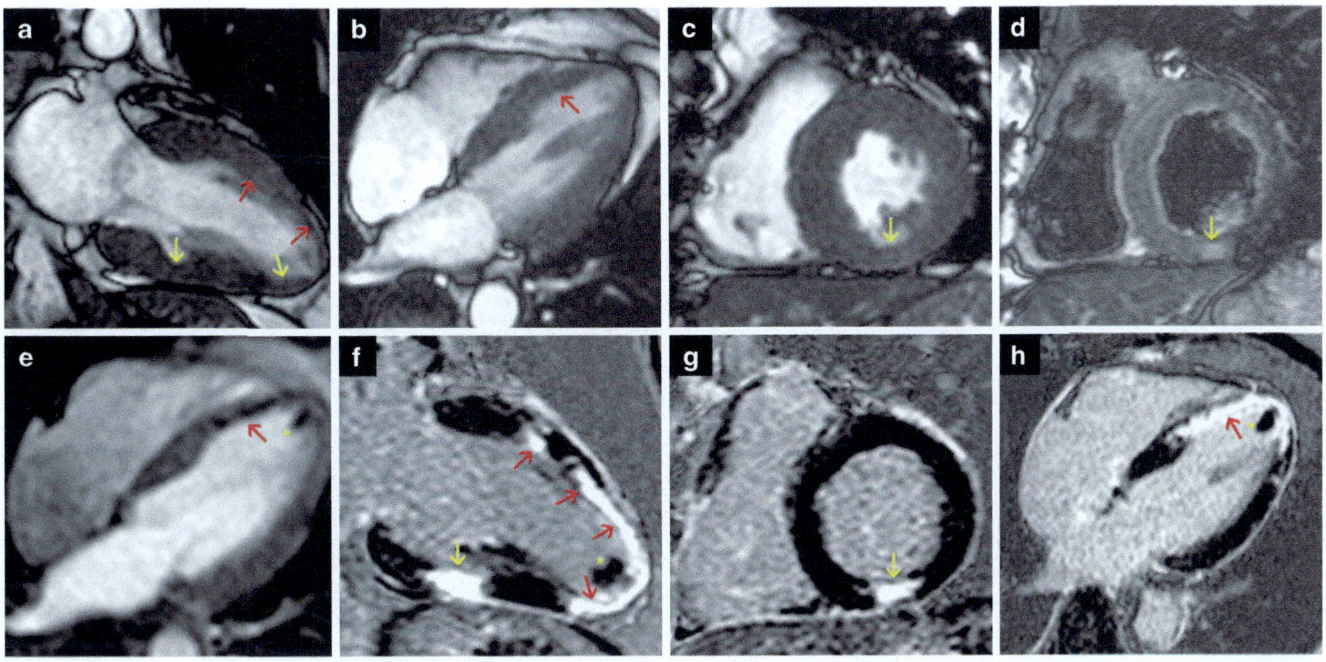

Findings and Interpretation

- He has non-dilated left ventricle (end-diastolic volume 63 ml/m^2), with a left ventricular ejection fraction of 42%.
- Systolic cine images (two-chamber, panel A; four-chamber, panel B; and short-axis, panel C) demonstrate hypokinetic mid/basal inferior and apical inferior segments (yellow arrows, in panels A and C), as well as of the anterior and septal mid and apical segments (red arrows, in panels A and B).
- T2-weighted mid-ventricular short-axis image (panel D) shows a focal area of transmural increased signal intensity (arrow), reflecting myocardial edema.
- First-pass myocardial perfusion images (panel E) demonstrated a septal perfusion defect (arrow) and an apical thrombus (*).
- Inversion-recovery images (two-chamber, panel F; short-axis, panel G; and four-chamber, panel H) demonstrate predominantly transmural late gadolinium enhancement (LGE) involving two different coronary artery territories: a large anterior wall myocardial infarction (red arrows in panels F and H) and a small inferior acute (with underlying myocardial edema) myocardial infarction (yellow arrow in panels F and G).
- After an acute myocardial infarction, myocardial edema evaluated with CMR using T2-weighted imagining is maximal and constant during the first week and starts to decrease at 15 days, being usually undetected at 6 months. On the contrary, acute LGE is a weak predictor of functional recovery compared with chronic LGE, since it can overestimate the extent of irreversible myocardial damage in the acute phase. Indeed, the extent of LGE decreases by 20% after 6 months.

Further Reading

Dall'Armellina E, Karia N, Lindsay AC, et al. Dynamic changes of edema and late gadolinium enhancement after acute myocardial infarction and their relationship to functional recovery and salvage index. Circ Cardiovasc Imaging. 2011;4:228–36.

Case 45

Complications of Myocardial Infarction

Clinical History

- Sixty-seven-year-old male.
- Coronary risk factors: hypertension, hypercholesterolemia, former smoking.
- Asymptomatic. He has a history of previous myocardial infarction 30 years ago, with no revascularization attempt.
- Referred for delayed-enhancement cardiac magnetic resonance (DE-CMR) to evaluate extent and patterns of myocardial necrosis.

Images

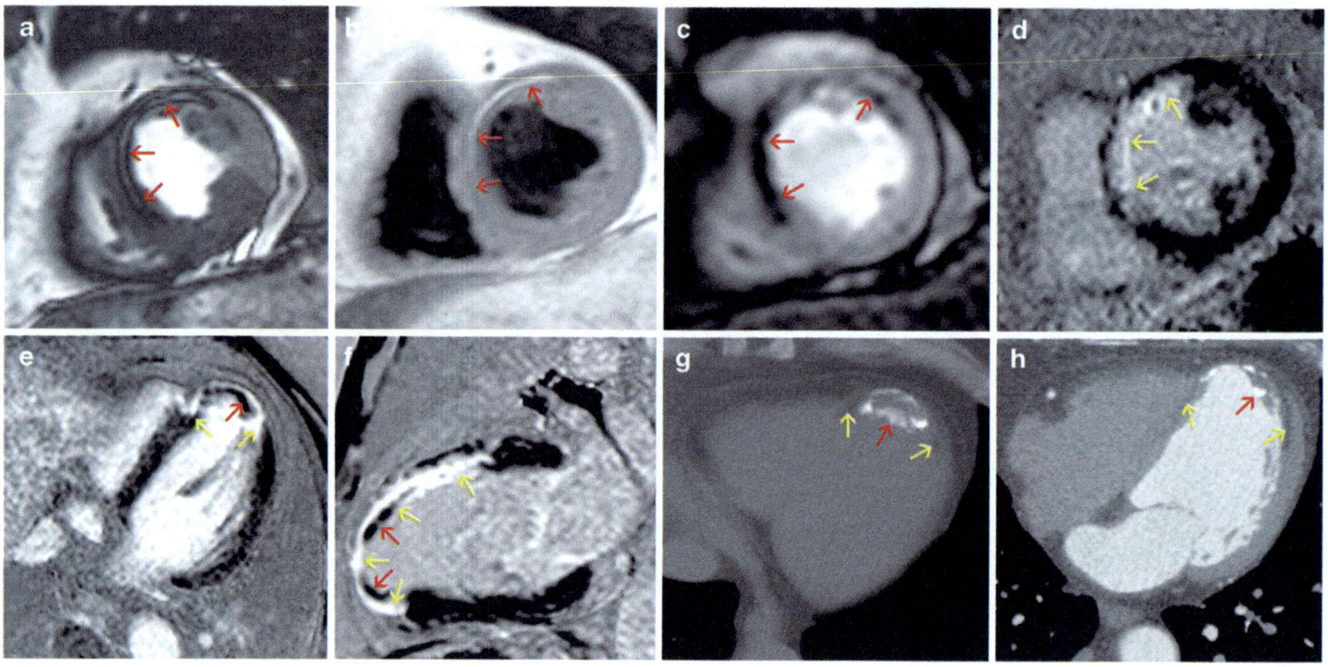

Findings and Interpretation

- The left ventricle has a normal size (end-diastolic volume 79 ml/m^2), with left ventricular ejection fraction of 43%.
- Systolic cine short-axis image demonstrates akinetic anterior and septal wall (arrows, in panel A), with low myocardial signal intensity and wall thinning.
- T1-weighted images show increased signal intensity of the aforementioned segments (arrows, in panel B), reflecting lipomatous metaplasia.
- Transmural myocardial perfusion defect is demonstrated at first-pass perfusion images (arrows, in panel C).
- Inversion-recovery images (short-axis, panel D; low four-chamber, panel E; and two-chamber, panel F views) demonstrate predominantly transmural late gadolinium enhancement (LGE, yellow arrows in panels D–F) involving the anterior, septal, and apical walls. Note the presence of laminar apical thrombus (red arrows).
- Non-contrast-enhanced cardiac computed tomography (CT, panel G) using a thick-slab reconstruction revealed the presence of a partially calcified mural apical thrombus (red arrow) and low-attenuation adjacent myocardium (yellow arrows), confirming the lipomatous metaplasia.
- Contrast-enhanced CT (panel H) showed similar findings, with organized thrombus (red arrow) and lipomatous metaplasia (yellow arrows).
- A large proportion of healed myocardial infarcts have evidence of adipose tissue, particularly those more than 1 year old. Indeed, the identification of lipomatous metaplasia, which can be easily detected with non-contrast-enhanced CT, is closely related to infarct age.

Further Reading

Rodríguez-Granillo GA, Rosales MA, Renes P, et al. Chronic myocardial infarction detection and characterization during coronary artery calcium scoring acquisitions. J Cardiovasc Comput Tomogr. 2010;4:99–107.

Su L, Siegel JE, Fishbein MC. Adipose tissue in myocardial infarction. Cardiovasc Pathol. 2004;13:98–102.

Case 46

Complications of Myocardial Infarction

Clinical History

- Sixty-seven-year-old male.
- Coronary risk factors: hypertension, hypercholesterolemia.
- Seventy-five days ago, he had an episode of prolonged chest pain, but did not consult the emergency department.
- Fifteen days later he was admitted with heart failure, and an evolved anterior wall myocardial infarction (MI) was diagnosed; being discharged with the following echocardiographic findings: mild left ventricular dilatation with severe ventricular dysfunction, associated with anterior wall thinning and akinesia, and mild pericardial effusion.
- One month later he was re-admitted with acute pulmonary edema. Echocardiography revealed a left ventricular ejection fraction of 20% and severe pericardial effusion. Pericardiocentesis revealed only mild hematic fluid. The patient underwent unsuccessful stenting of the left anterior descending artery.
- Referred for delayed-enhancement cardiac magnetic resonance (DE-CMR) for the evaluation of post-MI hemorrhagic pericardial effusion related to primary angioplasty.

Images

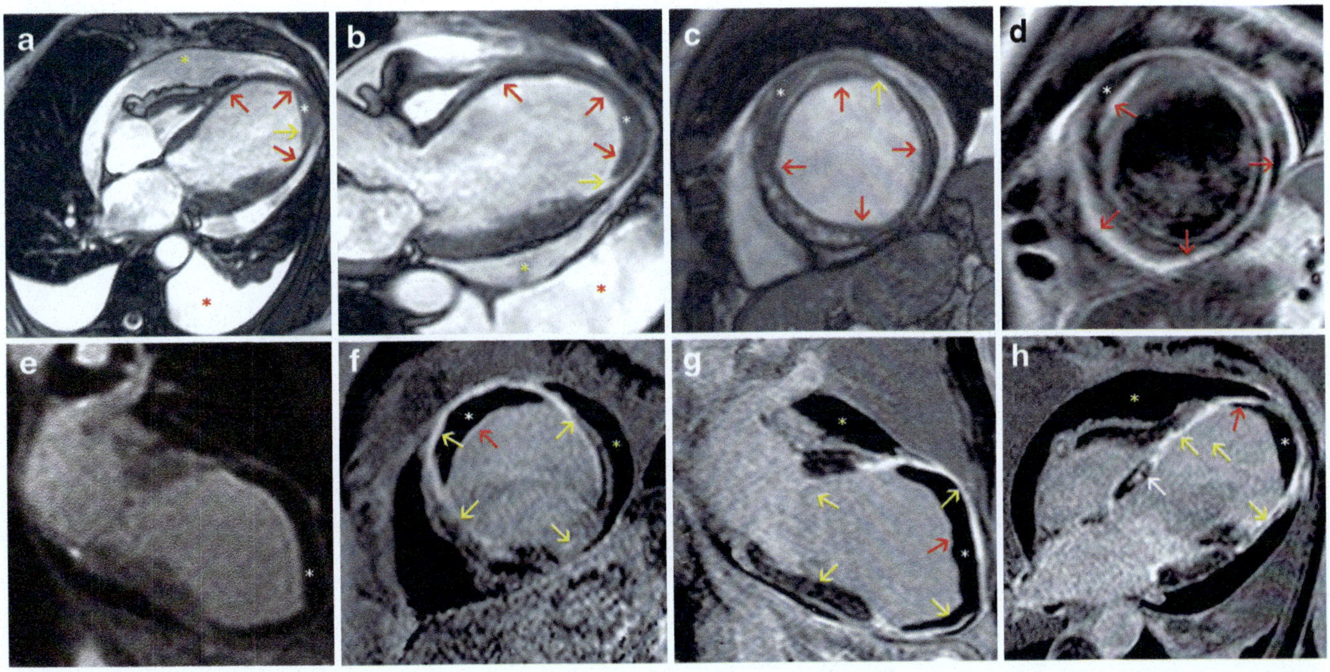

Findings and Interpretation

- Left ventricular aneurysm and severe left ventricular dilatation (end-diastolic volume 165 ml/m^2), with an ejection fraction of 12%.
- Systolic cine images (four-chamber, panel A; three-chamber, panel B; and short-axis, panel C) demonstrated a large left ventricular aneurysm, with dyskinetic wall motion (red arrows). An apical laminar filling defect (white asterisk) suggested mural thrombus, although a tear-like image was observed at the shoulder (yellow arrows).
- Moderate circumferential pericardial effusion (yellow asterisk in panels A and B), with partial diastolic right atrium collapse (not shown). Moderate pleural effusion was also observed (red asterisk in panel B).
- T2-weighted short-axis image (panel D) showed areas of increased regional signal intensity (red arrows) and areas of decreased myocardial signal intensity corresponding, respectively, to areas of edema and hemorrhage.
- First-pass myocardial perfusion images (panel E) showed an extensive perfusion defect of the anterior wall and an adjacent endocavitary mural mass with lack of gadolinium enhancement (*).
- Inversion-recovery images (short-axis, panel F; two-chamber, panel G; and four-chamber, panel H) demonstrated predominantly transmural late gadolinium

enhancement (yellow arrows F–H) of the anterior and apical segments. In these images, the presence of dissecting intra-myocardial hematoma is confirmed by demonstrating the triad comprised by a thin endocardial layer (red arrows), intramural thrombus (white asterisk), and LGE of the underlying myocardial wall (yellow arrows). Also note the presence of microvascular obstruction/no-reflow areas (white arrow in H). Pericardial effusion is denoted by yellow asterisks.

- The patient was managed with medical treatment for heart failure and received an implantable cardioverter defibrillator.
- This is a very rare but potentially fatal complication of acute MI, with high rates of mortality. Management of these patients is controversial, and a conservative approach can lead to spontaneous remission.

Further Reading

Galache Osuna JG, Marquina Barcos A, Cay Diarte E, et al. Conservative management of a post infarction intramyocardial dissecting hematoma. Intern Med. 2017;56:1067–70.

Leitman M, Tyomkin V, Sternik L, et al. Intramyocardial dissecting hematoma: two case reports and a meta-analysis of the literature. Echocardiography. 2018;35:260–6.

Case 47

Complications of Myocardial Infarction

Clinical History

- Sixty-year-old male.
- Six days ago he underwent primary angioplasty of the left anterior descending (LAD) artery due to an anterior wall ST-segment elevation acute myocardial infarction.
- He evolved with pleuritic chest pain.
- Referred for delayed-enhancement cardiac magnetic resonance (DE-CMR) to rule out post-myocardial infarction pericarditis.

Images

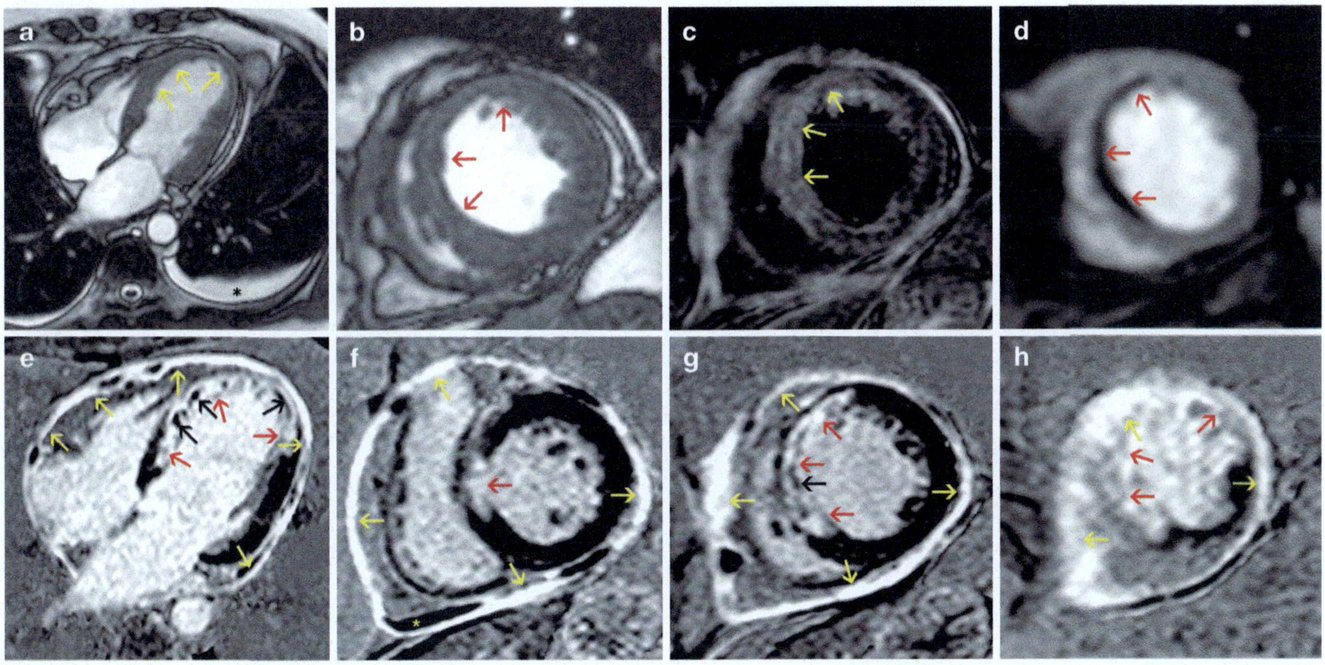

Findings and Interpretation

- The left ventricle had a normal size (end-diastolic volume 69 ml/m^2), with severe systolic dysfunction (left ventricular ejection fraction of 28%).
- Systolic cine images (four-chamber, panel A, and short-axis, panel B) demonstrate akinetic mid and apical anterior segments, with mild dyskinetic motion of the mid and apical anteroseptal segments (arrows, in panels A and B).
- T2-weighted mid short-axis images (panel C) show transmural increased signal intensity (arrows), reflecting myocardial edema.
- First-pass myocardial perfusion images (panel D) demonstrate transmural septal perfusion defect (arrows).
- Inversion-recovery images (four-chamber, panel E; short-axis, panels F–H) demonstrate large transmural late gadolinium enhancement (LGE, red arrows) involving the basal anterior segment (panel F), mid-anterior and anteroseptal segments (panel G), and apical anterior/lateral and septal segments (panel H). Note the presence of multiple areas of microvascular obstruction/no reflow (black arrows in panels E and G).
- Also, the pericardium has extensive LGE (yellow arrows in panels E–H), with minimal underlying effusion (*, in panel G).
- Mild pleural effusion is also noted (*, in panel A).
- Diagnosis of early post-infarction pericardial injury, a surrogate of extensive myocardial damage and a predictor of transmural necrosis, can sometimes be elusive. As shown in this patient, CMR is an excellent tool for the characterization of post-myocardial infarction pericardial injury.

Further Reading

Doulaptsis C, Goetschalckx K, Masci PG, et al. Assessment of early post-infarction pericardial injury by CMR. JACC Cardiovasc Imaging. 2013;6:411–3.

Case 48

Complications of Myocardial Infarction

Clinical History

- Seventy-nine-year-old female.
- Cardiovascular risk factors: hypertension and atrial fibrillation.
- Presents with acute chest pain and positive cardiac enzyme levels.
- Invasive coronary angiography showed a left main coronary artery anomaly with origin in the right coronary sinus without obstructive lesions.
- Cardiac magnetic resonance (CMR) was requested to evaluate cardiac structure and function.

Images

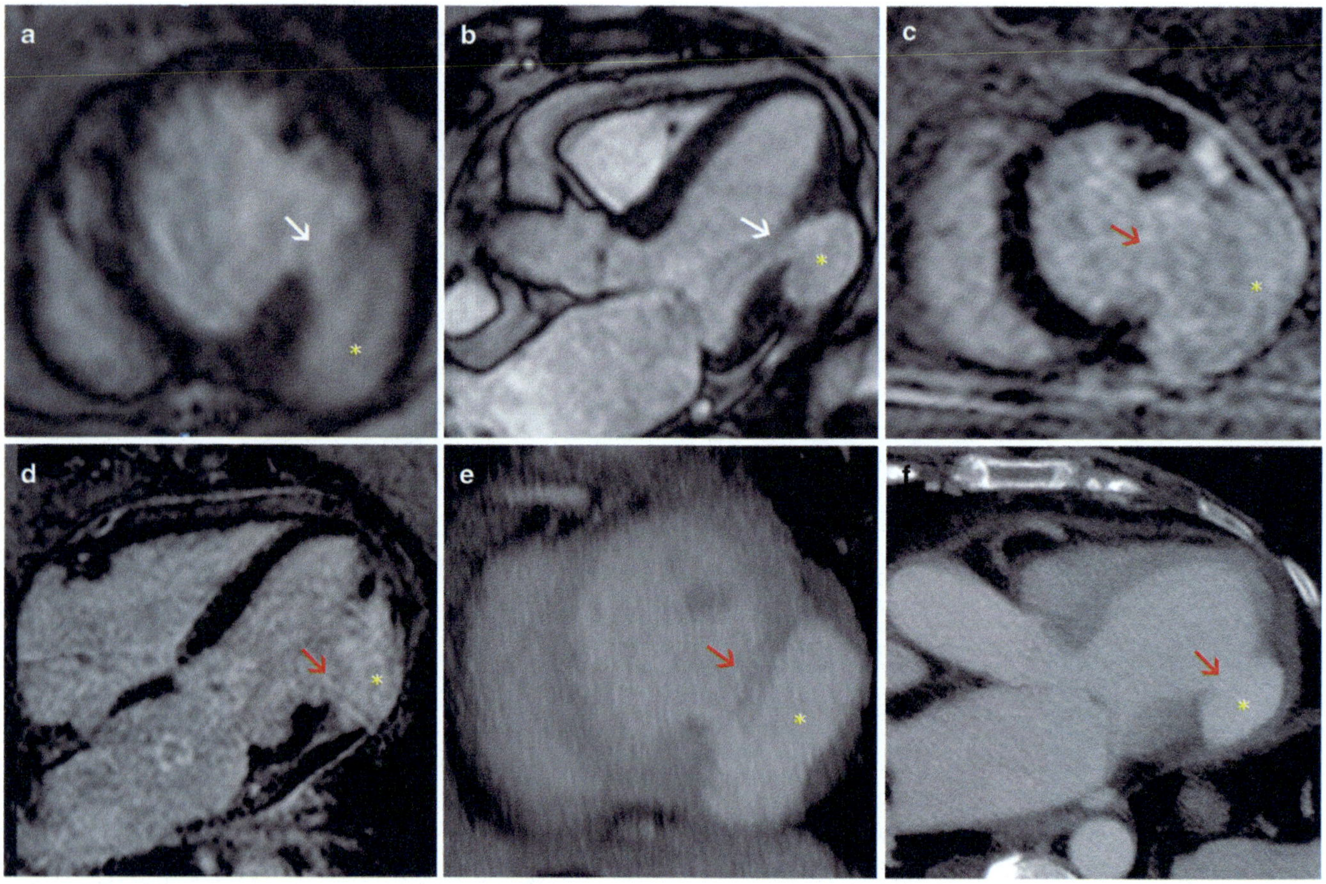

Findings and Interpretation

- Short-axis cine image at the midventricular level showing a lateral wall defect with a narrow neck (white arrow) and an adjacent pseudoaneurysm (asterisk) (panel A).
- Three chamber cine image showing the lateral defect (white arrow) and pseudoaneurysm (asterisk) (panel B).
- Late enhancement short-axis (panel C) and four-chamber views (panel D) showing similar findings.
- Cardiac CT in short-axis (panel E) and three-chamber views (panel F) illustrating similar findings than CMR.
- Left ventricular pseudoaneurysm is a rare but life-threatening complication that is frequently reported secondary to myocardial infarction or cardiac surgery.
- Clinical presentation can be nonspecific, including chest pain, congestive heart failure, dyspnea, or arrhythmia leading to a delay in the diagnosis.
- This outpouching is formed when cardiac rupture is contained by adherent pericardium or scar tissue, with no myocardial tissue. It tends to grow rapidly; for that reason early diagnosis and treatment are vital in these patients.
- Medical therapy can be considered in asymptomatic patients with small-sized outpouching (<3 cm) but is mandatory to perform a regular follow-up to determine the growth of this defect. Surgical approach is indicated when patients become symptomatic and when the aneu-

rysm increases the size considerably with risk of rupture. Recently, a new therapeutic approach is available by means of percutaneous closure.

Further Reading

Frances C, Romero A, Grady D. Left ventricular pseudoaneurysm. Am Coll Cardiol. 1998;32:557–61.

Inayat F, Ghani AR, Riaz I, et al. Left ventricular pseudoaneurysm: an overview of diagnosis and management. J Investig Med High Impact Case Rep. 2018;6:2324709618792025.

Weinstein D, Wait MA, McGuire DK, et al. Differentiating true versus pseudo left ventricular aneurysm: a case report and review of diagnostic strategies. Cardiol Rev. 2006;14:e27–30.

Myocardial Infarction with Nonobstructive Coronary Arteries (MINOCA)

3

Alejandro Deviggiano, Patricia M. Carrascosa, and Gastón A. Rodríguez-Granillo

Background

Myocardial infarction with nonobstructive coronary arteries (MINOCA) is a syndrome involving different etiologies; therefore it can sometimes be difficult to establish the definitive diagnosis. It is important to emphasize that invasive coronary angiography (ICA) must show normal or near-normal (stenosis less than 50%) coronary arteries. Performing a correct diagnosis has important prognostic and therapeutic implications for these patients. MINOCA represents between 5 and 25% of acute myocardial infarctions (AMI).

In patients with MINOCA, cardiac magnetic resonance (CMR) has shown to establish a definitive diagnosis in 70% of cases, providing a significant incremental impact on diagnosis and/or clinical management in 66% of patients. On the other hand, it should be noted that 30% of patients with MINOCA have normal CMR, related with a good remote prognosis.

CMR allows accurate evaluation of wall motion abnormalities using steady-state free precession cine imaging. It also determines the presence of myocardial edema using T2-weighted imaging and the identification of myocardial fibrosis through the late gadolinium enhancement (LGE) sequences.

In order to increase diagnostic performance of CMR, T2-weighted imaging should conveniently be performed early (within 2 weeks of the onset of symptoms), before myocardial edema resolves, being this particularly important in myocarditis and Takotsubo syndrome. The presence of myocardial LGE and its different distribution patterns provide the best CMR diagnostic performance.

Acute Myocardial Infarction

AMI represents 26% of MINOCA. It is recognized by the presence of wall motion abnormalities (hypokinesia, akinesia or dyskinesia), edema, and subendocardial or transmural LGE enhancement in segments related to a coronary artery territory (Fig. 3.1). Often, after the CMR diagnosis of an ischemic-necrotic lesion, a review of the ICA must be performed in search of unrecognized significant lesions or ostial occlusions of small coronary branches. Actually, computed tomography coronary angiography could be helpful in these cases.

Also, in the presence of images highly suspicious of embolic origin, exclusion of embolic sources such as patent foramen ovale, papillary fibroelastoma, and myxoma is required, aside from a possible prothrombotic state.

Acute Myocarditis

Myocarditis represents 27–33% of MINOCA. CMR provides high sensitivity and specificity for the diagnosis of myocarditis. Some patients may show regional (usually inferior/inferolateral) or global wall motion abnormalities, although such systolic dysfunction is not specific to inflammation. In T2-weighted imaging, myocardial edema can be

A. Deviggiano
Department of Cardiovascular Imaging, Diagnostico Maipu, Buenos Aires, Argentina

Cardiac CT and MRI Council of the Argentinian Society of Cardiology, Buenos Aires, Argentina

P. M. Carrascosa (✉)
Departments of CT, MR, and Research, Department of Cardiovascular Imaging, Diagnostico Maipu, Buenos Aires, Argentina

University of Buenos Aires, Buenos Aires, Argentina

Latin American Committee of the Society of Cardiovascular Computed Tomography, Buenos Aires, Argentina
e-mail: patriciacarrascosa@diagnosticomaipu.com.ar

G. A. Rodríguez-Granillo
Department of Cardiovascular Imaging, Department of Research, Diagnostico Maipu, Buenos Aires, Argentina

National Council of Scientific and Technical Investigations (CONICET), Buenos Aires, Argentina

P. M. Carrascosa et al. (eds.), *Clinical Atlas of Cardiac and Aortic CT and MRI*, https://doi.org/10.1007/978-3-030-03682-9_3

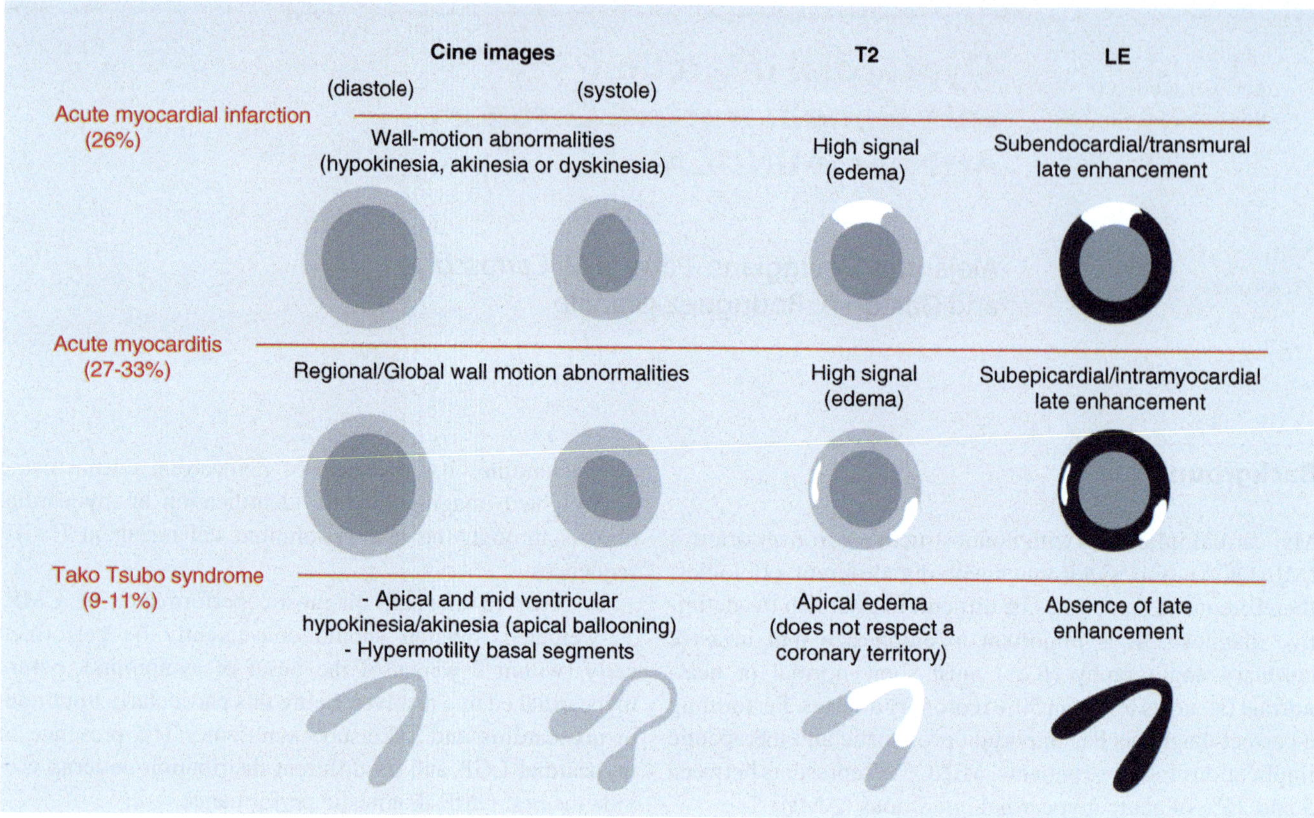

Fig. 3.1 Schematic representation of cardiac magnetic resonance findings among patients with MINOCA

localized or diffuse. Among these patients, LGE usually has two distinctive patterns: a patchy subepicardial/intramural pattern affecting the left ventricular lateral wall or less frequently an intramural (predominantly septal or even global) pattern (Fig. 3.1). As a general rule, the subendocardium is spared in patients with myocarditis, a feature that clearly differentiates this entity from myocardial infarcts.

Takotsubo Cardiomyopathy

Takotsubo cardiomyopathy is characterized by heart failure associated with a marked transient left ventricular dysfunction reversible in a period of days or weeks. It represents 9–11% of MINOCA and affects almost exclusively females who have recently suffered an episode of significant physical or emotional stress. In cine sequences, these patients show hypokinesia or akinesia of the mid- and apical segments (apical ballooning), usually with non-coronary distribution, and with hyperdynamic motion of basal segments. In T2-weighted sequences, transmural and circumferential myocardial edema at the mid- and apical level that does not respect a coronary territory coincides with dysfunctional segments. Another distinctive feature of takotsubo cardiomyopathy is the absence of perfusion defects at rest and lack of myocardial LGE (Fig. 3.1).

Further Reading

Agewall S, Beltrame JF, Reynolds HR, Niessner A, Rosano G, Caforio AL, et al. C working group position paper on myocardial infarction with non-obstructive coronary arteries. Eur Heart J. 2017;38:143–53.

Chopard R, Jehl J, Dutheil J, Genon VD, Seronde MF, Kastler B, et al. Evolution of acute coronary syndrome with normal coronary arteries and normal cardiac magnetic resonance imaging. Arch Cardiovasc Dis. 2011;104:509–17.

Dastidar AG, Rodrigues JC, Ahmed N, Baritussio A, Bucciarelli-Ducci C. The role of cardiac MRI in patients with troponin-positive chest pain and unobstructed coronary arteries. Curr Cardiovasc Imaging Rep. 2015;8:28.

Dastidar AG, Rodrigues JC, Baritussio A, Bucciarelli-Ducci C. MRI in the assessment of ischaemic heart disease. Heart. 2016;102:239–52.

Dastidar AG, Rodrigues JCL, Johnson TW, De Garate E, Singhal P, Baritussio A, et al. Myocardial infarction with nonobstructed coronary arteries: impact of CMR early after presentation. JACC Cardiovasc Imaging. 2017;10(10):1204–6.

Doltra A, Stawowy P, Dietrich T, Schneeweis C, Fleck E, Kelle S. Magnetic resonance imaging of cardiovascular fibrosis and inflammation: from clinical practice to animal studies and back. Biomed Res Int. 2013;2013:676489.

Fernandez-Perez GC, Aguilar-Arjona JA, de la Fuente GT, Samartin M, Ghioldi A, Arias JC, Sanchez-Gonzalez J. Takotsubo cardiomyopathy: assessment with cardiac MRI. AJR Am J Roentgenol. 2010;195:W139–45.

Friedrich MG, Sechtem U, Schulz-Menger J, Holmvang G, Alakija P, Cooper LT, et al. Cardiovascular magnetic resonance in myocarditis: a JACC white paper. J Am Coll Cardiol. 2009;53:1475–87.

Kim RJ, Fieno DS, Parrish TB, Harris K, Chen EL, Simonetti O, et al. Relationship of MRI delayed contrast enhancement to irreversible injury, infarct age, and contractile function. Circulation. 1999;100:1992–2002.

Laraudogoitia Zaldumbide E, Perez-David E, Larena JA, Velasco del Castillo S, Rumoroso Cuevas JR, Onaindia JJ, et al. The value of cardiac magnetic resonance in patients with acute coronary syndrome and normal coronary arteries. Rev Esp Cardiol. 2009;62:976–83.

Niccoli G, Scalone G, Crea F. Acute myocardial infarction with no obstructive coronary atherosclerosis: mechanisms and management. Eur Heart J. 2015;36:475–81.

Tornvall P, Gerbaud E, Behaghel A, Chopard R, Collste O, Laraudogoitia E, et al. Myocarditis or "true" infarction by cardiac magnetic resonance in patients with a clinical diagnosis of myocardial infarction without obstructive coronary disease: a meta-analysis of individual patient data. Atherosclerosis. 2015;241:87–91.

Case 49

Takotsubo Cardiomyopathy

Clinical History

- Fifty-year-old female.
- The patient presented acute chest pain related to an episode of emotional stress and was admitted in the emergency department with ST-segment elevation, elevated cardiac enzyme levels, and no evidence of obstructive coronary lesions at invasive coronary angiography.
- Echocardiogram showed mild left ventricular (LV) systolic dysfunction with anterior mid-ventricular and apical hypokinesia.
- Referred to cardiac magnetic resonance (CMR) to clarify the clinical scenario.

Images

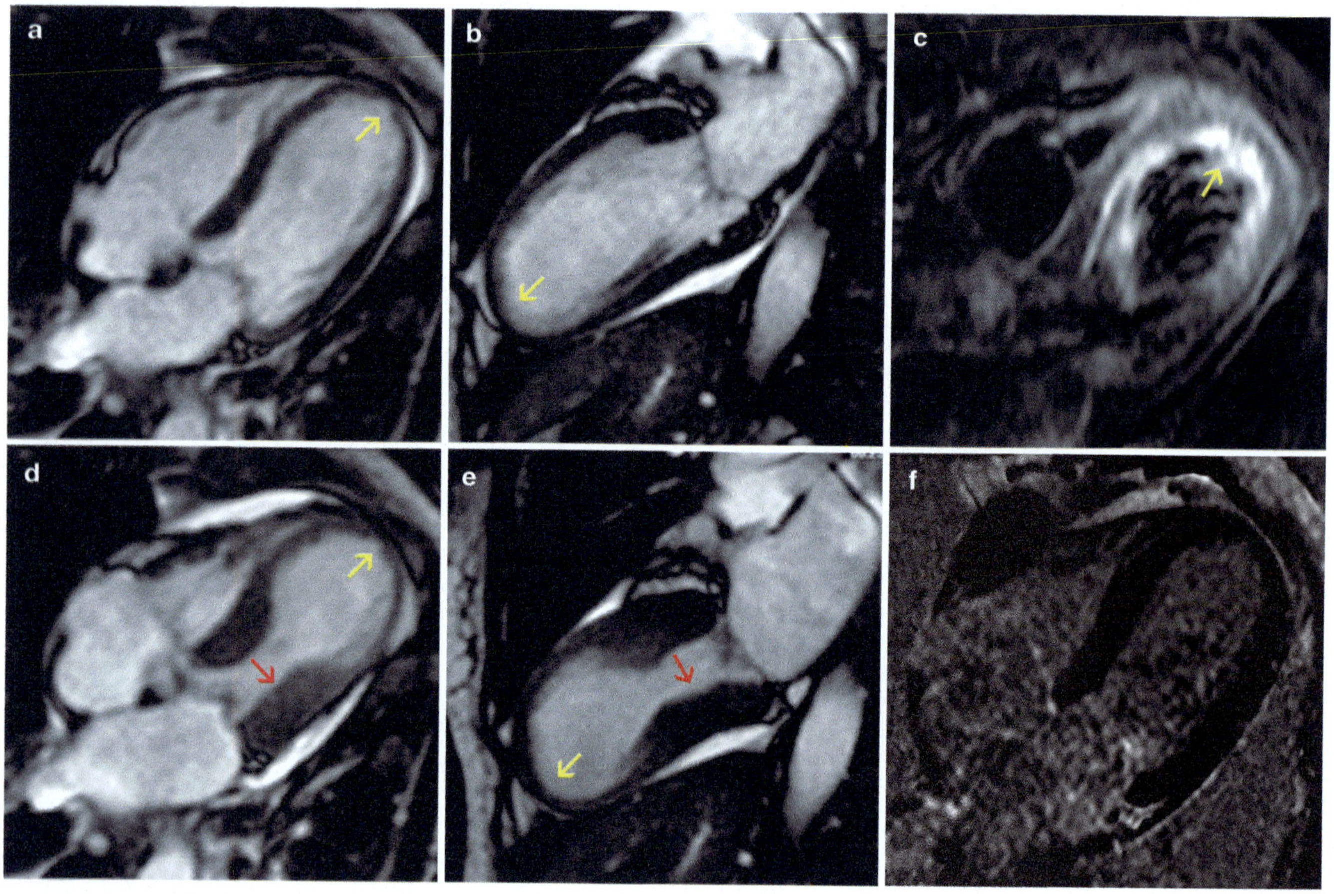

Findings and Interpretation

- Cine four-chamber and two-chamber views at end-diastole (panels A and B) and end-systole (panel D and E), respectively, demonstrating LV apical and mid-ventricular dyskinesia that extends beyond a single coronary artery territory also known as apical ballooning (yellow arrow), with hyperdynamic basal segments (red arrow).
- T2-weigthed image (panel C) with diffuse midventricular and apical LV edema (yellow arrow).
- Inversion recovery image shows no evidence of late gadolinium enhancement (panel F).
- Takotsubo cardiomyopathy is characterized by a transient, reversible ventricular wall motion abnormality that extends beyond a single coronary artery territory and typically presents with end-systolic apical ballooning that resembles its namesake, a Japanese octopus trap.

Further Reading

Stiermaier T, Lange T, Chiribiri A, et al. Left ventricular myocardial deformation in Takotsubo syndrome: a cardiovascular magnetic resonance myocardial feature tracking study. Eur Radiol. 2018. https://doi.org/10.1007/s00330-018-5475-2.

Case 50

Takotsubo Cardiomyopathy

Clinical History

- Sixty-five-year-old female.
- Admitted due to cardiogenic shock, cardiac enzyme elevation, and normal invasive coronary angiography. She did not respond to endovenous inotropic treatment.
- Echocardiogram showed left ventricular (LV) septal hypertrophy with dynamic obstruction of the outflow tract.
- Cardiac magnetic resonance (CMR) was required to discriminate between hypertrophic cardiomyopathy and Takotsubo cardiomyopathy.

Images

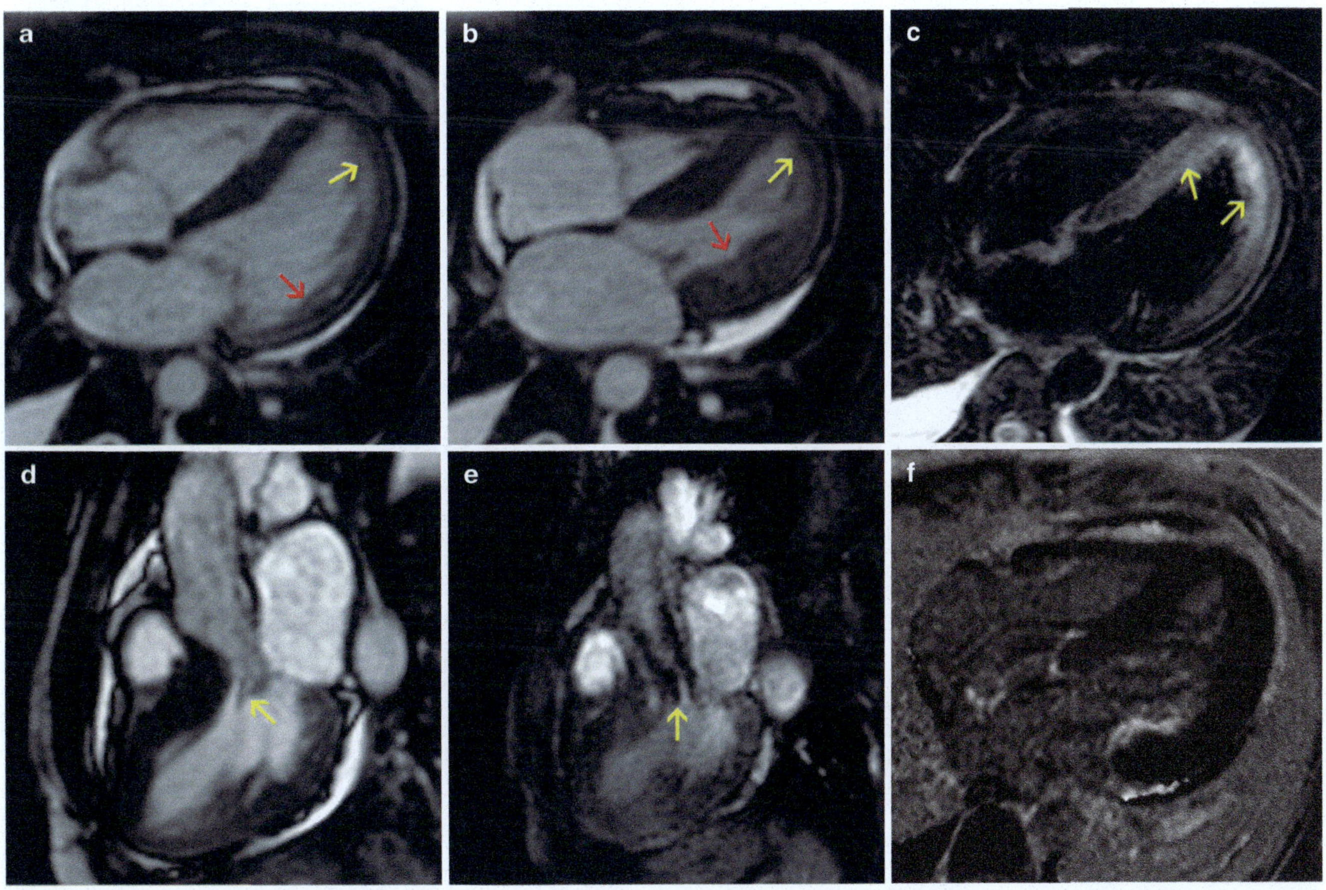

Findings and Interpretation

- Cine-CMR at end-diastole (panel A) and end-systole (panel B) demonstrating LV latero-apical hypokinesia (yellow arrow) with hyperkinesia of basal segments (red arrow).
- T2-weighted image showed diffuse mid and apical LV edema (arrow, panel C).
- Three-chamber views in cine and echo-planar imaging sequences (arrow, panels D and E, respectively) showing sigmoid septum with anterior systolic movement of the anterior leaflet of the mitral valve.
- There was no evidence of myocardial late gadolinium enhancement (panel F).
- Takotsubo cardiomyopathy is a phenomenon that can be triggered as a result of an emotional stress developing apical and mid-ventricular dyskinesia and usually associated with hyperkinetic basal segments, occasionally leading to LV outflow tract obstruction and mitral regurgitation.

Further Reading

Camastra GS, Sbarbati S, Danti M, et al. Cardiac magnetic resonance in patients with acute cardiac injury and unobstructed coronary arteries. World J Radiol. 2017;9:280–6.

Case 51

Myocarditis

Clinical History

- Thirty-five-year-old male.
- No history of cardiovascular disease.
- One month after flu symptoms, he had onset of acute chest dyspnea New York Heart Association functional class II. Four days later he was admitted to the emergency department with non-specific ventricular repolarization abnormalities and cardiac enzyme elevation.
- Transthoracic echocardiogram showed normal left ventricular (LV) function without regional wall motion abnormalities. The patient underwent invasive coronary angiography which showed normal coronary arteries.
- Referred to cardiac magnetic resonance (CMR) to clarify the clinical scenario.

Images

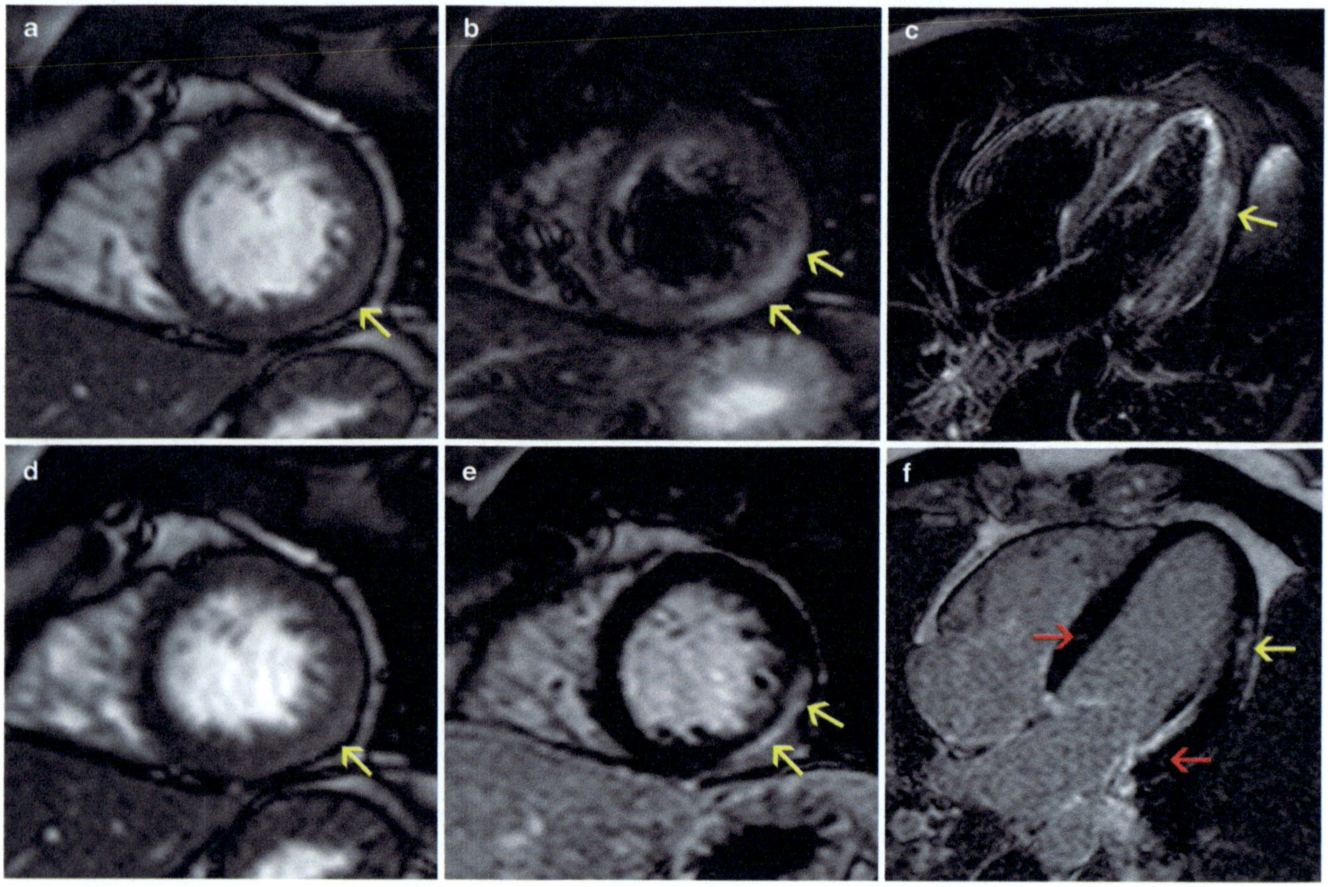

Findings and Interpretation

- Short-axis cine images at end-diastole (panel A) and end-systole (panel D) showed mild inferolateral hypokinetic wall and subepicardial area of increased signal intensity (yellow arrow). The LV ejection fraction was 55%. Short-axis and four-chamber T2-weighted images showed focal subepicardial edema (yellow arrows in panels B and C). Delayed enhancement (DE) images (panels E and F) demonstrated focal subepicardial (yellow arrows) and mid-wall (red arrows) late gadolinium enhancement.
- This case shows that CMR might have a greater impact than transthoracic echocardiogram in confirming the presence of acute myocarditis and evaluating the extent of myocardial involvement. T2-weighted edema imaging is routinely used as a tool for indicating the presence of acute myocardial inflammation. The value of DE imaging enables visualization of myocardial damage in patients with myocarditis after intravenous injection of gadolinium. DE imaging revealed two common patterns of intramural myocardial damage, frequently at the septal level and subepicardial distribution in the free LV lateral wall.

Further Reading

Kindermann I, Barth C, Mahfoud F, Ukena C, Lenski M, Yilmaz A, et al. Update on myocarditis. J Am Coll Cardiol. 2012;59:779–92.

Liu PP, Yan AT. Cardiovascular magnetic resonance for the diagnosis of acute myocarditis: prospects for detecting myocardial inflammation. J Am Coll Cardiol. 2005;45:1823–5.

Case 52

Myocarditis

Clinical History

- Fifty-seven-year-old male.
- Clinical history of smoking, hypertension, and previous myocardial infarction.
- One month after a pulmonary infection, he was admitted to the coronary unit with congestive heart failure and cardiac enzyme elevation that required inotropic drugs and mechanical respiratory assistance.
- Invasive coronary angiography showed a severe lesion in the ostium of the first diagonal and the obtuse marginal branch that did not justify the clinical setting.
- Cardiac magnetic resonance (CMR) was required in order to determine the etiology.

Images

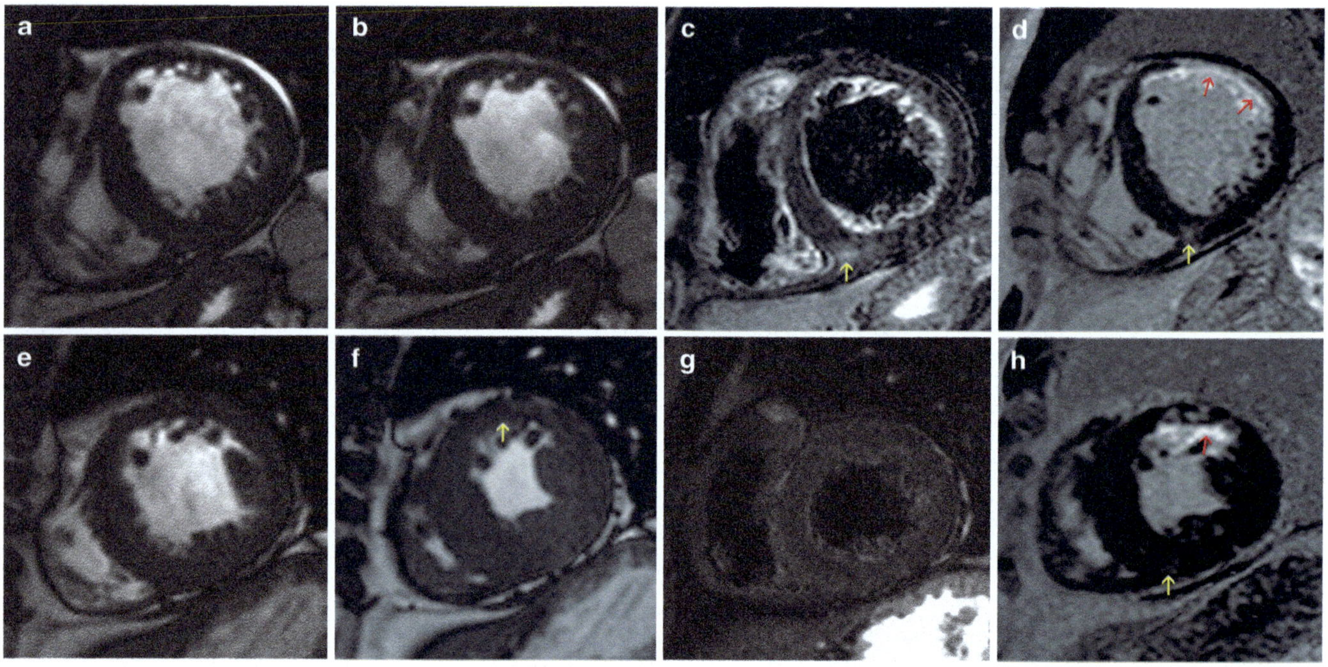

Findings and Interpretation

- Short-axis views (panels A and B). Cine images at end-diastole and end-systole, respectively, show diffuse hypokinetic left ventricular (LV) segments. LV ejection fraction (LVEF) was 23%. T2-weighted image with focal epicardial edema (arrow in panel C). Delayed enhancement images (panel D) showed focal late gadolinium enhancement (LGE, yellow arrow) and subendocardial/transmural LGE related to myocardial infarct (red arrow). Follow-up CMR was performed 4 months later.
- Cine images (panels E and F) at end-diastole and end-systole, respectively, illustrate anterior and lateral hypokinetic LV wall (arrow) and normal contraction of the other segments, with a LVEF of 60%. T2-weighted image (panel G) with no evidence of edema.
- Delayed enhancement images showed a persistent patchy subepicardial area of mild fibrosis (yellow arrow) and subendocardial fibrosis (red arrow panel H).
- Fulminant myocarditis is an inflammatory process that causes acute-onset heart failure. If patients with fulminant myocarditis are aggressively supported in a timely manner, most can have an excellent recovery.

Further Reading

Dastidar AG, Rodrigues JC, Ahmed N, Baritussio A, Bucciarelli-Ducci C. The role of cardiac MRI in patients with troponin-positive chest pain and unobstructed coronary arteries. Curr Cardiovasc Imaging Rep. 2015;8(8):28.

Gupta S, Markham DW, Drazner MH, Mammen PP. Fulminant miocarditis. Nat Clin Pract Cardiovasc Med. 2008;5:693–706.

Case 53

Myocarditis

Clinical History

- Twenty-five-year-old male.
- Admitted with typical chest pain, abnormal ECG findings, and elevated cardiac enzyme levels.
- He underwent invasive coronary angiography, without angiographic evidence of disease.
- Referred for delayed enhancement cardiac magnetic resonance (DE-CMR) for further evaluation.

Images

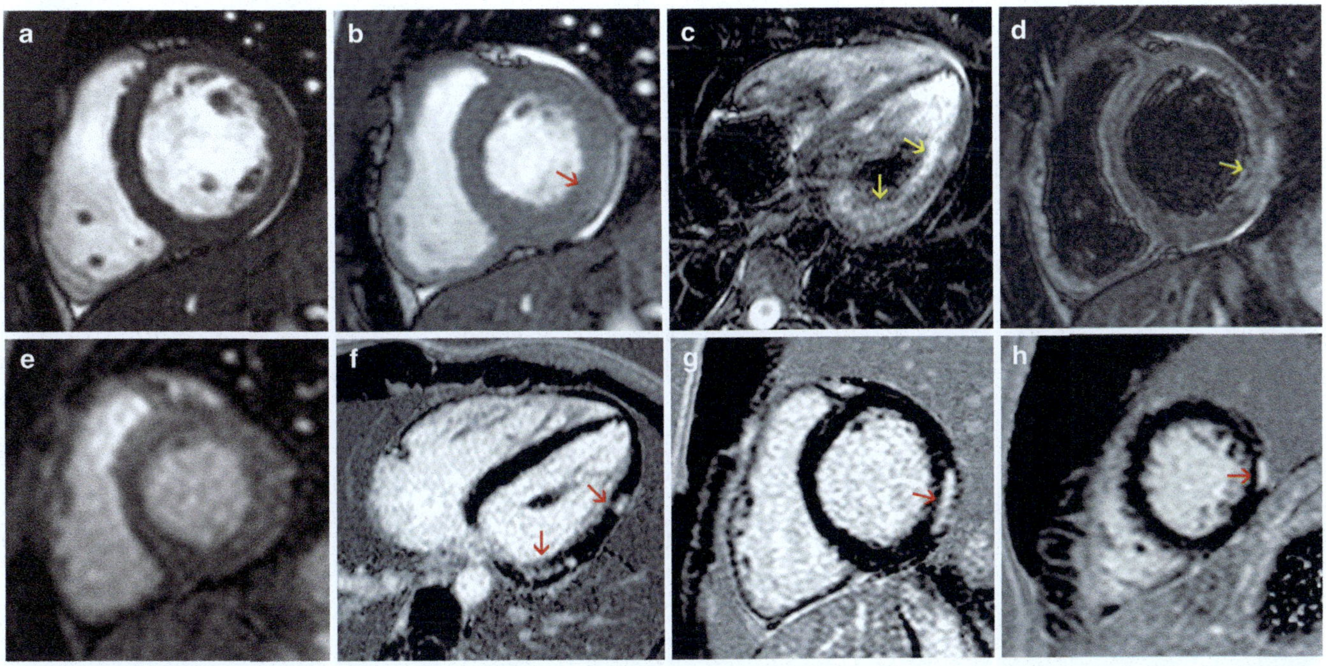

Findings and Interpretation

- Left ventricle (LV) dimensions were in the upper normal level (end-diastolic volume 90 ml/m^2), as was the global LV systolic function (ejection fraction 53%).
- Using basal cine short-axis views (panel A, end-diastolic; panel B, end-systolic), mild hypokinesia of the inferolateral basal wall (red arrow) was detected.
- The presence of patchy areas of intramural/subepicardial edema was reveled using T2-weighted imaging at four-chamber (panel C) and short-axis (panel D) views. Focal areas of increased myocardial signal intensity were detected (yellow arrows).
- Also, minimal and pericardial (panels A and B) effusion was noted.
- First-pass myocardial perfusion imaging (panel E) demonstrated the absence of perfusion defects.
- Inversion recovery images (panels F–H) demonstrated focal intramural and subepicardial areas of late gadolinium enhancement, sparing the endocardium.
- This is a typical case of acute myocarditis and shows the ability of DE-CMR to establish the diagnosis among patients presenting with acute coronary syndrome and nonobstructive coronary arteries.
- The absence of systolic dysfunction (ejection fraction <50%), sustained ventricular arrhythmias, or low cardiac output syndrome indicates a good prognosis among these patients.

Further Reading

Ammirati E, Cipriani M, Moro C, et al. Clinical presentation and outcome in a contemporary cohort of patients with acute myocarditis: the multicenter Lombardy registry. Circulation. 2018;138(11):1088–1099.

Case 54

Slow-Flow Phenomenon/Myocardial Infarction

Clinical History

- Fifty-one-year-old male.
- Coronary risk factors: hypercholesterolemia.
- Episodes of prolonged rest angina, relieved with nitroglycerin, with positive biomarker testing (troponin I) and negative T waves in precordial leads.
- Echocardiography was normal.
- He underwent invasive coronary angiography, revealing no evidence of obstructive lesions but the presence of tortuous vessels and slow phenomenon.
- Referred for delayed enhancement cardiac magnetic resonance (DE-CMR) to rule out acute myocarditis.

Images

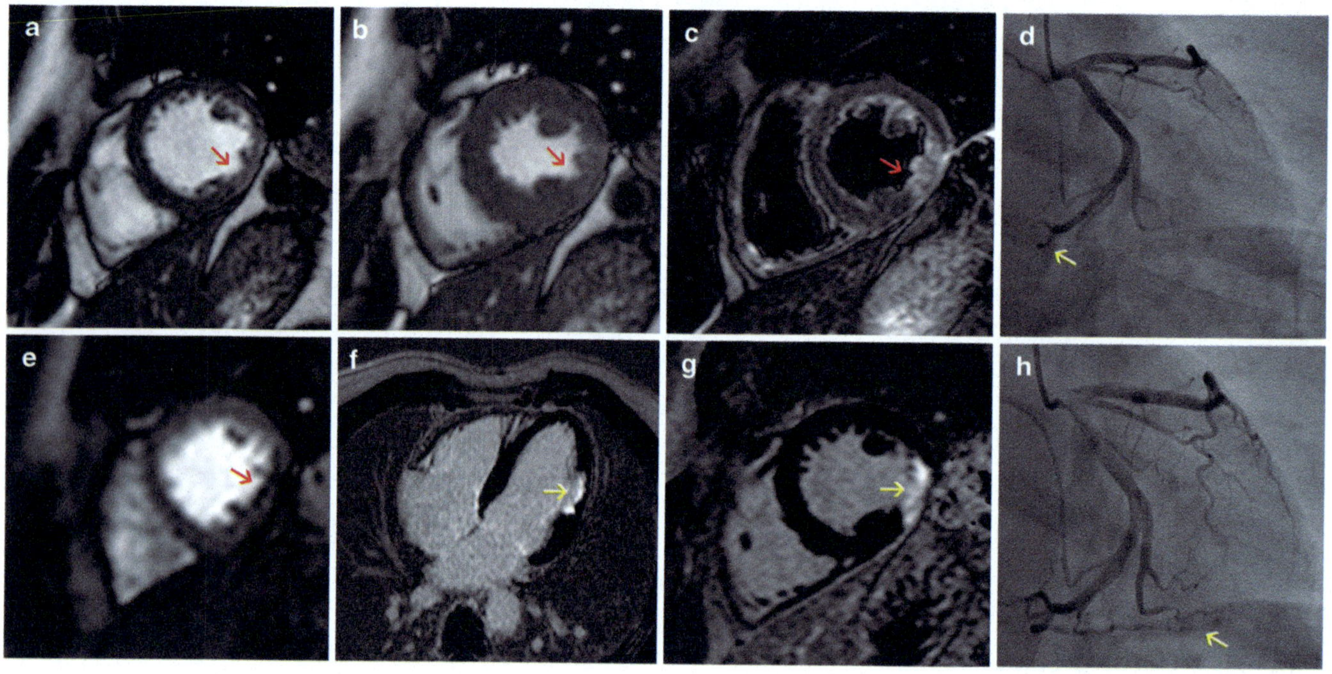

Findings and Interpretation

- Cine short-axis images (diastolic, A; systolic, B) demonstrate akinetic inferior lateral wall motion. Note the increased regional myocardial signal intensity, suggesting myocardial edema (arrows). The left ventricle was of normal size (end-diastolic volume 77 ml/m^2), with mild systolic dysfunction (left ventricular ejection fraction of 49%).
- T2-weighted images show increased regional signal intensity of the aforementioned segment (arrows in panel C), associated to myocardial edema.
- Subendocardial myocardial perfusion defect is demonstrated at first-pass perfusion images (arrow in panel E).
- Inversion recovery images (four-chamber, panel F and short-axis, panel G) demonstrate a small area of predominantly transmural late gadolinium enhancement (arrows in F and G) involving the inferior lateral mid-ventricular wall.
- Invasive coronary angiography measurement of coronary flow showed a slow progression of the dye in the coronary arteries. At 28 frame counts the most distal branch of last obtuse marginal (OM) artery is not visualized (arrow, in panel D). The rate at which the dye reaches to most distal branch of last OM is 39 frame counts (arrow, in panel H). Normal count of left circumflex artery is 22 ± 4.
- Coronary slow-flow phenomenon is an angiographic phenomenon characterized by the slow passage of contrast in the absence of obstructive coronary artery disease. Patients with coronary slow flow phenomenon frequently present with chest pain and ECG changes. A significant proportion present to the emergency department with features of an acute coronary syndrome and may have troponin elevations.

Further Reading

Beltrame JF, Limaye SB, Horowitz JD. The coronary slow flow phenomenon – a new coronary microvascular disorder. Cardiology. 2002;97:197–202.

Gibson CM, Cannon CP, Daley WL, Dodge JJ, Alexander BJ, Marble SJ, et al. TIMI frame count: a quantitative method of assessing coronary artery flow. Circulation. 1996;93:879–88.

Case 55

Myocardial Infarction/Small Vessel Disease

Clinical History

- Fifty-seven-year-old male.
- Coronary risk factors: hypercholesterolemia.
- Presented with acute chest pain with cardiac enzyme elevation and unspecific ECG changes.
- Echocardiography showed normal left ventricular (LV) ejection fraction, without regional wall motion abnormalities.
- He underwent invasive coronary angiography, revealing mild coronary stenosis in proximal left circumflex (LCX) artery.
- The patient was discharged from the emergency department with diagnosis of acute myocarditis.
- Cardiac magnetic resonance (CMR) was performed 1 week later to determine the extent of cardiac involvement.

Images

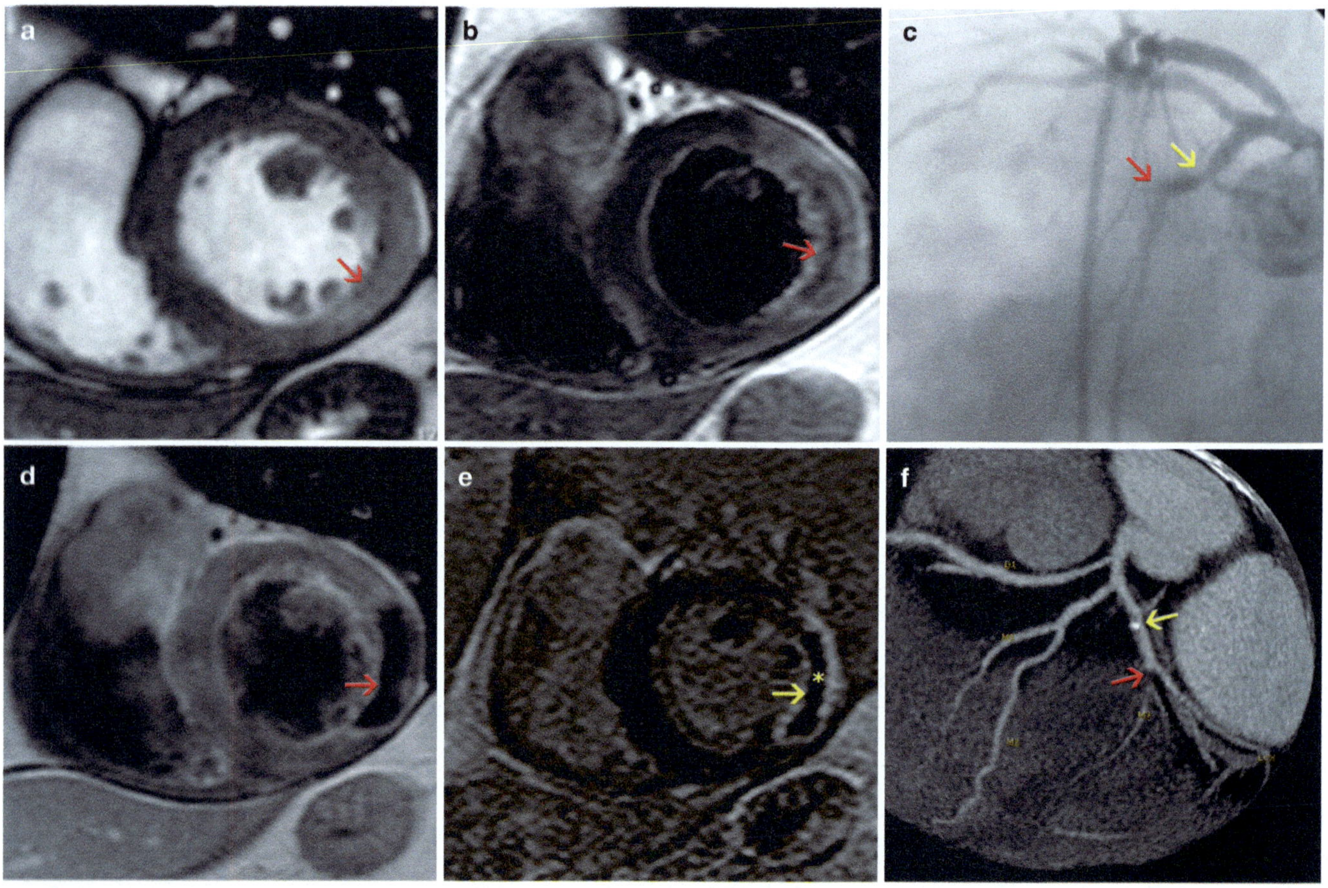

Findings and Interpretation

- Short-axis views (panels A, B, D, and E). Systolic cine-CMR image showing mid-ventricular inferolateral myocardial increased signal intensity coincident with akinetic segment (arrow in panel A).
- T2-weighted image showed myocardial edema in the same region associated with a core of mid-wall decreased signal intensity (arrow, panel B).
- In the early post-contrast T1-weighted image (panel D), transmural inferolateral decreased signal intensity was observed (arrow).
- At delayed enhancement images (panel E), peripheral late gadolinium enhancement (arrow) with a core of decreased signal intensity (asterisk) was identified, suggesting microvascular obstruction related with myocardial infarction (panel E).
- Invasive coronary angiography (panel C) showed mild proximal lesion in LCX artery (yellow arrow) and ostial obtuse marginal occlusion (red arrow). This last finding was not recognized in the initial evaluation.
- In panel F, computed tomography coronary angiography confirmed the obtuse marginal occlusion (red arrow) and mild proximal lesion in LCX artery (yellow arrow).

- The importance of the correct diagnosis of acute myocardial infarction due to coronary artery disease is that it allows a prompt initiation of treatment with aspirin, statins, and beta-blockers that provides a reduction in future cardiovascular events.

Further Reading

Niccoli G, Scalone G, Crea F. Acute myocardial infarction with no obstructive coronary atherosclerosis: mechanisms and management. Eur Heart J. 2015;36:475–81.

Case 56

Myocardial Infarction/Thrombophilia Disorders

Clinical History

- Thirty-six-year-old female.
- History of antiphospholipid syndrome, three consecutive miscarriages and migraine with visual aura.
- At 16 weeks of pregnancy, she had onset of epigastric pain, nausea, vomiting, proteinuria, and abnormal hepatogram.
- She was admitted to the emergency department with persistent pain and fetal death.
- Abdominal and brain computed tomography (CT) and magnetic resonance (MR) imaging showed liver embolic lesions and thrombosis of the sagittal sinus and right iliac vein. Anticoagulation treatment with enoxaparin was started.
- The patient evolved with heart failure with moderate left ventricular (LV) dysfunction and cardiac enzyme elevation. Invasive coronary angiography showed no obstructive lesions.
- A cardiac magnetic resonance (CMR) was performed to rule out myocarditis.

Images

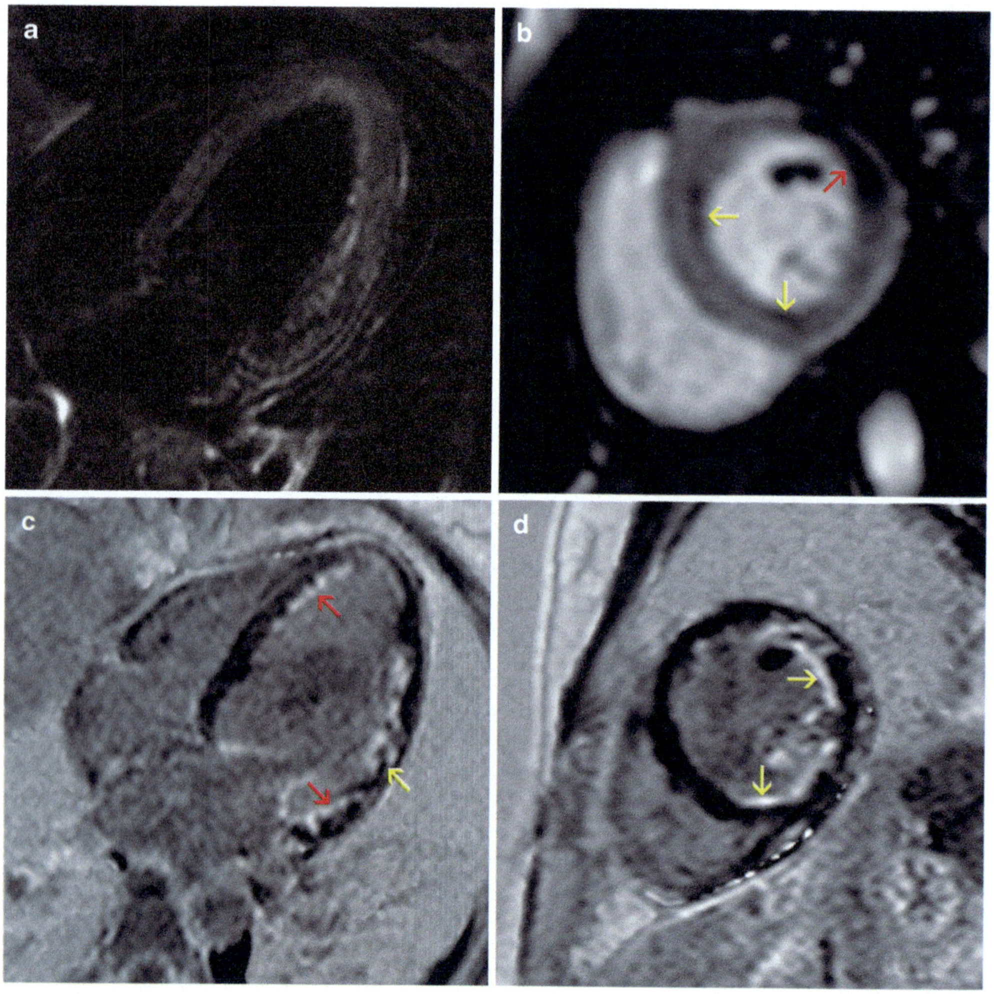

Findings and Interpretation

- Four chamber T2-weighted images showed medial diffuse myocardial edema (panel A).
- Short-axis rest first-pass perfusion image showed subendocardial septal defects and a transmural anterolateral defect (yellow and red arrows, respectively, in panel B).
- Delayed enhancement images in four-chamber (panel C) and short-axis (panel D) views illustrating subendocardial defects in the three coronary artery territories (red arrows) and focal areas of no-reflow pattern (yellow arrow in panel C).

- In the present case, involvement of the microvasculature with necrotic lesions is evident.
- Antiphospholipid syndrome is an autoimmune disease characterized by the presence of antiphospholipid antibodies. It can present with a variety of clinical phenotypes, including vein, artery, and microvasculature thromboses, as well as obstetrical complications.

Further Reading

Arachchillage DRJ, Laffan M. Pathogenesis and management of antiphospholipid syndrome. Br J Haematol. 2017;178:181–95.

Case 57

Myocardial Infarction in a Patient with Cardiac Amyloidosis

Clinical History

- Forty-six-year-old female.
- Coronary risk factors: diabetes and hypertension.
- History of rheumatoid arthritis and previous surgery for thyroid malignancy.
- She was admitted 15 days ago due to decompensated heart failure in the context of acute coronary syndrome (typical chest pain and elevated troponin levels).
- She underwent invasive coronary angiography, with no evidence of obstructive disease.
- Echocardiogram revealed marked concentric left ventricular (LV) hypertrophy with moderate systolic dysfunction, mild mitral regurgitation, moderate left atrium dilatation with restrictive filling pattern and markedly increased filling pressures (E/e´ 20), and pulmonary hypertension (46 mmHg). The septal wall showed a speckled appearance suggestive of amyloid heart disease.
- Referred for delayed enhancement cardiac magnetic resonance (DE-CMR) to define diagnosis.

Images

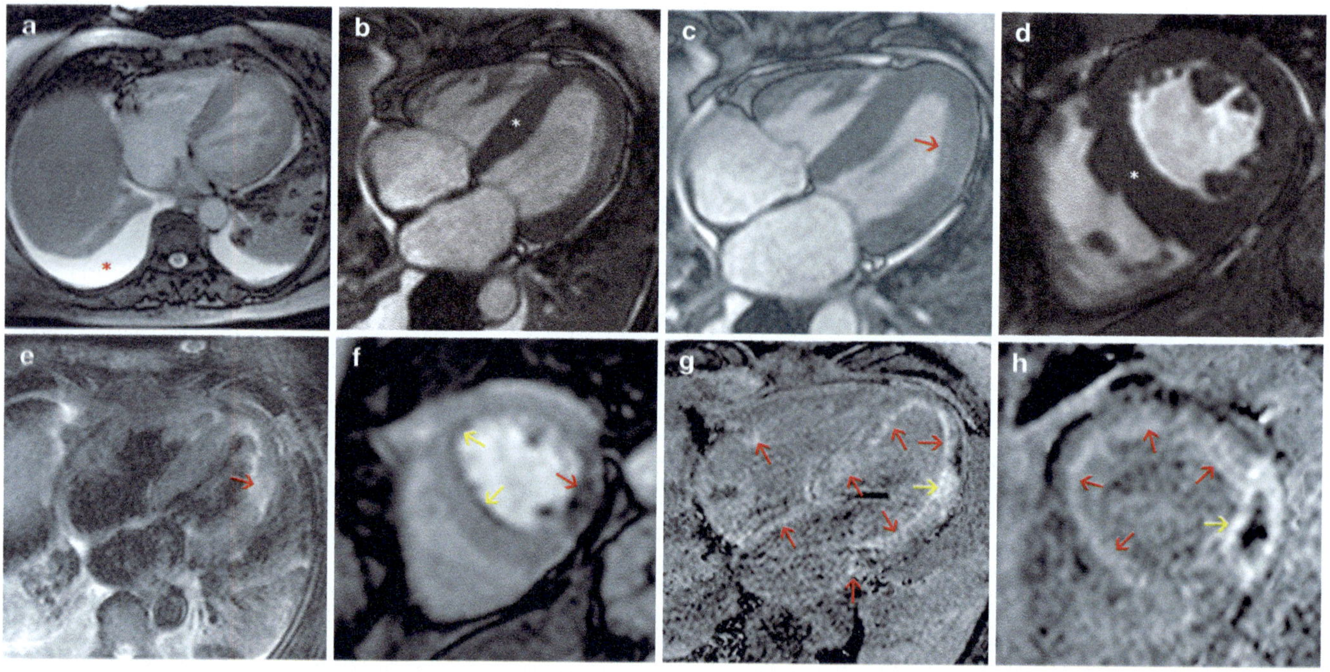

Findings and Interpretation

- LV dimensions were mildly incremented (end-diastolic volume 100 ml/m^2), with mild systolic dysfunction (ejection fraction 44%) and a left ventricular myocardial mass of 208 g.
- An axial scout view revealed mild to moderate pleural effusion (*, panel A).
- Diastolic (panel B) and systolic (panel C) cine four-chamber views demonstrated a thickened LV (*) predominantly involving the interventricular septal wall (17 mm), with a posterior wall thickness of 12 mm.
- Also, there was a mild increase in the right ventricular (RV) free wall thickness. Of note, a small area of myocardial wall hypokinesia was identified at the lateral mid-ventricular segment (arrow in panel C), coincident with mild increment in signal intensity. The left atrium was moderately dilated and there was minimal pericardial effusion.
- Diastolic cine mid-ventricular short-axis view (panel D) showing LV hypertrophy.
- T2-weighted imaging showed a focal transmural area of increased myocardial signal (arrow in panel E), suggesting edema.

- First-pass perfusion imaging (panel F) demonstrated transmural myocardial perfusion defect at the inferolateral wall (red arrow), as well as a minimal global subendocardial perfusion defect (yellow arrows).
- Inversion recovery images (four-chamber, panel G; and short axis, panel H) showed marked nulling of the blood pool and extensive, diffuse, and global late gadolinium enhancement (LGE) affecting multiple cavities including the interventricular septal wall from base to apex, as well as the basal right ventricle, the interatrial septum, and the left atrium (red arrows). Furthermore, a small area of transmural LGE at the inferolateral wall, with a hypointense core, suggestive of microvascular obstruction (yellow arrows).
- This is an atypical presentation of cardiac amyloidosis.
- A number of previous reports have demonstrated that amyloid deposits in the small intramyocardial arteries can lead to microvascular ischemia as well as to myocardial infarction. These patients commonly have normal invasive coronary angiography.
- Vascular involvement by amyloid infiltrates is more common in light-chain amyloidosis (AL) than in transthyretin amyloidosis (ATTR).
- Given patient's demographics (young female), clinical history (chronic inflammatory disease), the type of LV hypertrophy (concentric; septal wall to posterior wall ratio <1.5), and the LGE findings showing lack of basal/apical gradient, this is not likely to be a case of ATTR. Instead, secondary amyloidosis or AL should be excluded.

Further Reading

Boynton SJ, Geske JB, Dispenzieri A, et al. LGE provides incremental prognostic information over serum biomarkers in AL cardiac amyloidosis. J Am Coll Cardiol Imaging. 2016;9(6):680–6.

Cantwell RV, Aviles RJ, Bjornsson J, et al. Cardiac amyloidosis presenting with elevations of cardiac troponin I and angina pectoris. Clin Cardiol. 2002;25:33–7.

Dungu JN, Valencia O, Pinney JH, et al. CMR-based differentiation of AL and ATTR cardiac amyloidosis. JACC Cardiovasc Imaging. 2014;7:133–42.

George A, McClements B. Cardiac amyloidosis presenting as recurrent acute coronary syndrome with unobstructed coronary arteries: case report. Indian Heart J. 2015;67:570–73.

Nonischemic Cardiomyopathy

4

Gastón A. Rodríguez-Granillo, Cesar Nomura, Andrea Maria Giovannini Bercht, and Alejandro Deviggiano

Background: Definition and Classification

The term (nonischemic) cardiomyopathy comprises a heterogenous group of myocardial disorders that are not caused by hemodynamic disturbances such as hypertension, valve disease, obstructive coronary artery disease, or congenital heart disease and involves structural and/or functional myocardial abnormalities.

The European Society of Cardiology Working Group defines cardiomyopathies according to cardiac phenotype, as follows: (1) hypertrophic cardiomyopathy (HCM); (2) dilated cardiomyopathy (DCM); (3) arrhythmogenic right ventricular cardiomyopathy (ARVC); (4) restrictive cardiomyopathy (RCM); and (5) unclassified (mainly left ventricular non-compaction and Takotsubo cardiomyopathy). Furthermore, each one of the above will be discriminated between familial and non-familial and by the disease subtype and/or gene involved (or idiopathic). This classification is summarized in Table 4.1.

Cardiac magnetic resonance (CMR) has an important role in the diagnosis, classification, and risk stratification of patients with suspected or established cardiomyopathies and lacks the acoustic window limitations that can be observed with echocardiography in a number of patients. In particular, both the presence and extension of late gadolinium enhancement (LGE) are independent predictors of ventricular arrhythmia, systolic dysfunction, all-cause mortality, and sudden cardiac death. In parallel, cardiac computed tomography with late iodine enhancement offers an alternative to CMR among patients unsuitable or with contraindications for CMR, such as those with claustrophobia, non-compatible cardiac implants, obese, and end-stage renal failure. The main differences in late enhancement patterns are displayed in Fig. 4.1.

G. A. Rodríguez-Granillo (✉)
Department of Cardiovascular Imaging, Department of Research, Diagnostico Maipu, Buenos Aires, Argentina

National Council of Scientific and Technical Investigations (CONICET), Buenos Aires, Argentina

C. Nomura · A. M. Giovannini Bercht
Cardiovascular Magnetic Resonance and Computed Tomography Department, Heart Institute (InCor), University of Sao Paulo Medical School, Sao Paulo, Brazil

A. Deviggiano
Department of Cardiovascular Imaging, Diagnostico Maipu, Buenos Aires, Argentina

Cardiac CT and MRI Council of the Argentinian Society of Cardiology, Buenos Aires, Argentina

General Characteristics of the Main Groups

Dilated Cardiomyopathy (DCM)

Background Approximately half of patients have unknown etiology and 25% have affected family members. Peripartum cardiomyopathy is a form of DCM of unknown etiology (yet reported to be associated with a history of gestational hypertension, myocarditis, and non-compaction), presenting within the last month of pregnancy and the first 5 months from delivery. DCM is the leading cause of cardiac transplantation. Common complications include arrhythmia, thromboembolic events, and sudden death. Pathohistological findings include interstitial fibrosis. Coronary artery disease should be excluded to establish the diagnosis.

Main Imaging Findings Dilated left ventricle (LV) and rarely right ventricle (RV); mild myocardial wall thinning; global hypokinesia; LV dyssynchrony; myocardial edema (T2-weighted imaging); wall motion abnormalities discordant with the coronary territories; atrial dilatation; mitral and tricuspid regurgitation; incremented mitral-septal distance; intracavitary (apical or left atrial appendage) thrombus, pericardial, and pleural effusion; and mid-wall septal LGE.

P. M. Carrascosa et al. (eds.), *Clinical Atlas of Cardiac and Aortic CT and MRI*, https://doi.org/10.1007/978-3-030-03682-9_4

Table 4.1 Classification of most frequent cardiomyopathy subtypes

	Hypertrophic	Dilated	ARVC	Restrictive	Unclassified
Familial	HCM Unknown gene Sarcomeric mutations	Idiopathic	Unknown gene	Unknown gene	Left ventricular non-compaction Unknown gene Specific mutation
		Sarcomeric or cytoskeletal mutations	Disc protein mutations	Sarcomeric mutations	
		Muscular dystrophies (Duschenne, Becker)		Familial amyloidosis	
				Hemochromatosis	
				Anderson-Fabry	
				Glycogen storage disease	
	Glycogen storage disease (Pompe, Danon)			Cardiac amyloidosis (mutant-type ATTR)	
	Lysosomal storage disease (Anderson-Fabry)				
	Genetic syndromes (Friedreich's ataxia, Noonan's syndrome)				
	Other (familial amyloid)				
Non-Familial	Cardiac amyloidosis (AL, wild-type ATTR or other)	Myocarditis	Myocarditis?	AL, amyloidosis	Takotsubo cardiomyopathy
		Drugs Anthracyclines Drug abuse		Endomyocardial fibrosis Idiopathic Hypereosinophilic Drugs (serotonine, ergotamine)	
		Alcohol		Radiation	
		Endocrine Thyroid disease Other		Anthracyclines	
		Kawasaki disease		Carcinoid heart disease	
		Tachycardiomyopathy			
		Peripartum			
		Nutritional deficits			

HCM hypertrophic cardiomyopathy, *ARVC* arrhythmogenic right ventricular cardiomyopathy, *AL* light-chain amyloidosis, *ATTR* transthyretin amyloidosis

Hypertrophic Cardiomyopathy (HCM)

Background HCM is the most prevalent genetic cardiomyopathy (1:500 in the general population) and the first cause of sudden cardiac death in young adults. The main histological and structural abnormalities of patients with HCM include LV hypertrophy (LVH, defined as ≥15 mm and ≥13 mm in the case of a first-degree relative with diagnosis of HCM), disordered medial smooth muscle cell hyperplasia, and small intramural coronary artery dysplasia. Asymmetric LVH is the most common form, whereas in the apical form, of better prognosis, the apex has a spade-like shape and there is an inversion of the basal/apical wall thickness gradient. CMR offers advantages over echocardiography in the evaluation of HCM, related to the identification and quantification of myocardial fibrosis (LGE) and to a better diagnostic yield particularly in focal HCM. LGE reveals underlying myocardial fibrosis and arteriolar dysplasia and identifies patients at higher risk of ventricular tachyarrhythmia and sudden cardiac death, particularly those with LGE comprising more than 15% of the left ventricular mass. CMR also enables accurate differential diagnosis and better characterization of patients with positive genotype but negative phenotype (without LVH). Finally, CMR allows accurate discrimination from other causes of LVH (Table 4.2).

Main Imaging Findings LVH; LV outflow obstruction (approximately 50%) associated to systolic anterior motion of the anterior mitral leaflet suctioned into the outflow tract by a Venturi effect; normal or supranormal ejection fraction; dilated left atrium. Supporting findings, of outmost importance in patients with positive genotype (and abnormal ECG) but negative phenotype (without LVH), include ventricular crypts, papillary muscles abnormalities, mitral valve abnormalities (elongation, abnormal insertion), incremented myocardial trabeculation and/or ventricular bundles, and inversion or loss of the normal decreasing basal/apical wall thickness gradient.

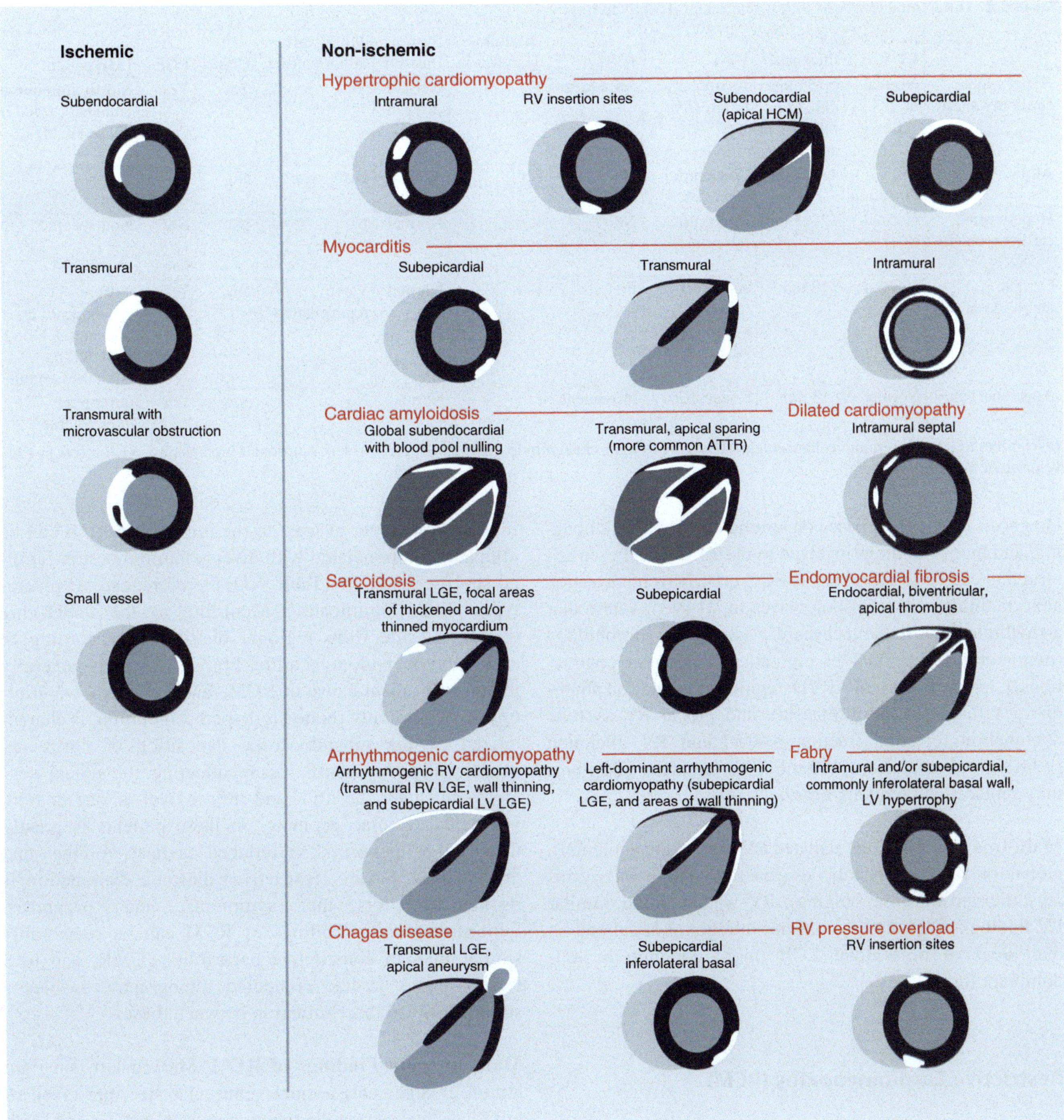

Fig. 4.1 Typical late gadolinium enhancement (LGE) patterns of ischemic and nonischemic cardiomyopathies. *HCM* hypertrophic cardiomyopathy, *LV* left ventricle, *RV* right ventricle, *ATTR* transthyretin cardiac amyloidosis

Arrhythmogenic Right Ventricular Cardiomyopathy (ARVC)

Background Despite some reports suggesting myocarditis as one of the possible underlying mechanisms, ARVC is mainly a genetic disease related to mutations in genes encoding desmosome structural proteins. In certain European regions, ARVC is one of the main causes of sudden cardiac death in young individuals. Histologically, ARVC involves a progressive replacement of RV (and occasionally the LV as well) myocardium with adipose and fibrous tissue, leading to chamber dilatation and wall motion abnormalities. When affecting mostly the LV (left-dominant arrhythmogenic cardiomyopathy), it can resemble the DCM phenotype.

Table 4.2 Differential diagnosis of left ventricular (LV) hypertrophy

	LV size	LV thickness	LVH	RVH	Diastolic dysfunction	Systolic function	Mitral valve abnormalities	Crypts	LGE	LGE pattern
Hypertrophic cardiomyopathy	Normal or ↓	≥15 mm (13–15 in relatives or apical)	Asymmetric, progressive	Infrequent	+	Normal or ↑	Yes	Yes	Yes	Mostly intramural (subendocardial in apical HCM)
Athlete's heart	Mild dilatation	12–15 mm	Concentric, reversible	No	No	Normal	No	No	No	
Hypertensive cardiomyopathy	Normal	12–15 mm	Concentric, reversible	No	+	Normal	No	No	No/ very rare	Non-specific
Cardiac amyloidosis	Normal	>13 mm	Asymmetric (can be symmetric in AL)	Frequent	+++	Normal or ↓	Valve regurgitation	No	Yes	Diffuse subendocardial, transmural, blood pool nulling, interatrial septum
Anderson-Fabry	Normal	>13 mm	Concentric	Infrequent	+	Normal	No	No	Yes	Intramural, inferolateral

LGE refers to late gadolinium enhancement; *AL* refers to light-chain amyloidosis; *LVH* refers to left ventricular hipertrophy; *RVH* refers to right ventricular hipertrophy

Diagnosis of ARVC is based on several clinical, ECG, imaging, and biopsy findings involved in the 2010 Task Force criteria that can be summarized as ECG criteria (repolarization abnormalities and/or Epsilon waves in V1–V3); ventricular arrhythmia [ventricular tachycardia with LBBB morphology (major criteria), >500/24hs premature ventricular contractions)]; family history of ARVD, regional wall motion abnormalities (akinesia or dyskinesia), and global RV systolic dysfunction (ejection fraction ≤40%) and RV dilatation (≥110 ml/m^2 in males, ≥100 ml/m^2 in females); and fibro-fatty replacement (endomyocardial biopsy).

Main Imaging Findings Dilated RV (global or segmental); global or regional systolic dysfunction; focal aneurysms (systolic and diastolic bulging); RV wall thinning; similar LV findings in left-dominant form; intramural or subepicardial areas of myocardial LGE (more common in left-dominant form).

Restrictive Cardiomyopathy (RCM)

Background RCM comprise a heterogeneous group of cardiac disorders (particularly endomyocardial fibrosis, cardiac amyloidosis, and hemochromatosis) that share the presence of right heart failure symptoms, predominantly diastolic dysfunction, and generally preserved systolic function (the latter at least in the initial phases). It can be idiopathic or associated with diverse familial or non-familial specific disorders (Table 4.1); therefore, cardiac phenotypes differ significantly according to the underlying etiology. Aside from regional distribution according to each subtype, endomyocardial fibrosis (EMF) is generally the most frequent cause of RCM. EMF, of unknown etiology and commonly related to hypereosinophilia, is characterized by the subendocardial deposition of fibrin and occasionally thrombotic tissue affecting the apical segments and later the mid- and inflow tract of one or both ventricles. Cardiac geometry in these patients is greatly distorted, with normal or reduced cavitary volumes and dilated atria. Severe (restrictive) diastolic dysfunction is responsible for the symptoms and prognosis. Echocardiographic findings of RCM can be remarkably similar than in constrictive pericarditis. CMR, and to a lesser degree cardiac computed tomography, enables a straightforward discrimination between these.

Main Imaging Findings of RCM Marked left and right atrium enlargement; normal ventricular size; preserved or mildly decreased systolic function; normal pericardium with absence of septal "bounce" or inspiratory flattening observed in constrictive pericarditis; apex obliteration (LGE/thrombus); increased ventricular wall thickness; mitral and tricuspid regurgitation; pericardial and/or pleural effusion; and vena cava dilatation.

Further Reading

Chan RH, Maron BJ, Olivotto I, et al. Prognostic value of quantitative contrast-enhanced cardiovascular magnetic resonance for the evaluation of sudden death risk in patients with hypertrophic cardiomyopathy. Circulation. 2014;130(6):484–95.

Elliott P, Andersson B, Arbustini E, et al. Classification of the cardiomyopathies: a position statement from the European Society of Cardiology working group on myocardial and pericardial diseases. Eur Heart J. 2008;29:270–6.

Ganesan AN, Gunton J, Nucifora G, et al. Impact of Late Gadolinium Enhancement on mortality, sudden death and major adverse cardiovascular events in ischemic and non-ischemic cardiomyopathy: A systematic review and meta-analysis. Int J Cardiol. 2018;254:230–7.

Marcus FI, McKenna WJ, Sherrill D, et al. Diagnosis of arrhythmogenic right ventricular cardiomyopathy/ dysplasia: proposed modification of the task force criteria. Circulation. 2010;121:1533–41.

Rodriguez-Granillo GA. Delayed enhancement cardiac computed tomography for the assessment of myocardial infarction: from bench to bedside. Cardiovasc Diagn Ther. 2017;7(2):159–70.

Case 58

Dilated Cardiomyopathy

Clinical History

- Thirty-three-year-old male.
- Coronary risk factors: smoking.
- One year ago he was hospitalized due to congestive heart failure and complete left bundle-branch block. He had normal cardiac enzyme levels and absence of obstructive lesions in the invasive coronary angiography, with a left ventricular (LV) ejection fraction of 31% (echocardiography).
- Referred for delayed-enhancement cardiac magnetic resonance (DE-CMR) to evaluate progression of disease and explore the presence and patterns of late gadolinium enhancement (LGE).

Images

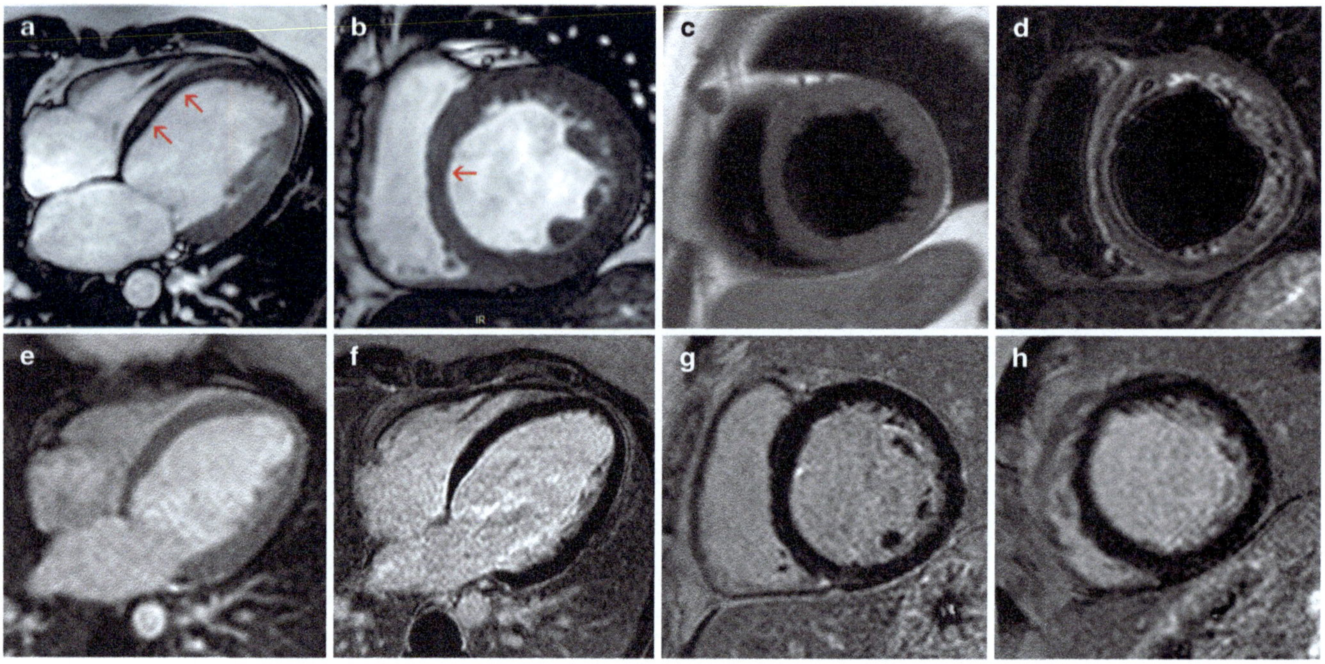

Findings and Interpretation

- Severe LV dilatation (end-diastolic volume 156 ml/m^2), with a LV ejection fraction of 30%.
- Systolic cine images (four-chamber, panel A; short-axis, panel B) demonstrated marked systolic dysfunction, mostly related to septal dyskinesia (red arrows) and diffuse hypokinesia of the remaining segments.
- T1-(panel C) and T2-(panel D) weighted images showed normal myocardial signal intensity, reflecting absence of fat infiltration or edema, respectively.
- First-pass perfusion image (panel E) revealed homogeneous myocardial perfusion.
- Inversion-recovery images (four-chamber, panel F; short-axis, panels G and H) did not show any evidence of LGE.
- The presence of LGE in patients with nonischemic cardiomyopathy, particularly of a mid-wall stria pattern, has been identified as the strongest independent predictor of sudden cardiac death (SCD) or appropriate implantable cardiac defibrillator therapy.
- Furthermore, patients with LGE have increased rates of all-cause mortality, heart failure hospitalization, and SCD/aborted SCD than patients without LGE.

Further Reading

Almehmadi F, Joncas SX, Nevis I, et al. Prevalence of myocardial fibrosis patterns in patients with systolic dysfunction: prognostic significance for the prediction of sudden cardiac arrest or appropriate implantable cardiac defibrillator therapy. Circ Cardiovasc Imaging. 2014;7:593–600.

Kuruvilla S, Adenaw N, Katwal AB, et al. Late gadolinium enhancement on cardiac magnetic resonance predicts adverse cardiovascular outcomes in nonischemic cardiomyopathy: a systematic review and meta-analysis. Circ Cardiovasc Imaging. 2014;7:250–8.

Case 59

Dilated Cardiomyopathy

Clinical History

- Thirty-year-old male.
- Coronary risk factors: hypercholesterolemia.
- He has a recent diagnosis of dilated cardiomyopathy. Echocardiography demonstrated severe left ventricular dilatation and dysfunction and elevated systolic pulmonary artery pressure (53 mmHg). Holter monitoring revealed an episode of non-sustained ventricular tachycardia.
- He was hospitalized 10 days ago with decompensated heart failure.
- Referred for outpatient delayed-enhancement cardiac magnetic resonance (DE-CMR) to evaluate progression of disease and explore the presence and patterns of late gadolinium enhancement (LGE).

Images

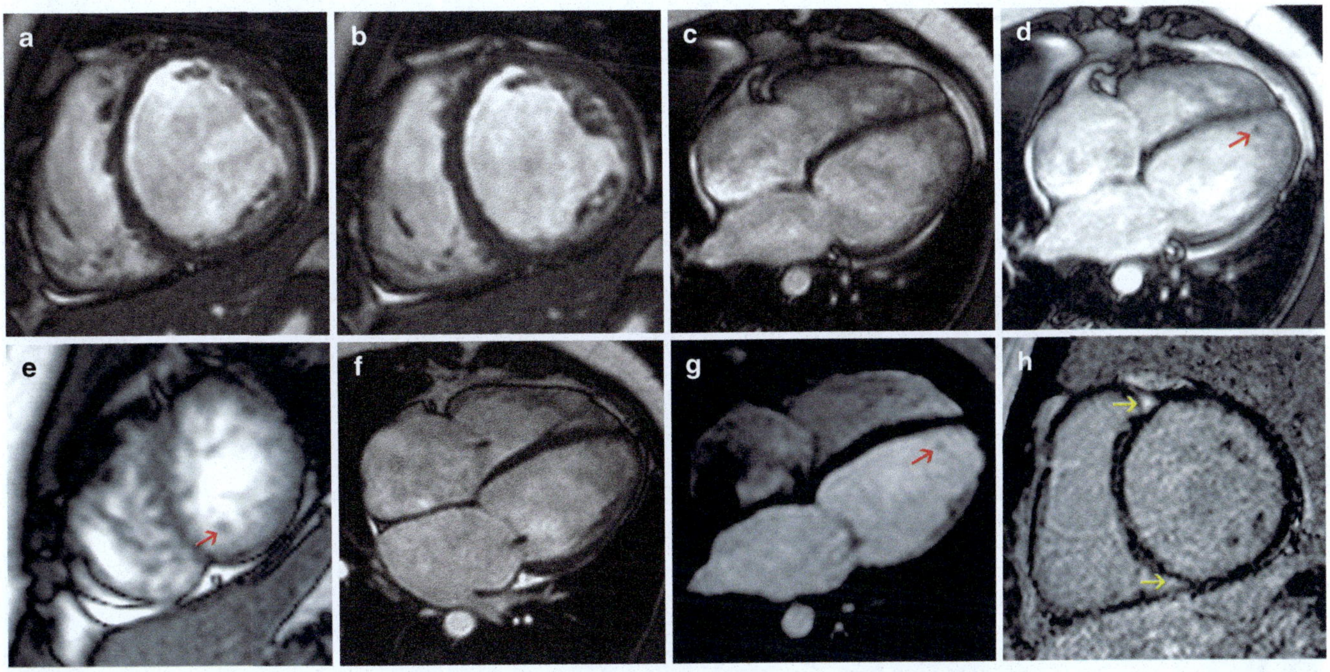

Findings and Interpretation

- Moderate LV dilatation (end-diastolic volume 139 ml/m^2, end-diastolic diameter 69 mm), with severe systolic dysfunction (ejection fraction of 15%). Furthermore, the right ventricle (RV) is dilated (end-diastolic volume 100 ml/m^2) and with moderate systolic dysfunction.
- Diastolic (panel A) and systolic (panel B) short-axis views demonstrate the severe wall motion abnormalities, with akinesia of most segments.
- End-diastolic cine four-chamber view (panel C) shows biventricular increment in myocardial trabeculae related to cardiac remodeling. Notably, unless window modifications and progression to early systolic phase are performed, a very small mobile thrombus adhered to trabeculae [red arrows in panels D, E, and G (first-pass perfusion)] would be missed.
- Moderate mitral and tricuspid regurgitation (panel F) and moderate dilatation of right and left atria are also noted.
- Short-axis inversion-recovery images demonstrate small subepicardial foci of LGE at the insertion sites of the right ventricle (RV) over the interventricular septum (yellow arrows in panel H). Such LGE pattern, possibly attributed to pulmonary hypertension, is not related to an incremental worse prognosis over the aforementioned cardiac findings.
- Severe forms of idiopathic dilated cardiomyopathy such as this have a poor prognosis, related not only to heart failure progression but also to ventricular arrhythmia and thromboembolic events. Given the presence of pulmonary hypertension, related to an increased incidence of death among this population of patients, this case does not seem to be of early onset.

Further Reading

Hirashiki A, Kondo T, Adachi S, et al. Prognostic value of pulmonary hypertension in ambulatory patients with non-ischemic dilated cardiomyopathy. Circ J. 2014;78:1245–53.

Swift AJ, Rajaram S, Capener D, et al. LGE Patterns in Pulmonary Hypertension Do Not Impact Overall Mortality. JACC Cardiovasc Imaging. 2014;7:1209–17.

Case 60

Peripartum Cardiomyopathy

Clinical History

- Thirty-five-year-old female.
- Presented to urgent care clinic 1 week after giving birth, reporting dyspnea and fatigue that had lasted 3 days.
- Medical history included obesity, but the patient was in good health until the recent hospitalization.
- Referred to cardiac magnetic resonance (CMR) for further assessment.

Images

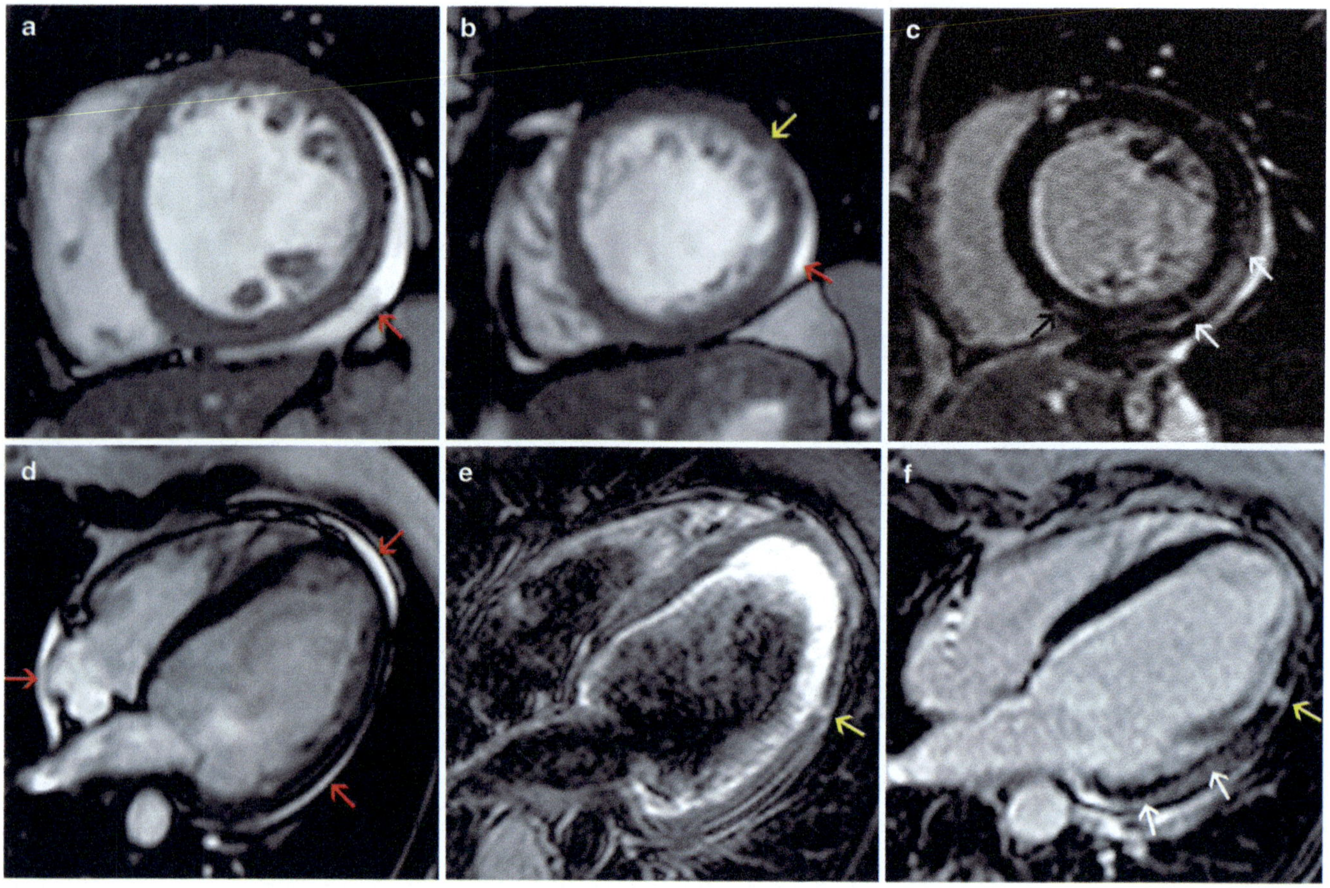

Findings and Interpretation

- Short-axis views (panel A and B) and four-chamber (panels D) cine images at end diastole showed left ventricular (LV) dilatation with mild pericardial effusion (red arrow). She had increased ventricular volumes and global hypokinesia with a severe systolic dysfunction (LV ejection fraction of 22%). There was a small myocardial ventricular crypt at LV lateral wall (yellow arrow in panel B).
- T2-weighted image with no evidence of edema (panel E). Lateral myocardial crypt mimics focal transmural edema (yellow arrow).
- Delayed-enhancement images (panels C and F) showed subepicardial late gadolinium enhancement (LGE) in basal and medial LV lateral wall (white arrow) and medial inferoseptal intramyocardial LGE (black arrow panel C) segment. Lateral myocardial crypt mimics focal transmural LGE (yellow arrow panel F).
- Peripartum cardiomyopathy is a potentially life-threatening pregnancy-associated disease that typically arises in the peripartum period and is marked by LV dysfunction and heart failure. Usually, patients with recovery of LV systolic function within the first 6 months have good prognosis.

Further Reading

Johnson-Coyle L, Jensen L, Sobey A. Peripartum cardiomyopathy: review and practice guidelines. Am J Crit Care. 2012;21:89–98.

Case 61

Hypertrophic Cardiomyopathy

Clinical History

- Forty-eight-year-old male.
- Coronary risk factors: none.
- He has high suspicion of hypertrophic cardiomyopathy (HCM), with deep negative T waves (V4–V6) and echocardiogram showing inconclusive findings including mild hypertrophy and hypokinetic apical segments, with normal diastolic function.
- Referred for delayed-enhancement cardiac magnetic resonance (DE-CMR) for further characterization and to confirm diagnosis.

Images

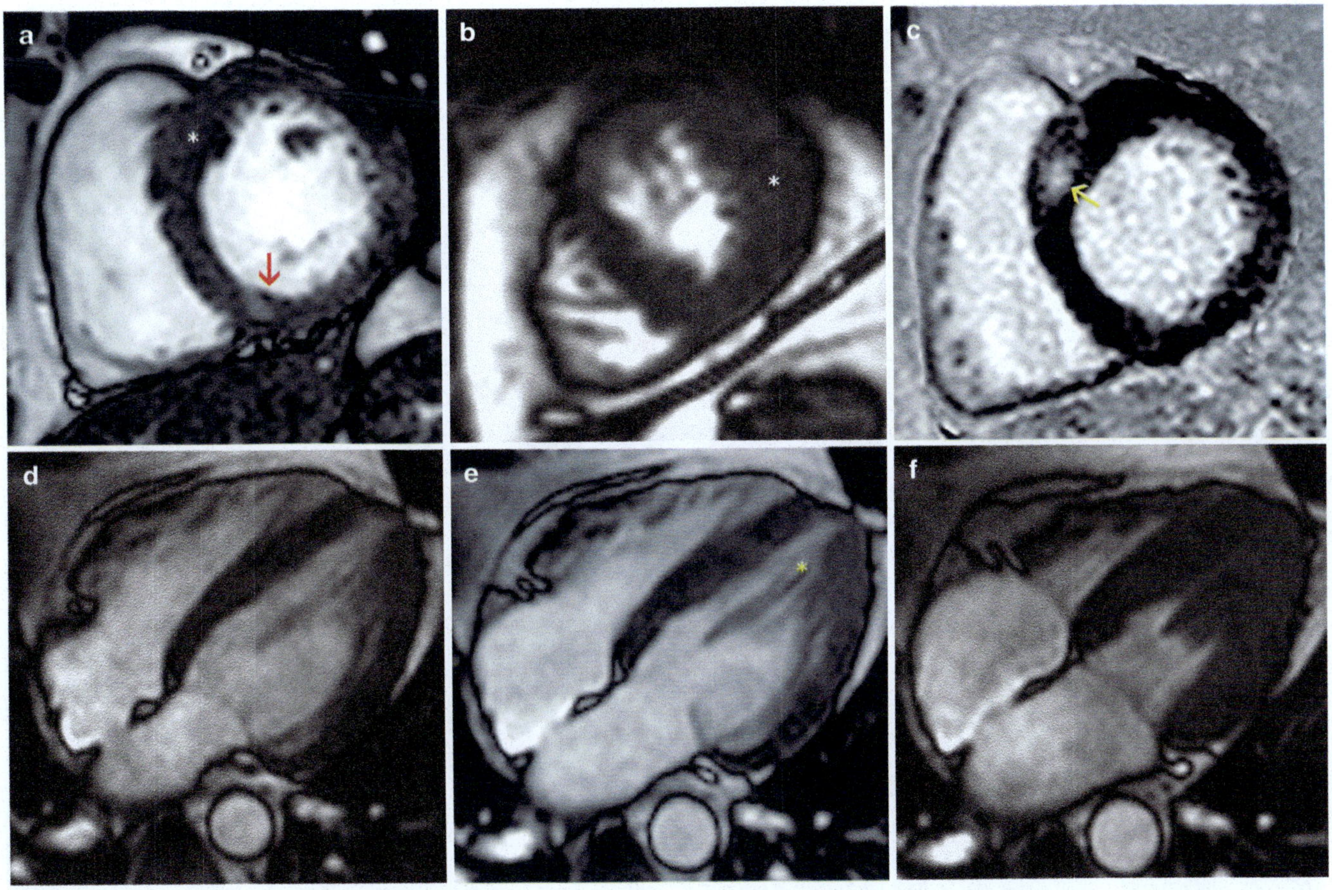

Findings and Interpretation

- Maximal septal wall thickness is 15.1 mm (*, in panel A). Notably, the apical lateral segment has a wall thickness of 13.4 mm (*, in panel B), and there is absence of the physiological basal/apical thickness gradient (four-chamber views in end diastole, proto-systole, and end systole, panels D–F, respectively).
- Furthermore, the presence of apical displacement of the papillary muscle (*, in panel E), a left ventricular crypt at the inferoseptal wall (arrow, in panel A), and mild left atrial enlargement (panel F) reinforce the diagnosis.
- Focal intramural late gadolinium enhancement at the anteroseptal basal wall reveals mild myocardial fibrosis (yellow arrow, panel C).
- This case highlights the great ability of CMR to characterize patients with HCM, especially those with mild phenotypic expression at echocardiography.

Further Reading

Cavalcante JL, Barboza JS, Lever HM. Diversity of mitral valve abnormalities in obstructive hypertrophic cardiomyopathy. Prog Cardiovasc Dis. 2012;54:517–22.

Maron MS, Olivotto I, Harrigan C, et al. Mitral valve abnormalities identified by cardiovascular magnetic resonance represent a primary phenotypic expression of hypertrophic cardiomyopathy. Circulation. 2011;124:40–7.

Case 62

Hypertrophic Cardiomyopathy

Clinical History

- Fifty-six-year-old male.
- Coronary risk factors: hypertension, former smoking.
- He has a 6-month history of palpitations. Holter monitoring revealed frequent monofocal premature ventricular beats.
- Doppler echocardiography reported mild septal hypertrophy (12 mm), papillary muscle hypertrophy, mild diastolic dysfunction (E/e 12) with left atrium dilatation, and the presence of mid-ventricular gradient (70 mmHg) with provocation maneuver (Valsalva).
- Referred for delayed-enhancement cardiac magnetic resonance (DE-CMR) for further characterization and to rule out the presence of myocardial fibrosis.

Images

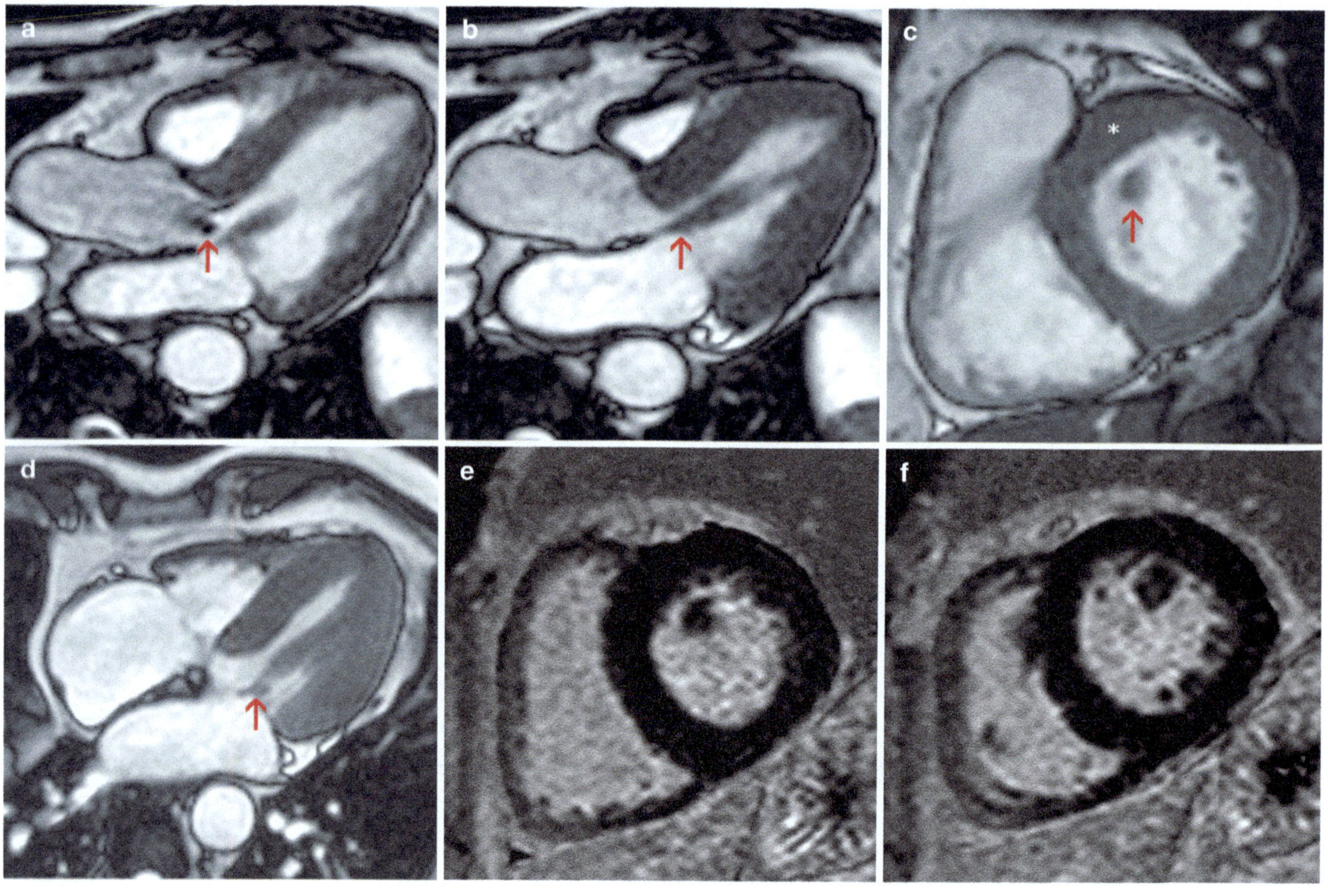

Findings and Interpretation

- Normal left ventricular size (end-diastolic volume 63 ml/m^2), with hyperdynamic systolic function (left ventricular ejection fraction of 75%).
- Cine images (panels A–D) demonstrate mild septal wall hypertrophy (13.1 mm, * in panel C). Of note, the anterior papillary muscle has an ectopic implant directly (without tendinae chord mediation) over the septal mitral annulus and anterior mitral leaflet (arrows in B–D). Systolic blood flow acceleration (gradient) is identified at the left ventricular outflow tract (arrow in panel A).
- Inversion-recovery images (panels E and F) show absence of late gadolinium enhancement (LGE).
- In patients with hypertrophic cardiomyopathy (HCM), LGE has been associated with myocardial fibrosis and arteriolar dysplasia. HCM patients with LGE, particularly if it involves more than 15% of the left ventricular myocardial mass, are at an increased risk of ventricular tachyarrhythmia, sudden cardiac death, and progression to heart failure. On the contrary, patients with absence of LGE have an excellent prognosis.

- Several abnormalities of the mitral apparatus can be present in patients with HCM, and a number of these can lead to outflow tract obstruction. This is particularly relevant among patients with positive genotype/negative phenotype or in those with mild phenotypic expression of the disease.

Further Reading

Cavalcante JL, Barboza JS, Lever HM. Diversity of mitral valve abnormalities in obstructive hypertrophic cardiomyopathy. Prog Cardiovasc Dis. 2012;54:517–22.

Chan RH, Maron BJ, Olivotto I, et al. Prognostic Value of quantitative contrast-enhanced cardiovascular magnetic resonance for the evaluation of sudden death risk in patients with hypertrophic cardiomyopathy. Circulation. 2014;130:484–95.

Maron MS, Olivotto I, Harrigan C, et al. Mitral valve abnormalities identified by cardiovascular magnetic resonance represent a primary phenotypic expression of hypertrophic cardiomyopathy. Circulation. 2011;124:40–7.

Weng Z, Yao J, Chan RH, et al. Prognostic Value of LGE-CMR in HCM. JACC Cardiovasc Imaging. 2016;9:1392–402.

Case 63

Hypertrophic Cardiomyopathy

Clinical History

- Fifty-year-old female.
- Coronary risk factors: none.
- He has a history of palpitations (premature ventricular beats); pathological Q waves in DII, DIII, AvF, and V3–V6 (with positive T waves); and a fragmented QRS complex.
- Echocardiography was normal, with maximum thickness of 10 mm and normal diastolic filling pattern.
- Referred for delayed-enhancement cardiac magnetic resonance (DE-CMR) to rule out arrhythmogenic right ventricular dysplasia (ARVD).

Images

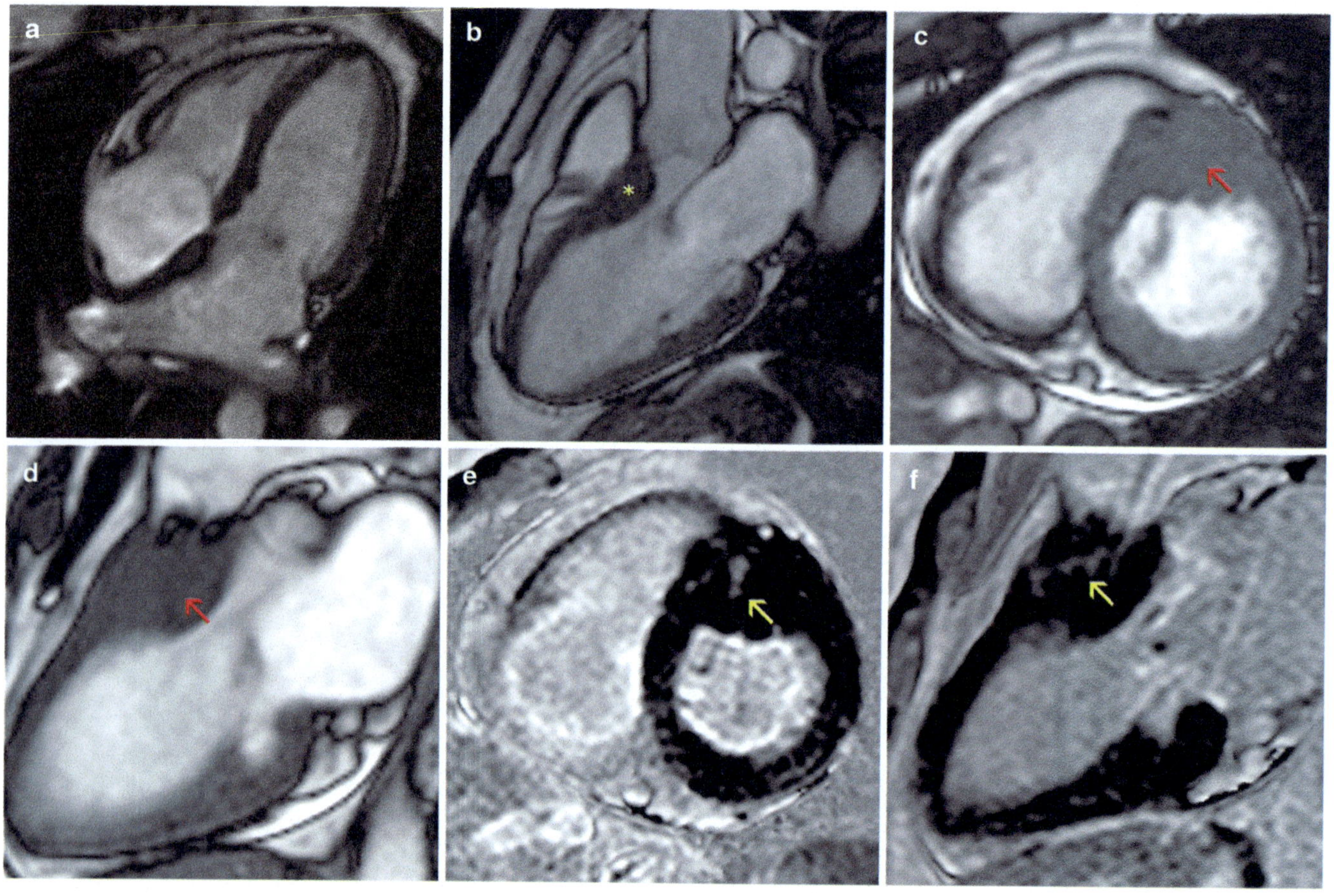

Findings and Interpretation

- Initial assessment using diastolic four-chamber (panel A) and left ventricular outflow tract (panel B) views revealed only a mild hypertrophy of the anterior-septal basal segment (*, in panel B).
- A basal short-axis view demonstrates a marked focal hypertrophy of the basal anterior (25 mm) and the antero-septal basal segments (red arrow in panel C).
- Same findings are detected using a two-chamber view (panel D).
- Inversion-recovery images (panels E and F) show minimal intramural/subepicardial late gadolinium enhancement (LGE).
- This case clearly depicts the benefits of CMR for the evaluation of patients with hypertrophic cardiomyopathy (HCM) as well as those with ventricular arrhythmia compared to the evaluation with echocardiography.
- False-negative echocardiographic findings among patients with HCM involve, among other, focal forms of HCM and apical HCM.

- In particular, focal HCM involving the basal anterior segment can be mistakenly overlooked using echocardiography.
- This case also underscores the importance of ECG findings among these patients.

Further Reading

Moon JC, Fisher NG, McKenna WJ, Pennell DJ. Detection of apical hypertrophic cardiomyopathy by cardiovascular magnetic resonance in patients with non-diagnostic echocardiography. Heart. 2004;90:645–9.

Prasad K, Atherton J, Smith G, McKenna G, Frenneaux M, Nihoyannopoulos P. Echocardiographic pitfalls in the diagnosis of hypertrophic cardiomyopathy. Heart. 1999; 82(Suppl 3):III8–III15.

Case 64

Hypertrophic Cardiomyopathy

Clinical History

- Sixty-year-old male.
- Coronary risk factors: hypertension.
- He has known hypertrophic cardiomyopathy (HCM). Asymptomatic. Holter monitoring with frequent premature ventricular beats.
- Referred for delayed-enhancement cardiac magnetic resonance (DE-CMR) for further characterization and to evaluate the presence and extent of myocardial fibrosis.

Images

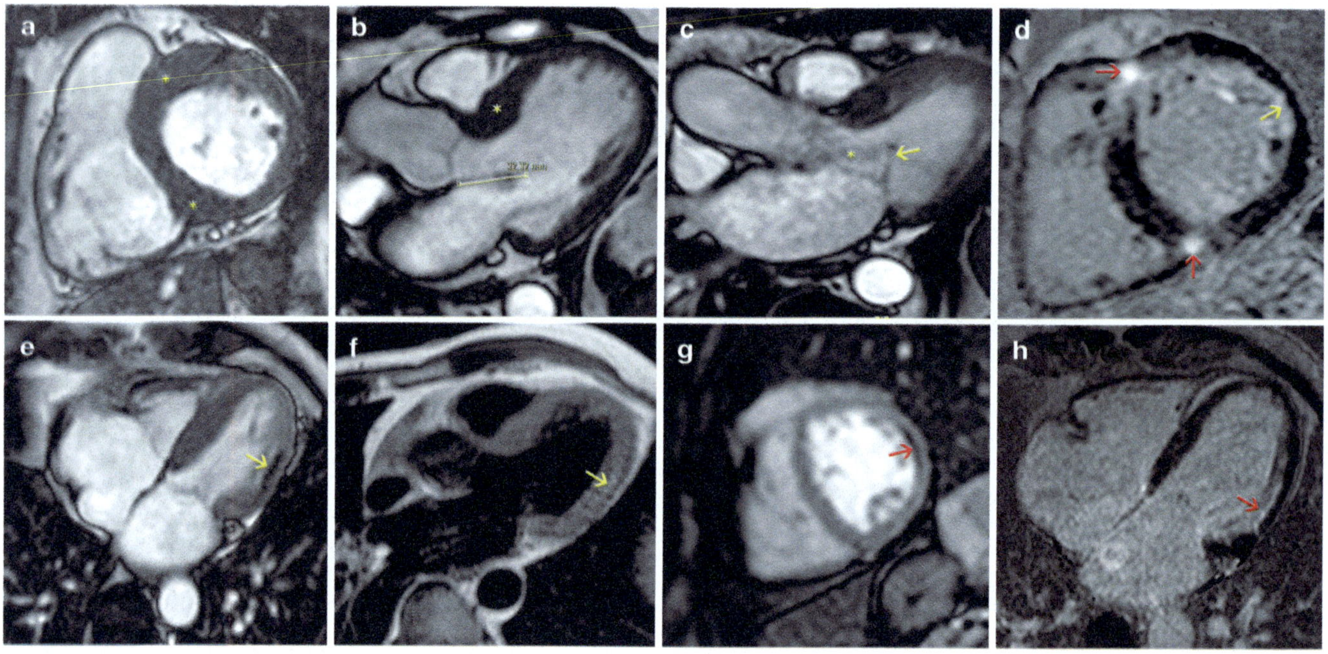

Findings and Interpretation

- Normal left ventricular dimensions, with end-diastolic volume of 69 ml/m^2. Maximal septal wall thickness is 17.5 mm (*, in panels A and B).
- The anterior mitral valve leaflet is elongated (32 mm, panel B) and has anterior systolic motion (yellow arrow in panel C), promoting a mild increment of systolic flow velocity at the left ventricular outflow tract (* in panel C).
- Inversion-recovery images (panel D) show typical late gadolinium enhancement (LGE) at the insertion sites of the right ventricle in the interventricular septum (red arrows in panel D). In addition, a different pattern (subendocardial) of LGE is also observed involving the left circumflex artery territory (yellow arrow).
- Systolic cine images at four-chamber view depict the presence of a small area of hypointense and hypokinetic myocardium at the lateral mid-ventricle (arrow in panel E).
- T1-weighted imaging confirms focal high signal intensity, revealing lipomatous metaplasia (panel F).
- First-pass myocardial perfusion (panel G) shows a subtle subendocardial perfusion defect in the same area. The presence of subendocardial LGE (arrow in panel H) confirms the diagnosis of a small myocardial infarct in the left circumflex territory.
- Patients with HCM and LGE only at the insertion sites of the right ventricle have in general a good prognosis, with very low rates of sudden cardiac death. However, this patient has a silent myocardial infarct, and therefore prognosis might be more related to this finding.

Further Reading

Bravo PE, et al. Late gadolinium enhancement confined to the right ventricular insertion points in hypertrophic cardiomyopathy: an intermediate stage phenotype? Eur Heart J Cardiovasc Imaging. 2016;17:293–300.

Chan RH, Maron B, et al. Significance of Late Gadolinium Enhancement at Right Ventricular Attachment to Ventricular Septum in Patients With Hypertrophic Cardiomyopathy. Am J Cardiol. 2015;116:436–41.

Qureshi WT, Zhang ZM, Chang PP, et al. Silent myocardial infarction and long-term risk of heart failure: The ARIC study. J Am Coll Cardiol 2018;71:1–8.

Case 65

Hypertrophic Cardiomyopathy

Clinical History

- Sixty-nine-year-old male.
- Coronary risk factors: none.
- Asymptomatic. He has an inconclusive diagnosis of hypertrophic cardiomyopathy (HCM), with maximal septal thickness of 13.2 mm at echocardiography.
- Referred for delayed-enhancement cardiac magnetic resonance (DE-CMR) for further characterization and to evaluate the presence and extent of myocardial fibrosis.

Images

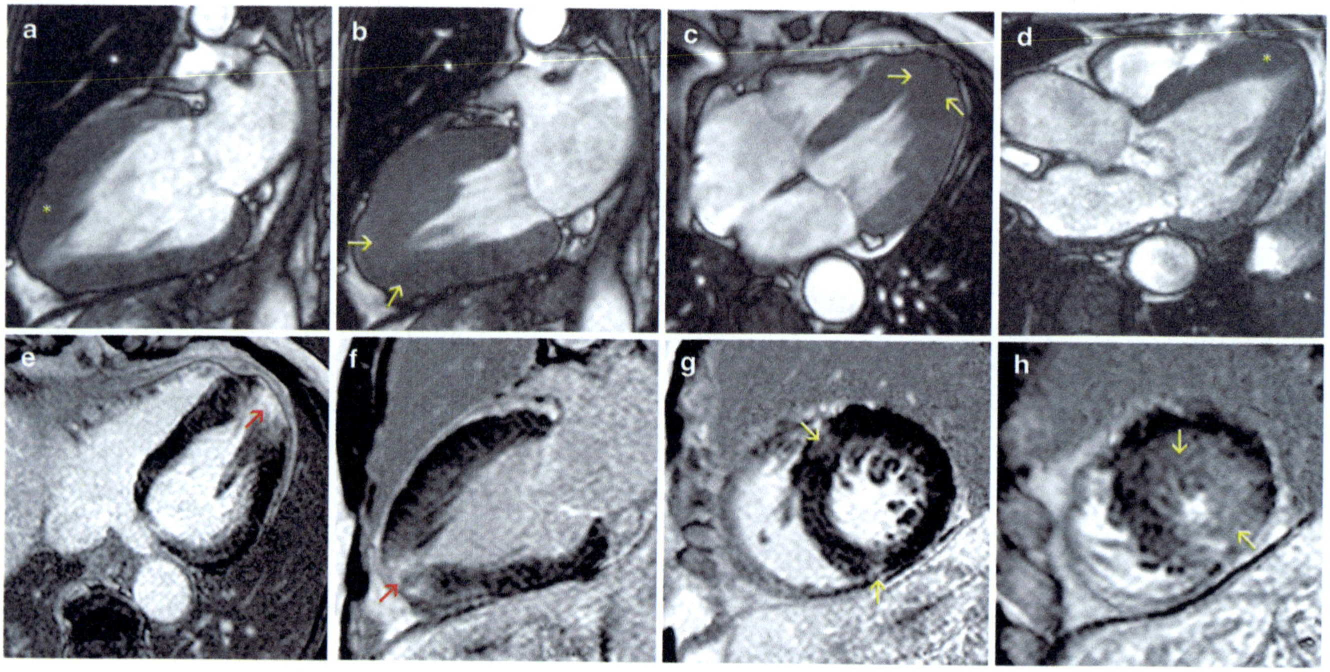

Findings and Interpretation

- Diastolic cine images demonstrate hypertrophy of apical segments (panels A–D), particularly of the anterior apical segment (*, in panels A and D), with systolic collapse of the apical cavity (yellow arrows in panels B and C).
- Note the inversion of the thickness gradient (greater in the apical compared to the basal segments). Maximal apical thickness is 15.8 mm.
- Inversion-recovery images (panels E–H) show late gadolinium enhancement (LGE) at the apical segments which is mostly subendocardial, and focal intramural LGE at the insertion sites of the right ventricle over the interventricular septum (panel G).
- This case depicts the ability of CMR to characterize patients with suspicion of apical MCH.

Further Reading

Flett AS, Maestrini V, Milliken D, et al. Diagnosis of apical hypertrophic cardiomyopathy: T-wave inversion and relative but not absolute apical left ventricular hypertrophy. Int J Cardiol. 2015;183:143–8.

Moon JC, Fisher NG, McKenna WJ, Pennell DJ. Detection of apical hypertrophic cardiomyopathy by cardiovascular magnetic resonance in patients with non-diagnostic echocardiography. Heart. 2004;90:645–9.

Case 66

Hypertrophic Cardiomyopathy

Clinical History

- Thirty-seven-year-old male.
- Coronary risk factors: none.
- He has recent diagnosis of hypertrophic cardiomyopathy (HCM), with typical ECG findings and a demonstration of obstructive HCM at Doppler echocardiography (resting gradient of 90 mmHg, increasing to 120 mmHg with Valsalva maneuver).
- Referred for delayed-enhancement cardiac magnetic resonance (DE-CMR) for further characterization and to evaluate the presence and extent of myocardial fibrosis.

Images

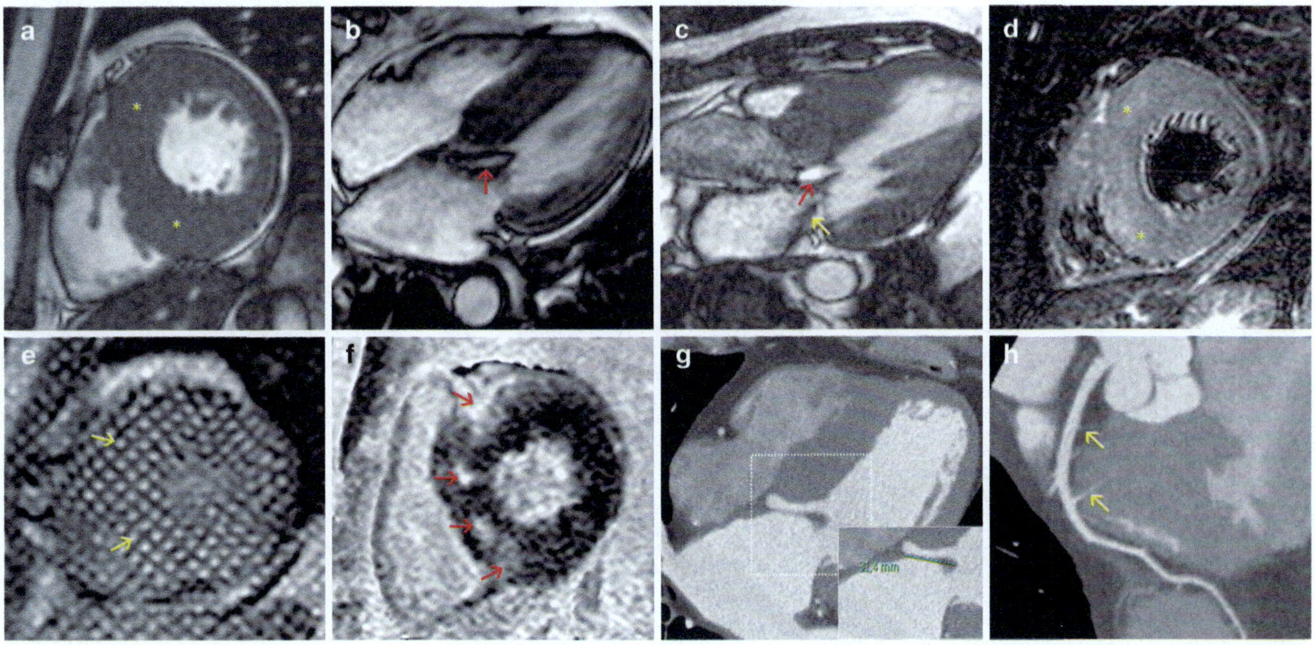

Findings and Interpretation

- Diastolic cine images demonstrate marked asymmetric septal hypertrophy, with maximal septal wall thickness of 26.8 mm (*, in panel A).
- Systolic cine images in four-chamber (panel B) and three-chamber (panel C) views demonstrate resting obstruction of the left ventricular (LV) outflow tract (red arrows). Also, eccentric mitral regurgitation is noted (yellow arrow in panel C).
- At T2-weighted imaging, intramyocardial and subepicardial hyperintense areas (*, in panel D) reflect myocardial edema, whereas myocardial tagging demonstrates significant reduction of systolic septal deformation (arrows, in panel E).
- Inversion-recovery images (panel F) show extensive late gadolinium enhancement (LGE) at the septal wall (arrows).
- The patient underwent computed tomography coronary angiography to evaluate the coronary tree before percutaneous septal ablation procedure (panels G and H). Mid-diastolic prospective ECG-gated acquisition demonstrates marked asymmetric septal hypertrophy, thickened and elongated anterior mitral leaflet, and normal coronary arteries. However, curve multiplanar reconstruction of the left anterior descending artery (panel H) revealed a submillimeter first septal branch and a larger (albeit very small) second septal branch. Therefore, this patient might not be suitable for percutaneous septal ablation.
- Patients with HCM and extensive LGE (particularly if larger than 20% of the LV myocardial mass) are at increased risk of progression to heart failure, ventricular tachyarrhythmia, sudden cardiac death, and all-cause mortality.

Further Reading

Chan RH, Maron BJ, Olivotto I, et al. Prognostic Value of Quantitative Contrast-Enhanced Cardiovascular Magnetic Resonance for the Evaluation of Sudden Death Risk in Patients With Hypertrophic Cardiomyopathy. Circulation. 2014;130:484–95.

Weng Z, Yao J, Chan RH, et al. Prognostic Value of LGE-CMR in HCM: A Meta-Analysis. JACC Cardiovasc Imaging. 2016;9:1392–402.

Case 67

Hypertrophic Cardiomyopathy

Clinical History

- Seventy-nine-year-old male.
- Coronary risk factors: none.
- Asymptomatic. Echocardiography with diagnosis of hypertrophic cardiomyopathy (HCM).
- Referred for delayed-enhancement cardiac magnetic resonance (DE-CMR) to evaluate the presence of myocardial fibrosis.

Images

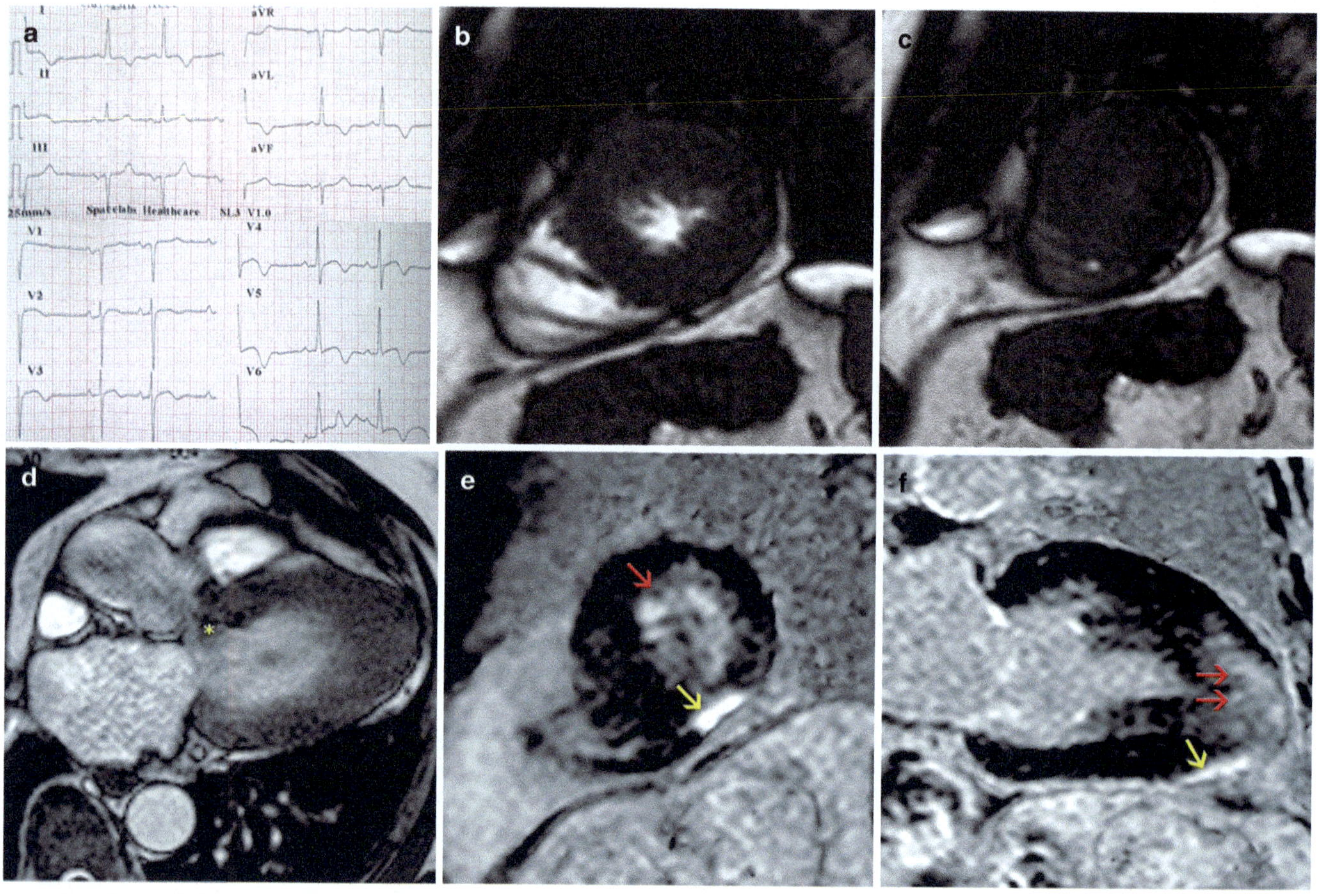

Findings and Interpretation

- Both the ECG (panel A) and left ventricular hypertrophy (panels B–D) have a mainly apical pattern (maximum thickness 17.5 mm, in panel B), with collapse of the apical cavity during systole (panels C and D).
- Anteroseptal wall thickness is 15.4 mm, with mild left ventricular outflow tract obstruction (*, in panel D).
- Inversion-recovery images demonstrate apical late gadolinium enhancement (LGE) with a heterogeneous pattern. Although predominantly subendocardial (red arrows in panels E and F), transmural and subepicardial patterns (yellow arrows) of different intensity levels are identified.
- The presence of heterogeneous LGE pattern is related to different forms of fibrosis. High intensity LGE reflects replacement fibrosis, whereas intermediate signal intensity LGE is related to interstitial fibrosis. Some studies suggest that intermediate LGE is a better predictor of ventricular tachyarrhythmias compared to high intensity LGE.

Further Reading

Appelbaum E, Maron BJ, Adabag S, et al. Intermediate-signal-intensity late gadolinium enhancement predicts ventricular tachyarrhythmias in patients with hypertrophic cardiomyopathy. Circ Cardiovasc Imaging. 2012;5:78–85.

Case 68

Arrhythmogenic Cardiomyopathy

Clinical History

- Twenty-seven-year-old male.
- Coronary risk factors: none.
- He refers occasional palpitations, with premature ventricular beats identified in a routine preoperative ECG.
- Holter monitoring (24 h) revealed high-density premature ventricular contractions (>17,000), with duplets, triplets, bigeminy, trigeminy, and runs of non-sustained ventricular tachycardia.
- Echocardiography showed dilated cardiac chambers, with moderate left ventricle (LV) systolic dysfunction and right ventricle (RV) systolic dysfunction.
- Referred for delayed-enhancement cardiac magnetic resonance (DE-CMR) to define etiology and evaluate the presence of late gadolinium enhancement (LGE).

Images

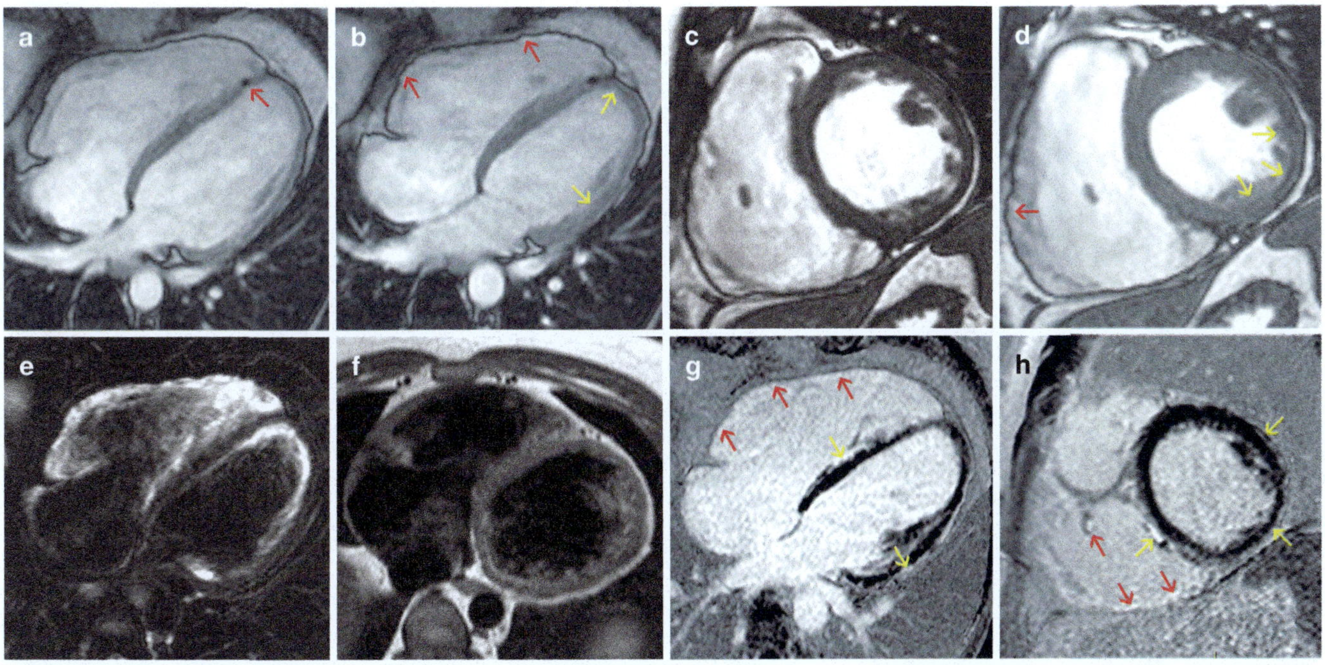

Findings and Interpretation

- Diastolic and systolic four-chamber (panels A and B) and short-axis (panels C and D) cine views show chamber size and systolic function. Severe RV dilatation (end-diastolic volume 210 ml/m^2) and moderate to severe LV dilatation (end-diastolic volume 152 ml/m^2, end-diastolic diameter 69 mm) are present, with severe RV systolic dysfunction (ejection fraction 20%) and moderate LV systolic dysfunction (ejection fraction 35%).
- The RV has a very thin myocardial wall, with focal dyskinetic areas (red arrows in panels B and D) corresponding to microaneurysms.
- Areas of myocardial wall thinning and akinesia are also observed at the LV wall (yellow arrows in panels B and D).
- T2 (panel E)- and T1 (panel F)-weighted images have normal myocardial signal intensity, reflecting absence of edema and fat infiltration, respectively. However, a small hypointense septal area suggestive of fibrous replacement is observed at the four-chamber view (red arrow, panel A).
- Inversion-recovery images (four-chamber, panel G; short-axis, panel H) show extensive LGE involving the RV free and inferior walls (red arrows), as well as patchy subepicardial areas of LGE involving the right aspect of the interventricular septum, and the inferior and lateral segments of the LV.
- Arrhythmogenic right ventricular cardiomyopathy (ARVC), which can also involve the LV (in up to 70% of patients as in this case), is a hereditary disorder with an estimated prevalence of 1:2000 to 1:5000 and is associated with a high risk of ventricular arrhythmias and sudden cardiac death. Mutation of several genes encoding desmosomes has been found in ARVD, leading to fibro-

fatty replacement of the myocardium, RV (and LV in the non-classical form) dilation, and systolic dysfunction. Diagnosis of arrhythmogenic cardiomyopathy is complex and based on several different aspects involved in the 2010 Task Force criteria that can be summarized as ECG criteria (repolarization abnormalities and/or Epsilon waves in V1–V3); ventricular arrhythmia [ventricular tachycardia with left bundle-branch block morphology (major criteria), >500/24hs premature ventricular contractions); family history of ARVD, regional wall motion abnormalities (akinesia or dyskinesia), and global RV systolic dysfunction (ejection fraction ≤40%) or RV dilatation (≥110 ml/m^2 in males, ≥100 ml/m^2 in females); and fibrofatty replacement (particularly in endomyocardial biopsy).

Further Reading

Akdis D, Brunckhorst C, Duru F, et al. Arrhythmogenic cardiomyopathy: electrical and structural phenotypes. Arrhythm Electrophysiol Rev. 2016;5:90–101.

Marcus FI, McKenna WJ, Sherrill D, et al. Diagnosis of arrhythmogenic right ventricular cardiomyopathy/ dysplasia: proposed modification of the task force criteria. Circulation. 2010;121:1533–41.

Case 69

Arrhythmogenic Cardiomyopathy

Clinical History

- Forty-six-year-old female.
- Coronary risk factors: hypercholesterolemia, smoking, family history of coronary artery disease.
- Chronic (3-year) heart failure, originally detected as dyspnea during exercise (hockey).
- Holter monitoring revealed high-density premature ventricular contractions.
- Echocardiography showed a dilated left ventricle (LV), moderate to severe systolic function (LV ejection fraction 35%), and normal right ventricular (RV) morphology and function.
- Referred for delayed-enhancement cardiac magnetic resonance (DE-CMR) to evaluate progression of dilated cardiomyopathy and explore the presence and patterns of late gadolinium enhancement (LGE).

Images

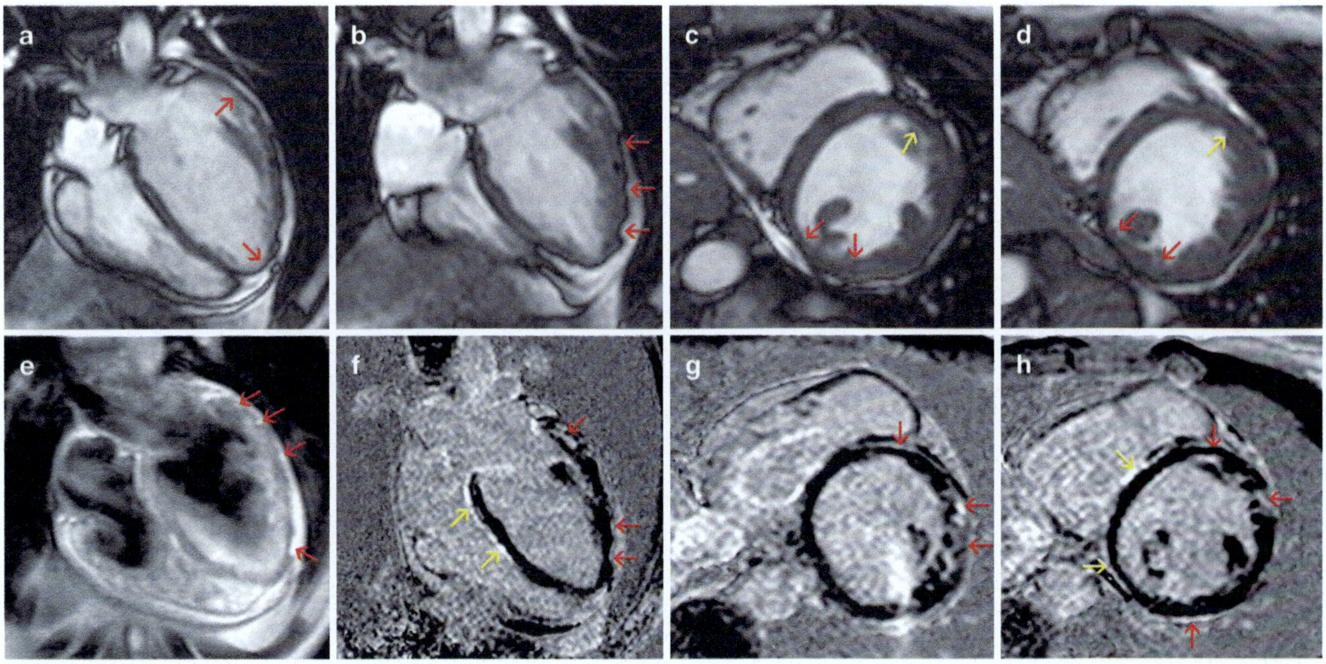

Findings and Interpretation

- Normal RV morphology and systolic function (end-diastolic volume 91 ml/m^2, ejection fraction 57%; panels A–D). Mild-moderate LV dilatation (end-diastolic volume 139 ml/m^2), with a LV ejection fraction of 36% and areas or regional akinesia [inferior wall, red arrows in panels C (diastole) and D (systole); anterior wall, yellow arrows in panels C (diastole) and D (systole)].
- The LV has an irregular shape, with areas of focal myocardial wall thinning (arrows in panel A) and subepicardial fatty infiltration (panel B), confirmed with T1-weighted imaging (panel E).
- Inversion-recovery images (four-chamber, panel F; short-axis, panels G and H) show predominantly subepicardial but also intramyocardial and transmural areas of LGE in multiple segments including the RV aspect of the interventricular septum (yellow arrows in panels F and H).
- Although genetic testing was not available and chronic myocarditis can sometimes share similar clinical presentation and cardiac phenotype, this seems a case of left-dominant arrhythmogenic cardiomyopathy.
- Regardless of the underlying etiology, patients with LGE have increased rates of all-cause mortality, heart failure hospitalization, and sudden cardiac death compared to those without LGE.
- Screening for family mutation carriers or at least CMR imaging in first-degree relatives is strongly suggested.

Further Reading

Kuruvilla S, Adenaw N, Katwal AB, et al. Late gadolinium enhancement on cardiac magnetic resonance predicts adverse cardiovascular outcomes in nonischemic cardiomyopathy: a systematic review and meta-analysis. Circ Cardiovasc Imaging. 2014;7:250–8.

Pilichou K, Mancini M, Rigato I, et al. Nonischemic left ventricular scar sporadic or familial? screen the genes, scan the mutation carriers. Circulation. 2014;130:e180–2.

Case 70

Endomyocardial Fibrosis

Clinical History

- Forty-nine-year-old female.
- Evaluated for restrictive cardiomyopathy associated with hypereosinophilia.
- Referred for delayed-enhancement cardiac magnetic resonance (DE-CMR) to define diagnosis.

Images

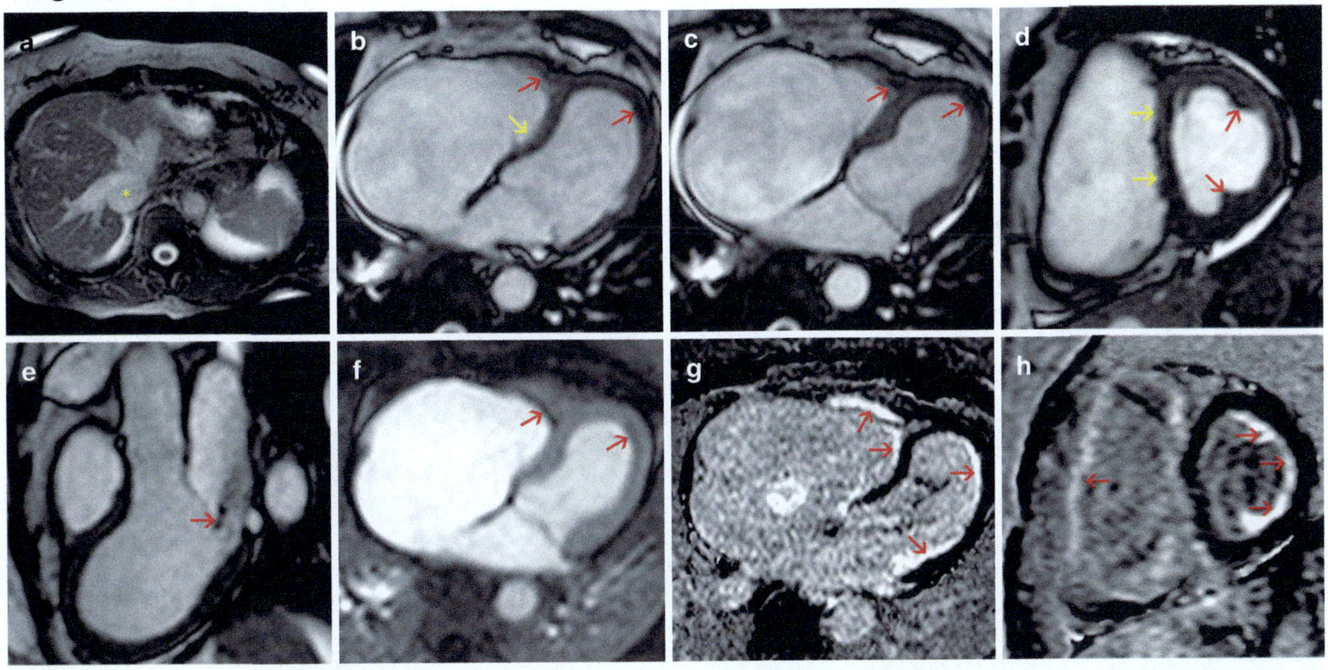

Findings and Interpretation

- Using conventional axial scout views, marked inferior vena cava and suprahepatic vein dilatation is noticed (*, panel A).
- Diastolic (panel B) and systolic (panel C) cine four-chamber views show normal left ventricular (LV) dimensions (end-diastolic volume 53 ml/m^2), with mild LV systolic dysfunction (ejection fraction 43%). Severe dilatation of the right atrium is clearly depicted, as well as mild pericardial effusion.
- Of note, the right ventricle (RV) is small, and the apical cavities of both ventricles seem to the occupied by a thin and linear hypointense tissue (red arrows in B and C). Also, the normal architecture of the LV papillary muscles is lost, showing a slurred triangular shape (red arrows in panel D).
- Protodiastolic septal excursion towards the left ventricle (yellow arrows in B and D) reveal increased filling pressures.
- Using the LV outflow tract view (panel E), moderate mitral regurgitation is identified (red arrow).
- First-pass perfusion images show a linear subendocardial defect involving the apical segments of both ventricles (panel F).
- Inversion-recovery images (four-chamber and mid-short-axis views, panels G and H) show subendocardial late gadolinium enhancement (LGE) affecting both ventricles, with significant involvement of the papillary muscles (panel H).
- Endomyocardial fibrosis is the most common cause of restrictive cardiomyopathy (systolic function is generally preserved). Commonly related to hypereosinophilia in the earlier stages, this condition of unknown etiology is characterized by subendocardial fibrin deposition involving the apical segments of one or both ventricles, later affecting the mid-segments and even the inflow tracts.
- These patients usually have a poor outcome, and surgical resection (though technically challenging and with high mortality rates) is the elective treatment.

Further Reading

Grimaldi A, Mocumbi AO, Freers J, et al. Tropical endomyocardial fibrosis natural history, challenges, and perspectives. Circulation 2016;133:2503–15.

Case 71

Endomyocardial Fibrosis

Clinical History

- Sixty-one-year-old female.
- Patient with hypothyroidism, dyslipidemia, and glucose intolerance.
- She has a 3-month history of palpitations and 6 months of dyspnea.
- An invasive coronary angiography carried out 8 years ago showed obliteration of the apices of both ventricles, more pronounced in the left ventricle and absence of significant coronary stenoses.
- A Doppler echocardiography performed a year later showed apical segment hypertrophy (16 mm) and hyperechogenic trabecular image with acoustic shadow in overlying endocardium causing obliteration of the cavity, left ventricular diastolic dysfunction, and hypertrophic right ventricle with preserved systolic function.
- Referred for cardiac magnetic resonance (CMR) for further assessment.

Images

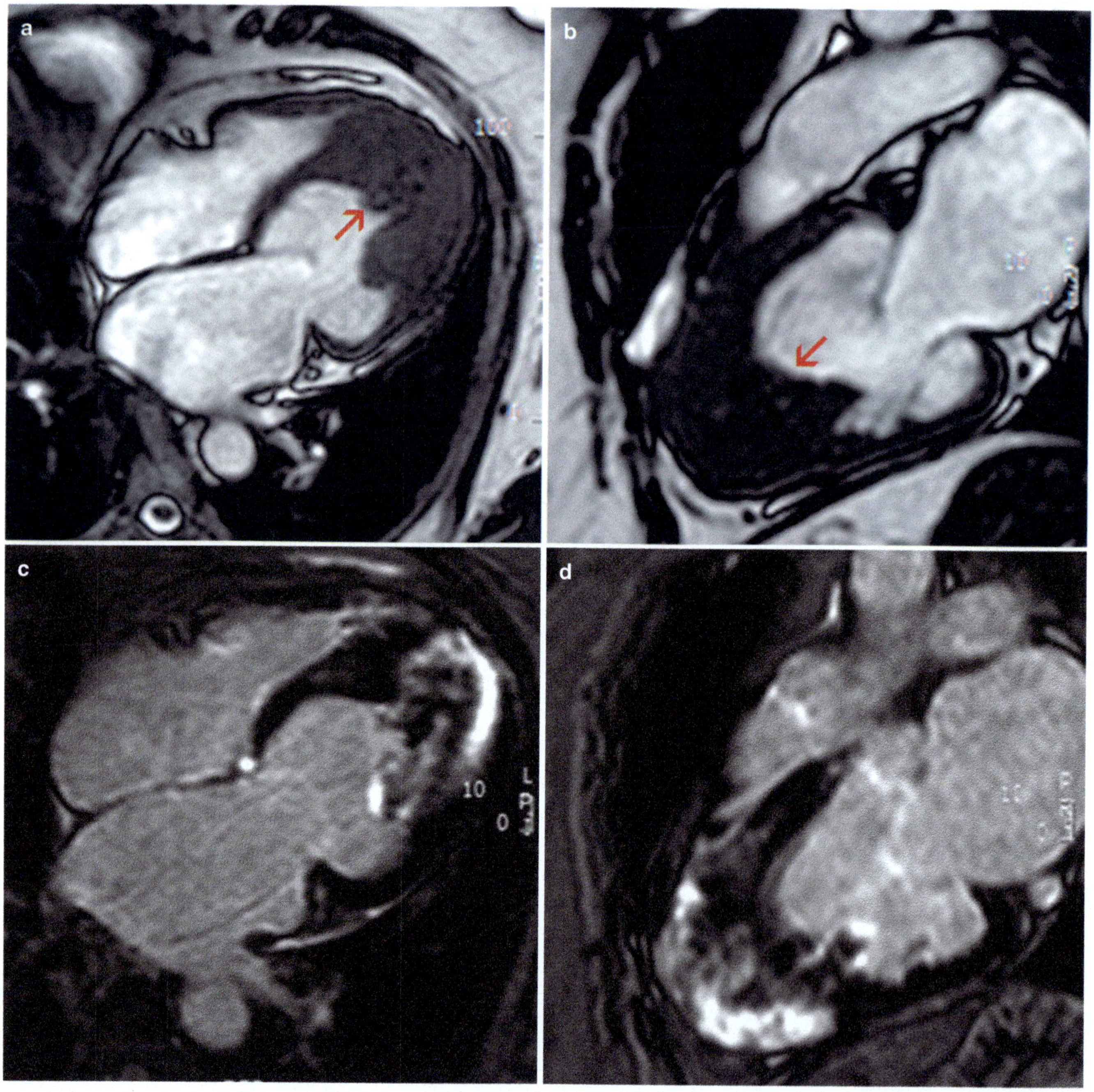

Findings and Interpretation

- Diastolic cine CMR in four-chamber (panel A) and two-chamber (panel B) views show biatrial dilatation and normal left ventricular size (end-diastolic volume 64 ml/m^2), with signs of endomyocardial fibrosis in the ventricular apices, with greater obliteration of the left ventricular apex (arrows in panels A and B).
- Inversion-recovery images at four-chamber (panel C) and two-chamber (panel D) views, depicting late gadolinium enhancement (LGE). Presence of heterogeneous LGE, suggesting area of fibrosis in the apical segments and apex. The subendocardial outer layer has high signal intensity corresponding to fibrosis, and the inner layer, in contact with the ventricular cavity, shows low signal intensity possibly corresponding to thrombus/calcification.
- Endomyocardial fibrosis (EMF)) is a form of endemic restrictive cardiomyopathy of unknown etiology. The clinical picture of EMF depends on the ventricle affected, the duration of disease, and the presence of signs of activity. Thrombosis and fibrosis are characteristically prominent in ventricular apices and at the posterior wall of the left ventricle, behind the posterior leaflet of the mitral valve, and most patients have mitral and tricuspid regurgitation.
- Right ventricular EMF is the most common form of presentation either in isolation or as part of biventricular disease. In left ventricular EMF, a soft and short systolic murmur confined to early systole is usually found. This is associated with a delayed opening snap and a loud pulmonary component of the second sound, indicating increased pulmonary pressures. In bilateral disease there is a combination of signs from left and right EMF.

Further Reading

Beaton A, Sable C, Brown J, Hoffman J, Mungoma M, Mondo C, et al. Genetic susceptibility to endomyocardial fibrosis Glob Cardiol Sci Pract. 2014;2014:473–81.

Bukhman G, Ziegler J, Parry E. Endomyocardial Fibrosis: Still a Mystery after 60 Years. PLoS Negl Trop Dis. 2008;2:e97.

Mocumbi AO. Endomyocardial fibrosis: a form of endemic restrictive cardiomyopathy. Glob Cardiol Sci Pract. 2012;2012:11.

Case 72

Endomyocardial Fibrosis

Clinical History

- Fifty-seven-year-old male.
- He has a history of right heart failure symptoms and hypereosinophilia.
- Doppler echocardiography revealed mild left ventricular (LV) dilatation with borderline systolic function, left atrium dilatation associated with a restrictive filling pattern, and an apical LV mural thrombus.
- Referred for delayed-enhancement cardiac magnetic resonance (DE-CMR) to confirm endomyocardial fibrosis.

Images

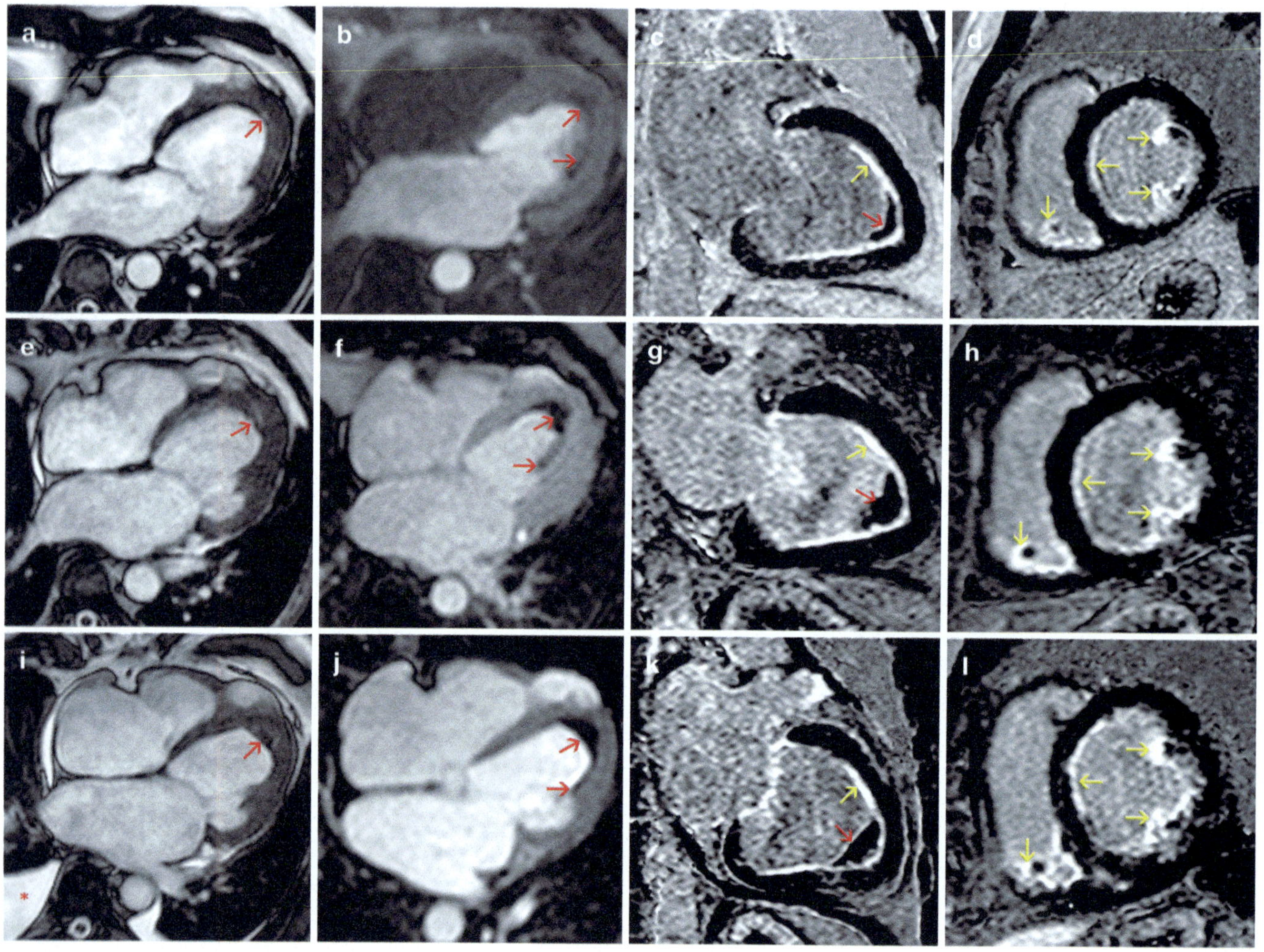

Findings and Interpretation

- In this case, DE-CMR was available for three consecutive years [upper (2015), mid (2016)-, and lower (2017) panels], enabling the assessment of the natural history of the disease and to have a glimpse on the extent of reproducible images provided by this technique.
- Serial images of diastolic cine four-chamber views (panels A, E, and I); first-pass perfusion (panels B, F, and J); and both two-chamber (panels C, G, and K) and short-axis (panels D, H, and L) inversion-recovery sequences are depicted.
- LV dimensions were in the upper normal limits, with mild basal and mid-diameter dilatation, and normal LV diastolic volumes.
- From 2015 to 2017, left and right atrial dimensions increased significantly; and the LV ejection fraction decreased from 46% in 2015 to 27% in 2017.
- Furthermore, right ventricular ejection fraction, which was normal in the first 2 years, decreased to 35% in 2017. The last follow-up also showed moderate pleural effusion (*, in panel I) and vena cava dilatation.

- In parallel, the size of apical LV thrombus (red arrows) showed a significant increment within the first 2 years.
- Panels D, H, and L show the typical impairment of the normal papillary muscles architecture, with extensive late gadolinium enhancement involving both ventricles and the LV papillary muscles (yellow arrows).

Further Reading

Grimaldi A, Mocumbi AO, Freers J, et al. Tropical endomyocardial fibrosis natural history, challenges, and perspectives. Circulation 2016;133:2503–15.

Case 73

Cardiac Amyloidosis

Clinical History

- Sixty-six-year-old male.
- Coronary risk factors: hypercholesterolemia.
- He has chronic atrial fibrillation and heart failure (NYHA functional class III–IV). He has a history of rheumatoid arthritis.
- Doppler echocardiogram revealed marked concentric left ventricular (LV) hypertrophy with borderline systolic function, moderate left atrium dilatation with restrictive filling pattern, and moderate mitral regurgitation.
- Invasive coronary angiography did not show evidence of obstructive disease.
- Referred for delayed-enhancement cardiac magnetic resonance (DE-CMR) to define diagnosis.

Images

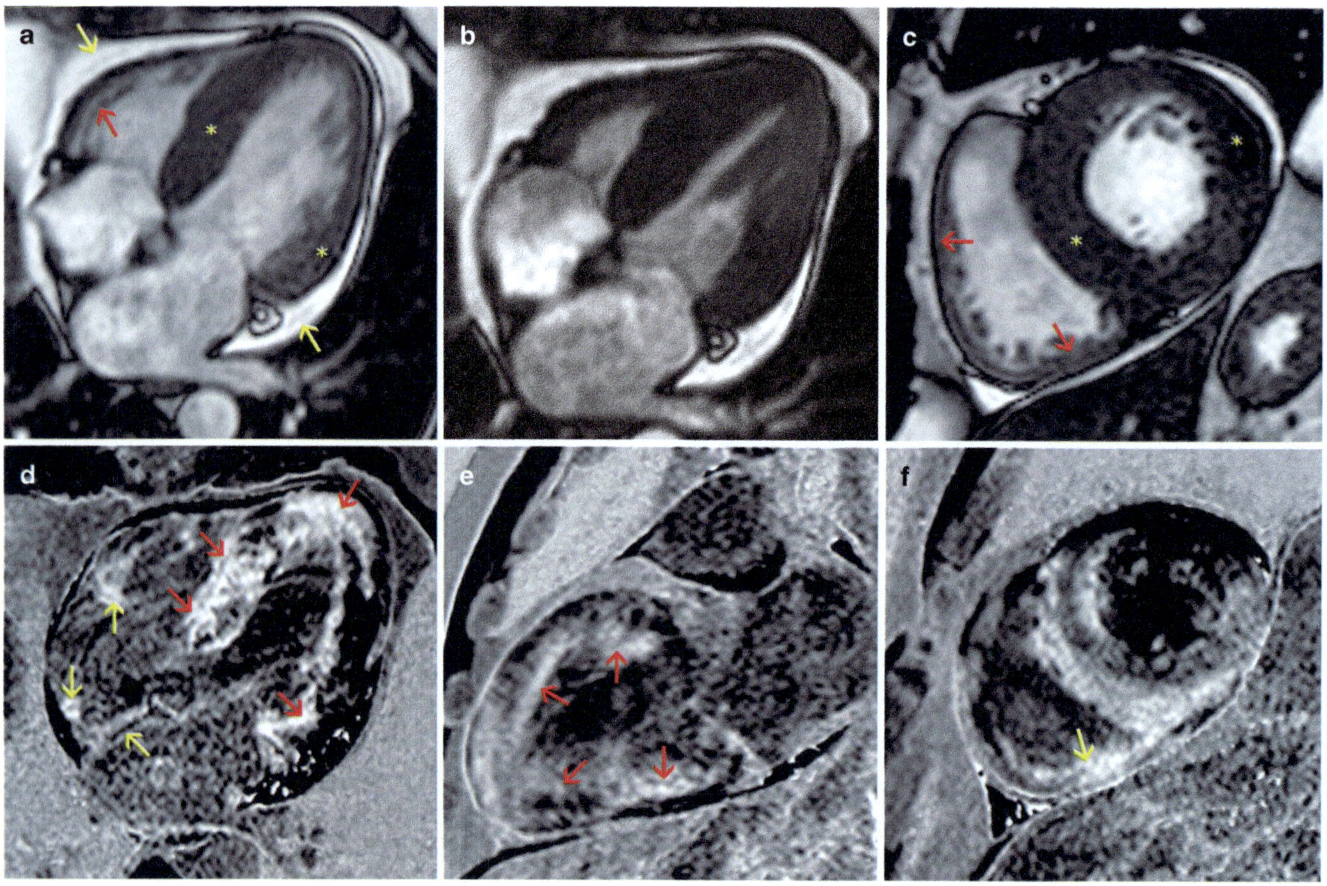

Findings and Interpretation

- LV dimensions were normal (end-diastolic volume 71 ml/m^2), with normal systolic function (ejection fraction 55%).
- Diastolic (panel A) and systolic (panel B) cine four-chamber views demonstrated markedly thickened LV (*) predominantly involving the interventricular septum (23 mm) and the basal lateral wall (17 mm). Also, there is an increase in the right ventricular (RV) basal wall thickness (red arrow in panel A). The left atrium is moderately dilated, and there is mild circumferential pericardial effusion (yellow arrows in panel A).
- Diastolic cine basal short-axis view (panel C) showed similar findings.
- Inversion-recovery images (four-chamber, two-chamber, and basal short-axis views, panels D–F) show marked nulling of the blood pool and extensive and diffuse late gadolinium enhancement (LGE) affecting multiple cavities including the interventricular septal wall from base to apex (red arrows in panels D and E), as well as the right ventricle, interatrial septum, and crista terminalis (yellow arrows in panel D).

- The extensive LGE involving the inferior wall of the right ventricle is clearly depicted in the short-axis view (panel F).
- This is a typical case of cardiac amyloidosis. Given the clinical history (chronic inflammatory disease) and the LGE findings showing lack of basal/apical gradient (actually, there is extensive apical LGE), this is not likely to be a case of ATTR amyloidosis. Instead, secondary amyloidosis or AL type should be excluded.

Further Reading

Boynton SJ, Geske JB, Dispenzieri A, et al. LGE Provides Incremental Prognostic Information Over Serum Biomarkers in AL Cardiac Amyloidosis. JACC. Cardiovascular imaging 2016;9:680–6.

Dungu JN, Valencia O, Pinney JH, et al. CMR-based differentiation of AL and ATTR cardiac amyloidosis. JACC Cardiovasc Imaging 2014;7:133–42.

Case 74

Cardiac Amyloidosis

Clinical History

- Eighty-six-year-old male, with a history of polyneuropathy and presyncopal episodes.
- Coronary risk factors: hypertension.
- Doppler echocardiogram (panels A and B) revealed concentric left ventricular (LV) hypertrophy, with preserved systolic function, normal pulmonary artery systolic pressure, and pseudonormal LV filling pattern (E/A ratio of 1.3; deceleration time 189 ms, and a E/e' ratio of 10, suggesting mildly incremented LV filling pressure).
- Referred for delayed-enhancement cardiac magnetic resonance (DE-CMR) with suspicion of cardiac amyloidosis.

Images

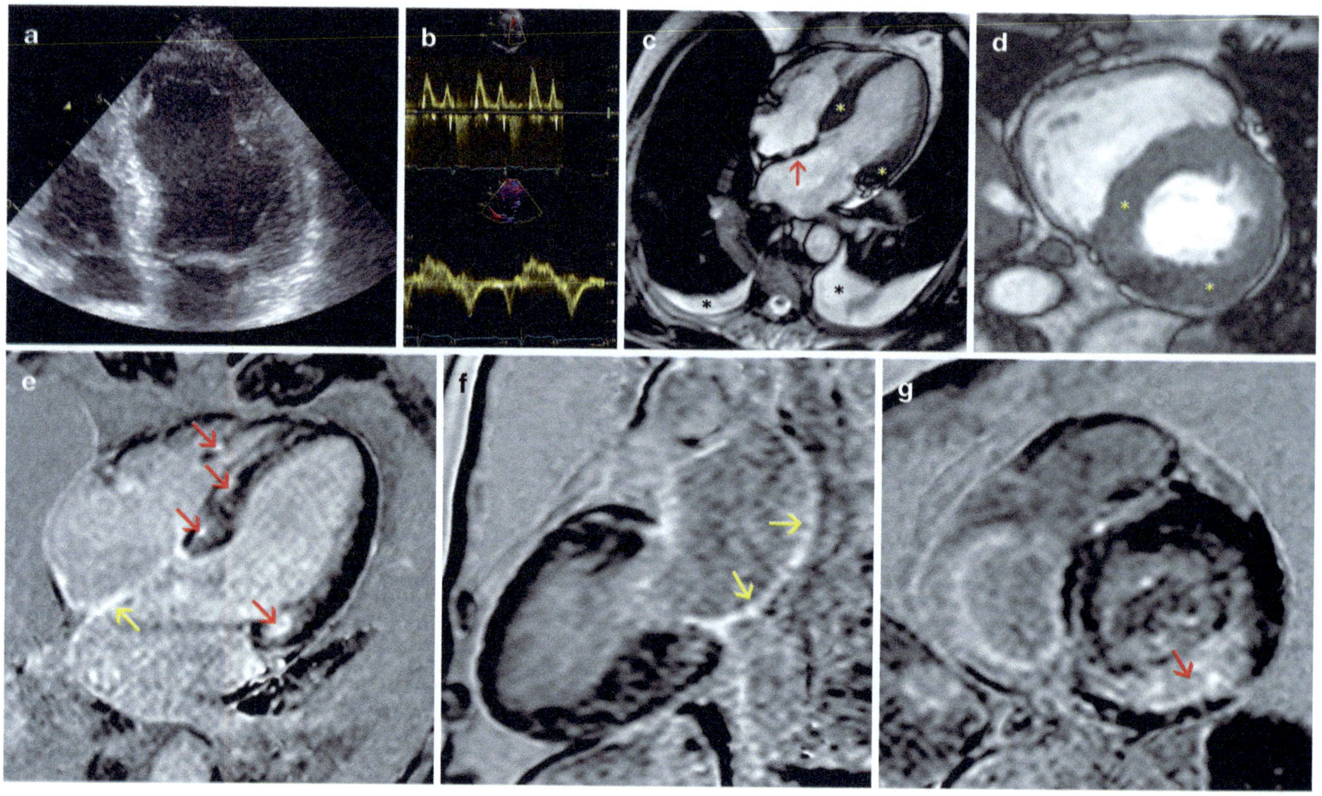

Findings and Interpretation

- LV dimensions were normal (end-diastolic volume 65 ml/m^2), with normal systolic function (ejection fraction 71%).
- Diastolic cine four-chamber view (panel C) demonstrated left atrial dilatation, moderate pleural effusion (black asterisks), and marked thickening of the LV basal segments (asterisks). Also, a thickened interatrial septum is noticed (red arrow).
- Diastolic cine basal short-axis view (panel D) showed a significant increment in wall thickness of the inferior septal (17.5 mm) and lateral (15.1 mm) basal segments.
- Inversion-recovery images (four-chamber, two-chamber, and basal short-axis views; panels E–G) showed intramural late gadolinium enhancement (LGE) affecting the interventricular septal wall and, partially, the right ventricle (panel E). Of note, diffuse and transmural LGE is observed at the inferior and lateral basal segments (panel G). Also, LGE is identified at the interatrial septum (yellow arrow in panel E) and left atrium (panel F).
- Finally, reinforcing the diagnosis of cardiac amyloidosis, nulling of the myocardial wall is suboptimal.
- Given the clinical presentation (octogenarian male with polyneuropathy and presyncopal episodes) and the cardiac phenotype (diastolic dysfunction, unexpected LV hypertrophy particularly affecting the basal segments, LGE involving multiple cavities with

transmural pattern at the inferolateral wall, and suboptimal myocardial nulling), it is likely that this patient has transthyretin amyloidosis (ATTR). Among other findings, apical sparing of LGE is particularly suggestive of ATTR.

- However, further noninvasive testing includes ruling out monoclonal protein in serum and/or urine and a positive bone scintigraphy (significantly higher myocardial retention in ATTR compared to AL).
- It has been reported that ATTR can be detected among up to 25% of autopsies in patients >85 years; up to 13% of >60-year-old patients with heart failure with preserved systolic function; up to 5% of patients with hypertrophic cardiomyopathy; up to 6% of patients with aortic valve stenosis undergoing surgery; and up to 16% of patients undergoing transcatheter aortic valve replacement (particularly in low-flow, low-gradient phenotype with mild systolic impairment). Accordingly, ATTR is far more common than expected.

Further Reading

Castaño A, Narotsky DL, Hamid N, Khalique OK, Morgenstern R, DeLuca A, et al. Unveiling transthyretin cardiac amyloidosis and its predictors among elderly patients with severe aortic stenosis undergoing transcatheter aortic valve replacement. Eur Heart J. 2017;38:2879–87.

Damy T, Costes B, Hagege AA, et al. Prevalence and clinical phenotype of hereditary transthyretin amyloid cardiomyopathy in patients with increased left ventricular wall thickness. Eur Heart J 2016;37:1826–34.

Dungu JN, Valencia O, Pinney JH, et al. CMR-based differentiation of AL and ATTR cardiac amyloidosis. JACC Cardiovasc Imaging 2014;7:133–42.

González-López E, Gallego-Delgado M, Guzzo-Merello G, de Haro-Del Moral FJ, Cobo-Marcos M, Robles C, et al. Wild-type transthyretin amyloidosis as a cause of heart failure with preserved ejection fraction. Eur Heart J. 2015;36:2585–94.

Case 75

Cardiac Amyloidosis

Clinical History

- Seventy-six-year-old male, with chronic atrial fibrillation and heart failure symptoms.
- Coronary risk factors: diabetes, hypercholesterolemia, hypertension.
- Doppler echocardiogram revealed concentric left ventricular (LV) hypertrophy, with preserved systolic function, left atrium dilatation, and restrictive LV filling pattern (E/A ratio of 5; deceleration time 79 ms).
- Referred for delayed-enhancement cardiac magnetic resonance (DE-CMR) with suspicion of cardiac amyloidosis.

Images

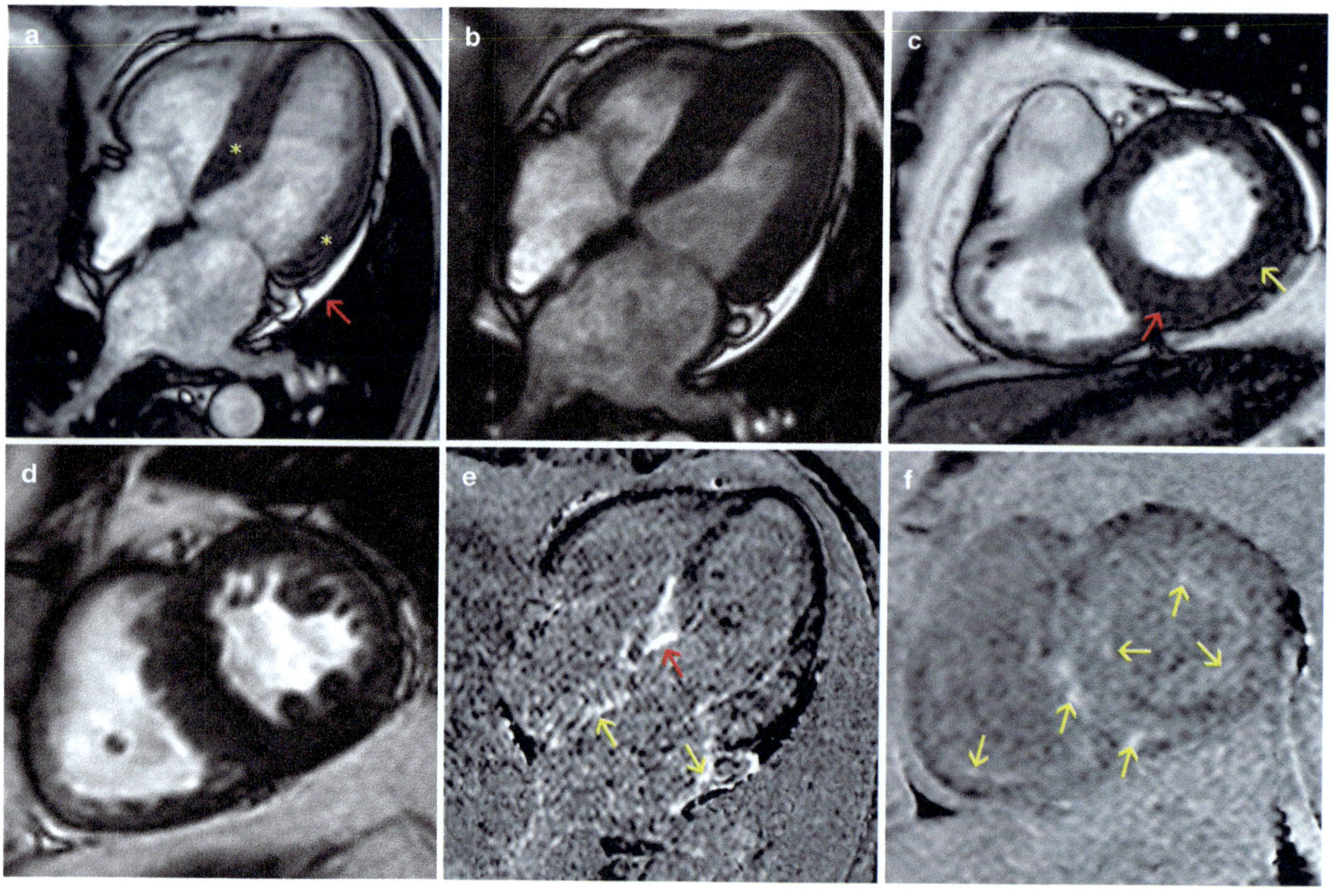

Findings and Interpretation

- LV dimensions were normal (end-diastolic volume 62 ml/m^2), with normal systolic function (ejection fraction 54%), left atrium dilatation (diastolic and systolic cine four-chamber views, panels A and B), thickened interatrial septum, and mild pericardial effusion (red arrow in panel A).
- Asymmetric LV hypertrophy, with marked thickening of the interventricular septal wall (red arrow, panel C) and basal inferolateral segment (yellow arrow, panel C). The maximal septal thickness was 17.5 mm.
- Inversion-recovery images (four-chamber and short-axis views; panels E and F) show the characteristic inadequate nulling of the myocardial wall and nulling of the blood pool (of high signal intensity in normal patients). Also, diffuse global subendocardial late gadolinium enhancement (LGE) affecting the basal and mid-segments of the LV and RV (panel F), as well a focal transmural LGE of the basal interventricular septum (red arrow in panel E). Finally, LGE affects the left atrium and the interatrial septum (yellow arrows in panel E).
- Cardiac amyloidosis is part of a systemic condition characterized by extracellular accumulation of insoluble

fibrillar proteins. In light-chain amyloidosis (AL; commonly related to plasma cell dyscrasia characterized by monoclonal production of kappa or lambda light chains by plasma cells), associated with a poor prognosis and a median <12 months of survival, amyloid fibrils derive from monoclonal immunoglobulin light chains. On the contrary, transthyretin-related amyloidosis (ATTR; a plasma protein mainly synthetized in the liver) is generally related with a better (median 2.5–3.5 year survival without treatment) outcome. ATTR can be senile, nonmutant type usually presenting as isolated cardiac amyloidosis and hereditary (autosomal dominant).

- There is some evidence that the presence of any segment with transmural LGE, as in this case, is more likely to be related to ATTR type. Furthermore, asymmetric LV hypertrophy is far more commonly observed in ATTR than in AL amyloidosis. Finally, another possible distinctive characteristic between these types is that ATTR type usually has a basal/apical gradient of LGE (panel E shows that LGE is clustered in the basal segments). Particularly, the apical segments are rarely involved in ATTR. Further noninvasive diagnostic algorithm to confirm ATTR warrants (1) ruling out monoclonal protein in serum and/or urine (including abnormal free light chain and immunofixation) and, if absent, (2) a positive bone scintigraphy (diphosphonates) and, if positive, (3) genetic testing to discriminate between wild-type and mutant ATTR.

Further Reading

Dungu JN, Valencia O, Pinney JH, et al. CMR-based differentiation of AL and ATTR cardiac amyloidosis. JACC Cardiovasc Imaging 2014;7:133–42.

Nativi-Nicolau J, Maurer MS. Amyloidosis cardiomyopathy: update in the diagnosis and treatment of the most common types. Curr Opin Cardiol. 2018;33:571–9.

Case 76

Cardiac Amyloidosis

Clinical History

- Seventy-year-old male.
- Coronary risk factors: hypertension.
- He has heart failure symptoms.
- Doppler echocardiogram revealed normal left ventricular (LV) size and systolic function, left atrial dilatation, and restrictive physiology (severe diastolic dysfunction).
- Referred for delayed-enhancement cardiac magnetic resonance (DE-CMR) for further assessment of restrictive cardiomyopathy.

Images

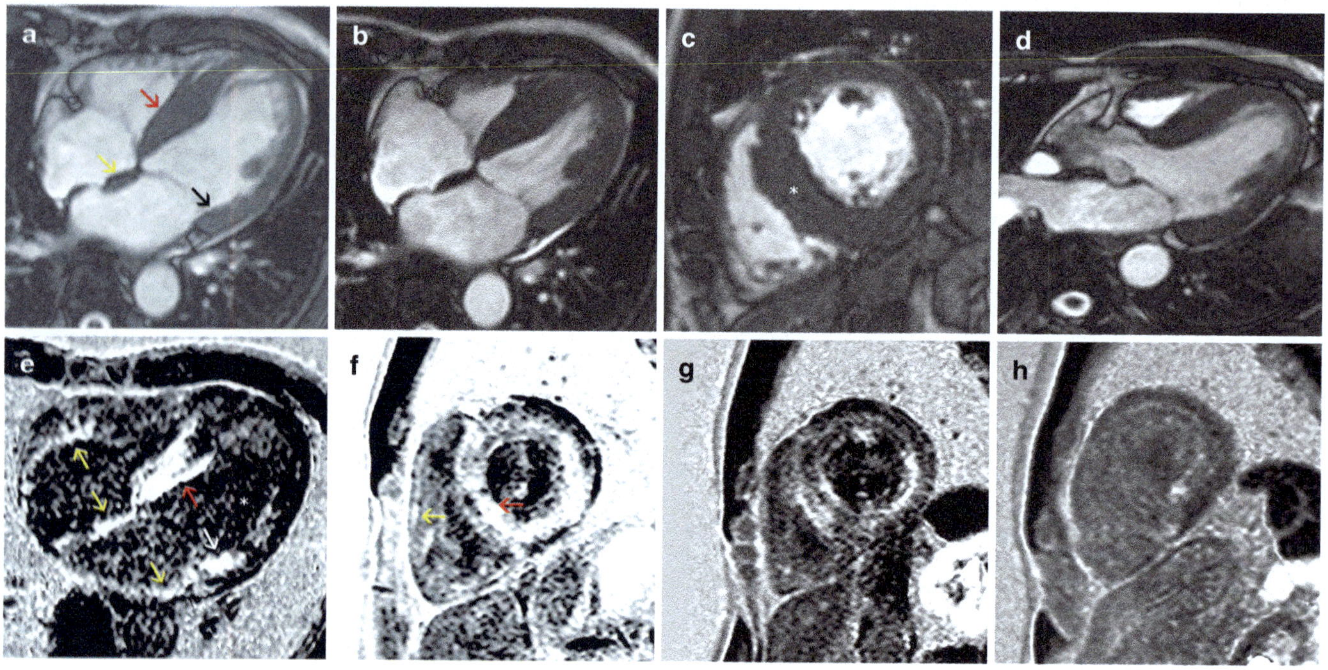

Findings and Interpretation

- Four-chamber end-diastolic (panel A) and end-systolic (panel B) cine CMR images showed normal LV dimensions, with systolic function within the lower normal threshold limit (ejection fraction 50%), mild left atrium dilatation, asymmetric LV hypertrophy (red arrow in panel A), and a thickened interatrial septum (yellow arrow in panel A).
- End-diastolic cine short-axis view (panel C) showed asymmetric hypertrophy (asterisk), despite mild lateral basal hypertrophy was also noted (black arrow in panel A).
- A systolic left ventricular outflow tract view demonstrated preserved opening of the aortic valve, ruling out aortic stenosis (panel D).
- Inversion-recovery images (four-chamber view, panel E; short-axis views from base to apex, panels F–H) showed the characteristic nulling of the blood pool (asterisk in panel E). Diffuse late gadolinium enhancement (LGE) involved predominantly the basal segments (panel E), with transmural LGE at the basal septal wall (red arrow in panels E and F) and subendocardial LGE in the basal lateral wall (white arrow in panel E) and in the mid- and mid- to apical segments (panels G and H).
- Both atria have extensive LGE (yellow arrows in panel E), and the right ventricle has mild LGE in the basal segments (yellow arrow in panel F).
- This is a typical case of cardiac amyloidosis, most likely of transthyretin amyloid cardiomyopathy (ATTR) given the sex, age, and phenotype (asymmetric hypertrophy, transmural LGE affecting mostly the basal segments with apical sparing).
- A number of clinical aspects should be explored in order to discriminate between AL and ATTR amyloidosis

including evidence of blood dyscrasia (AL amyloid), extracardiac symptoms (more related to ATTR, particularly peripheral nerve symptoms such as carpal tunnel syndrome), presence of serum free light chains and positive immufixation (AL amyloid), elevated troponine levels (more likely of AL amyloid), macroglossia and hepatomegaly (more likely AL amyloid), and bone scintigraphy (diphosphonate) with high-degree uptake (ATTR amyloid). Verification with biopsy (commonly subcutaneous fat) with immunohistochemical staining is desired.

- Such discrimination is critical since treatments differ completely, and median survival of ATTR without treatment is approximately 3 years compared to 6 months in AL.

Further Reading

Dungu JN, Valencia O, Pinney JH, et al. CMR-based differentiation of AL and ATTR cardiac amyloidosis. JACC Cardiovasc Imaging 2014;7:133–42.

Gertz MA, Benson MD, Dyck PJ, et al. Diagnosis, prognosis, and therapy of transthyretin amyloidosis. J Am Coll Cardiol. 2015;66:2451–66.

Case 77

Cardiac Sarcoidosis

Clinical History

- Forty-three-year-old female.
- No history of malignancy or known pathologies.
- Coronary risk factors: none.
- She was admitted with syncope related to complete atrioventricular block.
- Referred for delayed-enhancement cardiac magnetic resonance (DE-CMR) with high suspicion of cardiac sarcoidosis (no previous studies were provided).

Images

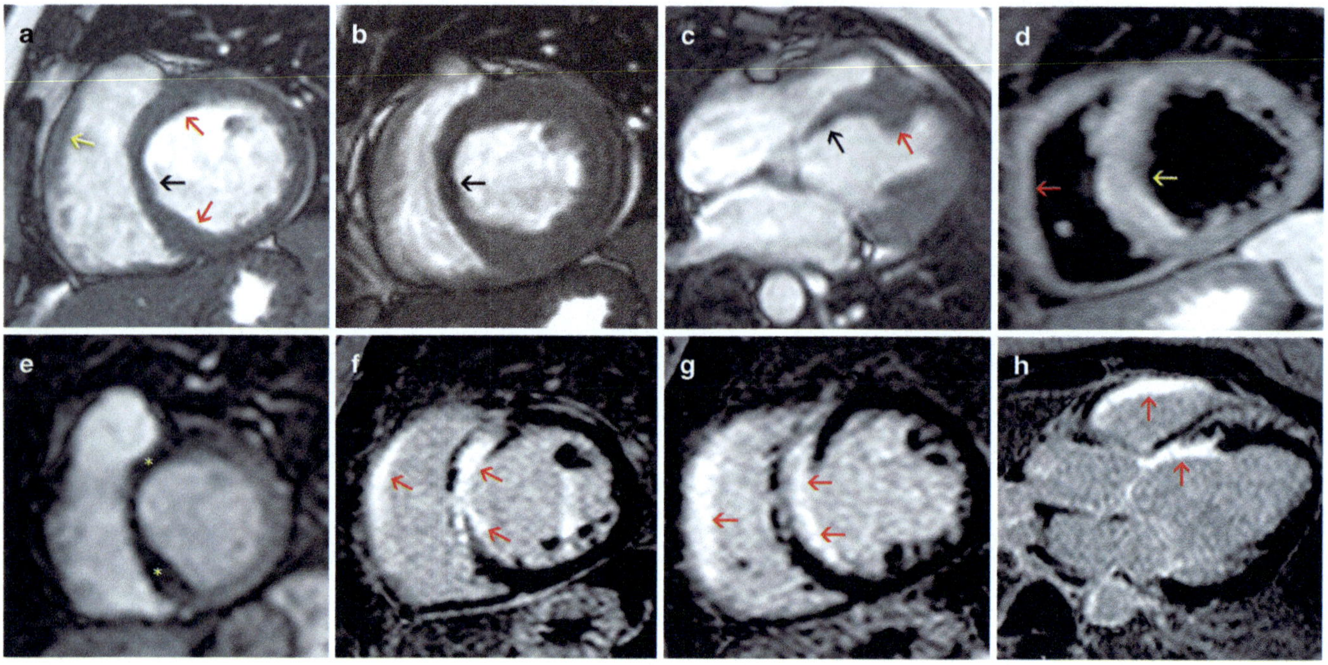

Findings and Interpretation

- Left ventricular (LV) dimensions were normal (end-diastolic volume 79 ml/m^2), with minimal LV systolic dysfunction (ejection fraction 49%).
- Cine images (diastolic basal short-axis, panel A; systolic basal short-axis, panel B; and systolic four-chamber view, panel C) demonstrate areas of myocardial wall thinning and akinesia (black arrows) and areas of increased wall thickness of the left (red arrows) and right (yellow arrow) ventricles.
- T2-weighted image (panel D) demonstrates increased myocardial signal intensity of the septal wall (yellow arrow) and of the right ventricular free wall (red arrow), reflecting myocardial edema.
- First-pass perfusion image (panel E) shows homogeneous transmural areas of hypoperfusion of the anterior and inferior septal wall (*).
- Inversion-recovery images (basal and mid-ventricular short-axis, panels F–G; LV outflow tract, panel H) show subendocardial and transmural areas of LGE (red arrows) involving the LV septal wall and the right ventricular outflow tract. Note that LGE is unrelated to any coronary artery territory.
- Sarcoidosis is a multisystemic inflammatory disease of unknown etiology that generally involves lymph nodes and formation of granulomas. Cardiac involvement is present in 5–10%, though higher in autopsy reports. Endomyocardial biopsy, as in most myocarditis, has a low diagnostic yield, and a combination of CMR and 18FDG PET-CT has recently been suggested as the reference standard.
- Indeed, the presence of LGE among patients with suspected cardiac sarcoidosis has been associated with an increased risk of all-cause death and arrhythmogenic events. The present case demonstrates how CMR can identify not only the presence of myocardial injury due to cardiac sarcoidosis but also to detect active disease using T2-weighted imaging.

Further Reading

Coleman GC, Shaw PW, Balfour PC, et al. Prognostic value of myocardial scarring on CMR in patients with cardiac sarcoidosis: a systematic review and meta-analysis. J Am Coll Cardiol Img 2017;10:411–20

Dweck MR, Abgral R, Trivieri MG, et al. Hybrid Magnetic Resonance Imaging and Positron Emission Tomography With Fluorodeoxyglucose to Diagnose Active Cardiac Sarcoidosis. J Am Coll Cardiol Img 2018;11:94–107

Greulich S, Deluigi CC, Gloekler S, et al. CMR imaging predicts death and other adverse events in suspected cardiac sarcoidosis. J Am Coll Cardiol Img 2013;6:501–11.

Case 78

Cardiac Sarcoidosis

Clinical History

- Thirty-nine-year-old male.
- No history of malignancy or known pathologies.
- Coronary risk factors: none.
- Admitted with syncope. He underwent an electrophysiological study reporting high risk of high-degree atrioventricular block.
- Referred for delayed-enhancement cardiac magnetic resonance (DE-CMR) with high suspicion of cardiac sarcoidosis.

Images

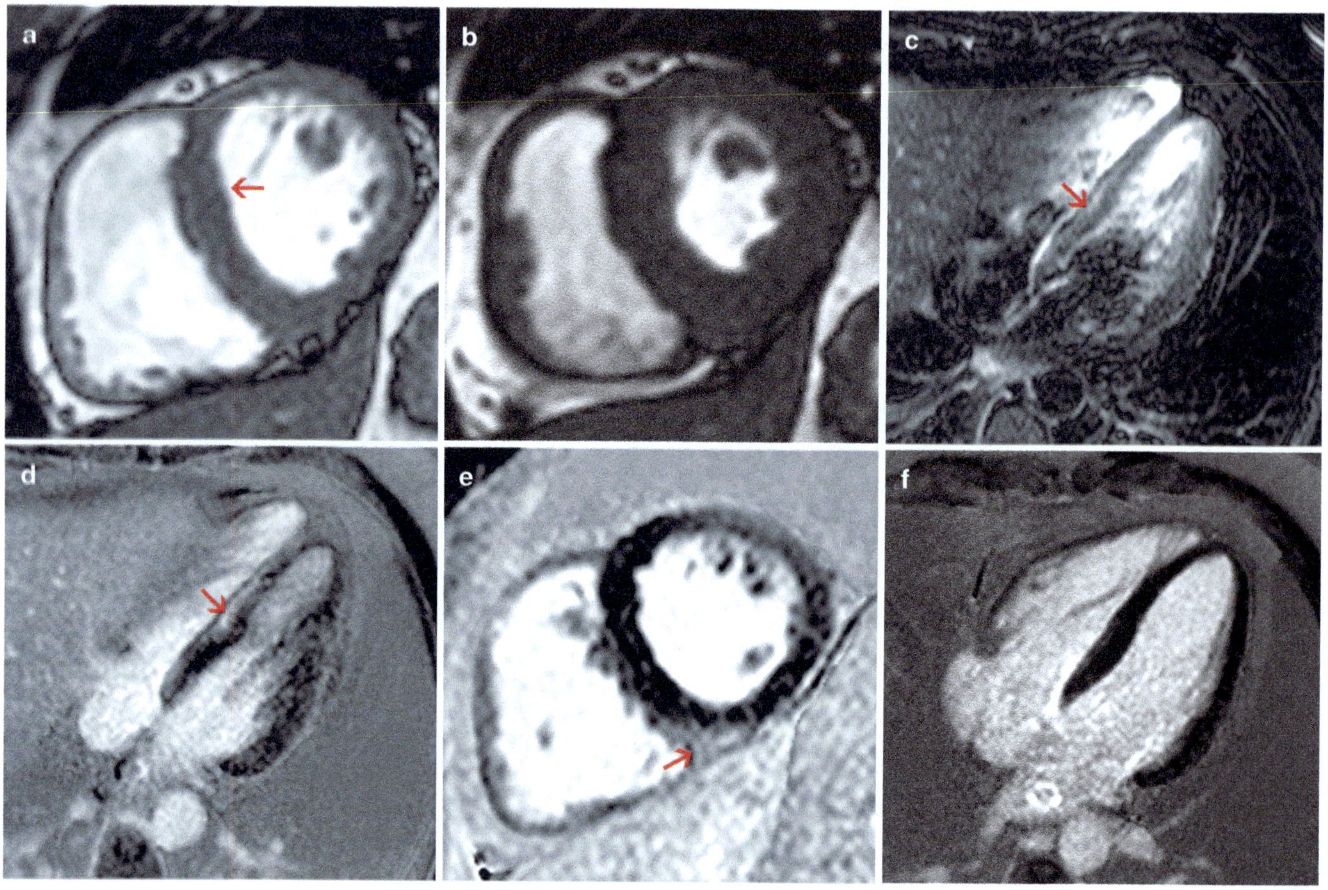

Findings and Interpretation

- Left ventricular (LV) dimensions were normal (end-diastolic volume 54 ml/m^2), with very mild LV systolic dysfunction (ejection fraction 47%) and LV dyssynchrony. The right ventricle also showed mild systolic dysfunction (ejection fraction 45%).
- Short-axis cine images (diastolic, A; systolic, B) demonstrated areas of increased wall thickness (arrow, A).
- T2-weighted images (low four-chamber view, panel C) demonstrate a small subepicardial area of increased myocardial signal intensity (arrow), reflecting myocardial edema.
- Inversion-recovery images (low four-chamber view, panel D) show subepicardial areas of late gadolinium enhancement (LGE, arrows in panels D and E). Note the absence of LGE in the mid (conventional)-four-chamber view (panel F).
- The presence of LGE in patients with high suspicion of cardiac sarcoidosis has been identified as an independent predictor of all-cause mortality and arrhythmogenic events.

Further Reading

Coleman GC, Shaw PW, Balfour PC, et al. Prognostic value of myocardial scarring on CMR in patients with cardiac sarcoidosis: a systematic review and meta-analysis. J Am Coll Cardiol Img 2017;10:411–20.

Greulich S, Deluigi CC, Gloekler S, et al. CMR imaging predicts death and other adverse events in suspected cardiac sarcoidosis. J Am Coll Cardiol Img 2013;6:501–11.

Case 79

Chagas Disease

Clinical History

- Forty-seven-year-old male.
- Last 6 months under assessment for moderate to severe ventricular dysfunction. In use of medications for heart failure.
- Dyspnea on minimal exertion and chest pain.
- Cardiac magnetic resonance (CMR) was required to evaluate etiology.

Images

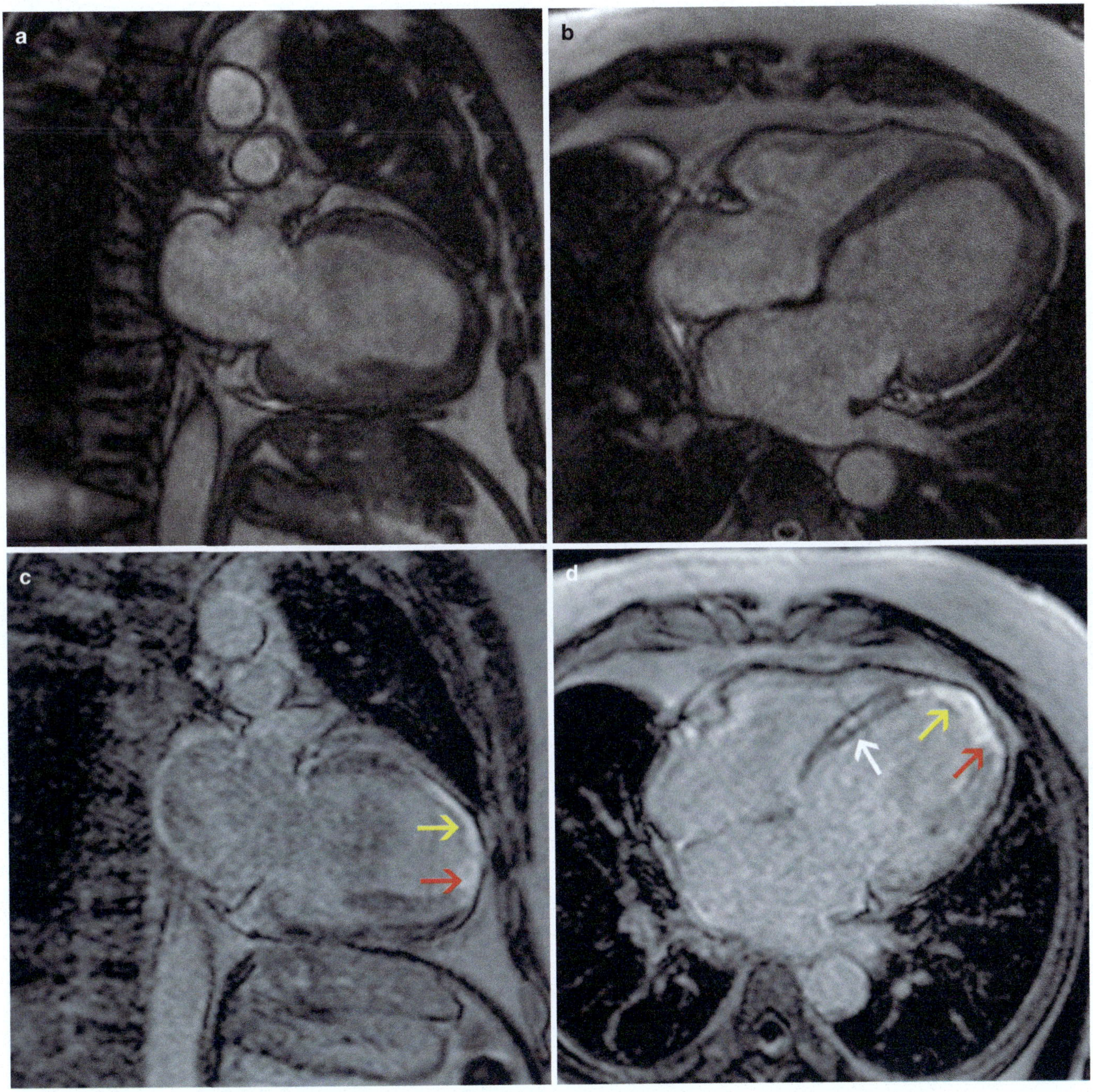

Findings and Interpretation

- Two-chamber (panel A) and four-chamber (panel B) cine images showing left atrium with increased dimensions (60 mL/m^2) as well as a dilated left ventricle (end-diastolic volume 108 mL/m^2). Significant left ventricular systolic dysfunction (ejection fraction 34%), at the expense of diffuse hypokinesia and apical dyskinesia, was present.
- Inversion-recovery images at two-chamber (panel C) and four-chamber (panel D) views showing transmural late gadolinium enhancement (LGE) predominantly affecting the apical segments (red arrows). Also, there is mid-septal intramural LGE (white arrow) and probable apical thrombus (yellow arrows).
- Presence of transmural nonischemic fibrosis, particularly if affecting the apical segments and when found in patients of endemic areas, is suggestive of Chagasic cardiomyopathy. The basal inferolateral segments are also a common location of LGE among these patients.

Further Reading

Torreão JA, Ianni BM, Mady C, Naia E, Rassi CH, Nomura C, et al. Myocardial tissue characterization in Chagas' heart disease by cardiovascular magnetic resonance. J Cardiovasc Magn Reson. 2015;17:97.

Uellendahl M, Menezes de Siqueira ME, Barros Calado E, Kalil-Filho R, Sobral D, Ribeiro C, et al. Cardiac Magnetic Resonance-Verified Myocardial Fibrosis in Chagas Disease: Clinical Correlates and Risk Stratification. Arq Bras Cardiol. 2016; 107:460–6.

Case 80

Chagas Disease

Clinical History

- Sixty-two-year-old male.
- He was raised in a Chagas disease-endemic area.
- Referred for cardiac magnetic resonance (CMR) due to ventricular arrhythmia and chronic heart failure symptoms.

Images

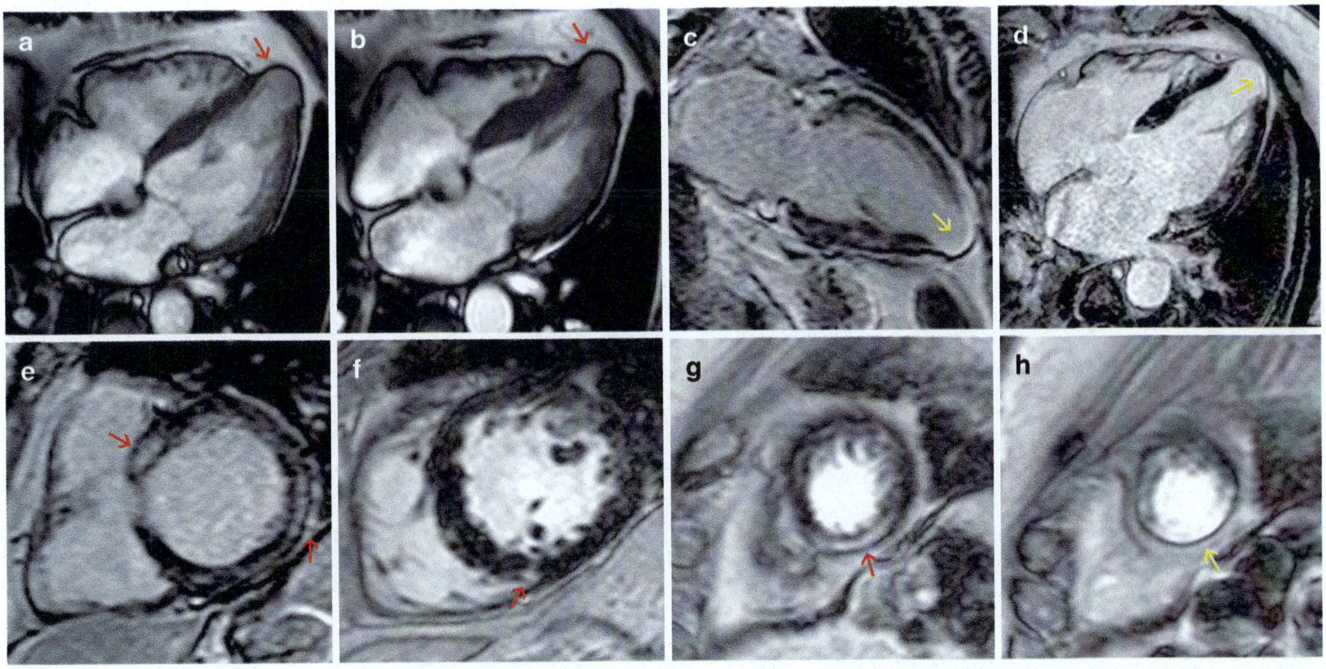

Findings and Interpretation

- Mild left ventricular dilatation (end-diastolic volume 100 ml/m^2). Using end-diastolic (panel A) and end-systolic (panel B) four-chamber cine images, a small apical aneurysm was detected (red arrows).
- Inversion-recovery images (panel C, two-chamber view; panel D, four-chamber view; and panels E to H, short-axis views from base to apex) show transmural late gadolinium enhancement (LGE) at the apical segments (yellow arrows), as well as intramural/subepicardial patchy areas of LGE at the inferolateral basal wall, interventricular septum, and inferior segments (red arrows).
- Chagas disease, also known as American trypanosomiasis, is a highly prevalent parasitic disease in certain endemic tropical areas of South America. The disease is caused by the *Trypanosoma cruzi* and is spread by a triatomine insect (vector). Approximately 20–30% of infected patients develop chronic cardiomyopathy (usually 15–30 years after the primo-infection), and vertical (pregnancy) and blood transfusions are also important sources of transmission.
- The most common complications of these patients are ventricular aneurysm, high-degree atrioventricular block, heart failure, thromboembolic complications, and sudden death.
- The two most common sites of LGE among these patients are the apical and inferolateral segments. Of note, the apical aneurysm in the current case is far too apical compared to the ischemic-necrotic etiology.
- Chronic patients can be treated with benznidazole.

Further Reading

Morillo CA, Marin-Neto JA, Avezum, et al. Randomized trial of benznidazole for chronic Chagas´ cardiomyopathy. N Engl J Med. 2015;373:1295–306.

Torreao JA, Ianni BM, Mady C, et al. Myocardial tissue characterization in Chagas´ heart disease by cardiovascular magnetic resonance. J Cardiovasc Magn Res 2015;17:97.

Case 81

Hemochromatosis

Clinical History

- Thirty-three-year-old male.
- Asymptomatic.
- He has prior diagnosis of hereditary hemochromatosis.
- Cardiac magnetic resonance (CMR) was indicated for further assessment of cardiac iron overload.

Images

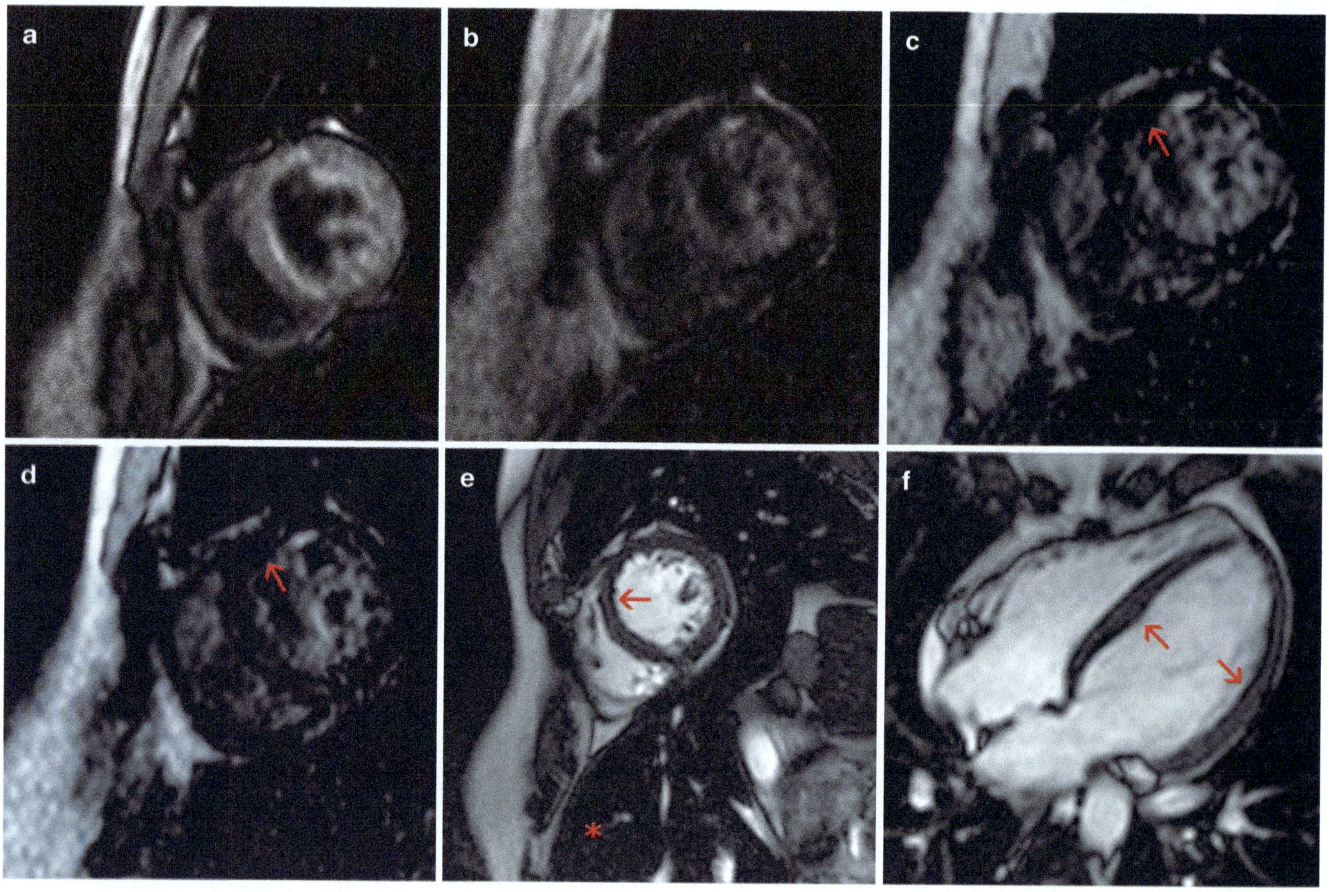

Findings and Interpretation

- Short-axis T2*-weighted images (panels A–D) were obtained at increasing echo times ranging from 3 to 21 milliseconds (ms). They show severe cardiac iron overload (T2* 6 ms). Note that iron overload tissues appear darker in the images (arrows).
- Short-axis (panel E) and four-chamber (panel F) cine images show normal ventricular dimensions and wall thickness (arrows). Note that iron overload tissues also appear darker in these sequences, including the liver (asterisk, panel E).
- Iron overload cardiomyopathy is defined as the presence of systolic or diastolic cardiac dysfunction secondary to increased deposition of iron in the heart independent of other concomitant processes. It's characterized in early stages by a restrictive cardiomyopathy with prominent early diastolic dysfunction which invariably progresses to an end-stage dilated cardiomyopathy.
- CMR is the only noninvasive method capable to quantitatively assess the myocardial iron load. In iron overload cardiomyopathy, the iron paramagnetic effect produces changes in CMR signal intensity susceptibility and shortens the relaxation time and darkens the image more quickly. Gradient echo T2*-weighted technique is used for quantification of cardiac iron content (T2* value 15–20 ms, mild iron overload; 10–15 ms, moderate iron overload; <10 ms, severe iron overload).

- Treatment differs according to the cause. In the case of this patient (primary hemochromatosis), the disorder is produced by increased intestinal iron absorption; therefore, phlebotomies are the treatment of choice. If the diagnosis is early, life expectancy is usually similar to the general population, and the iron depot normalization prevents the progression of the disease. However, in advanced stages of the disease, damage to organs such as the liver, pancreas, or heart usually occurs.

Further Reading

Gujja P, Rosing DR, Tripodi DJ, Shizukuda Y. Iron overload cardiomyopathy, better understanding of an increasing disorder. J Am Coll Cardiol 2010;56:1001–12.

Kremastinos DT, Farmakis D. Iron overload cardiomyopathy in clinical practice. Circulation 2011;124:2253–63.

Case 82

Anderson-Fabry Disease

Clinical History

- Fifty-nine-year-old female.
- Coronary risk factors: none.
- She has diagnosis of Anderson-Fabry disease (AFD), with cardiac, kidney, and skin involvement. Under enzyme replacement therapy for the last 12 months.
- Referred for delayed-enhancement cardiac magnetic resonance (DE-CMR) for further evaluation.

Images

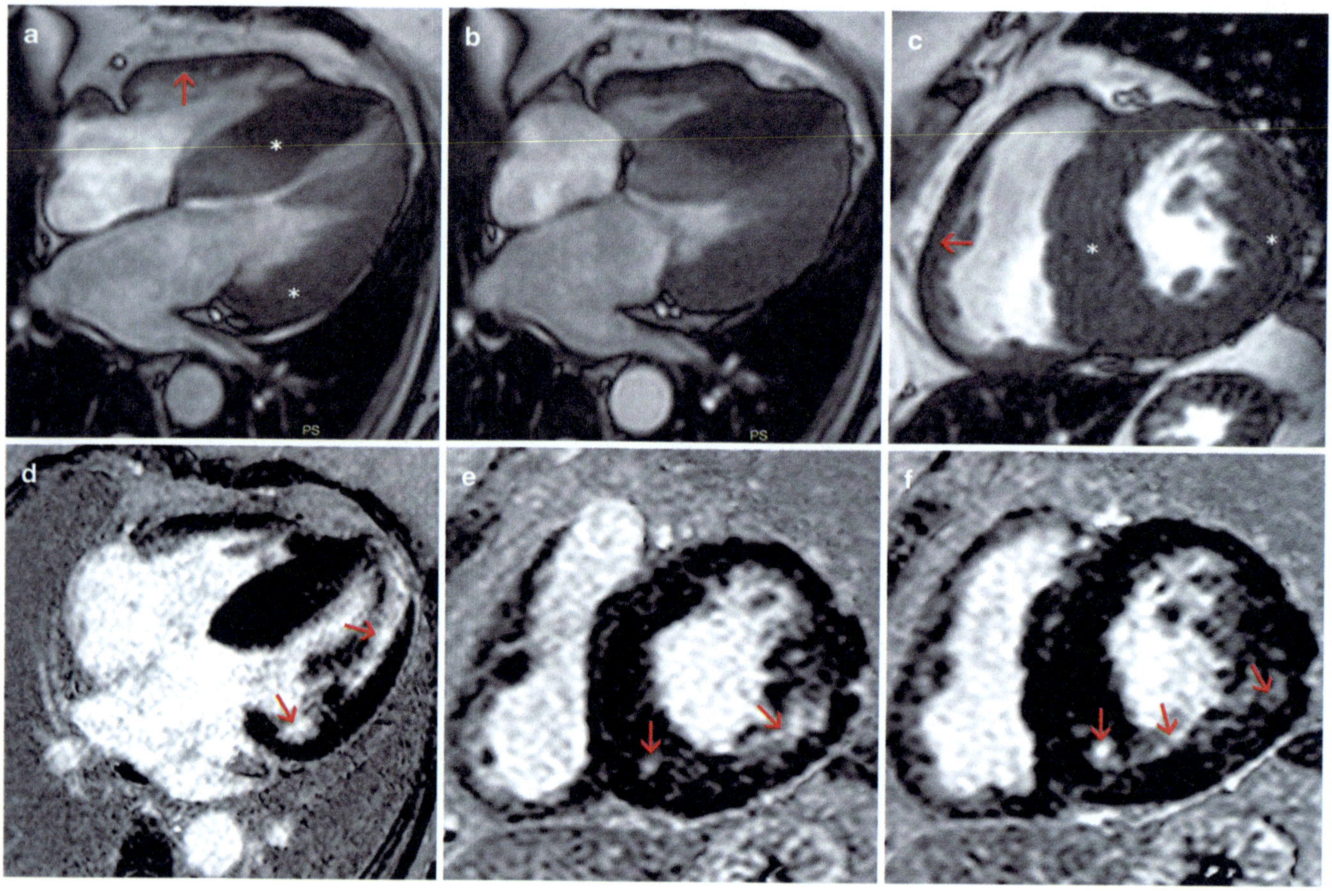

Findings and Interpretation

- The left ventricle (LV) has a reduced size (end-diastolic volume 61 ml/m^2, end-diastolic diameter 39 mm), with a normal systolic function (ejection fraction 63%).
- Diastolic (panels A and C) and systolic (panel B) cine views show marked left ventricular (LV) hypertrophy (*), with maximum septal thickness of 31 mm and maximum inferolateral and anteroapical thickness of 15 mm. The right ventricular free wall also has an increased thickness (red arrows in A and C).
- Inversion-recovery images (four-chamber, panel D; basal and mid-ventricular short-axis, panels E and F) demonstrate areas of predominantly intramyocardial late gadolinium enhancement (LGE, red arrows) involving inferolateral basal and mid segments and to a lesser extent the inferoseptal basal wall.
- Anderson-Fabry disease is a hereditary lisosomal storage disorder caused by an alfa-galactosidase-A (GLA) gene mutation located on the X chromosome (hemizygous males and heterozygous females can develop the disease, although males usually show the most severe forms), leading to a very similar cardiac phenotype to that of hypertrophic cardiomyopathy (HCM) associated with sarcomere gene mutation. Indeed, GLA mutations have been found in 3% of HCM patients without sarcomere mutations, and overall, it is estimated that around 1% of patients suspected of HCM have AFD. The main organs involved are the heart,

nerves, corneal deposits, and kidney. Cardiac manifestations include progressive LV hypertrophy that can be concentric, asymmetrical, or even apical, and the related complications are ventricular arrhythmia and diastolic heart failure. In these patients, enzyme replacement therapy has shown to be an effective means to reduce LV thickness.

- As shown in this case, some patients with AFD can mimic HCM; therefore, caution must be taken to avoid misinterpretations. One of the main differences in phenotypes between them is the fact that the basal inferolateral segment is almost never involved in HCM. Furthermore, hypertrophy in AFD is more frequently concentric or with mild asymmetry.

Further Reading

Havndrup O, Christiansen M, Stoevring B, et al. Fabry disease mimicking hypertrophic cardiomyopathy: genetic screening needed for establishing the diagnosis in women. Eur J Heart Fail. 2010;12:535–40.

Hsu TR, Hung SC, Chang FP, et al. Later onset fabry disease, cardiac damage progress in silence experience with a highly prevalent mutation. J Am Coll Cardiol 2016;68:2554–63.

Shah JS, Lee P, Hughes D, Thaman R, Sachdev B, Pellerin D, Mehta A, Elliott PM. The natural history of left ventricular systolic function in Anderson-Fabry disease. Heart 2005;91:533–4.

Case 83

Non-compacted Cardiomyopathy

Clinical History

- Forty-two-year-old male.
- Coronary risk factors: hypercholesterolemia, smoking.
- He has a positive family history (father and grandfather) for premature sudden death, and his sister has been recently diagnosed with non-compacted cardiomyopathy.
- He was admitted in the intensive care unit with heart failure symptoms and elevated pro-BNP levels.
- Echocardiography revealed a dilated left ventricle (LV) with global hypokinesia (ejection fraction 24%) and non-compacted myocardium.
- Referred for delayed-enhancement cardiac magnetic resonance (DE-CMR) to define diagnosis.

Images

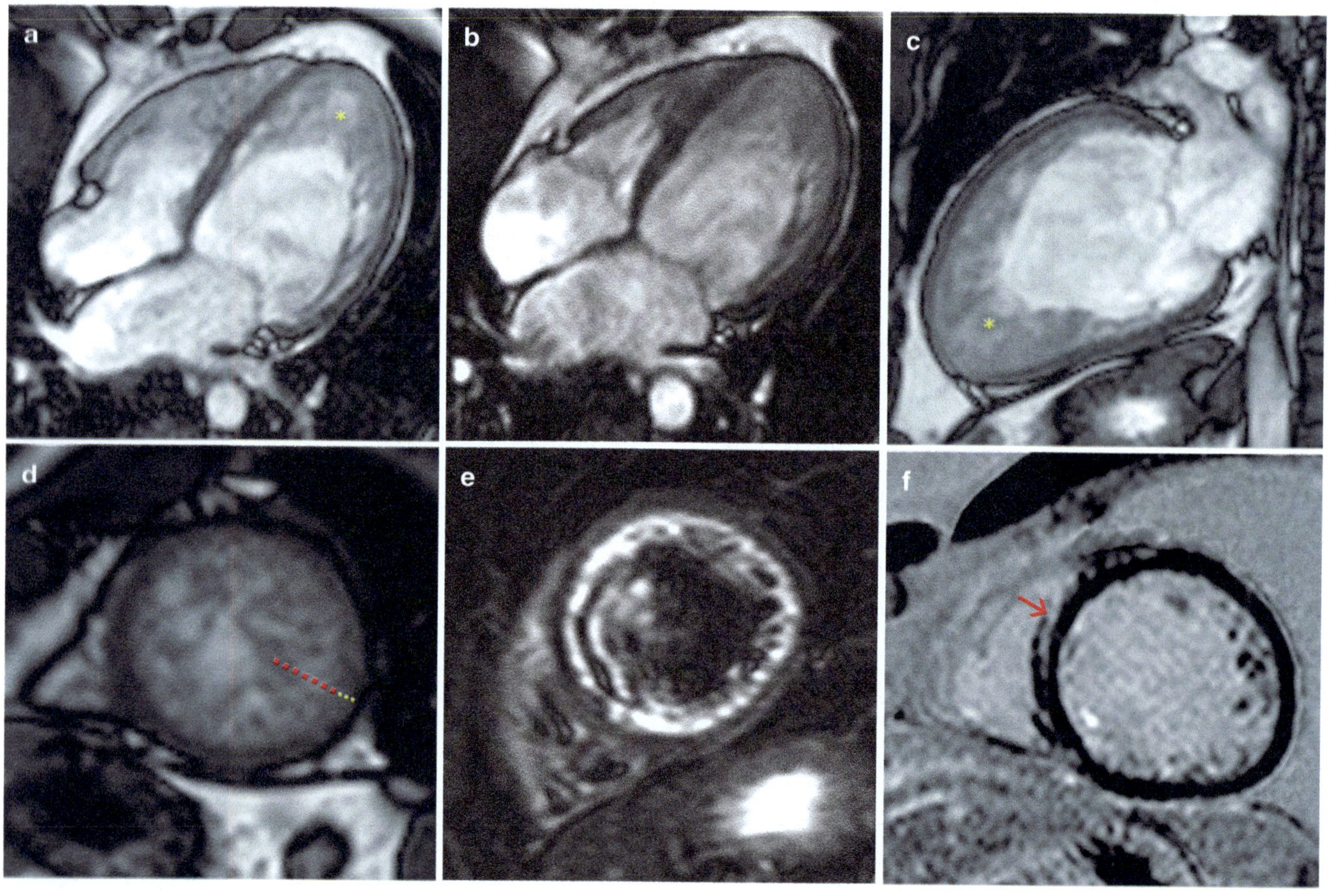

Findings and Interpretation

- LV dilatation (end-diastolic volume 131 ml/m^2), with severe systolic dysfunction (ejection fraction of 17%).
- Diastolic cine images (panels A and C) show marked apical, lateral, and anterior wall LV non-compaction (*), with a non-compacted (red)/compacted (yellow) ratio >3:1.
- Systolic cine images (four-chamber, panel B; short-axis, panel D) demonstrate the severe systolic dysfunction with akinetic segments. Also, very extensive myocardial trabeculae, with underlying wall thinning or the pars compacta, are clearly depicted.
- T2-weighted imaging (panel E) shows absence of myocardial edema.
- At short-axis inversion-recovery images, patchy subepicardial areas of late gadolinium enhancement are detected (arrow in panel F).
- This patient has a nonischemic cardiomyopathy, probably a case of isolated non-compacted cardiomyopathy.
- Rather than a cardiomyopathy itself, LV non-compaction might be better understood as a phenotypic expression of a wide range of disorders with different inherent prognosis.

- LV non-compaction is a genetically and clinically heterogeneous disorder that can be associated with multiple other conditions, such as multiple sarcomere and non-sarcomere mutations, hypertrophic cardiomyopathy, or myocarditis.

Further Reading

Karaca O, Cakal B, Cakal SD, Guler GB, Guler E. Which one is worse? acute myocarditis and co-existing non-compaction cardiomyopathy in the same patient. J Clin Diagn Res. 2015;9:OJ01.

Petersen SE, Selvanayagam JB, Wiesman F, et al. Left ventricular non-compaction insights from cardiovascular magnetic resonance imaging. J Am Coll Cardiol 2005;46:101–5

Rodriguez-Granillo GA. Non-compaction cardiomyopathy: a genetically and clinically heterogeneous disorder. Rev. Argent Cardiol. 2011;79:210–12.

Van Waning JI, Caliskan K, Hoedemakers YM, et al. Genetics, clinical features, and long-term outcome of non-compaction cardiomyopathy. J Am Coll Cardiol 2018;71:711–22

Case 84

Non-compacted Cardiomyopathy

Clinical History

- Fifty-nine-year-old male.
- Asymptomatic, with positive family history for non-compacted myocardium.
- Referred for assessment with cardiac magnetic resonance (CMR).

Images

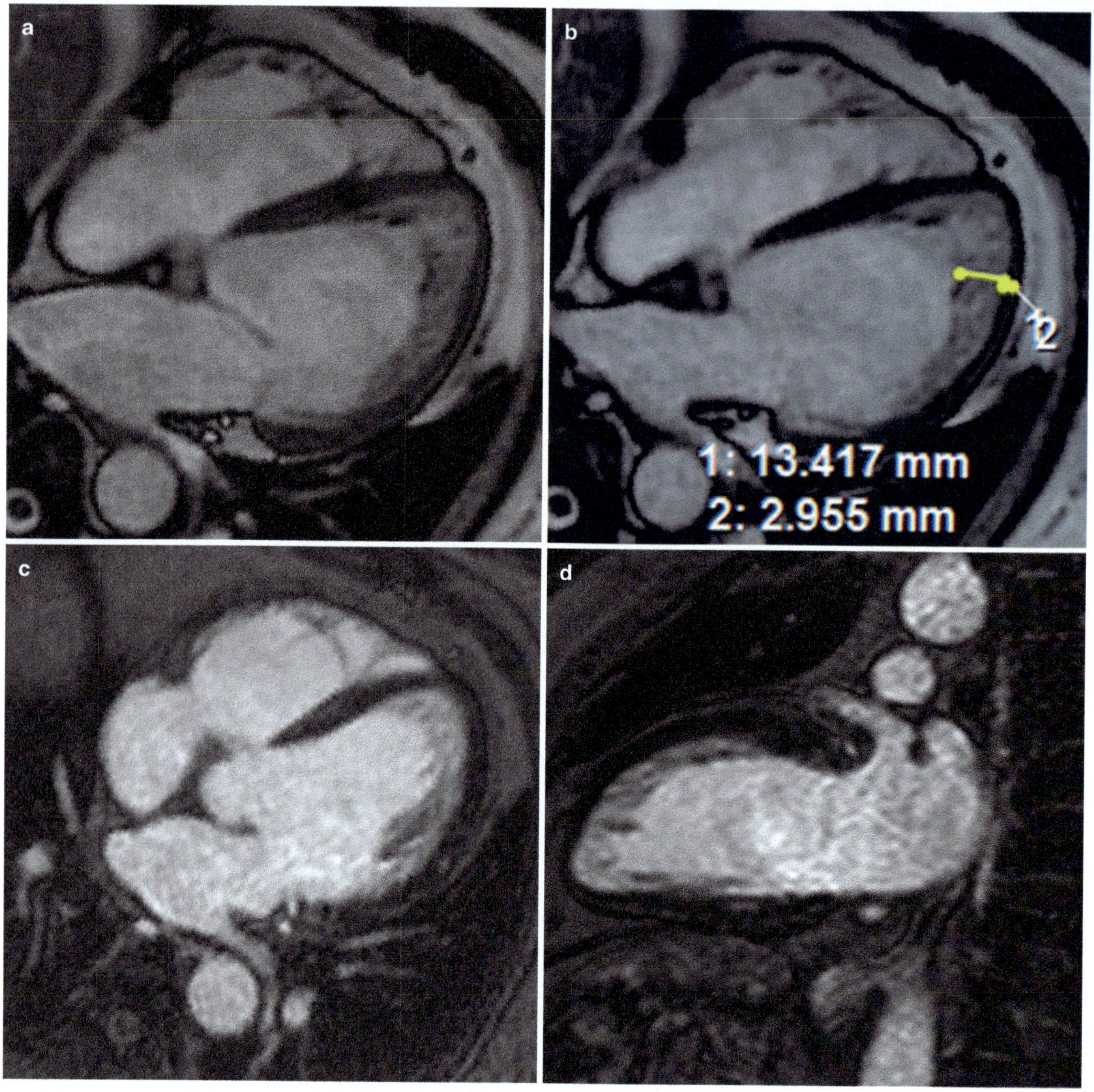

Findings and Interpretation

- The left ventricle is mildly dilated (panel A), and the systolic function is slightly impaired (ejection fraction 45%), with mild global hypokinesia.
- Increased left ventricular myocardial trabeculation is more evident in mid lateral wall and apical segments, with a non-compacted to compacted ratio of 4:1 (panel B).
- Absence of late gadolinium enhancement or intracavitary thrombus (panels C and D).
- These findings suggest incipient left ventricular non-compaction cardiomyopathy, with absence of myocardial fibrosis. This genetic cardiomyopathy has a low prevalence and can be related to several different mutations. In order to avoid false positives, a left ventricular trabecular mass above 20% (some authors even suggest above 35%) of the global myocardial mass has been proposed as more specific than the previous threshold of non-compacted to compacted ratio >2.3:1 in end diastole.
- Rather than a disease itself, left ventricular non-compaction is a phenotypical manifestation of multiple disorders. The prognostic markers related to ventricular arrhythmia, progression of heart failure, and thromboembolic events are hard to establish.

Further Reading

Anderson RH, Jensen B, Mohun TJ, Petersen SE, Aung N, Zemrak F, et al. Key Questions Relating to Left Ventricular Noncompaction Cardiomyopathy: Is the Emperor Still Wearing Any Clothes?. Can J Cardiol. 2017;33:747–57.

Choi Y, Kim SM, Lee SC, Chang SA, Jang SY, Choe YH. Quantification of left ventricular trabeculae using cardiovascular magnetic resonance for the diagnosis of left ventricular non-compaction: evaluation of trabecular volume and refined semi-quantitative criteria. J Cardiovasc Magn Reson. 2016;18:24.

Ivanov A, Dabiesingh DS, Bhumireddy GP, Mohamed A, Asfour A, et al. Prevalence and prognostic significance of left ventricular noncompaction in patients referred for cardiac magnetic resonance imaging. Circ Cardiovasc Imaging. 2017;10(9). pii: e006174.

Jacquier A, Thuny F, Jop B, Giorgi R, Cohen F, Gaubert JY, et al. Measurement of trabeculated left ventricular mass using cardiac magnetic resonance imaging in the diagnosis of left ventricular non-compaction. Eur Heart J. 2010;31:1098–104.

Kubik M, Dąbrowska-Kugacka A, Lewicka E, Daniłowicz-Szymanowicz L, Raczak G.Predictors of poor outcome in patients with left ventricular noncompaction: Review of the literature. Adv Clin Exp Med. 2018;27:415–22.

Case 85

Cardiotoxicity Related to Cancer Therapy

Clinical History

- Sixty-two-year-old female.
- Coronary risk factors: none.
- Three years ago she received cancer therapy with chemotherapy (anthracyclines) and radiation therapy for breast cancer, currently under remission.
- Forty-five days ago, a routine echocardiogram reported a mild systolic dysfunction (ejection fraction 47%) and severe mitral regurgitation.
- Referred for delayed-enhancement cardiac magnetic resonance (DE-CMR) for further evaluation.

Images

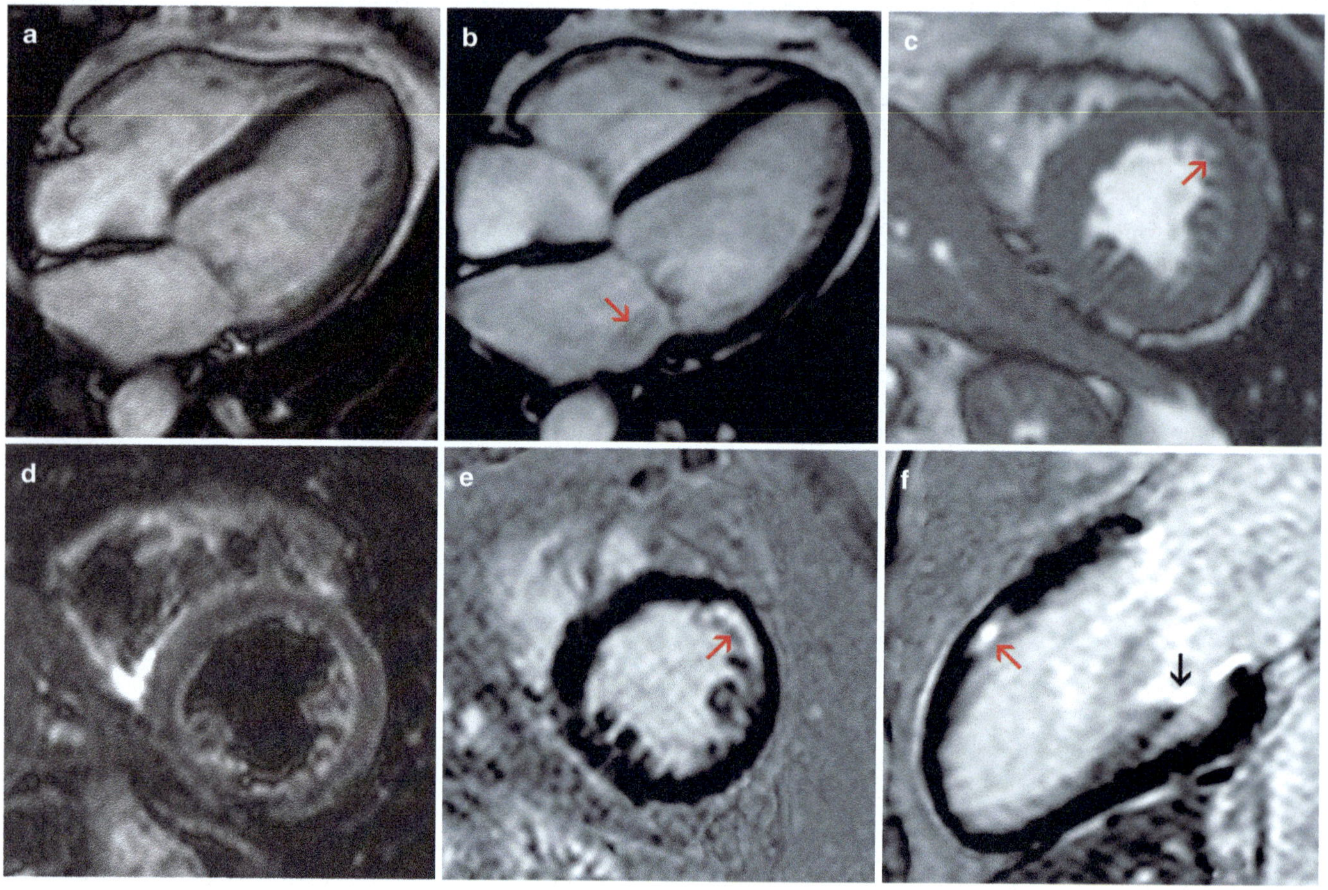

Findings and Interpretation

- The left ventricle (LV) has a normal size (end-diastolic volume 75 ml/m^2, panel A), with mild systolic dysfunction (ejection fraction 48%).
- Moderate mitral regurgitation is also detected (red arrow, in panel B).
- Systolic mid-ventricular short-axis view shows anterior wall hypokinesia (red arrow, in panel C).
- T2-weighted images (panel D) show absence of myocardial edema.
- Inversion-recovery images (mid-ventricular short-axis, panel E; two-chamber, panel F) demonstrate a small area of subendocardial late gadolinium enhancement (LGE) involving the anterior LV wall.
- Also, LGE involvement of the posterior papillary muscle is observed.
- Treatment of breast cancer is associated with various forms of cardiotoxicity, by means of multiple mechanisms.
- The pattern of LGE possibly reflects endothelial and microvascular/small vessel damage that has been related both to anthracyclines as well as to radiation therapy.

Further Reading

Mehta LS, Watson KE, Barac A, et al. Cardiovascular disease and breast cancer: where these entities intersect: A scientific statement from the American Heart Association. Circulation. 2018;137:e30–66.

Case 86

Cardiotoxicity Related to Cancer Therapy

Clinical History

- Sixty-year-old female.
- Coronary risk factors: none.
- She has a past history of previous malignancies under remission (breast and ovarian cancer), with radiotherapy and multiple chemotherapy cycles including anthracyclines, carboplatin, and paclitaxel.
- She was admitted due to heart failure symptoms progressing to acute pulmonary edema and referred a previous episode of uncharacteristic chest pain that was attributed to anxiety.
- ECG showed complete left bundle branch block (LBBB), and echocardiography revealed severe left ventricular dilatation and severe systolic dysfunction.
- Invasive coronary angiography did not demonstrate evidence of obstructive disease.
- Referred for delayed-enhancement cardiac magnetic resonance (DE-CMR) for further evaluation.

Images

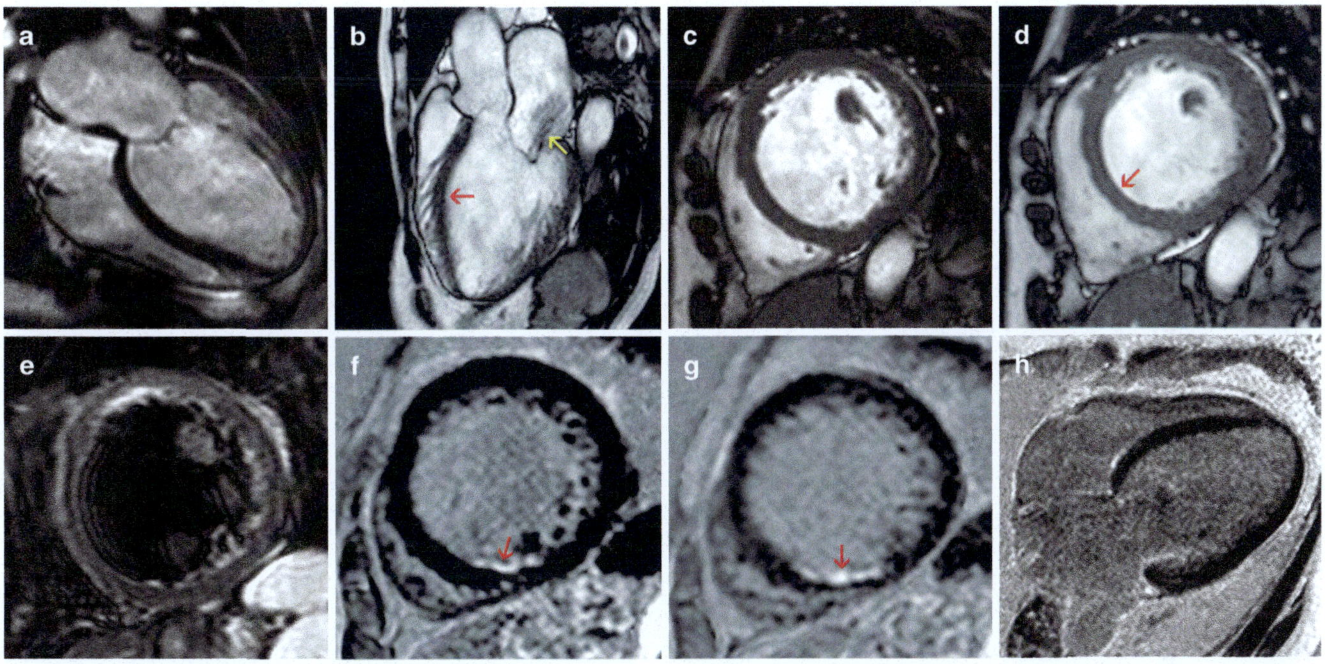

Findings and Interpretation

- Severe left ventricular (LV) dilatation (end-diastolic volume 208 ml/m^2, diameter 78 mm), with severe systolic dysfunction (LV ejection fraction 21%, end-systolic volume 163 ml/m^2).
- Cine images (four-chamber diastolic, panel A; three-chamber systolic, panel B; short-axis diastolic and systolic, panels C and D views) demonstrate these findings. Also, moderate mitral regurgitation (yellow arrow in B) and septal dyskinesia (red arrows in B and D) associated to LBBB are detected.
- T2-weighted imaging shows absence of myocardial edema (panel E).
- Inversion-recovery images (mid-ventricular and apical short-axis, panels F and G; four-chamber, panel H) show minimal subendocardial late gadolinium enhancement (LGE) involving the inferior septal (mid/apical) LV segments (red arrows).
- Cancer treatment can lead to various forms of early or late cardiotoxicity, ranging from LV dysfunction to ischemic disease, valvular disease, hypertension, arrhythmia, and pericarditis among other. Anthracyclines, commonly used agents in breast cancer, are particularly cardiotoxic through multiple mechanisms.
- In parallel, radiation therapy has been associated with accelerated atherosclerosis, microvascular dysfunction and endothelial damage, fibrosis, and oxidative stress, among others.
- Of note, latency period of cardiotoxicity related to chemotherapy or radiation therapy has been reported to appear as late as 30 years.

Further Reading

Mehta LS, Watson KE, Barac A, et al. Cardiovascular disease and breast cancer: where these entities intersect: A scientific statement from the American Heart Association. Circulation. 2018;137:e30–66.

Structural Heart Disease and Guidance of Percutaneous Procedures

5

Gastón A. Rodríguez-Granillo, Alejandro Zuluaga, Mariano L. Falconi, and Natalia Aldana Sepulveda

Role of Cardiac CT and MR for the Assessment of Valvular Heart Disease

Echocardiography has been largely established as the non-invasive reference standard for the evaluation of heart valve disease, allowing a safe, cheap, and accurate evaluation in most patients. Nonetheless, in selected patients with certain characteristics as we will address in this short introduction, as well as in those with suboptimal acoustic window, both cardiac computed tomography (CT) and cardiac magnetic resonance (CMR) emerge as useful tools for the diagnosis, follow-up, and prognosis of patients with native and prosthetic valve disease. Besides, these techniques, particularly CMR, allow improved evaluation of ventricular morphology and function, myocardial tissue characterization including patterns and extent of fibrosis, and more accurate evaluation of ventricular volumes. The latter is especially relevant for the assessment of the right ventricle, usually cumbersome with echocardiography.

Above all, cardiac CT and CMR, rather than alternatives to echocardiography, are complimentary diagnostic tools with different strengths and limitations. Indeed, cardiac CT is probably the best anatomic diagnostic tool, with excellent spatial resolution and nonrestricted volumetric imaging planes. Also, cardiac CT provides outstanding anatomic imaging for the guidance and follow-up of percutaneous and surgical valve replacement, aortic endovascular repair, and non-valvular cardiac devices.

In turn, the benefit of CMR in terms of valvular heart disease, aside from the reproducible and ionizing-free nature of this exam, is more related to the ability of CMR to quantify volumes (regurgitant volumes and fractions) and flow velocities using phase-encoding sequences, to enable differential diagnosis including specific cardiomyopathies, and to aid the determination of underlying mechanisms (for example, the identification of small myocardial infarct involving the posterior papillary muscle causing mitral regurgitation). For instance, recent studies suggest that a non-negligible portion of patients with low-flow, low-gradient aortic stenosis undergoing transcatheter aortic valve replacement have non-diagnosed cardiac amyloidosis.

Possibly the best scenario for CMR imaging regarding the assessment of valvular disease is among right-sided (particularly pulmonary) valve disease, of difficult assessment with echocardiography.

In brief, the relevant clinical scenarios for the role of CT and CMR imaging of valve disease involve:

- Suboptimal acoustic window
- Discordant echocardiographic findings

G. A. Rodríguez-Granillo (✉)
Department of Cardiovascular Imaging, Department of Research, Diagnostico Maipu, Buenos Aires, Argentina

National Council of Scientific and Technical Investigations (CONICET), Buenos Aires, Argentina

A. Zuluaga
Clinical Radiology Universidad CES, Medellín, Colombia

Clinical Radiology Universidad Pontificia Bolivariana, Medellín, Colombia

Radiology Residence Universidad Pontificia Bolivariana, Medellín, Colombia

CEDIMED, Body and Cardiovascular Imaging sections, Medellín, Colombia

M. L. Falconi
Universidad del Salvador, Buenos Aires, Argentina

Cardiology Specialist Career, Instituto Universitario Hospital Italiano, Buenos Aires, Argentina

Cardiovascular Imaging Unit, Cardiology Division, Hospital Italiano of Buenos Aires, Buenos Aires, Argentina

N. A. Sepulveda
Clinical Radiology Universidad CES, Medellín, Colombia

Clinical Radiology Universidad Pontificia Bolivariana, Medellín, Colombia

CEDIMED, Body and Cardiovascular Imaging sections, Medellín, Colombia

P. M. Carrascosa et al. (eds.), *Clinical Atlas of Cardiac and Aortic CT and MRI*, https://doi.org/10.1007/978-3-030-03682-9_5

- Low-gradient aortic valve stenosis
- Accurate location of the site of aortic stenosis: valvular, subvalvular, or supraaortic, as well as associated defects (aortic coarctation, ventricular septal defect, patent ductus arteriosus)
- Evaluation of the ascending aorta and surrounding structures
- Guidance of transcatheter aortic valve replacement (TAVR) and evaluation of the aortic annulus size and morphology
- Right valve disease, particularly in Ebstein's anomaly
- Quantification of regurgitant fraction and volumes in patients with inconclusive or borderline severe echocardiographic findings
- Accurate evaluation of right and/or left ventricular ejection fraction for clinical decision-making (particularly relevant in patients with mitral regurgitation)
- Accurate evaluation of end-diastolic volume for clinical decision-making (particularly relevant in patients with pulmonary regurgitation)
- Evaluation of myocardial viability, helpful for decision-making among patients with severe mitral regurgitation and low ejection fraction

Main CMR evaluation methods for valve assessment include:

- Multiplanar valve assessment using cine imaging, and valve area planimetry.
- Determination of maximum flow velocity and gradient [4 × velocity (m/s)]^2, as well as quantification of anterograde and retrograde flow using phase-encoding sequences perpendicular to flow direction immediately above the valve of interest.
- Using cine images, valve regurgitation and anterograde gradients are identified and can be qualitatively assessed and depicted as marked signal void related to turbulent flow-high velocity jets.
- One possible way to evaluate mitral valve regurgitation severity is by means of volumetric assessment, where the mitral regurgitant volume (MRV) is calculated as the total left ventricular systolic volume (end-diastolic minus end-systolic LV volume derived from cine imaging from base to apex) minus the anterograde aortic systolic volume (derived from phase-encoding sequence at the aortic root). And the mitral regurgitant fraction (%) is calculated as the MRV divided by the LV systolic volume × 100. This strategy can also be applied to right valve disease, adding a phase-encoding sequence at the pulmonary artery.
- Another straightforward way to evaluate right or left-sided regurgitant volumes, provided that there aren't other associated valve regurgitations, is by the difference between left and right (or right and left) ventricular systolic volumes.

Transcatheter Aortic Valve Replacement (TAVR)

Given the striking worldwide rise in TAVR and the pivotal role of cardiac CT as guidance and surveillance of TAVR procedures among diverse populations, this deserves to be specifically addressed.

Before performing TAVR, cardiovascular imaging studies are mandatory with two main objectives: to evaluate the "landing zone" (aortic annulus, leaflet anatomy, aortic root, and proximal ascending aorta) and the "access route" (access point to reach the vascular system and navigate to the aortic valve for accurate positioning of the prosthesis). Although different methods can be used, CT is one of the most commonly chosen as it can accurately evaluate both aspects in a single examination.

The landing zone is the portion of the LV outflow tract, aortic annulus, aortic root, and proximal ascending aorta where the percutaneous prosthesis will be deployed. In this area it is important to evaluate valve anatomy (tricuspid, bicuspid, or other morphology), severity, and symmetry of leaflet calcification; morphology and size of the annulus (diameters, area, perimeter, eccentricity) and presence and severity of calcifications (predictors of paravalvular regurgitation); coronary ostia position and height (a distance <10 mm is a risk factor for coronary occlusion during deployment); and size and morphology of the sinuses of Valsalva, sino-tubular junction, and proximal ascending aorta. Furthermore, information regarding the length of the membranous septum (anatomic surrogate of the distance between the annulus and the bundle of His) is important since a short membranous septum (<6 mm) has been related to a higher risk of mechanical compression of the conduction system. All this measurements and evaluation allow the right selection of the size and type of TAVR prosthesis to implant.

The other important aspect is the access evaluation, which includes the peripheral vascular anatomy including the femoral arteries, iliac arteries, and thoracic and abdominal aorta. In each of these sites, their size, tortuosity, presence of atherosclerotic disease, stenosis area and diameter, and previous prosthesis (surgical or stent) should be evaluated in order to establish the feasibility and safety for navigation with large catheters for valve introduction and deployment. In case femoral access is unsuitable, other access sites should be evaluated in the same CT scan (subclavian, ascending aorta, and transapical). The assessment of TAVR guidance using cardiac CT is succinctly depicted in the figure provided (Fig. 5.1).

When CT cannot be performed for any reason, for instance, in patients with renal dysfunction, other modalities can obtain similar information of the landing zone without contrast administration (transesophageal 3D echocardiography, CMR). Although valuable alternative methods, in most

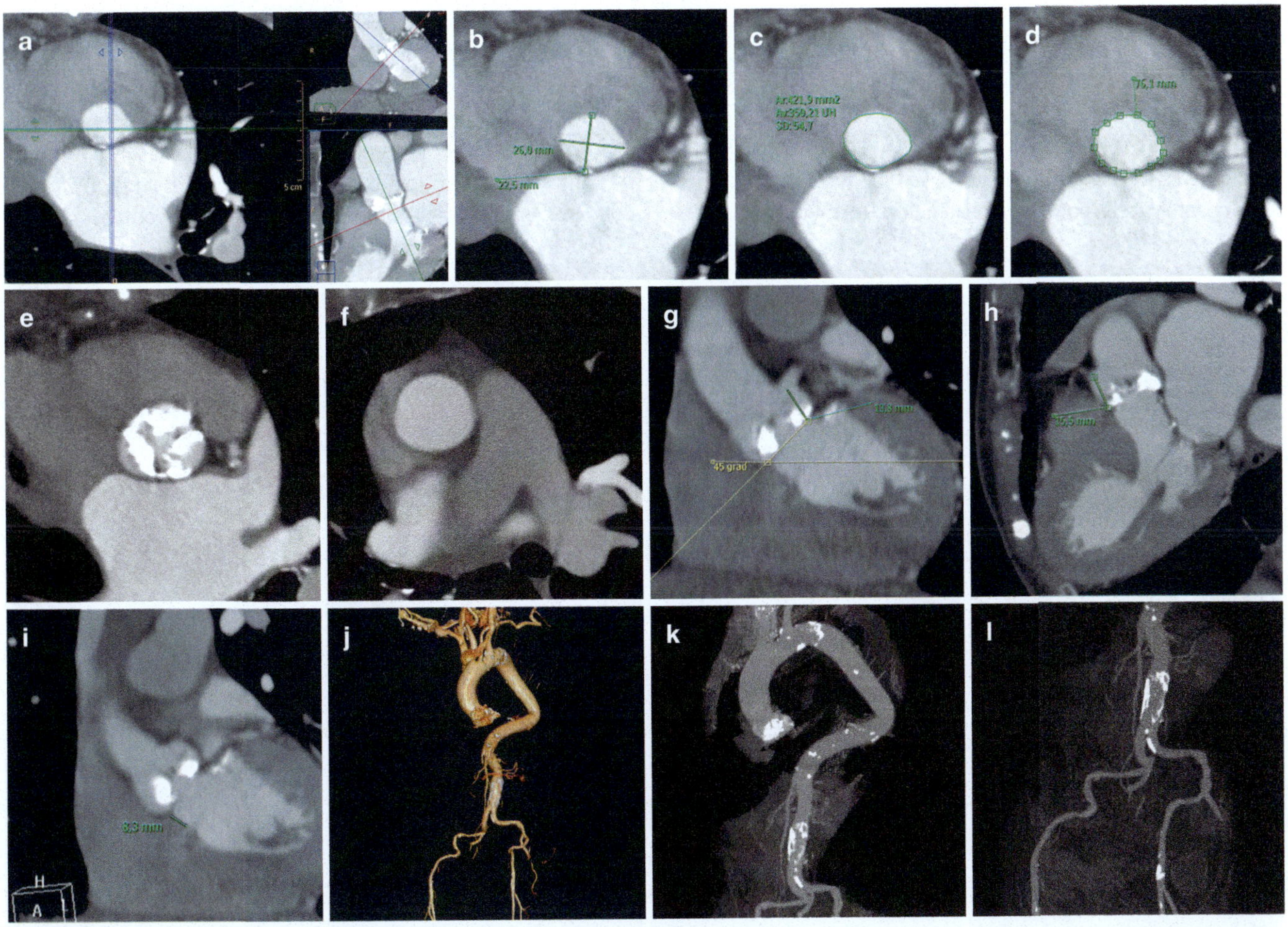

Fig. 5.1 This figure briefly describes the key measurements and findings that should be explored in patients undergoing cardiac CT as preoperatory evaluation of TAVR. Panel **A** shows how to obtain the aortic annulus orthogonal view that accurately corresponds to the insertion points of the valve cusps. Oblique coronal and sagittal multiplanar reformats are used for this purpose, as shown in the right side of panel **A**. Once the aortic annulus is displayed, aortic annulus minimum and maximum diameters (panel **B**), area (panel **C**), and perimeter (panel **D**) are calculated for accurate TAVR sizing. Slightly upward, the aortic valve is shown (panel **E**), and 40 mm further, the ascending aorta is displayed (panel **F**). The distance from the aortic annulus plane to the coronary artery ostia should be addressed, commonly using a coronal oblique plane for the left main (panel **G**, also used for the assessment of the angle between the diaphragm and the aortic annulus plane) and using a sagittal oblique plane for the right coronary artery (panel **H**). The length of the membranous septum is measured using an oblique coronal plane (panel **I**). Finally, the presence of significant aortic and iliofemoral tortuosity and atherosclerotic disease (panels **J**–**L**), as well as sizing of the common femoral and subclavian arteries, should be included in the report

institutions CT is the preferred one as it is fast, reproducible, and accurate and obtains all the information in a single examination.

Further Reading

Achenbach S, Delgado V, Hausleiter J, Schoenhagen P, Min JK, Leipsic JA. SCCT expert consensus document on computed tomography imaging before transcatheter aortic valve implantation (TAVI)/transcatheter aortic valve replacement (TAVR). J Cardiovasc Comput Tomogr. 2012;6(6):366–80.

Doherty JU, Kort S, Mehran R, Schoenhagen P, Soman P. ACC/AATS/AHA/ASE/ASNC/HRS/SCAI/SCCT/SCMR/STS 2017 Appropriate Use Criteria for Multimodality Imaging in Valvular Heart Disease: A Report of the American College of Cardiology Appropriate Use Criteria Task Force, American Association for Thoracic Surgery, American Heart Association, American Society of Echocardiography, American Society of Nuclear Cardiology, Heart Rhythm Society, Society for Cardiovascular Angiography and Interventions, Society of Cardiovascular Computed Tomography, Society for Cardiovascular Magnetic Resonance, and Society of Thoracic Surgeons. J Am Coll Cardiol. 2017;70(13):1647–72.

Case 87

Aortic Valve Stenosis

Clinical History

- Eighty-six-year-old female.
- Coronary risk factors: hypertension, former smoker.
- She has exertional dyspnea (New York Heart Association functional class III).
- Doppler echocardiography revealed a moderate aortic stenosis and a previous myocardial infarction.
- Referred for computed tomography coronary angiography (CTCA) to evaluate coronary and aortic valve anatomy as part of possible aortic valve replacement.

Images

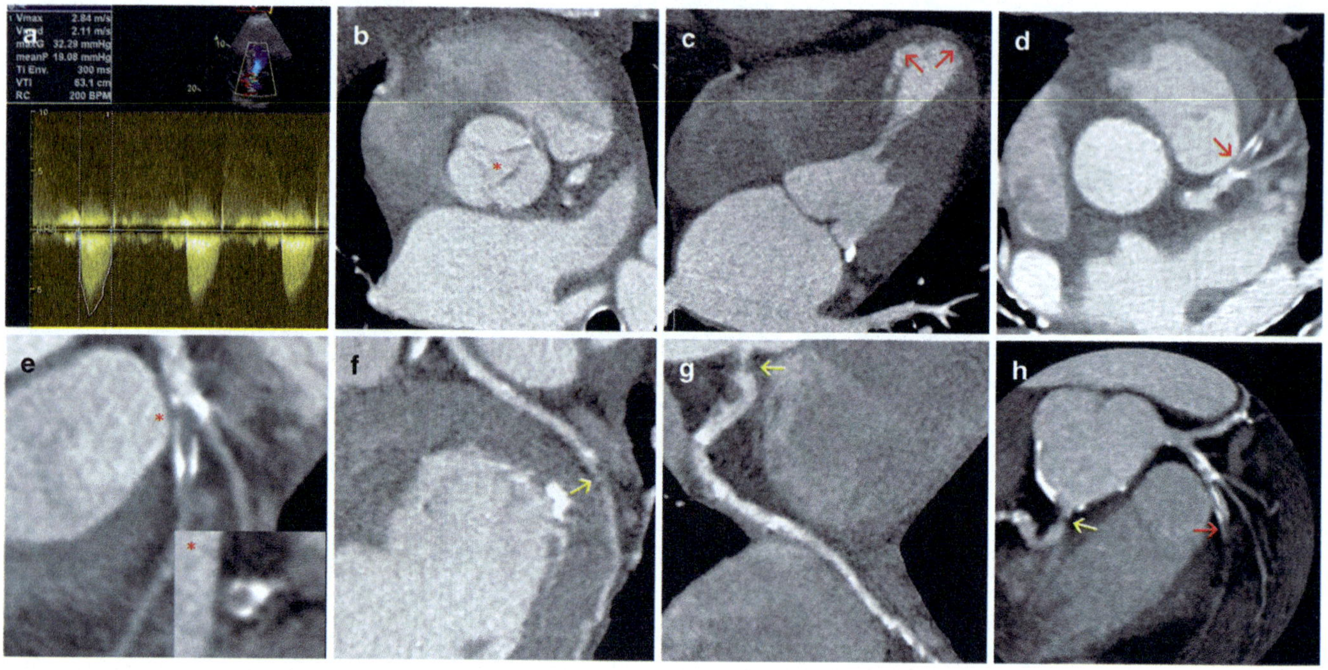

Findings and Interpretation

- Doppler echocardiogram (panel A) demonstrated moderate aortic stenosis (peak velocity 2.84 m/s; effective aortic orifice 1.15 cm^2). Left ventricular ejection fraction was 46%.
- CTCA allows an accurate assessment of non-coronary structures. In this case, a systolic orthogonal view of the aortic valve identified a moderate aortic valve stenosis (asterisk, in panel B), with an aortic valve area (planimetry) of 1.33 cm^2. Of note, only minimal aortic valve calcification was identified.
- In addition, a systolic four-chamber view was obtained to demonstrate an apical myocardial infarction (red arrows in panel C).
- The left anterior descending artery was totally occluded immediately after the takeoff of the first diagonal branch (panel D, arrow). The total occlusion had a short length with distal recanalization (panel E), and the entry site showed only peripheral calcification, clearly depicted using an orthogonal view (lower right quadrant in panel E).
- The left circumflex artery had a severe focal lesion at the distal segment (yellow arrow in panel F), whereas the right coronary artery had a tight focal lesion at the proximal segment (yellow arrows in panels G and H).
- This case shows that CTCA can be very useful to define treatment strategies in patients scheduled for potential valve surgery. In this patient, exertional dyspnea, initially mostly attributed to low-gradient aortic stenosis, turned out to be related to three-vessel disease.

Further Reading

Opolski MP, Staruch AD, Jakubczyk M, et al. CT angiography for the detection of coronary artery stenoses in patients referred for cardiac valve surgery systematic review and meta-analysis. J Am Coll Cardiol Img 2016;9:1059–70.

Case 88

Aortic Valve Stenosis

Clinical History

- Sixty-six-year-old male.
- Presented with severe, symptomatic aortic stenosis.
- Referred for non-contrast cardiac magnetic resonance (CMR) to evaluate aortic valve and annulus anatomy in order to plan surgical strategy.

Images

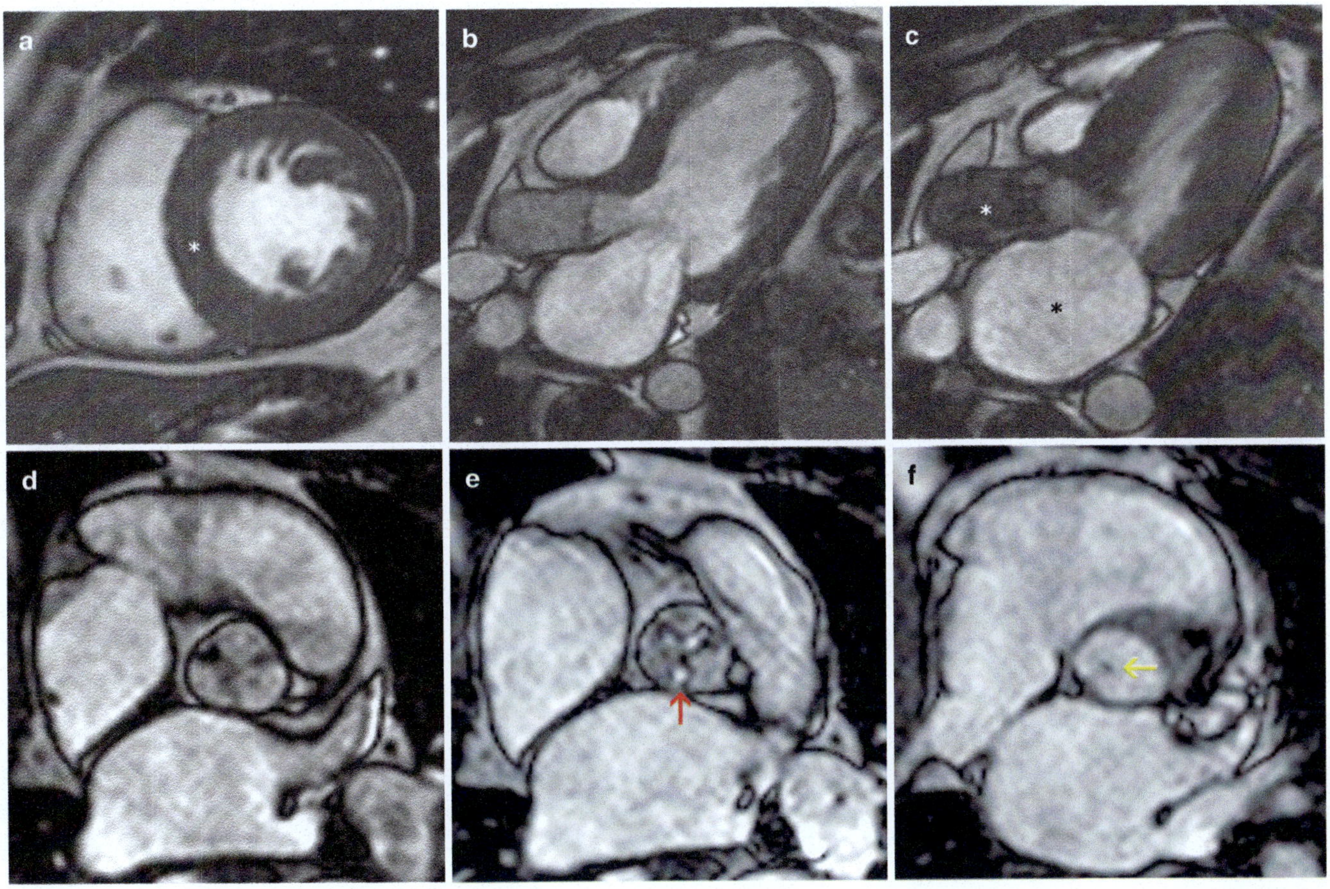

Findings and Interpretation

- End-diastolic cine short-axis view (panel A) showed normal left ventricular (LV) dimensions, with LV hypertrophy mainly involving the septal wall (asterisk).
- End-diastolic (panel B) and end-systolic (panel C) LV outflow tract views demonstrated marked signal void (surrogate of a high-velocity jet) immediately after the aortic valve (white asterisk) and a dilated left atrium (black asterisk).
- Orthogonal planes at the aortic valve (diastole, panel D; systole, panel E) enabled an accurate evaluation of the aortic valve (three cusps, degenerative, possibly with moderate calcification) and measurement of the valve area planimetry (0.78 cm^2).
- Using a lower orthogonal plane at the aortic annulus level (panel F), measurement of the aortic annulus diameters, area, and perimeter aid a correct sizing of the prosthetic valve. Mild aortic regurgitation is identi-

fied as a thin diastolic signal void (yellow arrow in panel F).
- This case shows how CMR enables accurate evaluation of patients with aortic valve disease even without the need of contrast. This might be useful among patients with poor echocardiographic window, as well as in those with renal failure.

Further Reading

Chambers JB, Myerson SG, Rajani R, Morgan-Hughes GJ, Dweck MR. Multimodality imaging in heart valve disease. Open Heart. 2016;3:e000330.

Case 89

Aortic Valve Stenosis

Clinical History

- Fifty-year-old male.
- Asymptomatic, with previous aortic valve replacement (biologic prosthesis) due to bicuspid valve disease.
- Referred for surveillance non-contrast cardiac magnetic resonance.

Images

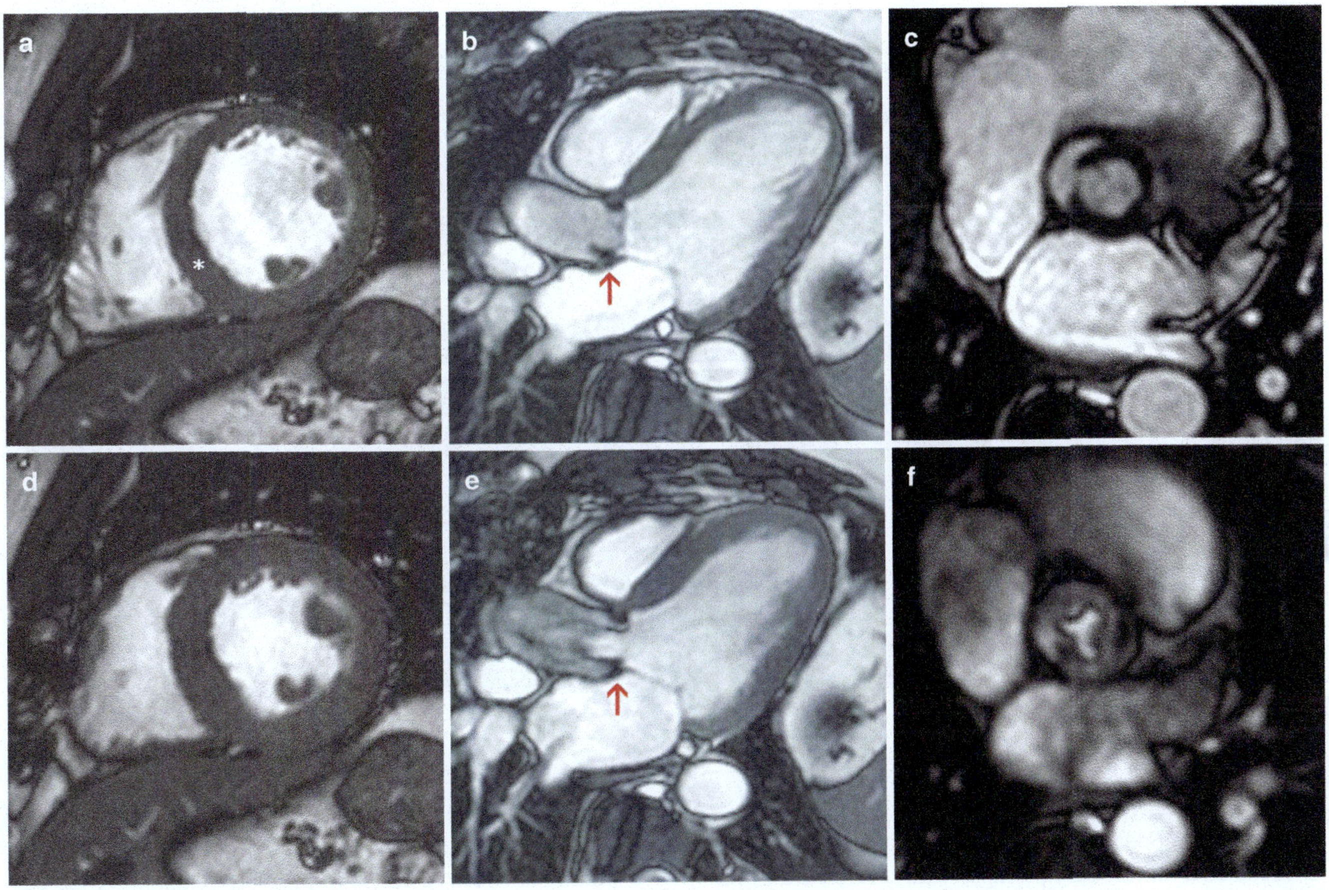

Findings and Interpretation

- End-diastolic (panel A) and end-systolic (panel D) cine short-axis views showed a dilated left ventricle (LV) and mild septal hypertrophy (asterisk).
- Using end-diastolic (panel B) and end-systolic (panel E) LV outflow tract views, the biologic prosthetic aortic valve is displayed (red arrow), with preserved opening and without evidence of regurgitation and/or periannular complications. Slightly increased transvalvular velocity is detected as a subtle distal signal void (panel E).
- Orthogonal planes at the aortic valve (diastole, panel C; systole, panel F) enabled an accurate evaluation of the aortic valve prosthesis, with normal thin valves and a small effective orifice area (1.25 cm^2).
- Patient-prosthesis mismatch refers to the presence of prosthetic valve with normal function but with an effective orifice area smaller than expected.

Further Reading

Chambers JB, Myerson SG, Rajani R, Morgan-Hughes GJ, Dweck MR. Multimodality imaging in heart valve disease. Open Heart. 2016;3:e000330.

Case 90

Mitral Valve Regurgitation

Clinical History

- Fifty-five-year-old male.
- Without coronary risk factors.
- He has palpitations and exertional dyspnea.
- Doppler echocardiography revealed mitral valve prolapse with severe regurgitation and a pulmonary artery systolic pressure of 38 mmHg.
- Referred for cardiac magnetic resonance (CMR) for further assessment.

Images

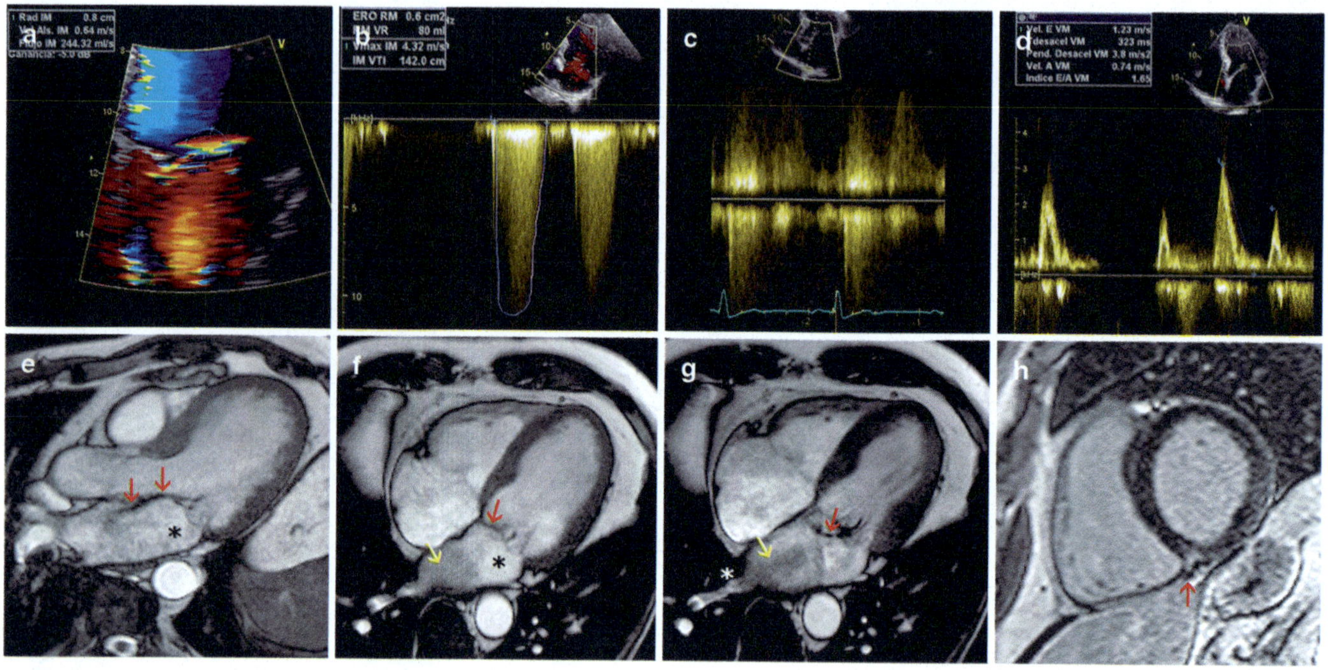

Findings and Interpretation

- Doppler echocardiographic findings (panels A to D) revealed a mitral valve prolapse with severe regurgitation. The regurgitating jet is eccentric and originated from the posterior valve (panel A), directed to the interatrial septum. The calculated effective regurgitant orifice area (panel B) was 0.6 cm^2 (severe regurgitation if larger than 0.4 cm^2). The identification of systolic pulmonary vein flow reversal (panel C) reinforces the severity of the regurgitating volume, as does the presence of a sharp and high-velocity early diastolic filling E wave (panel D).
- Cine CMR images (panels E to H). Systolic left ventricular outflow tract (panel E) and four-chamber (panels F and G) views demonstrated prolapse of the posterior mitral valve (asterisk in panels E and F), an eccentric regurgitating jet (red arrows) directed to the interatrial septum and adhered to the anterior mitral valve (Coanda effect phenomena).
- The regurgitating jet reaches the posterior wall of the left atrium (yellow arrow in panel G) and the inferior right pulmonary vein (asterisk in panel G), explaining the pulmonary vein flow reversal.
- At inversion-recovery imaging (panel H), subepicardial late gadolinium enhancement was identified at the insertion sites of the right ventricle over the septal wall (arrow), reflecting right ventricular pressure overload.
- Dilatation of the left atrium (31 cm^2) and the left ventricle (113 ml/m^2) were also noted, with preserved systolic function.
- Mitral valve prolapse is relatively common (approximately 2% of the population) and one of the main causes of primary mitral valve regurgitation requiring surgery. Mitral valve prolapse is also commonly associated with pulmonary artery hypertension. Indeed, pulmonary artery hypertension (particularly if larger than 50 mmHg) is a predictor of worse clinical outcome after valve repair.

Further Reading

Chambers JB, Myerson SG, Rajani R, Morgan-Hughes GJ, Dweck MR. Multimodality imaging in heart valve disease. Open Heart. 2016;3(1):e000330.

Parwani P, Avierinos JF, Levine RA, Delling FN. Mitral Valve Prolapse: Multimodality Imaging and Genetic Insights. Prog Cardiovasc Dis. 2017;60:361–369.

ung MH, Jung HO, Kim MJ, Lee JW, Youn HJ. Impact of prolapsing leaflet location on exercise pulmonary hypertension in mitral regurgitation. Eur Heart J Cardiovasc Imaging. 2017;18:576–583.

Wang J, Han J, Li Y, Xu C, Jiao Y, Yang B, et al. Preoperative risk factors of medium-term mitral valve repair outcome. Interact Cardiovasc Thorac Surg. 2014;19:946–54.

Case 91

Prosthetic Valves and Endovascular Aortic Repair

Clinical History

- Seventy-seven-year-old female.
- She has a history of aortic dissection treated with Bentall procedure with a prosthetic aortic tube and aortic valve replacement with a stented biological valve, plus thoracic endovascular aortic repair (TEVAR).
- Doppler echocardiography revealed a high transvalvular gradient (peak gradient 43 mmHg, mean gradient 24 mmHg) that seemed to be related to patient-valve mismatch. Also, moderate mitral and tricuspid regurgitation were detected, with a systolic pulmonary artery pressure of 55 mmHg.
- Referred for cardiac magnetic resonance (CMR) for further evaluation.

Images

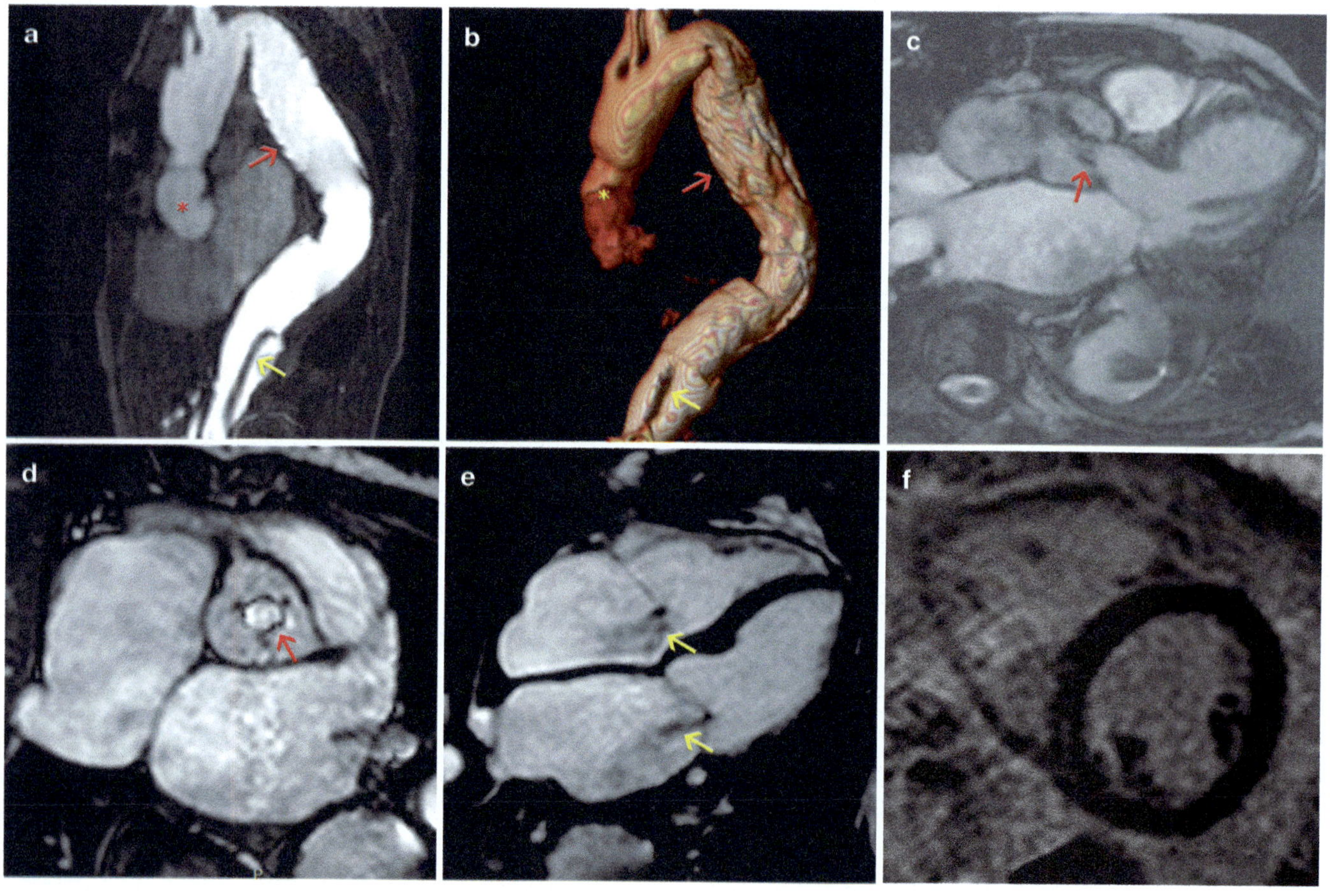

Findings and Interpretation

- Aortic angiogram shows the TEVAR endoprosthesis (red arrows in panels A and B) immediately distal to the left subclavian artery takeoff, without evidence of periprosthetic leak (panel A, maximum intensity projection; panel B, volume rendering). Persisting aortic dissection is detected distal to the endoprosthesis (yellow arrows in panels A and B).
- Also, a prosthetic aortic tube is observed (* in panels A and B).
- Using a systolic left ventricular outflow tract view (panel C), aortic valve opening is preserved though with a transvalvular systolic flow void suggestive of gradient of acceleration (red arrow). A phase-encoding sequence demonstrated a peak gradient of 29 mmHg.
- An orthogonal systolic view at the aortic valve level (panel D) demonstrated a preserved aortic valve opening, though with an effective valve area (using planimetry) of 0.99 cm^2 (0.71 cm/m^2).

- Four-chamber view (panel E) shows moderate mitral and tricuspid regurgitation (yellow arrows), related to annulus dilatation, as well as moderate left atrial dilatation (34 cm^2) and mild to moderate right atrial dilatation (27 cm^2).
- Ventricular size and systolic function were normal.
- Inversion recovery images (panel F) showed absence of myocardial late gadolinium enhancement.
- Patient-prosthesis mismatch, a concept referred to the presence of an effective orifice area smaller than expected for the body surface area, has been related to higher mortality rates.
- In parallel, the absence of late gadolinium enhancement rules out the presence of significant pulmonary artery hypertension.

Further Reading

Head SJ, Mokhles MM, Osnabrugge RLJ, et al. The impact of prosthesis–patient mismatch on long-term survival after aortic valve replacement: a systematic review and meta-analysis of 34 observational studies comprising 27186 patients with 133141 patient-years. Eur Heart J. 2012;33:1518–29.

Case 92

Transcatheter Aortic Valve Replacement (TAVR)

Clinical History

- Seventy-one-year-old female, with severe aortic stenosis scheduled for TAVR.
- Referred for gated computed tomography angiography (CTA) due to moderate to severe paravalvular aortic regurgitation.
- Pre-procedural and follow-up (6-month) CTA were performed.

Images

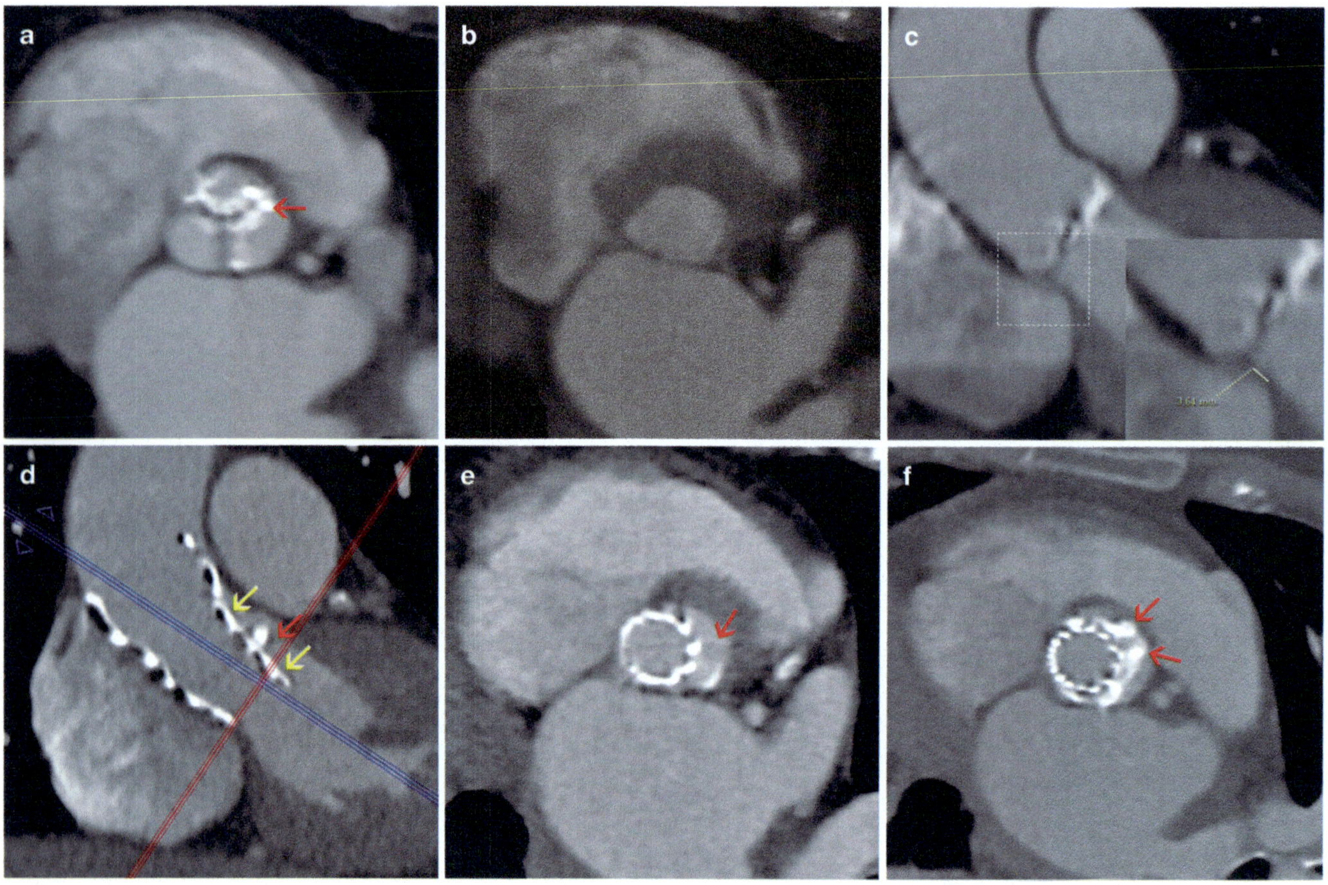

Findings and Interpretation

- Pre-procedural gated CTA (panels A–C) showed moderate but asymmetric calcification of the aortic valve cusps, predominantly involving the anterior-left commissure. The aortic annulus did not show calcifications (panel B).
- Using a coronal view (panel C), the presence of a short membranous septum (3.6 mm) is depicted.
- Follow-up CTA confirmed a suboptimal position of the device (panel D), including underexpansion (yellow arrows) and too high inflow position (red line). These could to be related to dense asymmetric calcification of the displaced commissure. Orthogonal views at the aortic annulus (panel E) and at the displaced cusps (panel F) revealed an incomplete apposition (arrow in panel E) related to the asymmetric calcification (arrows in panel F).
- In this case, the high position of the device might have been motivated by the likelihood of atrioventricular block among patients with a short (<6 mm) membranous septum length (the membranous septum length is a surrogate of the distance between the aortic annulus and the exit point of the bundle of His).

- The combination of a high position and asymmetric calcification resulted in underexpansion, incomplete circumferential apposition, and significant paravalvular aortic regurgitation. More than mild paravalvular aortic regurgitation greatly increases morbidity and mortality among patients with TAVR.

Further Reading

Blanke P, Schoepf UJ, Leipsic JA. CT in transcatheter aortic valve replacement. Radiology. 2013;269:650–69.

Hamdan A, Guetta V, Klempfner R, et al. Inverse relationship between membranous septal length and the risk of atrioventricular block in patients undergoing transcatheter aortic valve implantation. J Am Coll Cardiol Intv 2015;8:1218–28.

Sinning JM, Vasa-Nicotera M, Chin D, et al. Evaluation and management of paravalvular aortic regurgitation after transcatheter aortic valve replacement. J Am Coll Cardiol 2013;62:11–20.

Case 93

Transcatheter Aortic Valve Replacement (TAVR)

Clinical History

- Eighty-one year-old woman.
- History of hypertension and hyperlipidemia.
- Dyspnea and angina in the last 3 months, with no significant coronary artery lesions.
- Echocardiography showed a calcified aortic valve with peak gradient of 101 mmHg, mean gradient 71 mmHg, valve area 0.49 cm^2, and normal left ventricular systolic function.
- A computed tomography for TAVR planning was performed.

Images

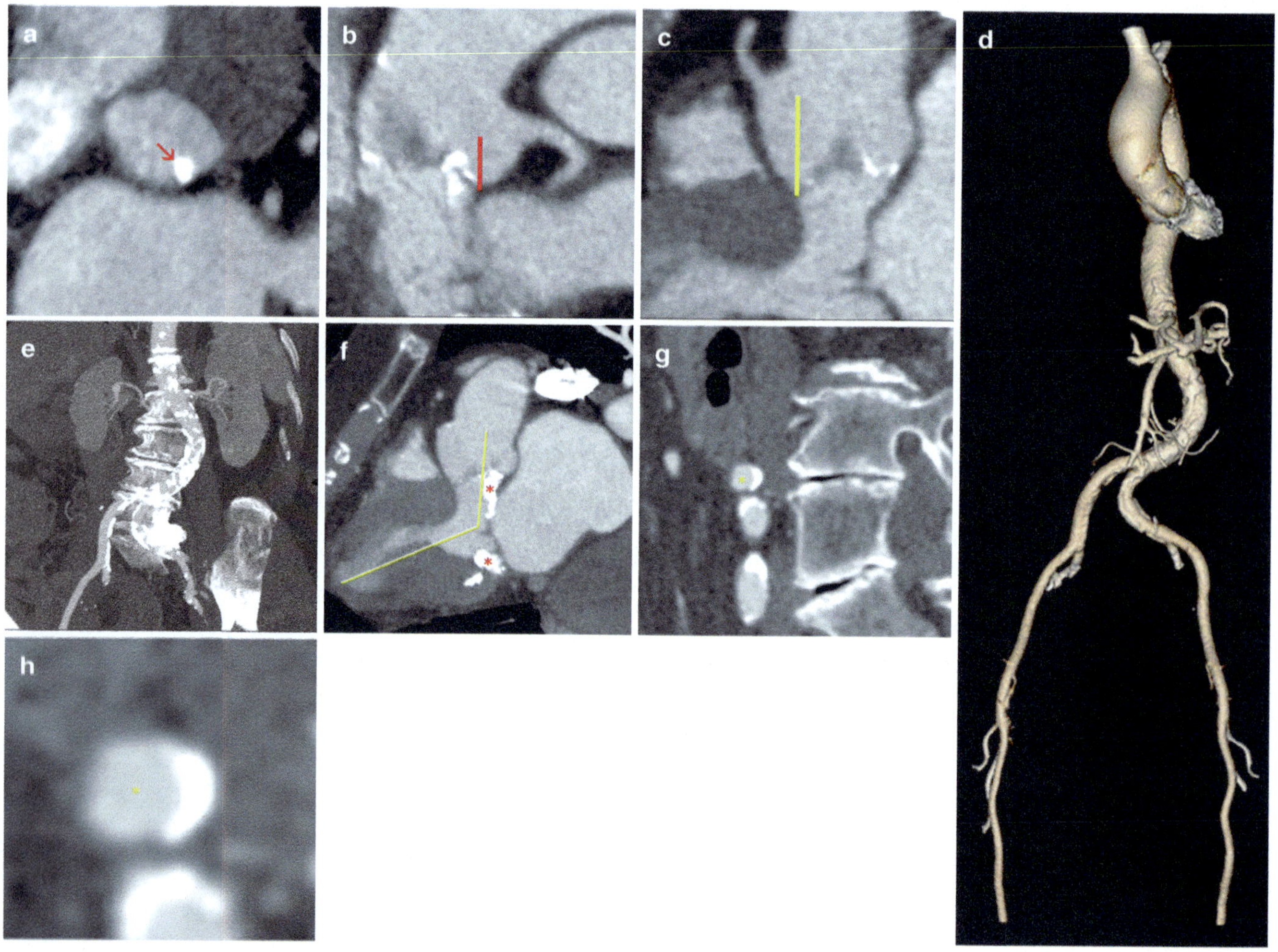

Findings and Interpretation

- Aortic annulus with oval morphology (orthogonal view, panel A) and a calcified nodule protruding to the cavity and extending to the left ventricular outflow tract. The presence of calcium protruding to the lumen >25% is a risk factor for paravalvular regurgitation after TAVR, as percutaneous prosthesis can remain unexpanded and/or not sealed to the annulus at this level. Eccentricity index (relation between major and minor axis of the annulus) is another risk factor related to paravalvular leak.
- Distance of the aortic annular plane to the coronary ostia: left (panel B) and right (panel C) coronary arteries are shown. Height of the left coronary ostia is approximately

10.5 mm. Risk of coronary occlusion (higher with Edwards valves) is high under 10 mm, and care should be taken between 10 and 12 mm (depending on prosthesis type and size and leaflet length and calcification). Right coronary artery height was nearly 21 mm, with low risk of coronary occlusion.

- Tortuous abdominal aorta (panel D, volume rendered; panel E, coronal view) results in more difficult vascular access and higher risk of vascular injury. Under this condition a transapical access was evaluated, but the angle between left ventricular apex and left ventricular outflow tract (Fig. F, yellow lines) was considered unfavorable. Calcification of the annulus with extension to the left ventricular outflow tract and calcification of the mitral annulus are clearly seen (red asterisks in panel F).
- Under this situation, and with an appropriate diameter and anatomy of right femoral and iliac arteries (yellow asterisks, panels G and H), the final decision was to perform a transfemoral approach.

Further Reading

Achenbach S, Delgado V, Hausleiter J, et al. SCCT expert consensus document on computed tomography imaging before transcatheter aortic valve implantation (TAVI)/transcatheter aortic valve replacement (TAVR). J Cardiovasc Comput Tomogr 2012;6:366–80.

Condado J, Corrigan F, Lerakis S, et al. Anatomical risk models for paravalvular leak and landing zone complications for balloon-expandable transcatheter aortic valve replacement. Catheter Cardiovasc Interv 2017;90:690–700.

Jilaihawi H, Makkar R, Kashif M, et al. A revised methodology for aortic-valvar complex calcium quantification for transcatheter aortic valve implantation. Eur Heart J Cardiovasc Imaging 2014;15:1324–32.

Kaneko H, Hoelschermann F, Tambor G, et al. Predictors of Paravalvular Regurgitation After Transcatheter Aortic Valve Implantation for Aortic Stenosis Using New-Generation Balloon-Expandable SAPIEN 3. Am J Cardiol. 2017;119:618–22.

Case 94

Transcatheter Aortic Valve Replacement (TAVR)

Clinical History

- Ninety-two-year-old male.
- Previous aortic valve replacement with biological prosthesis.
- History of dyspnea and dizziness, with an episode of loss of consciousness.
- Transthoracic echocardiography revealed high gradients, with findings suggestive of degenerative process of the surgical prosthesis.
- A TAVR procedure was performed with a valve-in-valve technique with low final gradients in the percutaneous aortic prosthesis (peak 22 mmHg, mean 11 mmHg).
- One month after the procedure, the patient referred dizziness episodes; a new transthoracic echocardiogram revealed high gradients in the percutaneous prosthesis (peak 76 mmHg, mean 48 mmHg), and transesophageal echocardiography showed thickened valves with reduced motion.

Images

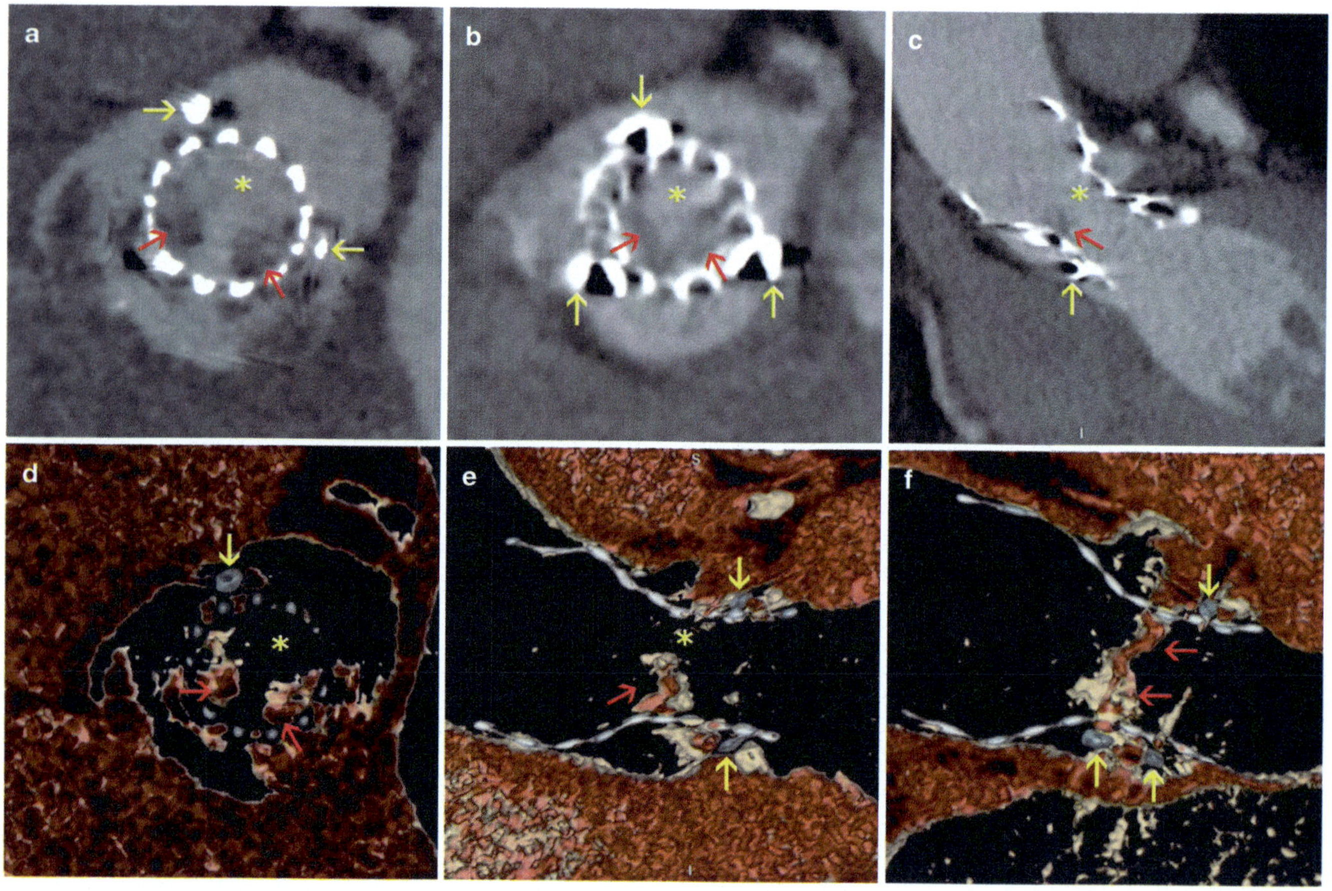

Findings and Interpretation

- Retrospective gated computed tomography (CT), aimed at reconstruction of the whole cardiac cycle.
- Axial images (panel A, diastole; panel B, systole) and coronal (panel C, systole) of the aortic prosthesis showing two of the three leaflets thickened, with a dense low-attenuated mass attached (red arrows), signs suggestive of thrombus. The third leaflet (yellow asterisk) is barely visible, a normal finding as this leaflet is not compromised by thrombus.

- The structure of the previous surgical prosthesis is visible outside the stent (yellow arrows).
- Volume rendering images (panels D–F) of the percutaneous prosthesis in diastole. In the orthogonal view (panel D), two leaflets are thickened by a mass (red arrows), while the third one is undetectable (yellow asterisk). In the coronal (panel E) and sagittal views (panel F), the mass is clearly seen attached to a thickened leaflet (red arrows). There is a free space corresponding to the non-affected leaflet (panel E, yellow asterisk). The previous surgical prosthesis is clearly seen outside the lower portion of the stent (yellow arrows).
- The combination of a soft tissue compromising the leaflets, a phenomenon called hypoattenuated leaflet thickening (HALT), with reduced leaflet motion (phenomena called RELM), is the hallmark for diagnosis of TAVR valve thrombosis in CT studies.

Further Reading

Jilaihawi H, Asch F, Manasse E, et al. Systematic CT Methodology for the Evaluation of Subclinical Leaflet Thrombosis. JACC Cardiovasc Imaging 2017;10:461–70.

Leetmaa T, Hansson N, Leipsic J, et al. Early aortic transcatheter heart valve thrombosis: diagnostic value of contrast-enhanced multidetector computed tomography. Circ Cardiovasc Interv. 2015;8:e001596.

Makkar RR, Fontana G, Jilaihawi H, et al. Possible Subclinical Leaflet Thrombosis in Bioprosthetic Aortic Valves. N Engl J Med. 2015;373:2015–24.

Soschynski M, Capilli F, Ruile P, et al. Post-TAVI Follow-Up with MDCT of the Valve Prosthesis: Technical Application, Regular Findings and Typical Local Post-Interventional Complications. Rofo. 2018;190:521–30.

Testa L, Latib A. Assessing the Risk of Leaflet Motion Abnormality Following Transcatheter Aortic Valve Implantation. Interv Cardiol. 2018;13:37–9.

Case 95

Transcatheter Aortic Valve Replacement (TAVR)

Clinical History

- Eighty-one-year-old female.
- Coronary risk factors: hypertension.
- History of long-standing atrial fibrillation treated with oral anticoagulant therapy.
- Shortness of breath, long-standing aortic stenosis.
- Doppler echocardiography showed calcified aortic valve, peak gradient 88 mmHg, mean gradient 54 mmHg, and aortic valve area 0.8 cm^2. Left ventricular ejection fraction 74%.
- Referred for computed tomography for TAVR planning.

Images

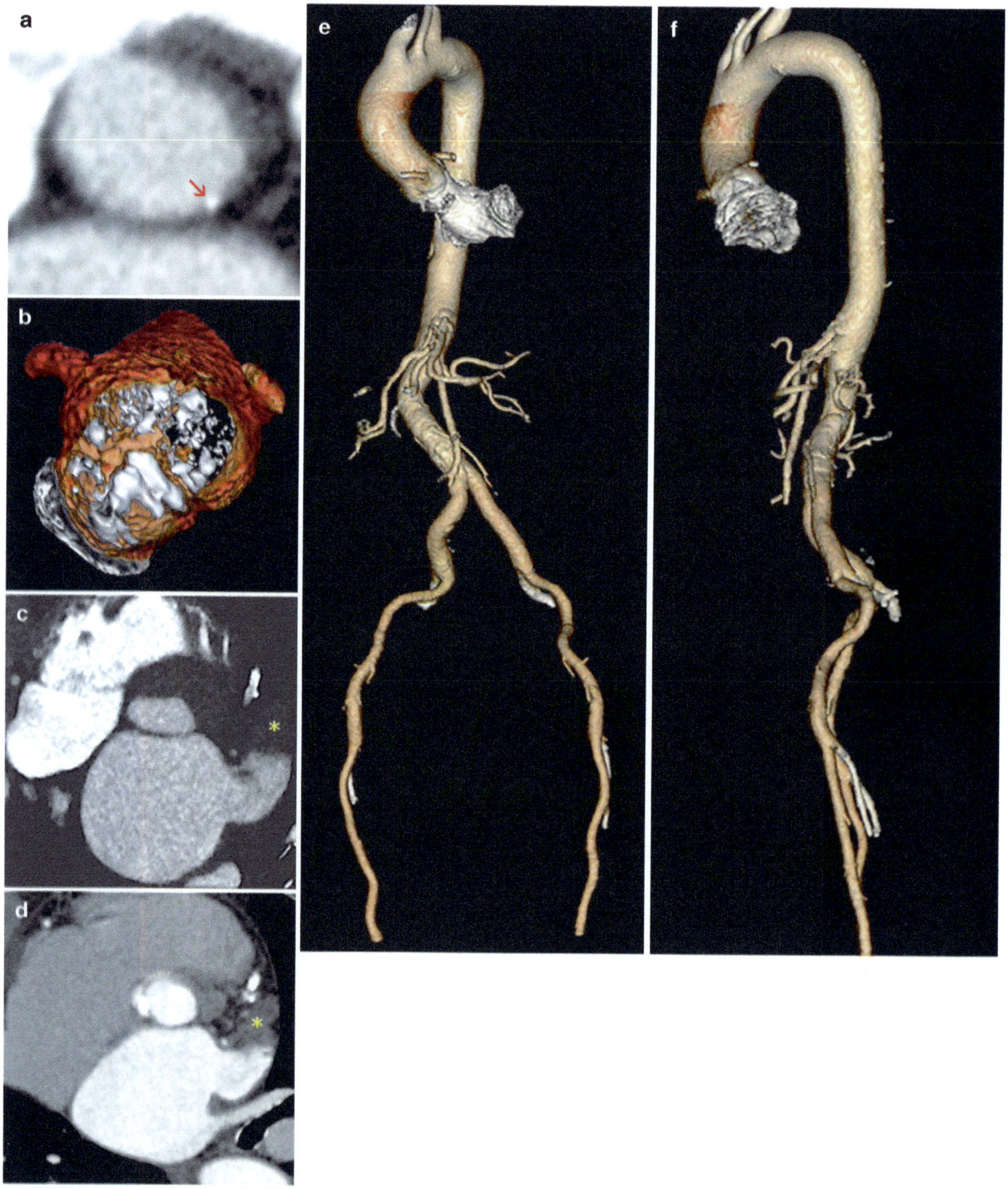

Findings and Interpretation

- Orthogonal view of the aortic annulus with a small spot of calcium down the left coronary sinus (panel A).
- Volume rendering of the aortic valve (panel B), showing a tricuspid, heavily calcified aortic valve, a common finding in degenerative aortic stenosis. In this case, asymmetric calcification of the leaflets predisposes to paravalvular leak: the non-coronary leaflet (NC) shows more amount of calcium than the right (RC) and left (LC) coronary leaflets.
- Presence of a filling defect within the left atrial appendage detected at different timepoints (panels C and D), suggesting thrombus (yellow asterisks). The presence of left atrial thrombus in this population is a frequent finding (up to 10% in selected cases) and can be detected with high accuracy with cardiac computed tomography.
- Volume rendered images (panels E and F) of thoracic and abdominal aorta showing appropriate vascular access, without significant tortuosity or vascular disease, favorable for transfemoral approach.

Further Reading

Lenders G, Paelinck B, Wouters K, et al. Transesophageal echocardiography for cardiac thromboembolic risk assessment in patients with severe, symptomatic aortic valve stenosis referred for potential transcatheter aortic valve implantation. Am J Cardiol 2013;111:1470–74.

Pathan F, Hecht H, Narula J, et al. Roles of transesophageal echocardiography and cardiac computed tomography for evaluation of left atrial thrombus and associated pathology. J Am Coll Cardiol Img 2018;11:616–27.

Case 96

Transcatheter Aortic Valve Replacement (TAVR)

Clinical History

- Eighty-eight-year-old man.
- History of hypertension, type II diabetes mellitus, and hyperlipidemia.
- Previous revascularization with percutaneous coronary angioplasty (drug eluting stent to left anterior descending coronary artery).
- Dyspnea in the last 9 months, coronary angiography without significant coronary lesions.
- Echocardiographic evaluation showed aortic stenosis with calcified aortic valve, peak gradient 91 mmHg, mean gradient 44 mmHg, valve area 0.64 cm^2, and normal left ventricular systolic function.
- A computed tomography for TAVR planning was performed.

Images

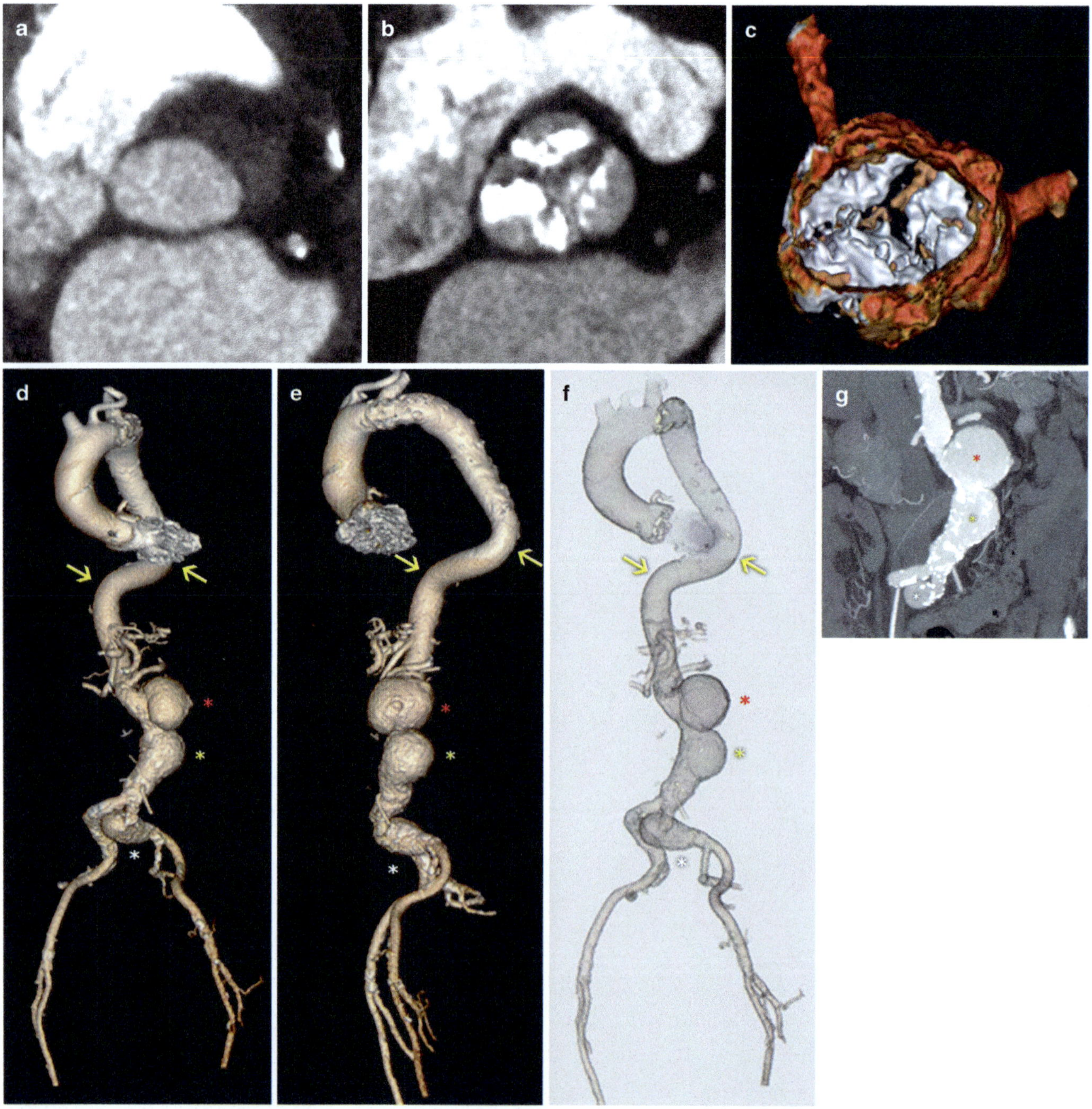

Findings and Interpretation

- Oval annulus without calcification (panel A). This is a common finding: aortic annulus is usually oval. The long and short diameter, area, and circumference should be measured as prostheses are selected according to these measurements. The absence of calcification at the level of the annulus is a favorable finding, as it reduces the risk of paravalvular regurgitation.
- Heavily calcified tricuspid aortic valve (panels B and C). It is important to define valve anatomy, presence, and severity of calcification, as it has been related to paravalvular leak and risk of coronary occlusion after implantation.
- A tortuous, markedly angulated thoracic aorta was found (volume rendered images, panels D–F). The presence of acute angles (yellow arrows) makes navigation difficult and exposes to vascular injury.
- The presence of aneurysms in the abdominal aorta is another negative finding in this patient (volume rendered images, panels D–F; coronal view, panel G): a saccular infrarenal aortic aneurysm (red asterisk), followed by a second fusiform aneurysm (yellow asterisk) and an aneurysm in the left common iliac artery (white asterisk), increases the risk of vascular complications. The presence of aneurysmatic and tortuous aorta made this patient unsuitable for transfemoral access (the preferable access). A transapical approach was selected.

Further Reading

Achenbach S, Delgado V, Hausleiter J, et al. SCCT expert consensus document on computed tomography imaging before transcatheter aortic valve implantation (TAVI)/transcatheter aortic valve replacement (TAVR). J Cardiovasc Comput Tomogr 2012;6:366–80.

O'Sullivan C, Stortecky S, Buellesfeld L, et al. Preinterventional screening of the TAVI patient: how to choose the suitable patient and the best procedure. Clin Res Cardiol 2014;103:259–74.

Toggweiler S, Leipsic J, Binder R, et al. Management of vascular access in transcatheter aortic valve replacement: part 1: basic anatomy, imaging, sheaths, wires, and access routes. JACC Cardiovasc Interv 2013;6:643–53.

Case 97

Pulmonary Veins: Normal Variants

Clinical History

- Forty-eight-year-old male.
- Symptomatic (palpitations and poor exercise tolerance) paroxysmal atrial fibrillation, with no response to adequate medical treatment.
- Referred to cardiac computed tomography (CT) for left atrium (LA) and pulmonary veins (PVs) evaluation before the ablation procedure.

Images

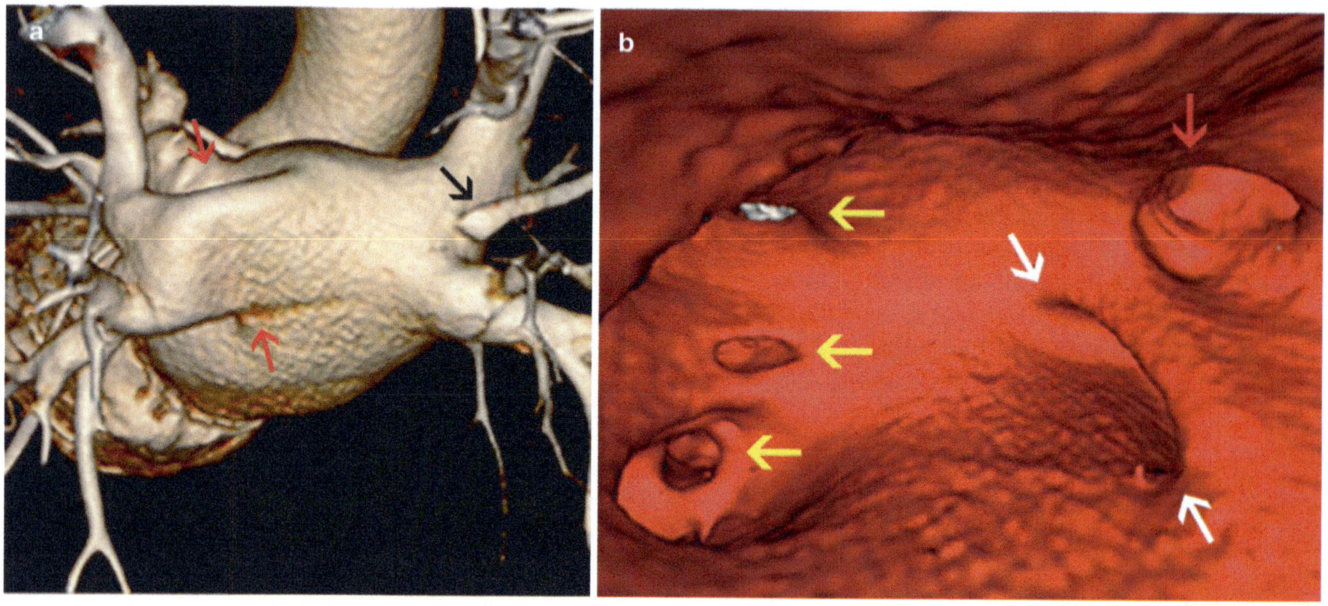

Findings and Interpretation

- Three-dimensional volume rendering CT image of posterior aspect of the LA (panel A) shows variant anatomy including a right accessory mid PV (black arrow) and common trunk of left-sided PVs, defined as joint ostia of superior and inferior PVs of >5 mm, before entering left atrium (red arrows).
- Endoluminal CT view of LA (panel B) shows three distinct right-sided pulmonary venous ostia (yellow arrows), common trunk of left-sided pulmonary veins (white arrows), and left atrial appendage ostium (red arrow).
- Most patients have four PVs, two superior and two inferior with independent ostia draining separately into the LA; this normal arrangement is found in 56–81% of the general population.
- A number of variations have been described in the literature, the commonest of which are left common ostium (up to 30% of patients) and a separate origin for the right middle PV (up to 27% of patients). A single ostium on the left side is larger than the most circular mapping catheters; therefore, segmental isolation is sometimes not possible in the presence of this variant. A right mid vein, draining the right mid lobe of the lung, if unrecognized, poses higher risk of trauma during the ablation procedure and later of pulmonary vein stenosis.
- Modification of ablation technique may be required in the presence of a right mid vein, because a *figure-of-eight* ablation is not possible, and the rim of intervening tissue between veins may not be adequate to stably support the ablation catheter. Owing to the smaller ostial diameter, the right middle PV may be overlooked during the ablation procedure, leading to the recurrence of AF or becoming a consistent source of arrhythmogenic ectopy.
- Although prior knowledge of the diameter of the PVs is useful in the sizing of circular mapping catheters, it is essential if balloon-based ablation (cryoablation) catheters are to be used, as a close approximation of the balloon to the PV ostia is required for successful isolation.

Further Reading

Cronin P, Sneider MB, Kazerooni EA, et al. MDCTof the left atrium and pulmonary veins in planning radiofrequency ablation for atrial fibrillation: a how-to-guide. AJR Am J Roentgenol 2004, 183:767–78.

Mansour M, Holmvang G, Sosnovik D, et al. Assessment of pulmonary vein anatomic variability by magnetic resonance imaging: implications for catheter ablation techniques for atrial fibrillation. J Cardiovasc Electrophysiol 2004;15:387–93.

Marom, E. M., Herndon, J. E., Kim, et al. Variations in pulmonary venous drainage to the left atrium: implications for radiofrequency ablation. Radiology 2004;230:824–29.

Sarabanda AV, Bunch TJ, Johnson SB, et al. Efficacy and safety of circumferential pulmonary vein isolation using a novel cryothermal balloon ablation system. J Am Coll Cardiol 2005;46:1902–12.

Scharf, C., Sneider, M., Case, I., et al. Anatomy of the pulmonary veins in patients with atrial fibrillation and effects of segmental ostial ablation analyzed by computed tomography. Jof Cardiovasc Electrophysiol 2003;14:150–5.

Wood MA, Wittkamp M, Henry D, et al. A comparison of pulmonary vein ostial anatomy by computerized tomography, echocardiography, and venography in patients with atrial fibrillation having radiofrequency catheter ablation. Am J Cardiol 2004;93:49–53.

Case 98

Catheter-Based Pulmonary Vein Isolation

Clinical History

- Sixty-four-year-old male.
- History of persistent atrial fibrillation (AF) treated with radiofrequency ablation 3 years ago.
- The patient presents with recurrent AF.
- Referred to cardiac magnetic resonance (CMR) to rule out post-ablation line gaps.

Images

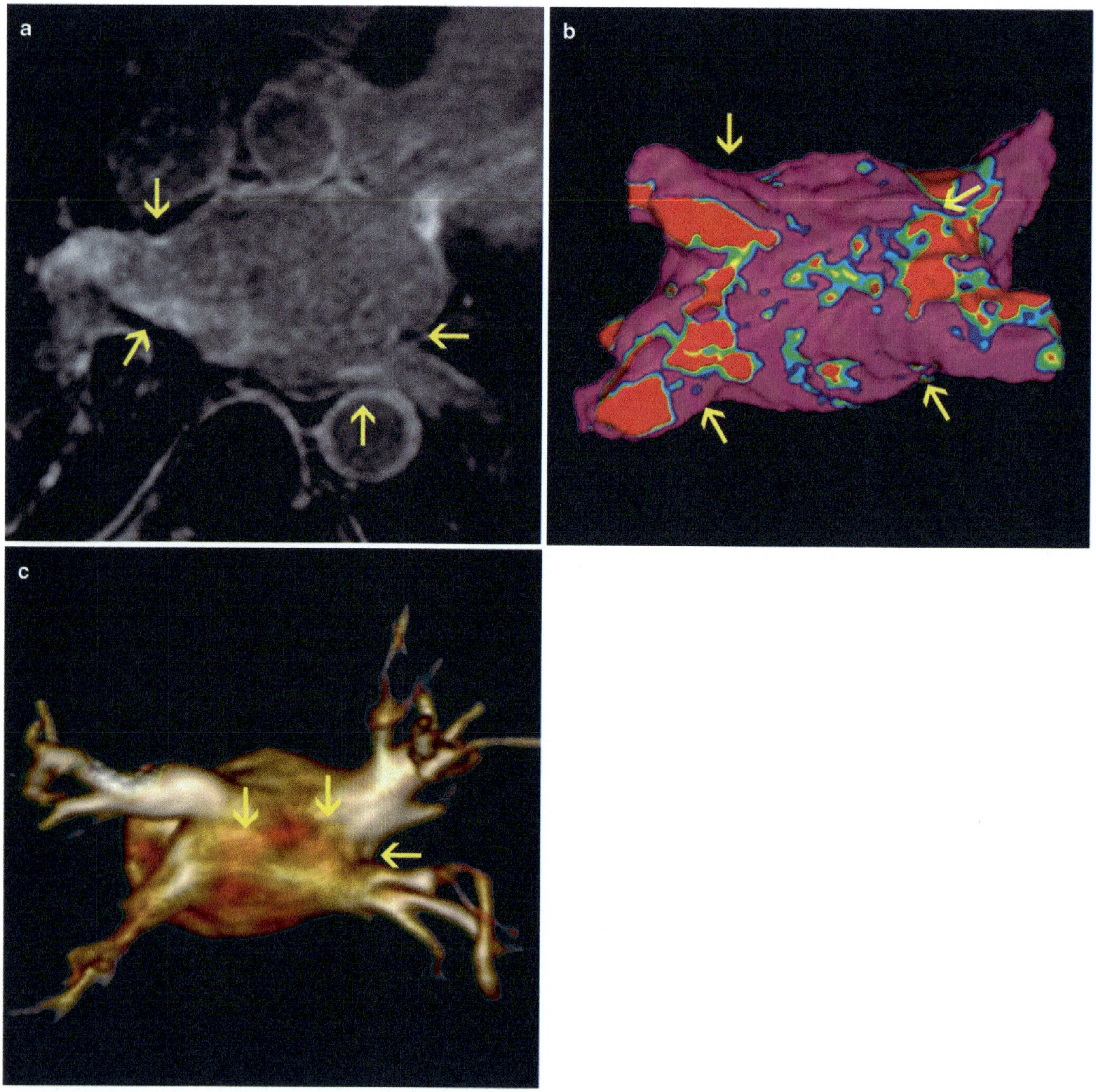

Findings and Interpretation

- Axial plane of a 3D delayed enhancement image (panel A) at the atrial level, showing areas of late gadolinium enhancement (LGE) around the ostium of the pulmonary veins (yellow arrows) that corresponds to the ablation lines.
- In a three-dimensional shell derived from 3D LGE-CMR (panel B), the purple tissue corresponds to normal myocardial tissue and the red tissue to fibrotic ablation lines. Ablation gaps (yellow arrows) can be observed using this 3D delayed enhancement CMR reconstruction.
- Three-dimensional volume rendered image from a 3D CMR angiography of the posterior aspect of left atrium (panel C) shows remodeling around the ostium of the pulmonary veins (mainly the lower ones) with indentation of the contour in the sites of previous ablation (yellow arrows) that correlates with the ablation lines (red tissue in panel B).
- Structural, contractile, or electrical alterations are associated with the onset and the perpetuation of AF. Fibrosis is the hallmark of atrial structural remodeling; it results from an excessive deposition of extracellular matrix to replace degenerating atrial myocytes. Fibrotic tissue can be detected in left atrium of AF patients with identifiable cardiac disease and in lone AF and is one of the major risk factors for AF progression.
- CMR imaging with LGE allows the detection and quantification of fibrotic tissue by slow washout kinetics of gadolinium in diseased tissue. While ventricular fibrosis assessment has achieved excellent results with CMR imaging, the challenge of atrial fibrosis assessment remains open due to limited image resolution and the thinness (1–2 mm) and unpredictable shape of the LA wall. However, several recent studies managed to assess the feasibility of LGE-CMR in detecting both pre-existing and post-ablation-induced atrial fibrosis, showing promising findings. The extent of the baseline LGE has emerged as the strongest independent predictor of AF recurrence after ablation and a good tool for selecting the appropriate patients and procedural strategy.
- With regard to ablation-induced fibrosis, LGE-CMR is a powerful tool to identify LA wall injury caused by radiofrequency energy delivery in the myocardium, to recognize ablation line gaps, and even to guide the ablation procedure, both in animal models and in humans, by integrating the CMR model into the navigation system. Pulmonary vein reconnection is considered the main cause for ablation failure, and discontinuities in previous ablation sets are a common underlying mechanism for resumption of conduction. Recent studies showed that delayed enhancement CMR is a reliable tool to precisely depict gaps in prior ablation and to guide reablation procedures targeting the ablation line gaps.

Further Reading

Badger TJ, Daccarett M, Akoum NW, et al. Evaluation of left atrial lesions after initial and repeat atrial fibrillation ablation: lessons learned from delayed-enhancement MRI in repeat ablation procedures. Circ Arrhythm Electrophysiol 2010;3:249–59.

Bisbal F, Guiu E, Cabanas-Grandio P, et al. CMR-guided approach to localize and ablate gaps in repeat AF ablation procedure. JACC Cardiovasc Imaging. 2014;7: 653–63.

Halbfass PM, Mitlacher M, Turschner O, et al. Lesion formation after pulmonary vein isolation using the advance cryoballoon and the standard cryoballoon: lessons learned from late gadolinium enhancement magnetic resonance imaging. Europace 2015;17:566–73.

Ranjan R, Kholmovski EG, Blauer J, et al. Identification and acute targeting of gaps in atrial ablation lesion sets using a real time MRI system. Circ Arrhythm Electrophysiol 2012;5:1130–5.

Siebermair J, Kholmovski EG, Marrouche N. Assessment of Left Atrial Fibrosis by Late Gadolinium Enhancement Magnetic Resonance Imaging. Methodology and Clinical Implications. ACC Clin Electrophysiol. 2017;3: 791–802.

Case 99

Pulmonary Vein Isolation

Clinical History

- Fifty-four-year-old female.
- History paroxysmal atrial fibrillation treated with radiofrequency ablation 1 year ago.
- The patient presents to the emergency room with dyspnea, cough, hemoptysis, and chest pain.
- Referred to cardiac computed tomography (CT) to rule out pulmonary vein stenosis.

Images

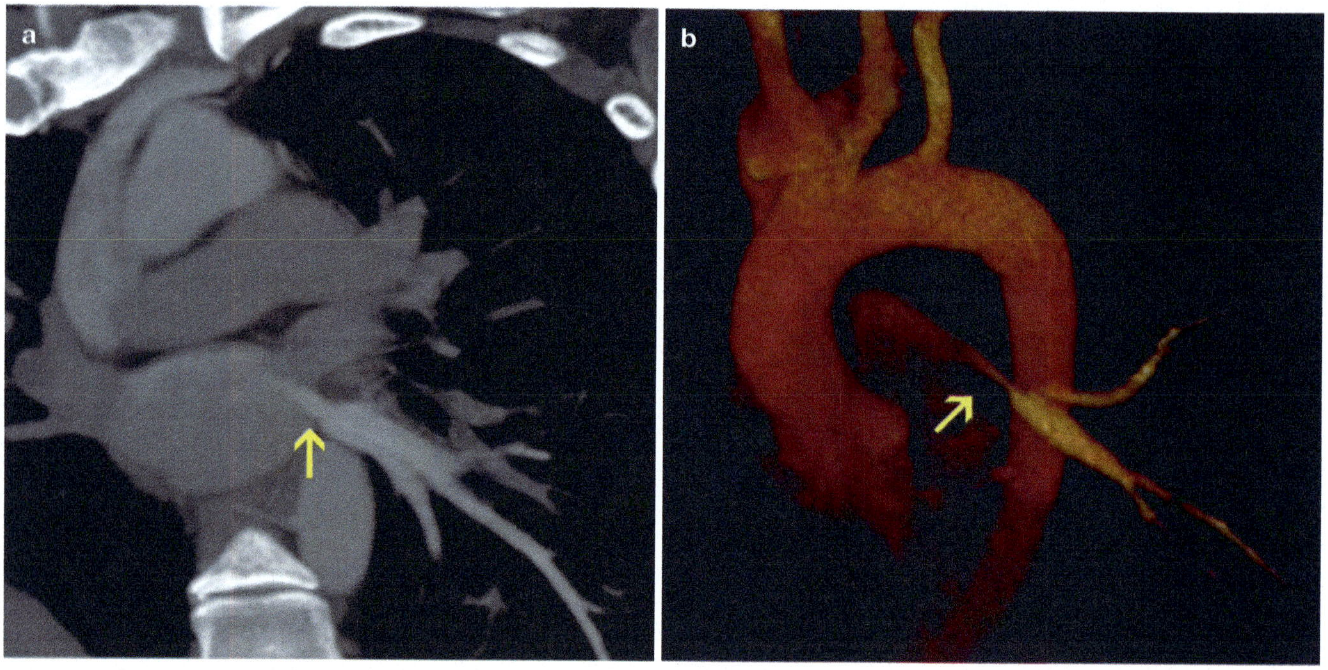

Findings and Interpretation

- Oblique coronal multiplanar maximum intensity projection (MIP) reconstruction of the left atrium (panel A) demonstrates significant stenosis of the left inferior pulmonary vein (arrow).
- In a three-dimensional volume rendering reconstruction, oblique view (panel B), the inferior pulmonary vein shows a symmetric severe narrowing (arrow) as the vein joins the left atrium.
- A well-recognized complication of atrial fibrillation ablation is pulmonary vein stenosis. This complication usually presents within a year after the ablation procedure with dyspnea and other findings sometimes reminiscent of pulmonary embolus.
- Diagnosis of pulmonary vein stenosis can be challenging, as patients may be asymptomatic or may present with nonspecific symptoms. CT or magnetic resonance imaging is required to confirm the diagnosis. There is discordant data in the literature concerning the incidence of iatrogenic pulmonary vein stenosis after atrial fibrillation ablation, ranging from 0 to 42%.
- Contrast-enhanced CT can enable the diagnosis by directly depicting the stenosis and other associated features, such as pulmonary parenchymal septal thickening caused by localized pulmonary venous hypertension, peripheral opacities caused by infarctions, and increased attenuation of mediastinal fat adjacent to the stenosis.

Further Reading

Cappato R, Calkins H, Chen SA, et al. Worldwide survey on the methods, efficacy, and safety of catheter ablation for human atrial fibrillation. Circulation. 2005;111(9):1100–5.

Packer DL, Keelan P, Munger TM, et al. Clinical presentation, investigation, and management of pulmonary vein stenosis complicating ablation for atrial fibrillation. Circulation 2005;111:546–54.

Saad EB, Rossillo A, Saad CP, et al. Pulmonary vein stenosis after radiofrequency ablation of atrial fibrillation: functional characterization, evolution, and influence of the ablation strategy. Circulation 2003;108:3102–7.

Case 100

Left Atrial Diverticula

Clinical History

- Forty-two-year-old female.
- Symptomatic (shortness of breath) paroxysmal atrial fibrillation.
- No response to adequate medical treatment.
- Scheduled for catheter ablation.
- Referred to cardiac computed tomography (CT) for left atrium (LA) and pulmonary veins evaluation before the ablation procedure.

Images

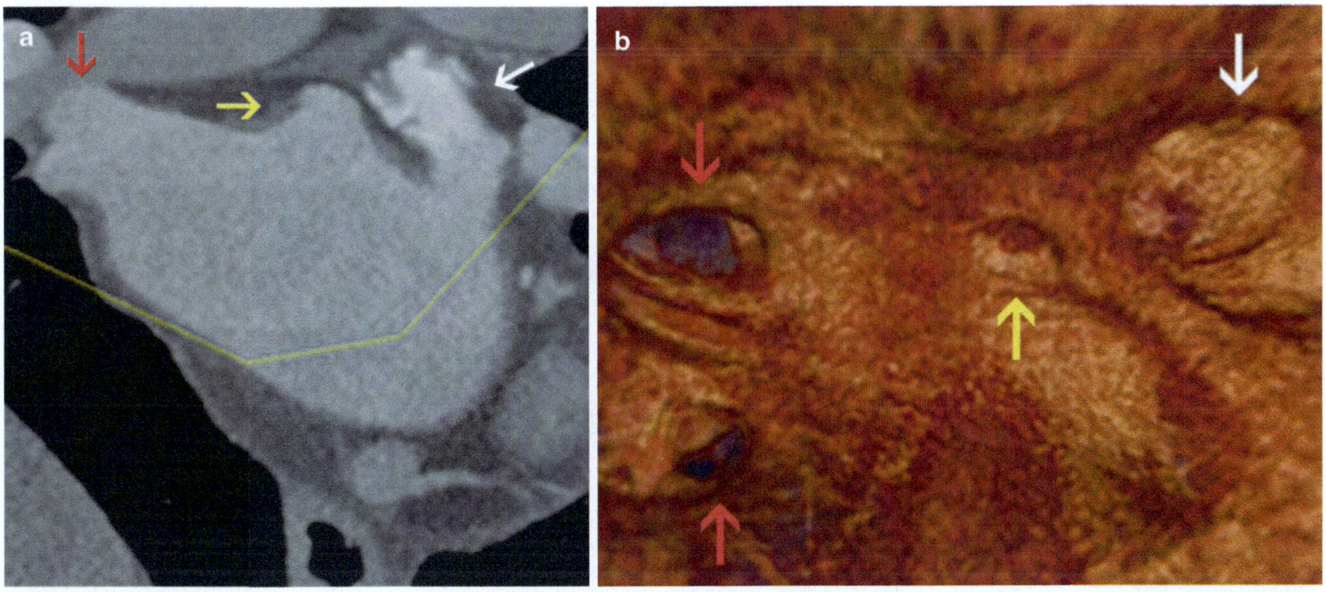

Findings and Interpretation

- Oblique multiplanar CT reconstruction of the LA (panel A) demonstrates the presence of a LA diverticulum arising from the superior wall (yellow arrow). Note the saclike shape of the diverticula with a broad-based ostium and a smooth contour of its body, the LA appendage (white arrow), and the right superior pulmonary vein (red arrow).
- Endoluminal CT view of the LA shows the LA diverticula ostia (yellow arrow), the LA appendage ostia (white arrow), and the right pulmonary veins ostia (red arrows).
- Accessory LA appendages and atrial diverticula have an incidence of 10–46%. Diverticula are significantly more common than accessory LA appendages. An accessory appendage has a discernible ostium at the LA with a neck and body that displayed irregular contours suggestive of the presence of pectinate muscles. An atrial diverticulum has a saclike shape with a broad-based ostium and a smooth contour of its body. The structures described appear to represent anatomic variants rather than pathologic findings.

Further Reading

Abbara S, Mundo-sagardia JA, Hoffmann U, Cury RC. Cardiac CT assessment of left atrial accessory appendages and diverticula. Am J Roengenol 2009;193:807–12.

Troupis J, Crosset M, Scneider-Kolsky M, Nandurkar D. Presence of accessory left atrial appendage/diverticula in a population with atrial fibrillation compared with those in sinus rhythm: a retrospective review. Int J Cardiovasc Imaging 2012;28:375–80.

Wan Y, He Z, Zhang J, et al. The anatomical study of left atrium diverticulum by multidetector row CT. Surg Radiol Anat 2009;31:191–8.

Case 101

Left Atrial Appendage Thrombus

Clinical History

- Fifty-eight-year-old male.
- Symptomatic (palpitations and syncope) persistent atrial fibrillation, with no response to adequate medical treatment.
- Risk factors: hypercholesterolemia, smoking, and hypertension.
- Non diagnostic transesophageal echocardiography (TEE).
- Referred to cardiac computed tomography (CT) for left atrium (LA) and pulmonary veins evaluation before the ablation procedure.

Images

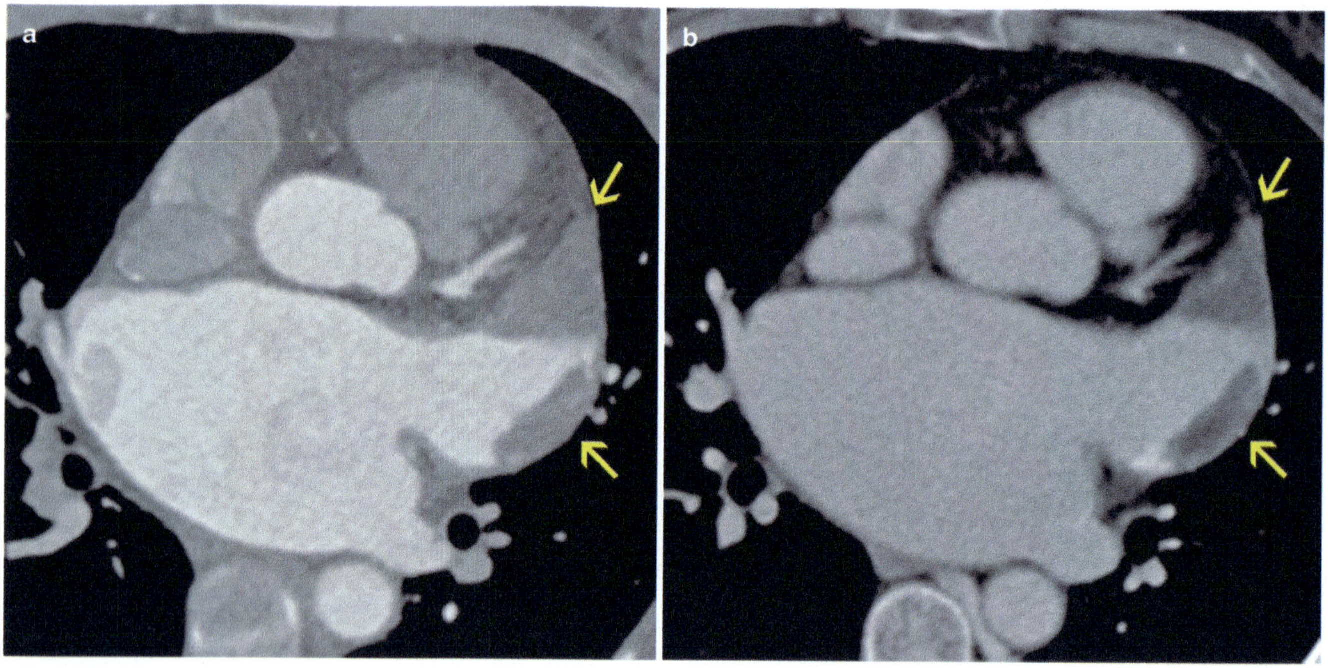

Findings and Interpretation

- Initial retrospective ECG gated CT axial image (panel A) demonstrates filling defects in the left atrial appendage (yellow arrows).
- Delayed non-gated axial image (panel B) show persistent filling defects during the delayed phase acquired after 2 min, confirming the presence of thrombus (yellow arrows).
- Left atrial thrombi are a common phenomenon in patients with atrial fibrillation (AF) with a prevalence of 13–15%, most frequently affecting the left atrial appendage (LAA). Left atrial thrombi represent a potential source for thromboembolic events necessitating treatment with anticoagulants. Screening for the presence of atrial thrombus is mandatory prior to atrial fibrillation ablation for patients at risk, as catheter manipulation could dislodge a thrombus with the potential for embolic complications, and its presence is a contraindication for catheter ablation. TEE serves as the clinical reference imaging modality with a high diagnostic accuracy. Since cardiac CT is a static study and the images are captured a few seconds after arrival of contrast to the left heart, it can be difficult to differentiate thrombus from sluggish flow (incomplete mixing of contrast and blood due to slow flow). The addition of delayed imaging allows a better distinction between both conditions. Cardiac CT, particularly when delayed imaging is performed, is a reliable alternative to TEE for the detection of LA thrombi/clot, avoiding the discomfort and risks associated with TEE, with sensitivity and specificity of 100% and 99%, respectively, and a positive predictive value and negative predictive value of 92% and 100%, respectively.

Further Reading

Fuster V, Ryde'n LE, Cannom DS, et al. ACC/AHA/ESC 2006 guidelines for the management of patients with atrial fibrillation: full text. Europace. 2006;8:651–745.

Oral H, Chugh A, O'zaydin M, et al. Risk of thromboembolic events after percutaneous left atrial radiofrequency ablation of atrial fibrillation. Circulation. 2006;114:759–65.

Romero J, Husain SA, Kelesidis L, et al. Detection of left atrial appendage thrombus by cardiac computed tomography in patients with atrial fibrillation: a meta-analysis. Circ Cardiovasc Imaging. 2013;6:185–94.

Case 102

Left Atrial Appendage with Suspected Thrombus

Clinical History

- Forty-four-year-old male.
- Symptomatic (syncope) paroxysmal atrial fibrillation, with no response to adequate medical treatment.
- Referred to cardiac computed tomography (CT) for left atrium (LA) and pulmonary veins evaluation before the ablation procedure.

Images

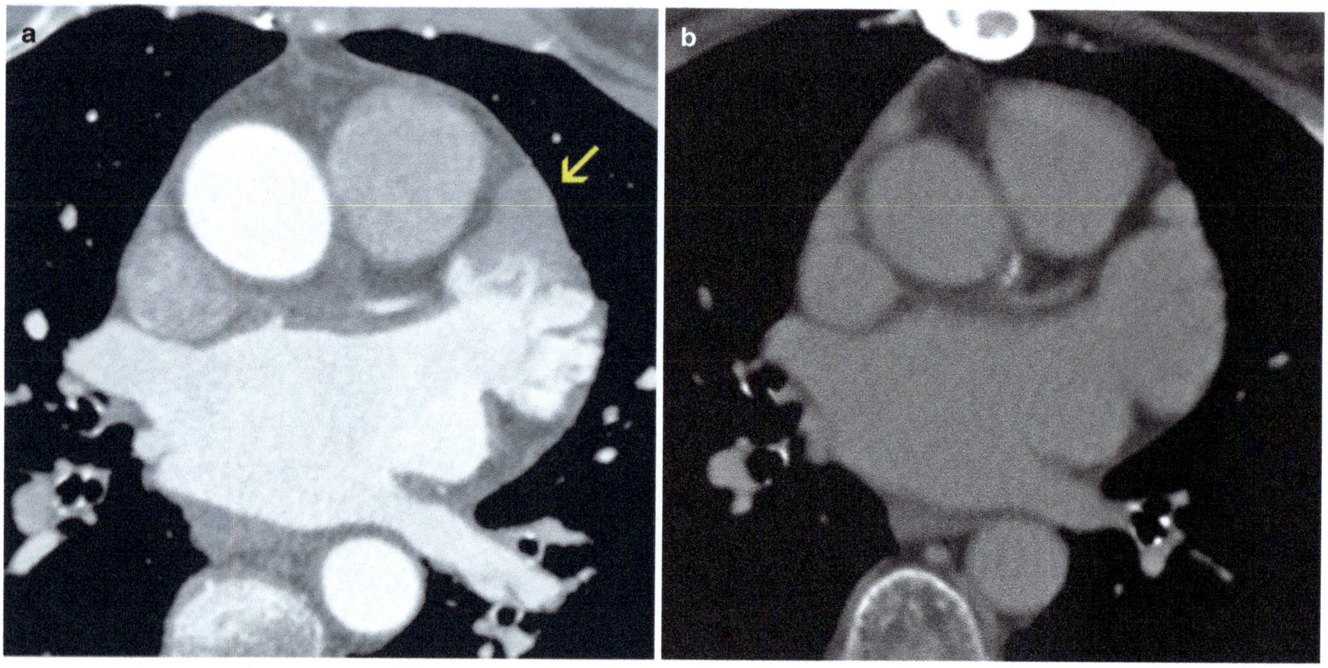

Findings and Interpretation

- Initial contrast-enhanced cardiac CT with retrospective ECG gating (panel A) demonstrates a filling defect in the left atrial appendage (yellow arrow).
- Delayed non-gated axial image (panel B) demonstrates complete contrast opacification and resolution of the filling defect in the left atrial appendage.
- Cardiac CT has an excellent diagnostic accuracy for the detection of left atrial appendage thrombus in patients with atrial fibrillation, allowing a safe alternative imaging method among patients non-suitable for transesophageal echocardiogram or for institutions where the latter is not available.
- In the presence of a filling defect of the left atrial appendage during contrast-enhanced cardiac CT, a negative delayed acquisition allows ruling out thrombus. However, such mismatch (positive early defect, negative late defect) implies blood stasis/slow flow and has been related to a high risk of thromboembolic events.

Further Reading

Romero J, Husain SA, Kelesidis I, Sanz J, Medina HM, Garcia MJ. Detection of left atrial appendage thrombus by cardiac computed tomography in patients with atrial fibrillation: a meta-analysis. Circ Cardiovasc Imaging. 2013;6:185–94.

Wang L, Kadiyala M, Koss E, Yarramaneni A, Rapelje K, Kampfer S, et al. CTA Detection of Left Atrial Stasis and Thrombus in Patients with Atrial Fibrillation. Pacing Clin Electrophysiol. 2016;39:1388–93.

Zabalgoitia M1, Halperin JL, Pearce LA, Blackshear JL, Asinger RW, Hart RG. Transesophageal echocardiographic correlates of clinical risk of thromboembolism in nonvalvular atrial fibrillation. Stroke Prevention in Atrial Fibrillation III Investigators. J Am Coll Cardiol. 1998;31:1622–6.

Case 103

Guidance of Percutaneous Closure of Left Atrial Appendage

Clinical History

- Forty-eight-year-old male.
- Symptomatic (palpitations and poor exercise tolerance) paroxysmal atrial fibrillation (AF).
- No response to adequate medical treatment.
- Referred to cardiac computed tomography (CT) for left atrium (LA) and pulmonary veins evaluation before the ablation procedure.

Images

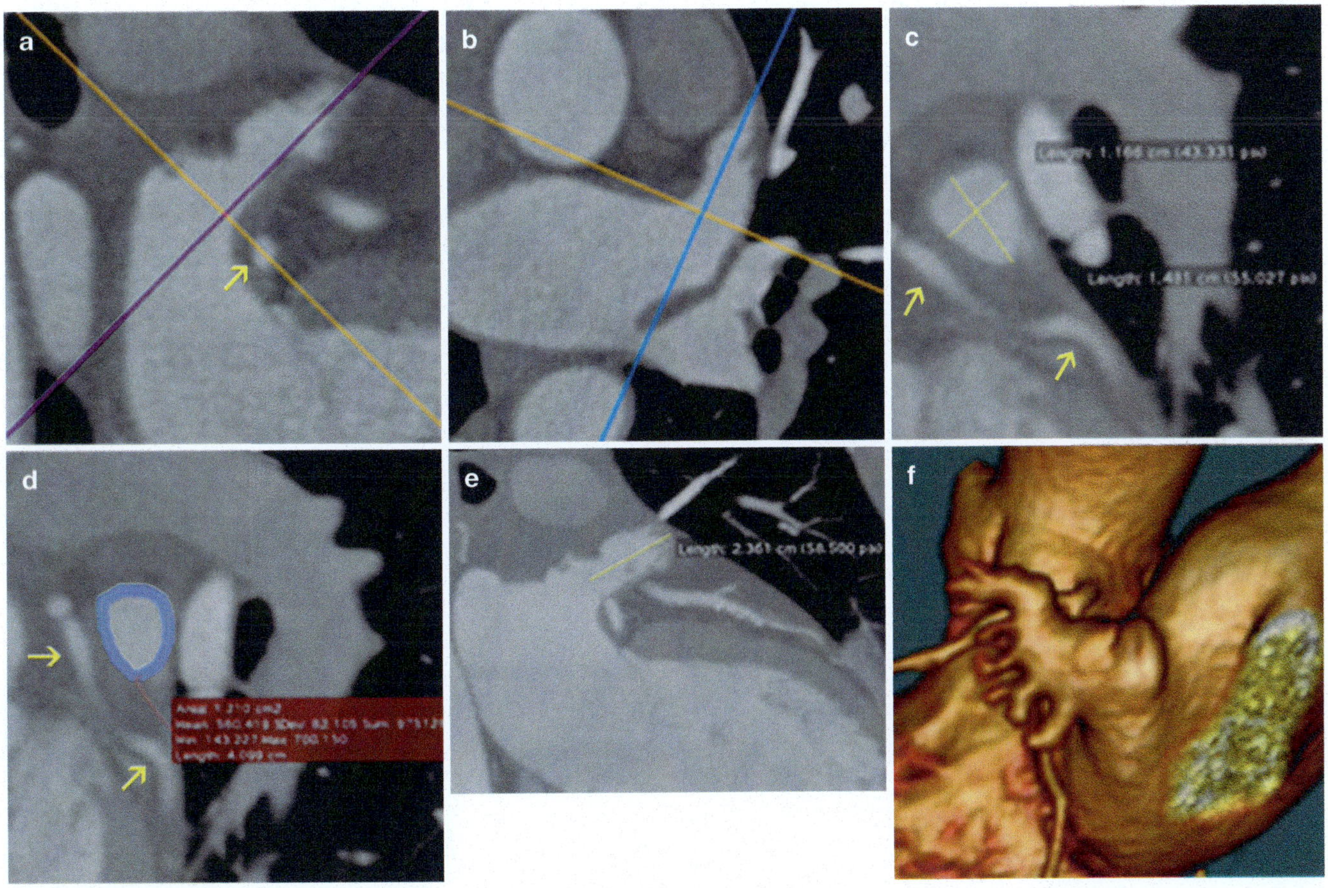

Findings and Interpretation

- Two different long axis planes of the LA appendage (LAA) (panels A and B) are used to obtain an ostial orthogonal plane (panel C) at the level of the left circumflex coronary artery (yellow arrows). This orthogonal plane is used to calculate the LAA ostia diameters (panel C) and perimeter (panel D).
- LAA length is calculated using a long axis plane (panel E).
- Three-dimensional volume rendering LAA reconstruction (panel F) demonstrating its configuration. LAA measurements and 3D imaging at cardiac CT for LAA occluder device must be done 1 cm deeper than LAA ostium, demonstrating the resulting landing zone.
- The LAA is the source of thrombi formation in more than 90% of strokes in patients with non-valvular AF. Anticoagulation treatment reduces the risk of stroke. However, it has a narrow therapeutic range and carries a significant bleeding hazard with low compliance to treatment leading to clinical utilization in only 50–60%. LAA occlusion is becoming an accepted procedure for AF patients with contraindications to anticoagulation therapy. Recently, several devices have been developed for percutaneous LAA occlusion. The wide variation of its size and morphology makes percutaneous occlusion especially challenging. Incorrect device choice and sizing may necessitate multiple device insertion or procedure failure.

- Cardiac CT provides high spatial resolution three-dimensional data of the LAA and may help to achieve a more appropriate sizing of the LAA occluder device and after the procedure to confirm that the appendage has been excluded from the circulation. The length/depth of the LAA should also be measured to ensure a landing zone that exceeds the maximal ostium diameter.
- For the assessment of the LAA morphology in three-dimensional volume rendering images, LAA are categorized into four different types: chicken wing (a single curved central lobe, with no more than one secondary lobe), windsock (dominant central lobe, with secondary lobes in other direction), cauliflower (complex structure, with several secondary fork-like lobes), and cactus (short, with a central lobe and several secondary superior and inferior lobes) or more straightforward and clinically relevant as chicken wing or non-chicken wing. It has been reported that chicken wing LAA morphology is less likely to have an embolic event.

Further Reading

Di Biase L, Santangeli P, Anselmino M, et al. Does the left atrial appendage morphology correlate with the risk of stroke in patients with atrial fibrillation? Results from a multicenter study. J Am Coll Cardiol. 2012;60:531–8.

E Gul E, Boles U, Haseeb S, Flood J, Bansal A, Glover B, et al. Left Atrial Appendage characteristics in patients with Persistent Atrial Fibrillation undergoing catheter ablation (LAAPAF Study). J Atr Fibrillation. 2017;9:1526.

Goitein O, Fink N, Hay I, et al. Cardiac CT Angiography (CCTA) predicts left atrial appendage occluder device size and procedure outcome. Int J Cardiovasc Imaging. 2017;33:739–747.

J Van Rosendael P, Katsanos S, W.V. van den Brink O, et al. Geometry of left atrial appendage assessed with multidetector-row computed tomography: implications for transcatheter closure devices. EuroIntervention 2014;10:364–71.

Congenital Heart Disease

6

Fernando Abramzon, Maria Jose Bosaleh, Pablo Pollono,
Ezequiel Levy Yeyati, Juan Wolcan,
and Gastón A. Rodríguez-Granillo

Background

Congenital heart disease (CHD) is the most common cause of major congenital anomalies (approximately 28%), representing a major global health problem. In the past 80 years, this statistic has increased due to improved diagnostic methods and facilitated patient access. Currently, the difference in CHD incidence found between high-income (with higher prevalence) and low-income countries also partially illustrates this asymmetric situation.

In parallel, improvements in cardiothoracic surgical and endovascular treatments have also determined a marked increase in the prevalence of CHD in adults, related to a significant increase in survival of patients with severe heart defects. These adult patients will need long-term expert medical care which represents high healthcare-related costs.

CHD has an estimated incidence of 0.8% of all new live births globally and a global prevalence of 0.4% in adults.

Cardiac magnetic resonance (CMR) and CT play an important role in the diagnosis and surveillance, planification of surgical strategies, and follow-up of patients who undergo surgical or percutaneous repair of CHD. Cardiac CT enables an unsurpassed evaluation of the anatomy of patients with complex CHD, with nonrestricted volumetric imaging planes. In turn, CMR provides accurate, reproducible, and ionizing-free data particularly useful for the evaluation of valves and shunts, including precise anterograde and retrograde volume quantification. CMR is particularly useful for the evaluation of the right ventricular morphology and function and for right-sided valvular disease.

Classification

Several classifications have been proposed for CHD. We prefer to use a classification that facilitates comprehension and detection by the nonspecialized reader, emphasizing the most frequent variants in routine obstetric and newborn studies (Table 6.1).

These frequencies are modified among adults mainly due to evolving self-resolution, therapeutic practices, and changing mortality statistics. In adulthood, imaging tools play an

Table 6.1 Classification of congenital heart disease (CHD)

Classification of most frequent CHD in newborns		
Acyanotic		Cyanotic
Left-to-right shunts	**Obstructive**	Tetralogy of Fallot (10%)
Ventricular septal defect (40%)	Aortic coarctation (5%)	Transposition of the great arteries (7%)
Atrial septal defect (10%)	Aortic stenosis (4%)	Tricuspid atresia (1%)
Patent ductus arteriosus (7%)	Pulmonary stenosis (8%)	Truncus arteriosus (1%)
Partial anomalous pulmonary venous return (0.5%)		Total anomalous pulmonary venous return (0.1%)

F. Abramzon
Cardiovascular Imaging, Department of Radiology, Hospital de Trauma y Emergencias "Dr. Federico Abete", University of Buenos Aires, Buenos Aires, Argentina

M. J. Bosaleh
Department of Pediatrics, Pediatric Cardiology Section, Department of Radiology, Section of CT and MR, Hospital Nacional Alejandro Posadas, Buenos Aires, Argentina

P. Pollono · J. Wolcan
Department of Non-Invasive Cardiovascular Imaging, Hospital del Cruce, Florencio Varela, Buenos Aires, Argentina

E. Levy Yeyati
Cardiovascular Imaging, Department of Radiology, Hospital Municipal de Merlo "Eva Perón", University of Buenos Aires, Buenos Aires, Argentina

G. A. Rodríguez-Granillo (✉)
Department of Cardiovascular Imaging, Department of Research, Diagnostico Maipu, Buenos Aires, Argentina

National Council of Scientific and Technical Investigations (CONICET), Buenos Aires, Argentina

P. M. Carrascosa et al. (eds.), *Clinical Atlas of Cardiac and Aortic CT and MRI*, https://doi.org/10.1007/978-3-030-03682-9_6

even more preponderant role in the surveillance of these patients, especially to guide and follow up percutaneous or surgical treatment. In addition, among adults, other etiologies and factors should be taken into consideration such as Ebstein's anomaly and Eisenmenger's syndrome. The latter (also known as tardive cyanosis), a type of physiology rather than an etiology itself, consists in a reversal of a long-standing left-to-right shunt (generally caused by large atrial septal defect, ASD, or ventricular septal defect, VSD) into a cyanotic right-to-left shunt due to significant pulmonary hypertension.

General Characteristics of the Main Groups (Also See Fig. 6.1.)

Acyanotic CHD CHD that initially do not interfere with the amount of oxygenated blood in the systemic circulation

- *(Left-to right) shunts*: Most frequent. Usually non-symptomatic until advanced disease (with pulmonary hypertension or systolic failure) or Eisenmenger's syndrome develops. Murmurs commonly detected by pediatricians on scheduled control appointments.

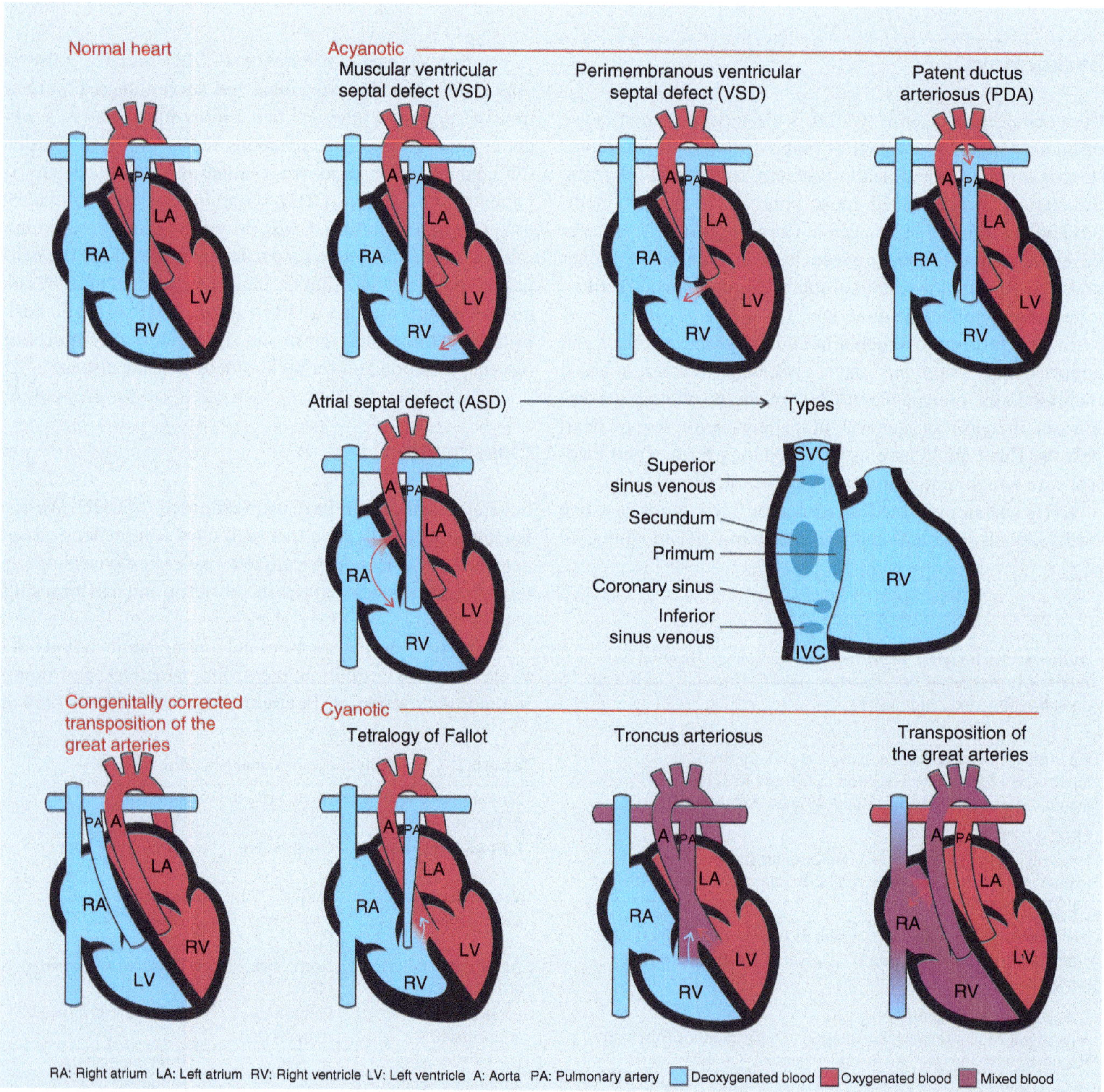

Fig. 6.1 Graphical representation of the characteristics of some of the main defects with acyanotic and cyanotic CHD (aortic coarctation is not represented given the simple evaluation of this defect)

Although VSDs are the most common CHD in newborns, almost 70% of all VSDs undergo spontaneous closure within the first years of life; therefore ASD is generally the most frequent CHD in adults. VSDs, commonly associated with other CHD [patent ductus arteriosus (PDA), bicuspid aortic valve, aortic coarctation, among others], are classified according to their location, being the most frequent type perimembranous VSD and less frequently muscular VSD. They are further classified as restrictive, defect size <1/3 of the aortic root, pulmonary to systemic flow ratio (Qp/Qs)<1.5:1, with high velocity jet and normal pulmonary artery systolic pressure; moderately restrictive, defect size of approximately 50% of the aortic root, Qp/Qs between 1.5 and 2:1, and normal or mild increment in pulmonary artery systolic pressure; and non-restrictive VSD, defect size >50% of the aortic root, Qp/Qs>2:1, low-velocity jet and pulmonary hypertension. VSDs are also classified as small (<3 mm and most frequent type), medium (3–6 mm), and large (>6 mm).

ASDs are more frequently found in women and are classified as ostium secundum (accounts for >75% cases and are the only type suitable for percutaneous closure, at the fossa ovalis level), ostium primum (adjacent to the atrioventricular valves), and sinus venosus (superior or inferior). ASD, particularly sinus venosus ASD, can be associated with anomalous pulmonary vein return. When evaluated by CMR or cardiac CT, evaluation of ASD warrants the assessment of the size and exact location of the defect (including distance from venous structures and the aortic root), as well as the estimation of the Qp/Qs ratio (closure indicated if >1.5:1, implying a pulmonary blood flow 50% greater than the systemic), and the size and systolic function of the right ventricle (RV). RV overload is typically identified a dilated and/or hypertrophic RV, with flattening of the interventricular septum, late enhancement at the insertion points of the RV over the septum, and dilated pulmonary artery.

- *Obstructive*: Unless severe, they are usually detected in the adulthood. Left ventricular outflow tract (LVOT) obstruction can be valvular, subvalvular, or supravalvular or even a combination of the above. Indeed, the Shone's complex is a very rare CHD that consists in the presence of multiple left-sided obstructive defects. The most common underlying etiology of LVOT obstruction is bicuspid aortic valve, with an estimated prevalence of 1–2% of the general population. Supravalvular aortic stenosis is much less common and can present as an hourglass narrowing, as a diffuse stenosis, or (less frequently) as a fibrous diaphragm. Supravalvular stenosis can be as present as part of the Williams syndrome. Subaortic stenosis is usually detected as a thin fibromuscular narrowing proximal to the aortic valve.

Pulmonary stenosis, usually detected during adulthood, is generally related to the fusion of pulmonary valves.

Coarctation of the aorta (CoA) has an estimated prevalence of 5–8% of all CHD and has a strong association with bicuspid aortic valve and other stenotic left-sided defects. Stenosis in these patients can present as discrete or as a diffuse hipoplastic segment. Also, CoA can be ductal, pre-ductal, post-ductal and, though very rarely, ectopic (descending aorta or abdominal aorta).

Cyanotic CHD These CHD interfere with the amount of oxygenated blood in the systemic circulation (arterial desaturation). Most cyanotic CHD require surgical correction immediately or soon after birth due to high mortality rates. Except from Ebstein's anomaly, nonsurgically corrected adults with cyanotic CHD are difficult to find in developed countries.

Tetralogy of Fallot (ToF) is the most common cyanotic CHD, particularly among >1-year-old (comprising approximately 10% of all CHD). In brief, this defect involves different degrees of the following: (1) aorta overriding the septum, (2) nonrestrictive VSD, (3) RV outflow tract obstruction (valvular, subvalvular, with or without pulmonary branch stenosis), and (4) RV hypertrophy. Frequent associated defects can be found such as ASD, right aortic arch, and coronary artery anomalies, among others. Given the good prognosis of ToF repair, adult patients with this defect are common in cardiovascular imaging departments. The most common late complications are pulmonary regurgitation, RV dilatation and systolic dysfunction, residual RV outflow tract obstruction, residual VSD, aortic root dilatation and regurgitation (this common complication is believed to be related to congenital cystic medial necrosis of the aorta), and sudden cardiac death (QRS > 180 ms risk factor). Supportive imaging findings for pulmonary valve replacement in ToF include left ventricular dysfunction, RV end-diastolic volume > 140 ml/m^2, RV systolic pressure > 60 mmHg, and/or severe pulmonary regurgitation (regurgitation fraction <20%, mild; 20–40%, moderate; >40%, severe).

Transposition of the great arteries (TGA), also known as D-TGA, is the most frequent cyanotic CHD in neonates, with mortality rates over 90% without treatment and commonly associated with other CHD defects. Usually, patients survive until surgery due to the presence of shunts (PDA, patent foramen ovale, ASD, VSD). These patients have atrioventricular concordance and ventricular-arterial discordance, since the pulmonary artery arises from the left ventricle and the aorta from the RV. Accordingly, the vessels are in a parallel position (with the aorta in an anterior right position). Surgical treatment can be an arterial switch (Jatene's surgery) or atrial switch (Senning/Mustard procedure). The most frequent complication of atrial switch is the presence of RV dysfunction given that this ventricle, which serves as the systemic, is not designed to tolerate systemic pressures. Also, significant tricuspid regurgitation can be found in these patients. One important role of CMR is to identify the patency of the intra-atrial conduits or baffles.

In congenitally corrected TGA (L-TGA), there is both atrioventricular and ventriculo-arterial discordance. In brief, the ventricles are inverted. Accordingly, the aorta arises from the RV (systemic ventricle, functionally left) in an anterior position, whereas the pulmonary artery arises from the left ventricle (pulmonary ventricle, functionally right) in a posterior position. These patients are usually diagnosed as adults and commonly have associated defects that dictate the natural history. Typically, the RV (systemic ventricle) ends up developing systolic dysfunction. Definitive corrective surgery involves double switch (atrial and arterial switch).

Finally, we have to mention the concept of the univentricular heart. This concept involves a wide spectrum of different defects, including tricuspid atresia, hypoplastic right or left heart syndrome, pulmonary atresia with intact interventricular septum, double inlet RV or LV, or even undefined forms. What these defects have in common is the fact that there is a simple functional ventricle that receives both pulmonary and systemic vein return; and the surgical treatment generally involves the generation of cavopulmonary anastomosis that enables a passive flow from the caval veins to the pulmonary arteries. This is accomplished by the anastomosis of the superior vena cava to the pulmonary artery (Glenn surgery) and also from the inferior vena cava usually through an extracardiac conduit (Fontan) in a second stage.

Further Reading

Dolk H, Loane M, Garne E, for the European Surveillance of Congenital Anomalies (EUROCAT) Working Group. Congenital heart defects in Europe: prevalence and perinatal mortality, 2000 to 2005. Circulation. 2011;123:841–9.

Elizabeth Brickner M, David Hillis L, Richard A. Lange congenital heart disease in adults. N Engl J Med. 2000;342:256–63.

ECG guidelines for the management of grown-up congenital disease (new version 2010): the Task Force on the management of grown-up congenital disease of the European Society of Cardiology (ESC). Eur Heart J. 2010;31(23):2915–57.

Gupta SK, Juneja R, Anderson RH, Gulati GS, Devagorou V. Clarifying the anatomy and physiology of totally anomalous systemic venous connection. Ann Pediatr Cardiol. 2017;10(3):269–77.

Hoffman JI, Kaplan S. The incidence of congenital heart disease. J Am Coll Cardiol. 2002;39:1890.

Khairy P, Ionescu-Ittu R, Mackie AS, Abrahamowicz M, Pilote L, Marelli AJ. Changing mortality in congenital heart disease. J Am Coll Cardiol. 2010;56:1149–57.

Kreutzer C, Kreutzer J, Kreutzer GO. Reflections on five decades of the fontan kreutzer procedure. Front Pediatr. 2013;1:45.

Mercer-Rosa L, Yang W, Kutty S, Rychik J, Fogel M, Goldmuntz E. Quantifying pulmonary regurgitation and right ventricular function in surgically repaired tetralogy of Fallot: a comparative analysis of echocardiography and magnetic resonance imaging. Circ Cardiovasc Imaging. 2012;5(5):637–43.

Reller MD, Strickland MJ, Riehle-Colarusso T, Mahle WT, Correa A. Prevalence of congenital heart defects in metropolitan Atlanta, 1998-2005. J Pediatr. 2008;153:807–13.

The World Bank Group. World Bank Income groups distribution 2008. Available at: http://www.enterprisesurveys.org/Methodology/EconomyRegionIncomeGroupList.aspx. Accessed 16 Dec 2010.

van der Linde D, Konings EEM, Slager MA, Witsenburg M, Helbing WA, Takkenberg JJM, Roos-Hesselink JW. Birth prevalence of congenital heart disease worldwide. J Am Coll Cardiol. 2011;58(21):2241–7. https://doi.org/10.1016/j.jacc.2011.08.025.

Case 104

Atrial Septal Defect

Clinical History

- Seventy-year-old female.
- Asymptomatic, with a known atrial septal defect (ASD).
- Echocardiography revealed an ASD, with mild right and left atrial dilatation and a pulmonary artery systolic pressure of 39 mmHg.
- Referred to cardiac magnetic resonance (CMR) for further evaluation of the venous return anatomy and to evaluate the interatrial septum.

Images

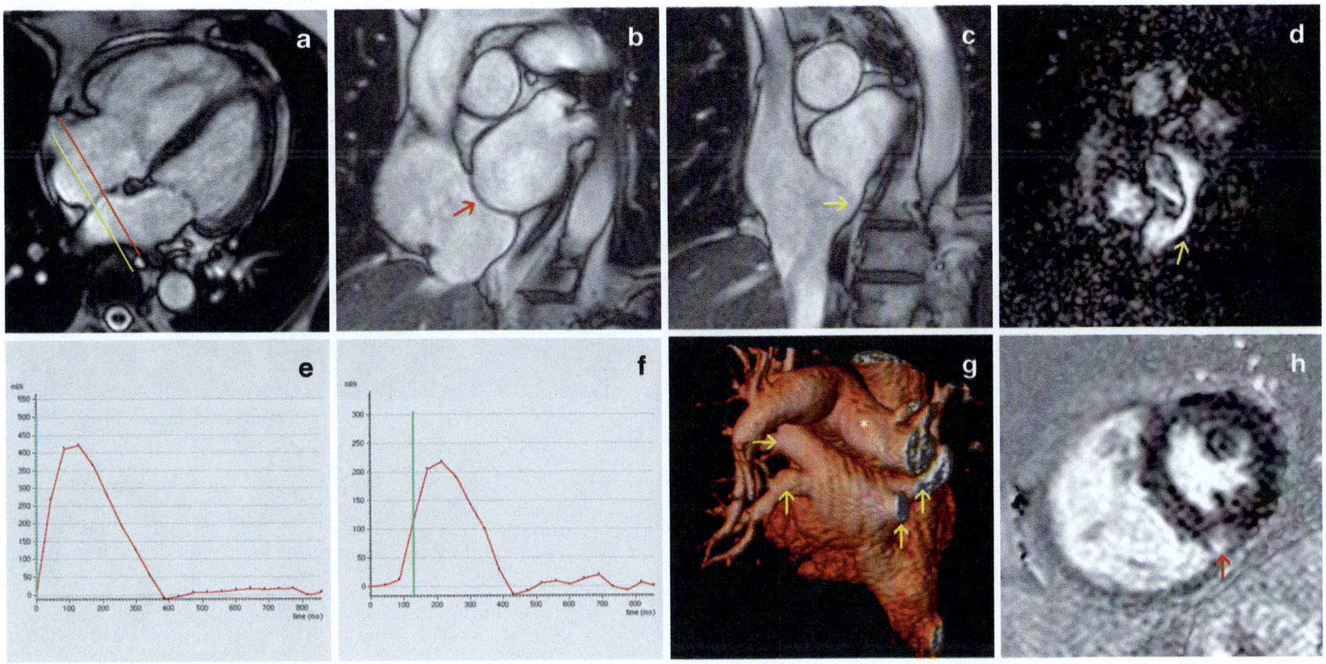

Findings and Interpretation

- As shown in an end-diastolic cine four-chamber view (panel A), the right ventricle (RV) is mildly dilated, and at first sight the interatrial septum is complete, hypermobile, and displaced to the right atrium.
- A basal short-axis view at the fossa ovalis level (panel B, at red line in panel A) shows similar findings. However, few millimeters backward to the posterior wall (panel C, at yellow line in panel A), a sinus venosus ASD is detected (arrow in panel C). The presence of a left-to-right shunt is nicely depicted in the same view using a phase-encoding sequence (arrow in panel D).
- Using phase-encoding sequences in orthogonal planes located at pulmonary artery trunk (panel E) and ascending aorta (panel F) level, a pulmonary to systemic flow ratio (Qp/Qs) of 2.1:1 was calculated.
- Three-dimensional MR angiogram (panel G) demonstrated normal pulmonary vein return (arrows) and a dilated pulmonary artery (*).
- Inversion-recovery images (panel H) revealed small areas of late gadolinium enhancement (LGE) coincident with the RV insertion points at the septal wall (arrow).
- Inferior sinus venosus ASD is one of the least common ASD types, with a prevalence of <1% of all ASDs, compared to ostium secundum (70%), ostium primum (15%), and superior sinus (5%) ASD.
- Superior sinus venosus ASD is more commonly associated with abnormal pulmonary vein return.
- The presence of a dilated pulmonary artery along with typical LGE reflects the presence of pulmonary hypertension.
- Given the age, lack of symptoms, and low likelihood of percutaneous closure, a conservative management would probably be better in this patient despite the presence of a significant left-to-right shunt.

Further Reading

ECG guidelines for the management of grown-up congenital disease (new version 2010): the Task Force on the management of grown-up congenital disease of the European Society of Cardiology (ESC). Eur Heart J. 2010;31(23):2915–57.

Case 105

Atrial Septal Defect

Clinical History

- Thirty-nine-year-old female.
- She has previous diagnosis of an atrial septal defect (ASD). Currently symptomatic (dyspnea New York Heart Association functional class II).
- Transesophageal echocardiography revealed a dilated right ventricle (RV) and an ostium secundum atrial septal defect (ASD) of approximately 15 mm diameter, with a significant left-to-right shunt (pulmonary to systemic flow ratio of 2.5:1).
- Referred to cardiac magnetic resonance (CMR) for further evaluation of the venous return anatomy.

Images

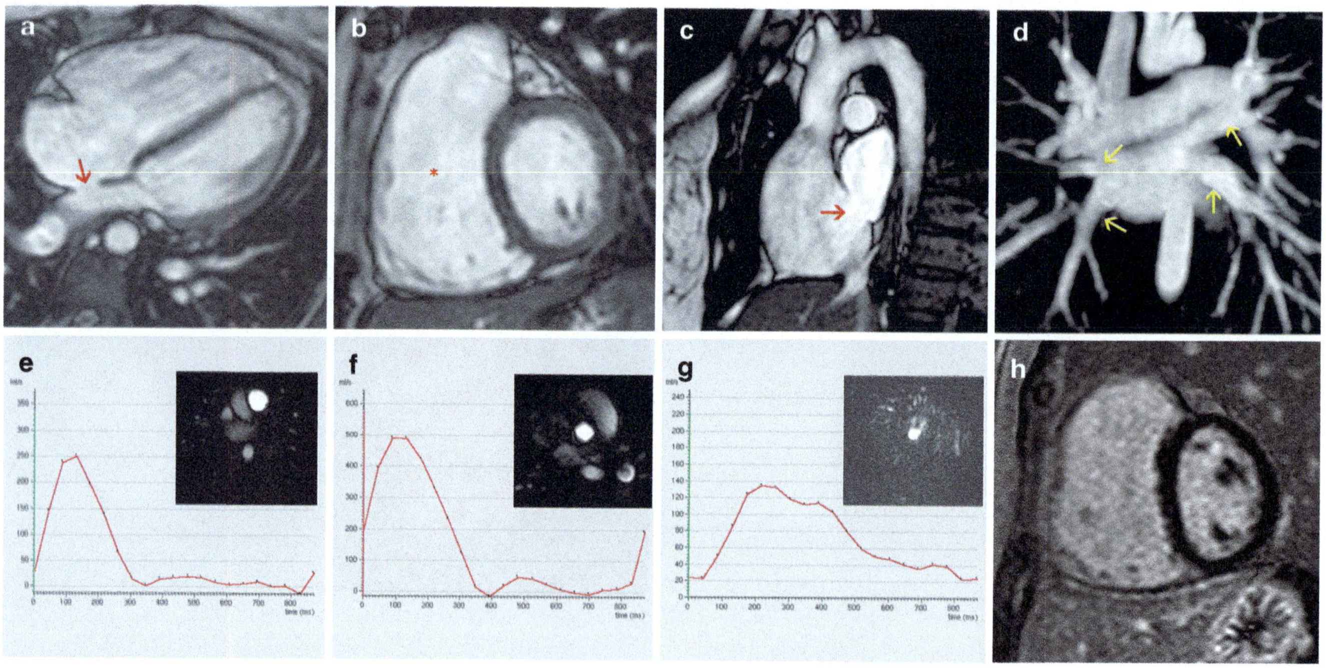

Findings and Interpretation

- End-diastolic cine four-chamber view (panel A) demonstrated a dilated RV (end-diastolic volume 106 ml/m^2) and right atrium (25 cm^2), with a clear defect of the interatrial septum at the level of the fossa ovalis (ostium secundum ASD, red arrow in panel A).
- A basal short-axis view (panel B) shows significant RV dilatation (*).
- A short-axis view at the fossa ovalis level (panel C) depicts a medium-sized (12 mm × 17 mm) ostium secundum ASD, with left-to-right shunt (red arrow in panel C).
- Maximum intensity projection MR angiography (panel D) demonstrates normal pulmonary vein return (yellow arrows in panel D).
- Using phase-encoding sequences in orthogonal planes located at pulmonary artery trunk (panel E) and the ascending aorta (panel F) level, a pulmonary to systemic flow ratio (Qp/Qs) of 2.45:1 was calculated. Also, a phase-encoding sequence was obtained passing through the fossa ovalis (panel G), nicely depicting the morphology of the defect and calculating a 63 ml left-to-right shunt.
- Inversion-recovery images (panel H) did not show any late gadolinium enhancement.
- Ostium secundum ASD is the commonest type of ASD (>75%). Percutaneous closure is the treatment of choice in these patients particularly if <38 mm in diameter and if it has a sufficient rim (≥5 mm) towards the aorta.
- Furthermore, the absence of pulmonary hypertension (normal pulmonary artery size and lack of late gadolinium enhancement) suggests a good prognosis after the procedure.

Further Reading

ECG guidelines for the management of grown-up congenital disease (new version 2010): the Task Force on the management of grown-up congenital disease of the European Society of Cardiology (ESC). Eur Heart J. 2010;31:2915–57.

Case 106

Atrial Septal Defect

Clinical History

- Twenty-one-year-old female.
- Dyspnea New York Heart Association functional class III.
- Past medical history of syncope.
- Transthoracic echocardiogram showed severe pulmonary hypertension and severe dilation of the right chambers.
- Cardiac computed tomography (CT) was required to rule out congenital heart disease.

Images

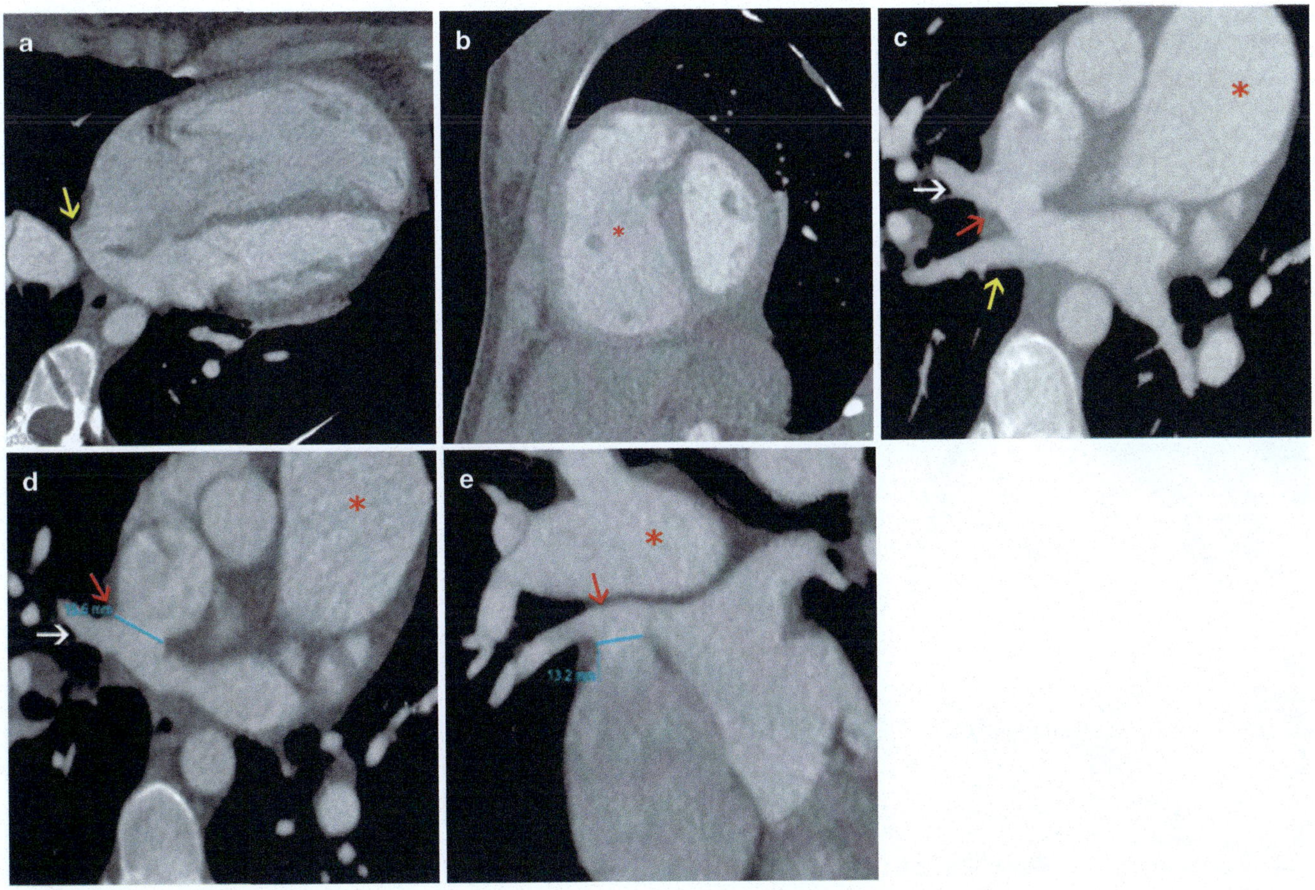

Findings and Interpretation

- Four-chamber view (panel A) showing severe dilation of right chambers and a superior sinus venosus atrial septal defect (ASD, arrow).
- In a short-axis view (panel B), the right ventricle is dilated (asterisk) with normal left ventricle.
- Severe dilation of pulmonary artery is detected using multiple views (asterisk in panels C–E).
- Multiplanar reconstructions (panels C–E) illustrating the presence of a superior sinus venosus ASD (red arrows) and the right superior pulmonary vein connecting into the superior dome of the right atrium at the level of the cavo-atrial junction (white arrows). Left pulmonary veins drain normally in the left atrium (yellow arrow in panel C).
- This patient was discarded for surgery as was deemed eligible for heart transplantation.

Further Reading

Amat F, Le Bret E, Sigal-Cinqualbre A, Coblence M, Lambert V, Rohnean A, et al. Diagnostic accuracy of multidetector spiral computed tomography for preoperative assessment of sinus venosus atrial septal defects in children. Interact Cardiovasc Thorac Surg. 2011;12:179–82.

Case 107

Ventricular Septal Defect

Clinical History

- Sixty-three-year-old male.
- With recurrent atrial fibrillation.
- Echocardiography revealed a small (3 mm) restrictive (high-velocity, 4.3 m/s) perimembranous ventricular septal defect (VSD). Pulmonary artery systolic pressure was normal (30 mmHg).
- Referred to cardiac magnetic resonance (MR) to evaluate pulmonary vein catheter ablation.

Images

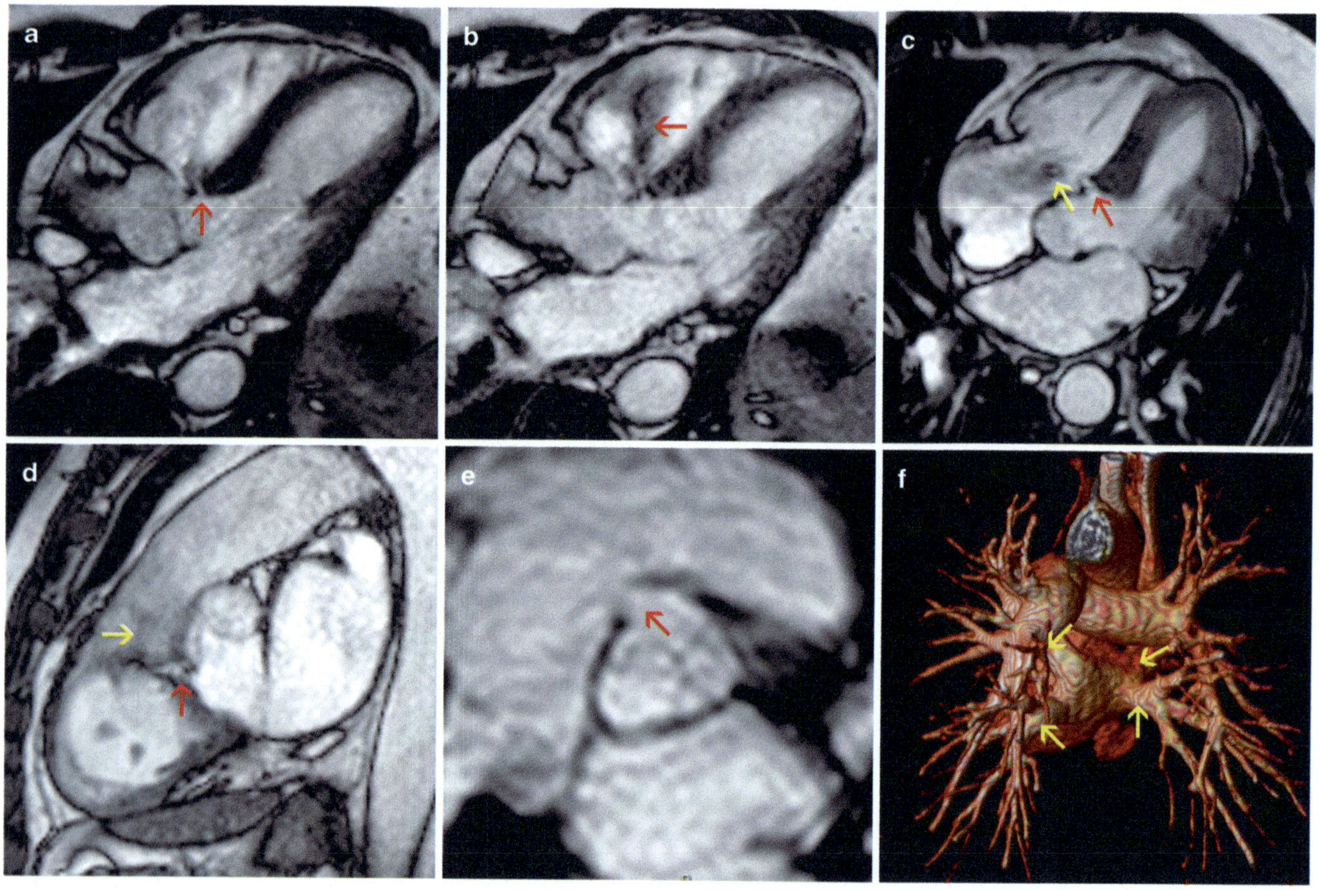

Findings and Interpretation

- As shown using left ventricular outflow tract views (panel A, end-diastolic; panel B, systolic), left ventricular dimensions were normal (end-diastolic volume 79 ml/m^2), with mild septal hypertrophy (13.5 mm) and preserved systolic function.
- A small perimembranous VSD was detected (arrows in panels A, C, D, and E), with a left-to-right shunt (arrow in panel B).
- A sagittal (panel D) and an orthogonal view at the aortic valve level (panel E) further aid the evaluation of the defect.
- Mild pulmonary (yellow arrow in panel D) and moderate tricuspid regurgitation (yellow arrow in panel C) were also identified, the latter associated with the VSD.
- Three-dimensional volume rendering MR angiography showed normal pulmonary vein anatomy (yellow arrows in panel G).

- Given that this patient was referred to evaluation of the pulmonary veins, and the fact that the VSD was small and not associated to significant hemodynamic impact (normal size of cardiac chambers, lack of pulmonary hypertension, defect size <1/3 of the aortic root, high-speed jet), phase-encoding sequences were not performed to quantify the shunt.
- VSD is the most frequent congenital heart disease in newborns, although up to 70% have spontaneous closure within the first years of life.

Further Reading

ECG guidelines for the management of grown-up congenital disease (new version 2010): the Task Force on the management of grown-up congenital disease of the European Society of Cardiology (ESC). Eur Heart J. 2010;31:2915–57.

Case 108

Ventricular Septal Defect

Clinical History

- Thirty-eight-year-old male.
- Asymptomatic, without coronary risk factors.
- He has a family history (mother and sister) of hypertrophic cardiomyopathy.
- Echocardiography revealed asymmetric septal hypertrophy (15 mm) and mild diastolic dysfunction.
- Referred to cardiac magnetic resonance for further assessment.

Images

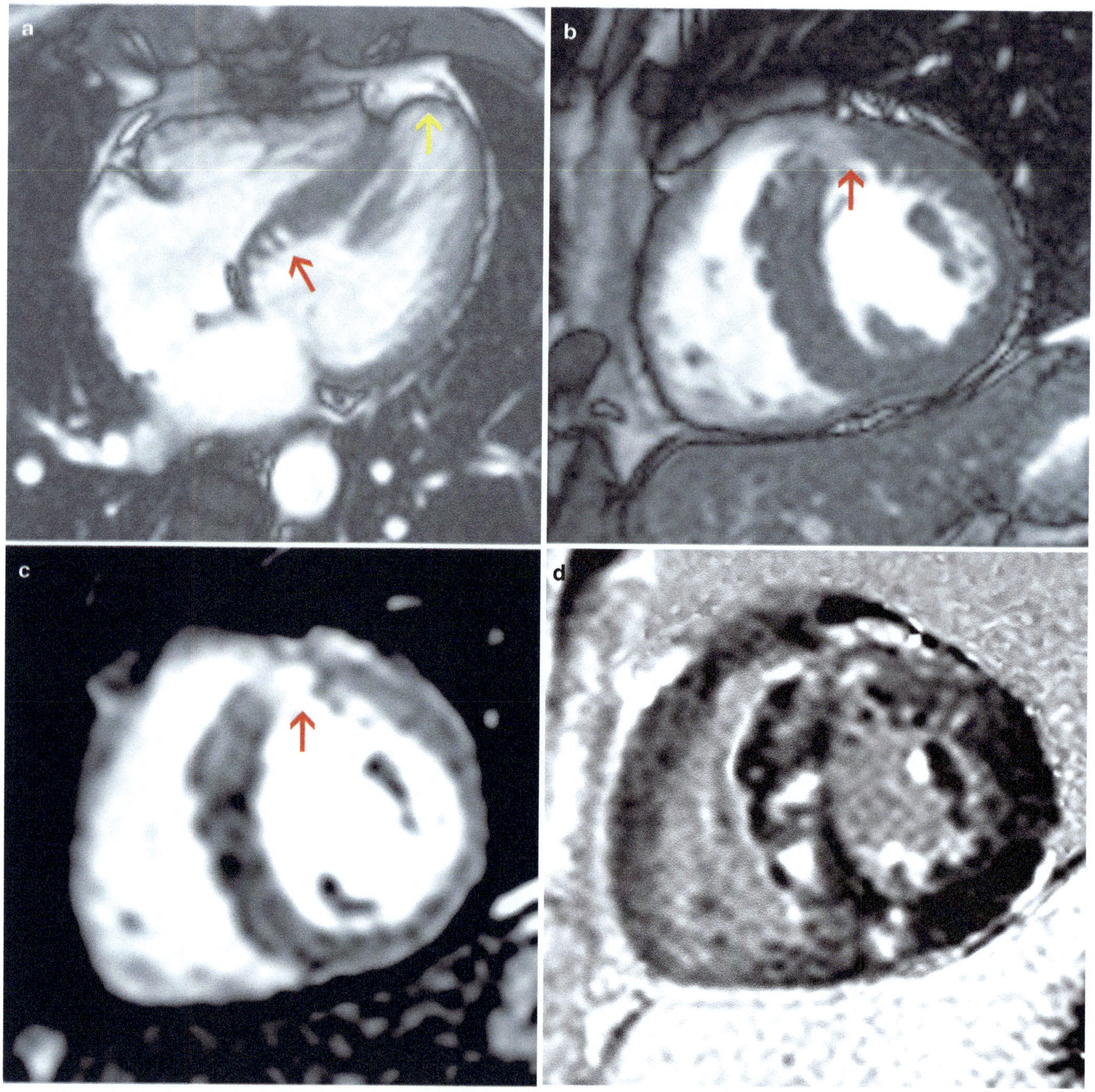

Findings and Interpretation

- Left ventricular dimensions were normal, with mild asymmetric septal hypertrophy (maximum septal thickness of 13.0 mm, panels A and B) and areas of myocardial wall thinning (yellow arrow in panel A).
- Using a low four-chamber view (panel A), small inferior septal ventricular crypts were identified (arrow in panel A).
- At the mid-ventricular level, a muscular ventricular septal defect (VSD) was detected (red arrow in panel C), with only minimal left-to-right shunt given the high position (thus with systolic closure) and the interposition of a portion of the moderator band.
- At first-pass perfusion imaging, myocardial perfusion was normal, with interrupted perfusion at the VSD.
- Inverse-recovery images showed extensive late gadolinium enhancement (panel D), as a reflection of diffuse myocardial fibrosis.
- VSDs are the most common congenital heart defect at birth detected as an isolated finding, and spontaneous closure is very frequent. VSD also can be associated with multiple defects.
- The prevalence of VSD is higher among patients with HCM. Although this is not the case, this relationship has been particularly reported among patients with Noonan´s syndrome.

Further Reading

Reddy ST, Paladino Filho AT, Williams RB, et al. Simultaneous hypertrophic cardiomyopathy and muscular ventricular septal defect in an adult patient. Echocardiography. 2012;29:110–11.

Case 109

Patent Ductus Arteriosus

Clinical History

- Twenty-four-year-old male.
- Preterm birth, with maternal history of mumps and measles during pregnancy. Heart murmur. Strabismus with amaurosis of the right eye. Hearing loss. Repetitive pneumonia during childhood.
- Consulted for dyspnea and palpitations.
- ECG showed right axis deviation with signs of right ventricular (RV) hypertrophy and incomplete right bundle branch block.
- Transthoracic echocardiography confirmed RV hypertrophy. Systolic function of the RV was in the lower normal range. He had signs of pulmonary hypertension: rectification of the interventricular septum, dilated pulmonary artery, mild pulmonary insufficiency, with mean pulmonary pressure of 105 mmHg, and nonconclusive persistent ductus arteriosus (PDA).
- Transesophageal echocardiography with bubbles confirmed the presence of right-to-left shunt.
- Referred computed tomography (CT) angiography of the aorta to confirm the presence of PDA.

Images

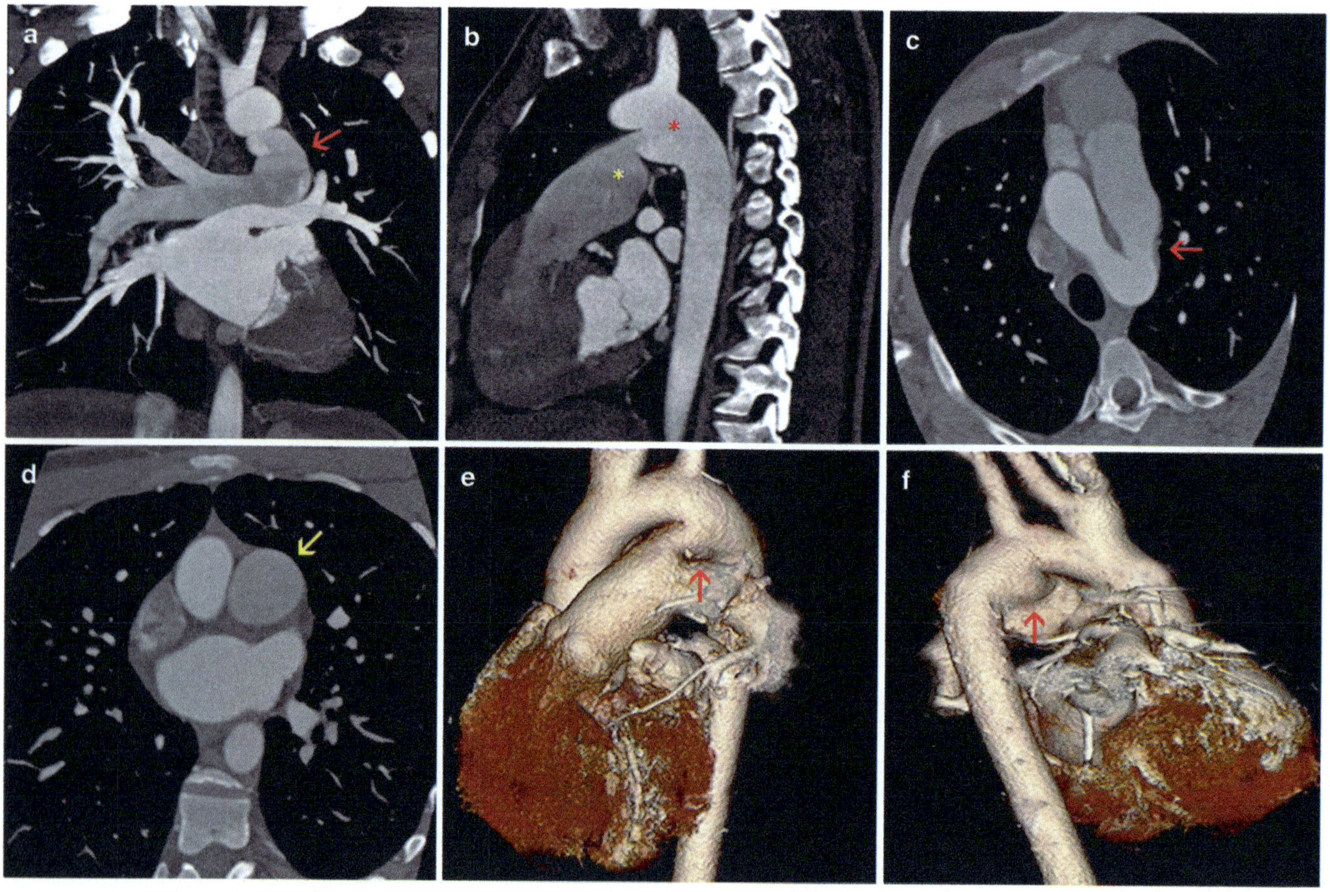

Findings and Interpretation

- CT angiography confirmed the presence of PDA (panels A–C, E, and F) with a maximum diameter of 17 mm (red arrow in panel A and C). In panels E and F, the red arrows show the three-dimensional reconstruction of the large PDA.
- Measurements of the aortic (22 mm) and pulmonary (13 mm) ends were estimated (red and yellow asterisk, respectively, in panel B).
- Dilatation of the pulmonary artery, with a maximum diameter of 35 mm (yellow arrow in panel D).
- With this study it was possible to confirm the presence of PDA that caused pulmonary hypertension in order to complete the hemodynamic evaluation and guide percutaneous or surgical closure.

Further Reading

Parekh D, Krajcer Z. Patent ductus arteriosus and pulmonary arterial hypertension: is it closer to closure?. Catheter Cardiovasc Interv. 2017;89:726–72.

Yan C, Zhao S, Jiang S, Xu Z, Huang L, Zheng H, et al. Transcatheter closure of patent ductus arteriosus with severe pulmonary arterial hypertension in adults. Heart. 2007;93:514–8.

Zhang CJ, Huang YG, Huang XS, Huang T, Huang WH, Xia CL, et al. Transcatheter closure of large patent ductus arteriosus with severe pulmonary arterial hypertension in adults: immediate and two-year follow-up results. Chin Med J (Engl). 2012;125:3844–50.

Zhang DZ, Zhu XY, Lv B, Cui CS, Han XM, Sheng XT, et al. Trial occlusion to assess the risk of persistent pulmonary arterial hypertension after closure of a large patent ductus arteriosus in adolescents and adults with elevated pulmonary artery pressure. Circ Cardiovasc Interv 2014;7:473–81.

Case 110

Patent Ductus Arteriosus

Clinical History

- Sixty-two-year-old female.
- Abdominal ultrasound imaging was performed in the setting of acute abdominal pain. A 4.8 cm abdominal aortic aneurysm was diagnosed.
- Medical history did not provide evidence of any cardiovascular risk factors.
- The patient was referred for thoracic computed tomography (CT) angiography to exclude thoracic aortic aneurysm.

Images

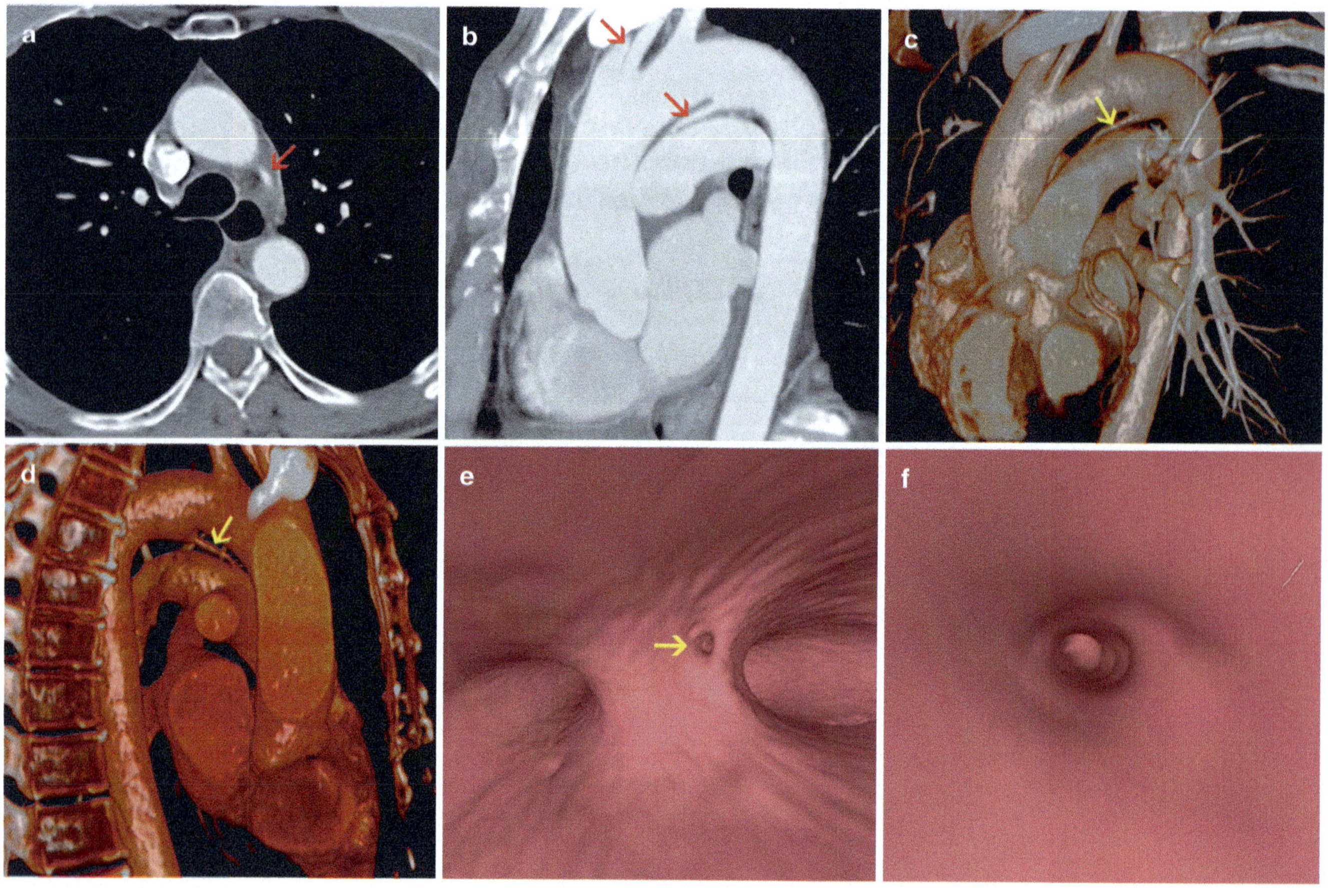

Findings and Interpretation

- CT angiography of the aorta shows a normal thoracic aortic diameter. The presence of unknown patent ductus arteriosus (PDA) was determined.
- Axial and sagittal multiplanar reconstructions (panels A, B) and 3D volume rendering image, left and right lateral views (panels C, D), show a tubular PDA connecting the proximal left pulmonary artery to the descending aorta just distal to the left subclavian artery. Virtual endoscopy view from the roof of the aortic arch (panel E) shows the aortic foramen of the patent ductus. PDA virtual endoscopy view (panel F).
- PDA is a relatively common congenital defect, with an incidence as high as 1 in 1,500 and a female-to-male ratio of 2:1. It results from a failure in spontaneous closure of the ductus arteriosus, usually occurring within the first 48 h of life.
- The ductus arteriosus may persist in an infinite variety of shapes and sizes. Both characteristics are important determinants of the degree of shunting and physiological impact. Large ductus may cause high-magnitude left-to-right shunt, resulting over time in impairment of systemic cardiac output and pulmonary artery hypertension.

- Angiographic classification typically recognizes five types of PDA:
  - Type A, conical ductus
  - Type B, window ductus
  - Type C, tubular ductus
  - Type D, complex ductus
  - Type E, elongated ductus
- Echocardiography is considered as the gold standard for diagnosing a PDA, characterizing the anatomy as well as the physiology of the PDA. CT angiography gives excellent image quality of the vascular anatomy.

Further Reading

Cassidy HD, Cassidy LA, Blackshear JL. Incidental discovery of a patent ductus arteriosus in adults. J Am Board Fam Med. 2009;22:214–8.

Krichenko A, Benson LN, Burrows P, Möes CA, McLaughlin P, Freedom RM. Angiographic classification of the isolated, persistently patent ductus arteriosus and implications for percutaneous catheter occlusion. Am J Cardiol. 1989;63:877–80.

Schneider DJ. The patent ductus arteriosus in term infants, children, and adults. Semin Perinatol. 2012;36:146–53.

Case 111

Aortic Coarctation Associated with Bicuspid Aortic Valve

Clinical History

- Seventy-four year-old male.
- Aortic root dilatation and bicuspid aortic valve diagnosed by routine echocardiography.
- Adult aortic coarctation was discovered incidentally on computed tomography (CT) angiography of the thoracic aorta.
- Past medical history indicates persistent atrial fibrillation under anticoagulation therapy and recent diagnosis of arterial hypertension.
- Neither surgical nor endovascular repair of aortic coarctation was performed.
- Referred for follow-up contrast-enhanced magnetic resonance angiography (MRA) of the thoracic aorta.

Images

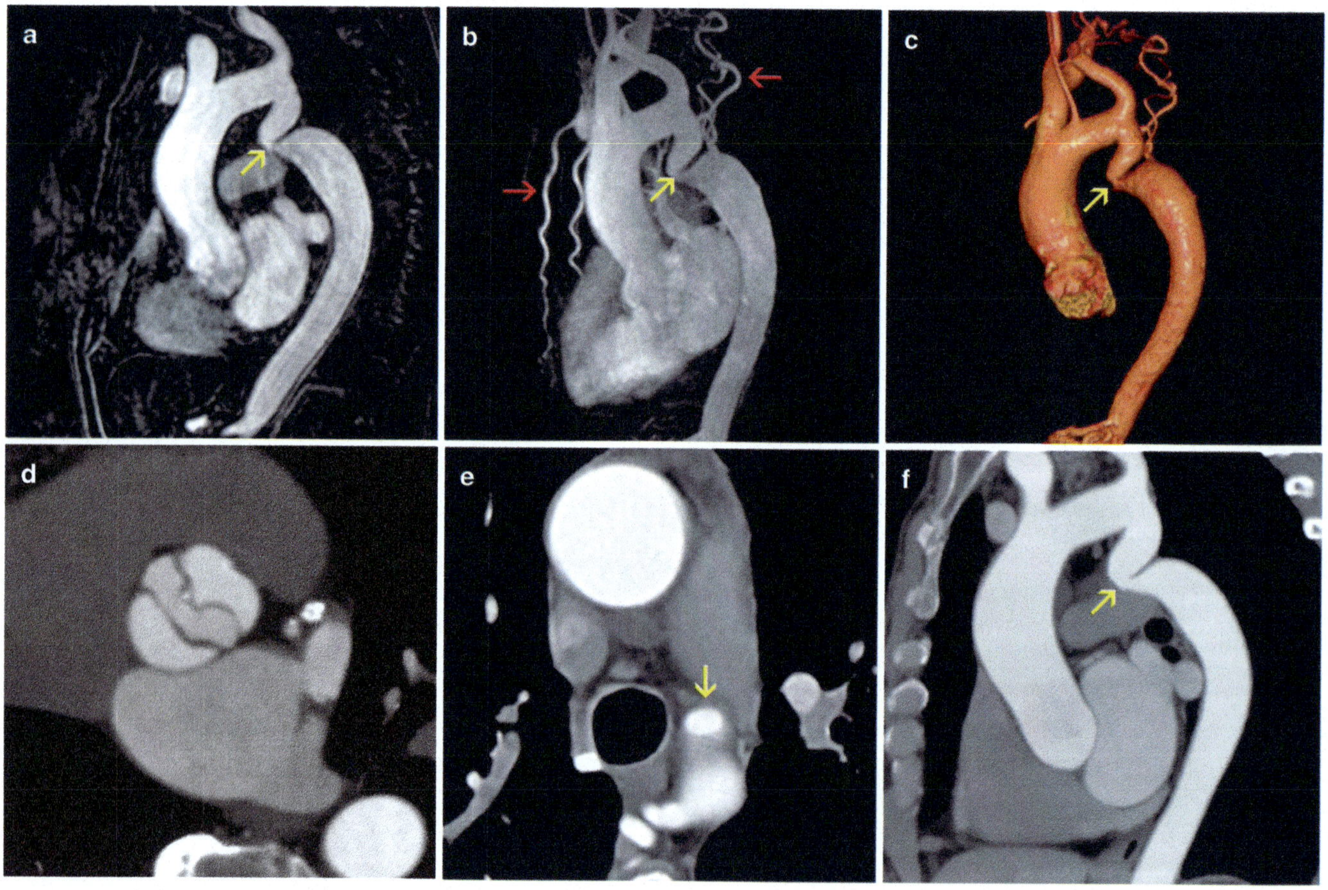

Findings and Interpretation

- Current follow-up contrast-enhanced MRA (panels A–C) and CT angiography performed 3 years earlier (panels D–F) show the presence of an adult-type coarctation distal to the left subclavian artery.
- Sagittal oblique MR image (panel A), sagittal maximum intensity projection (MIP) image (panel B), and volume rendering image (panel C) of the thoracic aorta demonstrate a severe aortic narrowing (yellow arrow) distal to the left subclavian artery with mild poststenotic dilatation. MRA also demonstrates enlarged internal mammary arteries and dilated right posterior intercostal arteries (collateral circulation, red arrows).
- CT angiography shows a bicuspid aortic valve (panel D) and the presence of a shelflike isthmic stenosis of the thoracic aorta distal to the origin of the left subclavian artery, as seen in the axial CT image (panel E) in a perpendicular plane at the level of narrowing of the thoracic aorta (arrow) and in the sagittal oblique CT MIP image (panel F). Note a mild dilatation of the tubular portion of the ascending aorta.

- Coarctation of the aorta is a congenital narrowing of the thoracic aorta, representing the 5–10% of all congenital heart disease, being more frequently in males. In cases remaining undiagnosed until adulthood, it constitutes an important cause of secondary systemic hypertension. Accelerated coronary heart disease, stroke, aortic dissection, and congestive heart failure are also common complications in the natural history of unrepaired aortic coarctation.
- Cross-sectional imaging techniques such as CT and MR angiographies provide excellent anatomic resolution. Since MR imaging does not use ionizing radiation, it may be considered for the follow-up of these patients.

Further Reading

Abbruzzese PA, Aidala E. Aortic coarctation: an overview. J Cardiovasc Med (Hagerstown). 2007;8:123–8.

Maldonado JA, Henry T, Gutiérrez FR. Congenital thoracic vascular anomalies. Radiol Clin N Am. 2010;48(1):85–115.

Pemberton J, Sahn DJ. Imaging of the aorta. Int J Cardiol. 2004;97 Suppl 1:53–60.

Szkutnik M, Sulik S, Fiszer R, Chodor B, Głowacki J, Bialkowski J. Native aortic coarctation stenting in patients ≥46 years old. Postepy Kardiol Interwencyjnej. 2017;13:302–6.

Case 112

Aortic Coarctation

Clinical History

- Nineteen-year-old male.
- He has known aortic coarctation.
- Referred for aortic computed tomography (CT) angiography to define surgical strategy.

Images

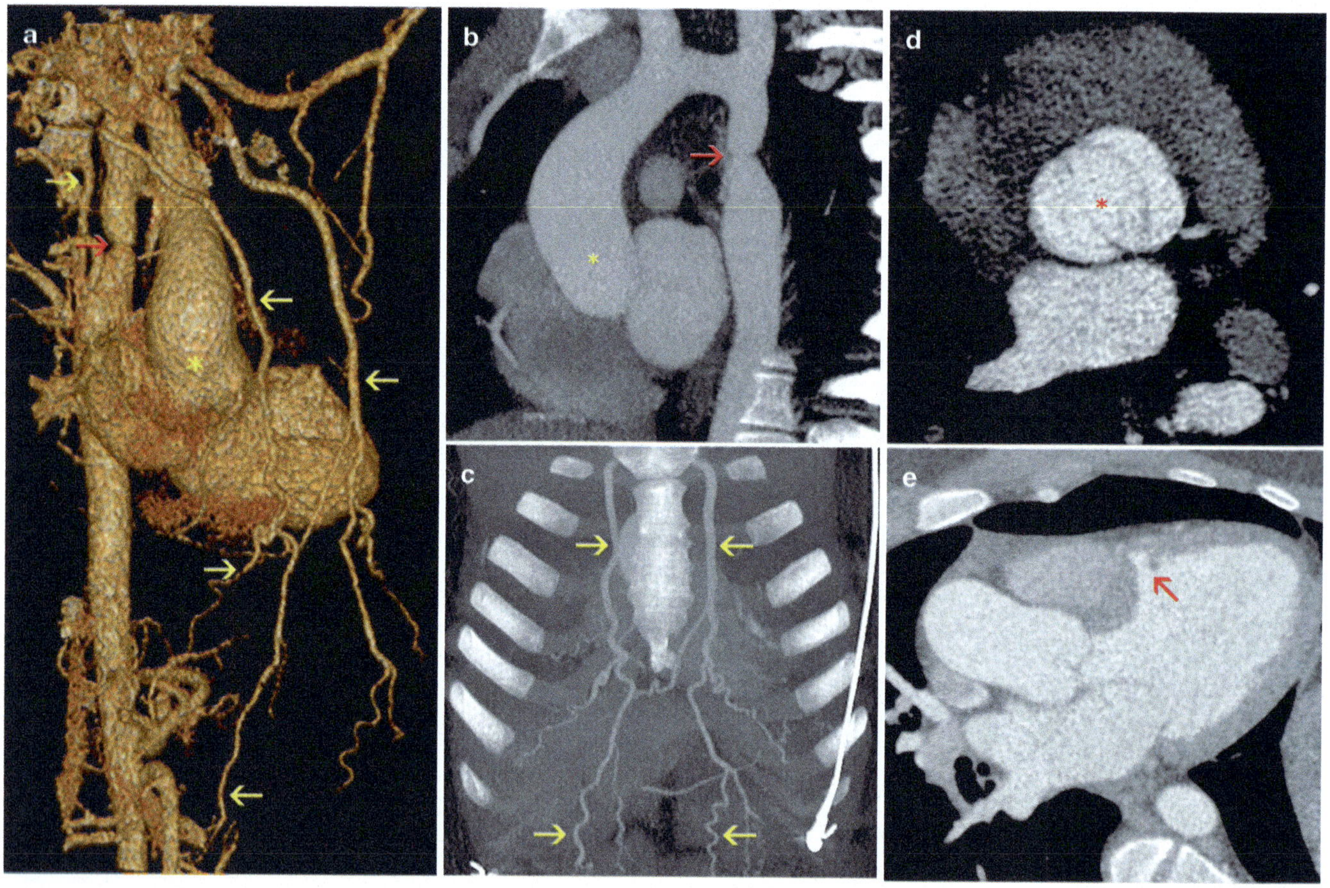

Findings and Interpretation

- Thoracic CT angiography demonstrated a severe post-ductal aortic coarctation (red arrow in panels A and B), distal to the ligamentum arteriosus.
- Both internal mammary arteries are enlarged, with extensive collateral circulation from intercostal, vertebral, and epigastric arteries (yellow arrows in panels A and C).
- The sinus and the proximal tubular portions of the ascending aorta are markedly dilated (asterisk in panels A and B), being this related to the presence of a previously unrecognized bicuspid aortic valve (panel D).
- A left ventricular outflow tract view also shows a spontaneously closed muscular ventricular septal defect (red arrow in panel E).
- Aortic coarctation is among the most prevalent congenital heart disease subtypes, representing approximately 5–8% of all cardiac anomalies. A substantial proportion of patients with aortic coarctation have concomitant bicuspid aortic valve. These patients are at significantly higher risk of aortic dissection compared with patients with non-complex (isolated) aortic coarctation.

Further Reading

Van der Linde D, Konings EEM, Slager MA, Witsenburg M, Helbing WA, Takkenberg JJ, et al. Birth prevalence of congenital heart disease worldwide a systematic review and meta-analysis. J Am Coll Cardiol. 2011;58:2241–7.

Warnes CA. Bicuspid aortic valve and coarctation: two villains part of a diffuse problem. Heart. 2003;89:965–6.

Case 113

Aortic Coartaction

Clinical History

- Twenty-five-year-old male.
- Marfan's phenotype, with loose joints and aortic enlargement.
- Underwent surgery due to aortic coarcation at 18 months and required reoperation when he was 19 years old due to recoarctation.
- Transthoracic echocardiogram demonstrated a dilated ascending aorta with no signs of recoartaction and normal ventricular function.
- Cardiac computed tomography (CT) was performed to evaluate anatomy due chest and abdominal murmur.

Images

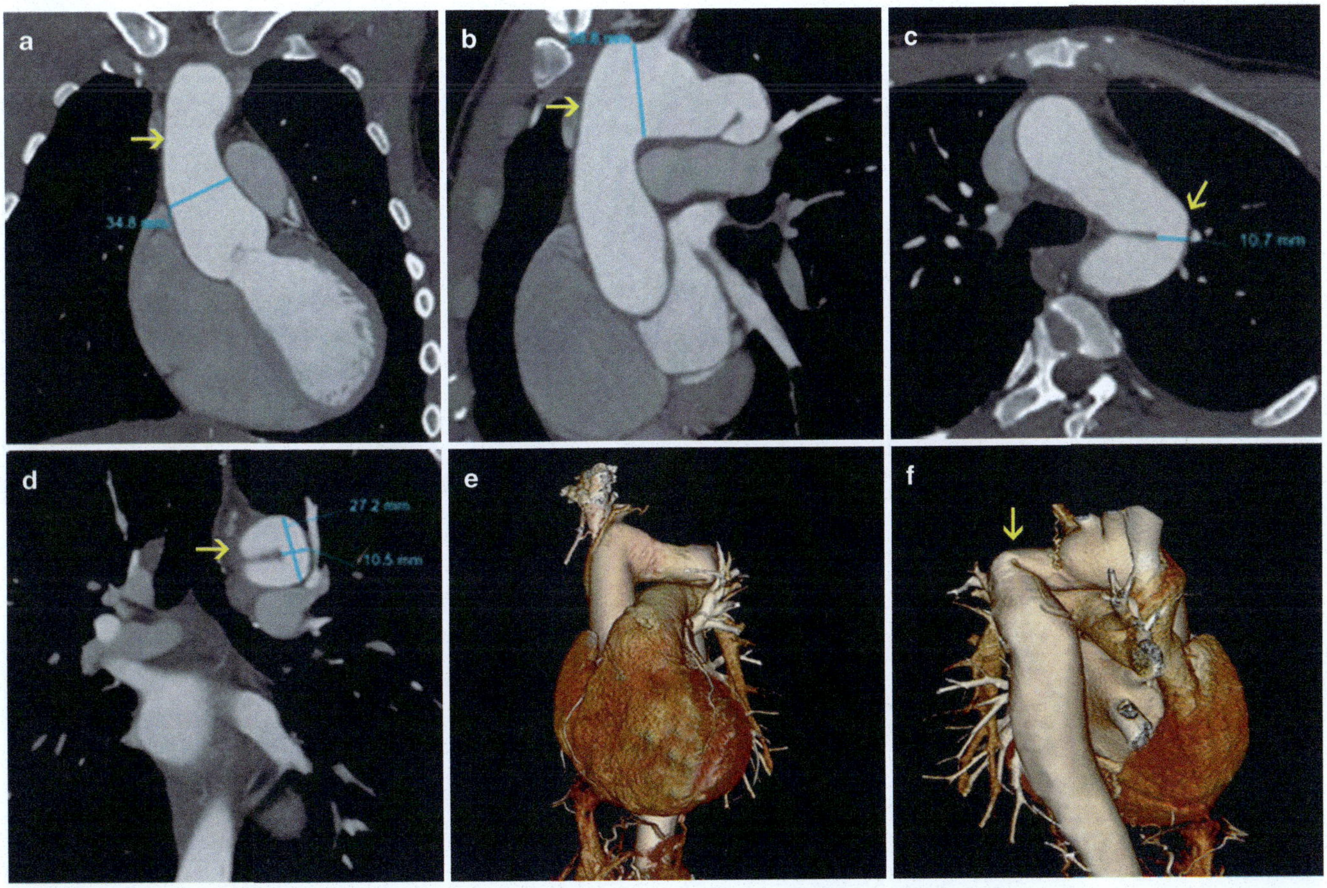

Findings and Interpretation

- Coronal and oblique reconstructions showing a dilated ascending aorta and aortic arch (arrows) (panels A and B).
- Axial image and coronal reformats (panels C and D respectively) illustrating kinking at the level of previous surgery (arrow) that is generating a pseudocoarc tation.
- Volume rendering reconstructions (panels E and F) showing the dilated aorta and the area where the bend is present (arrow in panel F).

Further Reading

Anagnaostopoulos–Tzifa A. Management of aortic coarctation in adults: endovascular versus surgical therapy. Hellenic J Cardiol. 2007;48:290–5.

Baumgartner H, Bonhoeffer P, De Groot NM, et al. ESC Guidelines for the management of grown-up congenital heart disease (new version 2010). Eur Heart J. 2010;31: 2915–57.

Jurcu R, Daraban AM, Lober A, et al. Coarctation of the aorta in adults: what is the best treatment? Case report and literature review. J Med Life. 2011;4:189–95.

Case 114

Aortic Coarctation

Clinical History

- Thirty-one-year-old female.
- History of arterial hypertension diagnosed 3 years ago, with resistant hypertension (high blood pressure despite full pharmacologic treatment with beta-blocker, ACE inhibitors, and diuretics).
- No history of cardiac disease or family history of hypertension.
- Clinical exam showed a blood pressure of 150/90 mmHg in the right arm and 140/90 mmHg in the left arm. Both radial pulses were palpable, but no pulse was palpable at the femoral arteries or distal to that level.
- Posteroanterior (PA) chest X-ray showed a normal cardiothoracic index and bilateral rib notching.
- Referred for chest magnetic resonance angiography (MRA).

Images

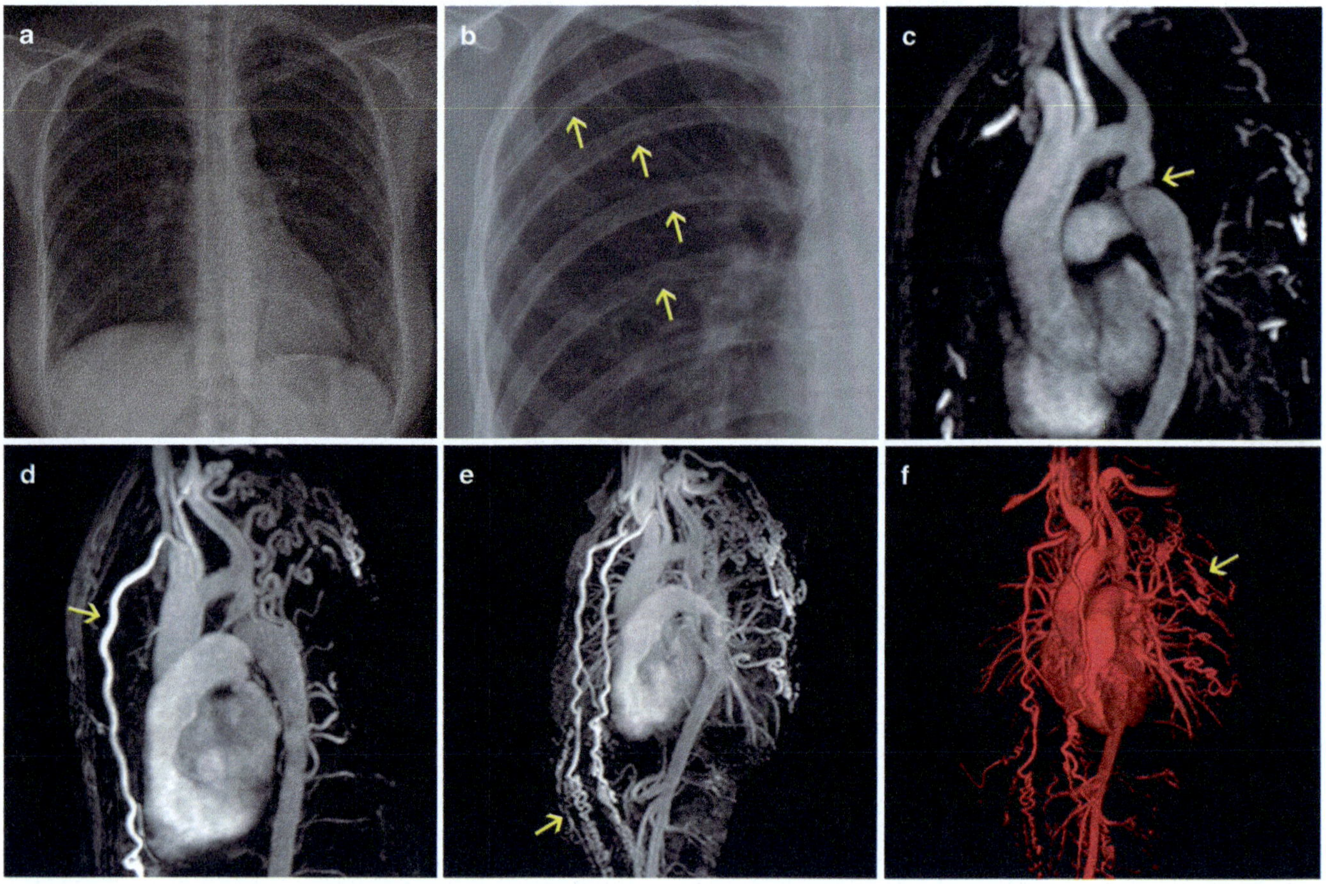

Findings and Interpretation

- PA chest X-ray (panel A, and panel B, close view) shows bilateral rib notching involving the inferior surface of the posterior fourth to eight ribs. These imaging findings are the result of enlarged collateral intercostal arteries (arrows) due to increased blood flow.
- MRA shows the presence of an adult-type coarctation with a typical "shelflike" lesion distal to the left subclavian artery. Sagittal multiplanar reformatted image (panel C), sagittal maximum intensity projection images (panels D, E) and coronal volume rendering image (panel F) show the severe aortic narrowing (yellow arrow) distal to the left subclavian artery with poststenotic dilatation. MRA also demonstrates the extent of collateral circulation, with the presence of enlarged internal mammary arteries (panel D), enlarged superior epigastric arteries (panel E), and dilated post-coarctation collateral intercostal arteries (panel F).
- Coarctation of the aorta represents 7% of congenital heart disease, with a male-female ratio of 1.5:1. Its clinical con-

sequences range from being life-threatening in childhood to remaining undiagnosed until adulthood. Among the latter, it constitutes an important cause of secondary hypertension.

- Typically, coarctation of the aorta is a focal constriction of the thoracic aorta just distal to the left subclavian artery. However, the narrowing may be proximal to the left subclavian artery or rarely in the abdominal aorta; it may also present as a long segment or a tubular hypoplasia (infantile-type coarctation).
- Cross-sectional imaging techniques such as CT and MR angiographies provide excellent anatomic detail, location of the narrowing of aortic lumen, and evaluation of collateral vessels, as well as cardiac chamber and cardiac valve assessment (bicuspid aortic valve is found in up to 85% of the cases).

Further Reading

Maldonado JA, Henry T, Gutiérrez FR. Congenital thoracic vascular anomalies. Radiol Clin N Am. 2010;48:85–115.

Pemberton J, Sahn DJ. Imaging of the aorta. Int J Cardiol. 2004;97 Suppl 1:53–60.

Sebastià C, Quiroga S, Boye R, Perez-Lafuente M, Castellà E, Álvarez-Castells A. Aortic stenosis: spectrum of diseases depicted at multisection CT. Radiographics. 2003;23 Spec No:S79–91.

Tanous D, Benson LN, Horlick EM. Coarctation of the aorta: evaluation and management. Curr Opin Cardiol. 2009;24:509–15.

Case 115

Aortic Coarctation

Clinical History

- Twenty-three-day-old male.
- Left sternal border systolic ejection murmur.
- Decreased lower extremity pulses.
- Referred for computed tomography (CT) angiography for evaluation of the aorta.

Images

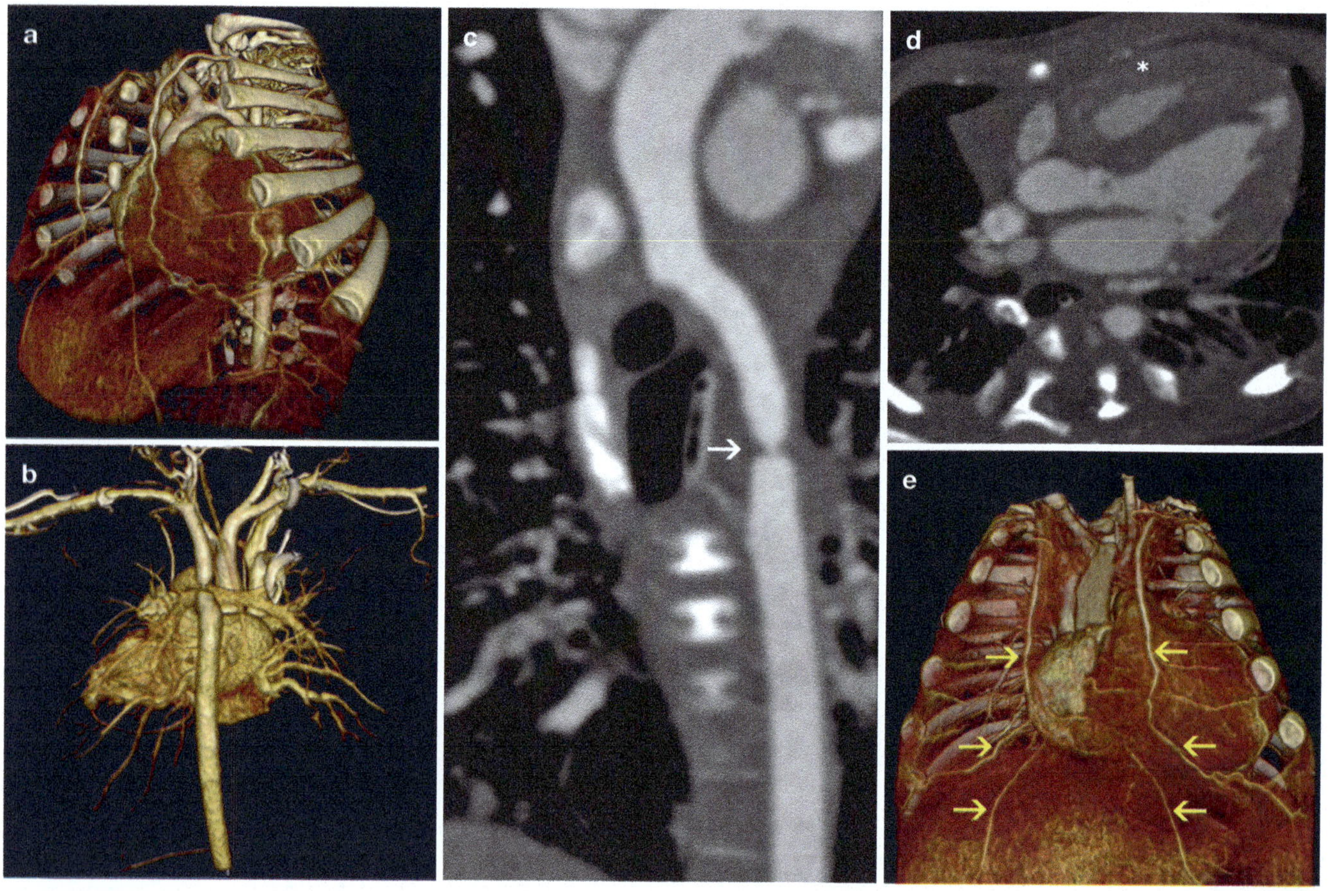

Findings and Interpretation

- Volume-rendered three-dimensional CT reconstructions using sagittal (panel A) and posterior (panel B) views show narrowing of the aortic lumen distal to the origin of the left subclavian artery at the junction of the aortic arch and the descending aorta and large internal thoracic arteries.
- Curved multiplanar reconstruction of the thoracic aorta (panel C) showing the site and the degree of the stenosis (white arrow).
- Axial CT scan (panel D) shows both left ventricular and right ventricular (asterisk) hypertrophy.
- Volume-rendered three-dimensional reconstruction of the thorax, frontal view (panel E), shows enlarged internal thoracic arteries arising from the subclavian arteries and connecting with the descending aorta via the intercostal arteries (3–8°) and with the external iliac arteries via superior and inferior epigastric arteries (yellow arrows).
- Aortic coarctation represents approximately 7% of all congenital heart disease. Since the right ventricle is the systemic ventricle during fetal life, this leads to right ventricle pressure overload in the presence of aortic coarctation and to the presence of biventricular hypertrophy as in this case.

Further Reading

Hanneman K, Newman B, Chan F. Congenital variants and anomalies of the aortic arch. RadioGraphics. 2017;37:32–51.

Maldonado JA, Henry T, Gutiérrez FR. Congenital thoracic vascular anomalies. Radiol Clin North Am. 2010;48:85–115.

Case 116

Aortic Arch Hypoplasia

Clinical History

- One-month-old patient.
- Full-term newborn with appropriate weight.
- No family history of congenital heart disease.
- Genetic syndrome in study. History of mechanical ventilation due to sepsis that required inotropic support in the first days of life.
- Symptomatic for arterial hypertension.
- Transthoracic echocardiography revealed dilatation of the ascending aorta, high suspicion of aortic coarctation, and dilatation of the supraoartic vessels.
- Referred for thoracic computed tomography (CT) angiography to define anatomy.

Images

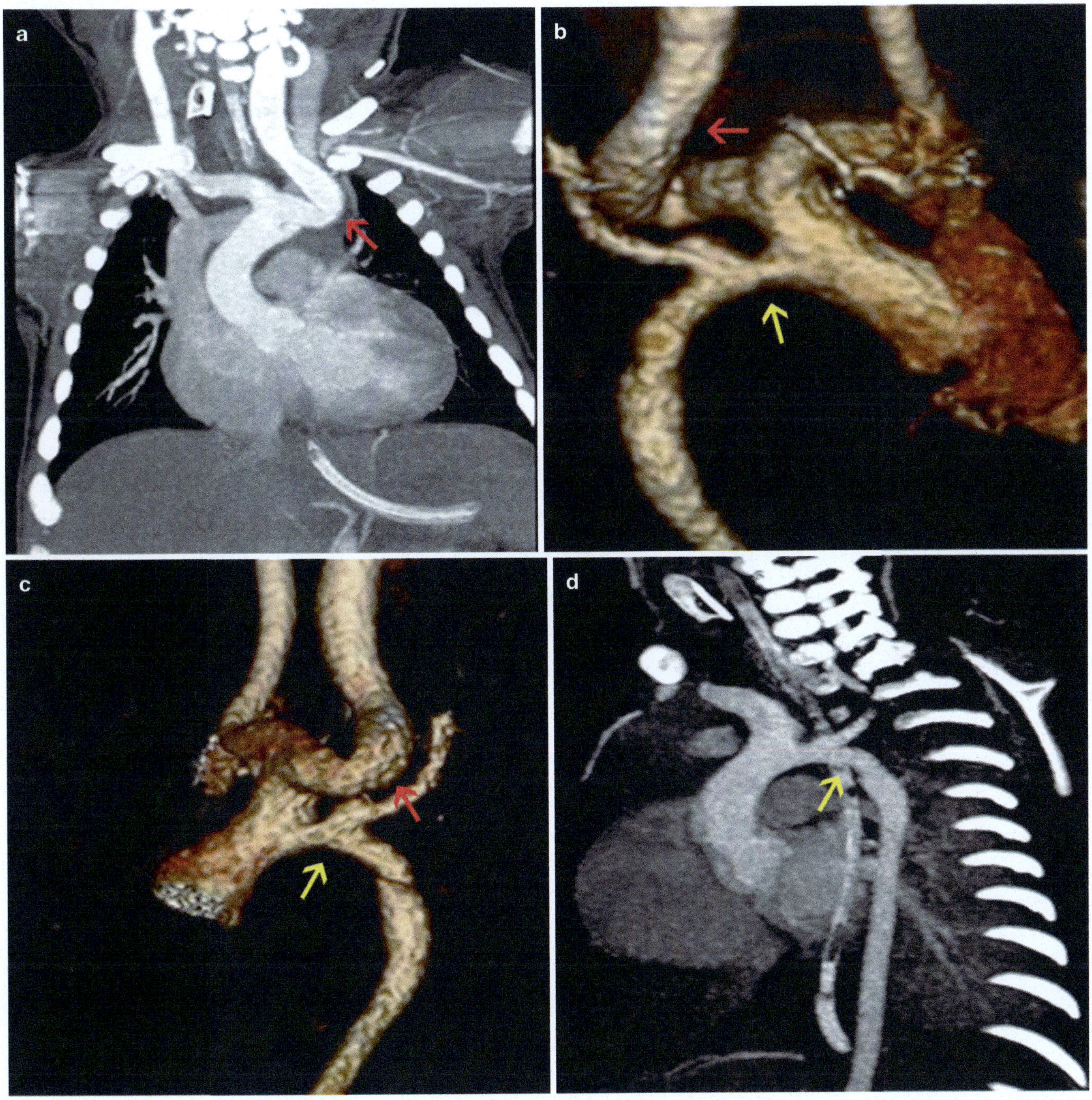

Findings and Interpretation

- Common origin of innominate trunk and left common carotid artery are detected. The latter is dilated and tortuous and has an acute bending at an approximate 8 mm distance from its origin, reaching a maximum diameter of 8.5 mm at the neck level (red arrow in panels A–C).
- Hypoplasia and coarctation of the aortic arch (yellow arrow in panels B–D) after the origin of the common trunk. An abrupt decrease of the aortic caliper is observed, with a minimum diameter within the mid-arch portion of 4.9 mm (z-score − 4). Thereafter and until the proximal descending aorta at the ductal ampulla level, the aortic caliper remains diminished.
- Aortic arch hypoplasia can be defined by the following: (1) size of the arch in mm is less than the patient's weight in kg +1; (2) aortic arch diameter z-score is <−2; and (3) ratio of the diameter of the transverse arch to the descending aorta is <50%.
- Surgical repair or reconstruction of the hypoplastic segment has been recommended in symptomatic patients with hypoplastic aortic arch. The type of surgical repair depends on the age of the patient, imaging findings, and operative findings.

Further Reading

Langley SM, Sunstrom RE, Reed RD, Rekito AJ, Gerrah R. The neonatal hypoplastic aortic arch: decisions and more decisions. Semin Thorac Cardiovasc Surg Pediatr Card Surg Annu. 2013;16:43–51.

Singh S, Hakim FA, Sharma A, Roy RR, Panse PM, Chandrasekaran K, et al. Hypoplasia, pseudocoarctation and coarctation of the aorta – a systematic review. Heart Lung Circ. 2015;24:110–8.

Case 117

Interrupted Aortic Arch

Clinical History

- Neonate with loss of appetite, tired and weak appearance.
- Tachycardia.
- Pale with a weak pulse due to insufficient blood flow.
- Referred for thoracic computed tomography tomography (CT) angiography for further assessment.

Images

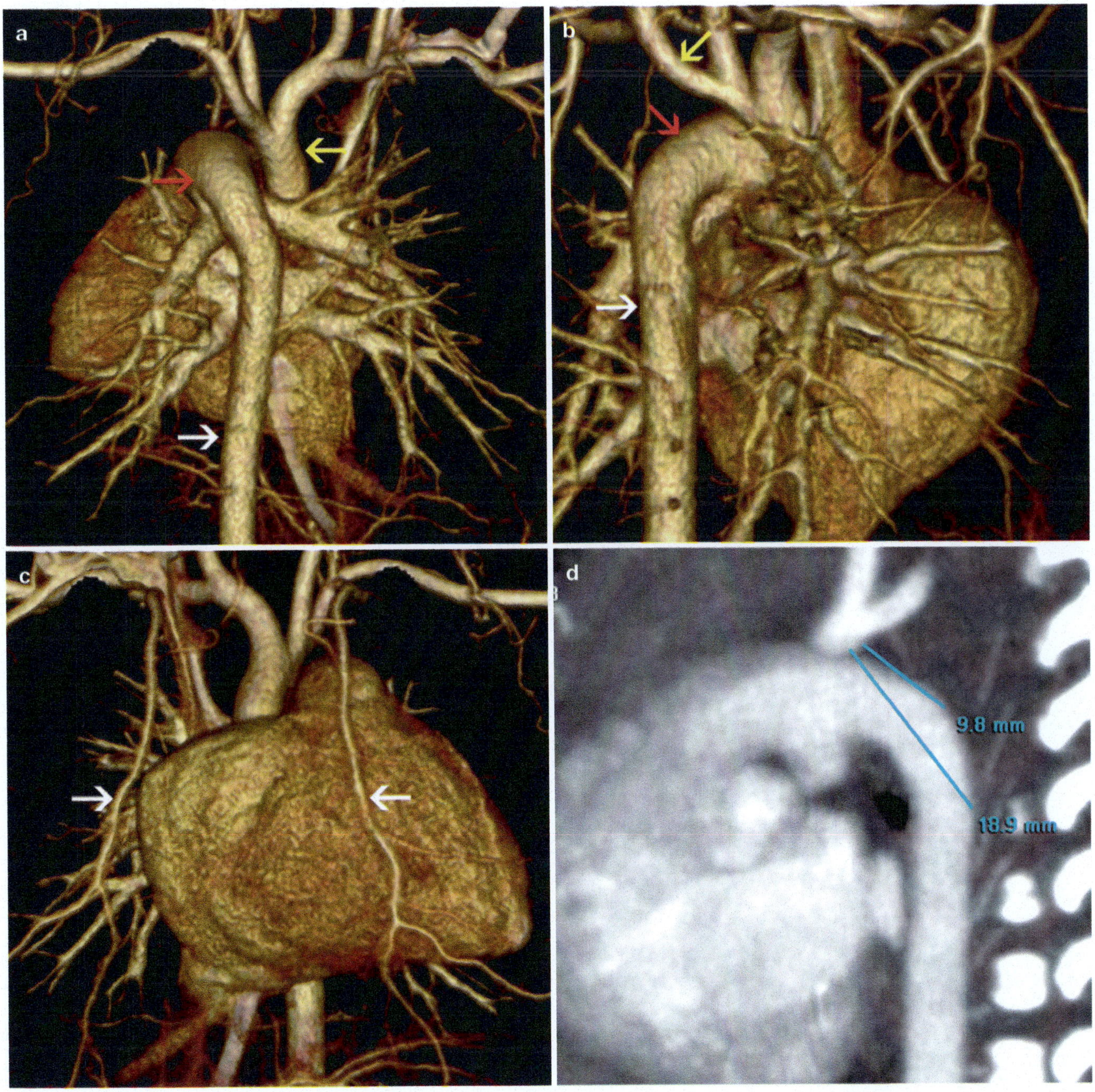

Findings and Interpretation

- Three-dimensional volume rendering reconstruction using posterior view (panel A) and posterior oblique view (panel B) shows a descending aorta (white arrow) communicating with the pulmonary trunk through a large ductus arteriosus (red arrow). Interruption of the aortic arch just beyond the left subclavian artery (yellow arrow).
- There is a complete discontinuity of the aortic lumen between the aortic arch and the descending aorta. This is a type A interrupted aortic arch because the site of the interruption is distal to the subclavian artery.
- Three-dimensional volume rendering reconstruction using anterior view (panel C) shows the ascending aorta giving rise to the innominate artery, the left carotid, and left subclavian arteries. Note the enlargement of internal thoracic or mammary arteries (white arrow).
- Sagittal maximum intensity projection image (panel D) shows continuity of the descending aorta with the main pulmonary artery through a large patent ductus arteriosus. Different distance between the discontinuous segments and the size of the ductus are helpful for preoperative planning.
- This is a very rare congenital heart anomaly, where the aorta is not fully developed. The classification depends on the site of the interruption: type A (after the left subclavian artery), type B (between the left common carotid and left subclavian), and type C (between the innominate artery and the left common carotid). A large percent of these patients have other associated congenital heart defects. Surgery is indicated.

Further Reading

Maldonado JA, Henry T, Gutiérrez FR. Congenital thoracic vascular anomalies. Radiol Clin North Am. 2010;48:85–115.

Case 118

Subvalvular Aortic Stenosis

Clinical History

- Fifty-seven-year-old male.
- Under evaluation due to exertional dyspnea.
- Doppler echocardiography revealed pulmonary hypertension (58 mmHg) with normal size of right chambers and mild left atrium dilatation, preserved systolic function, mild aortic regurgitation, and incremented left ventricular filling pressures (E/e´16).
- Referred to cardiac magnetic resonance to rule out anomalous pulmonary vein return.

Images

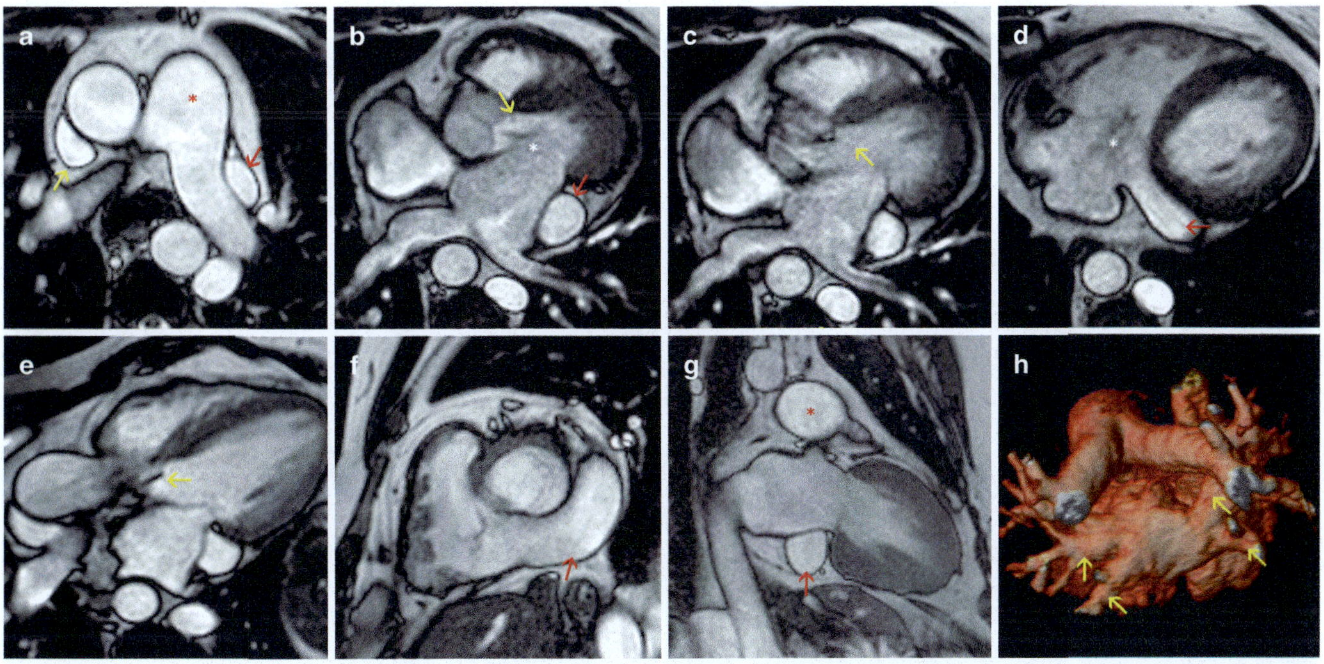

Findings and Interpretation

- Among patients with suspected congenital anomalies, performing cine axial views from the aortic arch to the diaphragm (panels A–D) is highly valuable. In this regard, superior axial cine views identified a persistent left superior vena cava (red arrows in panels A and B), draining at an enlarged coronary sinus (red arrow in panel D). The presence of an enlarged coronary sinus is clearly depicted also using a basal short-axis (panel F) and a two-chamber view (panel G). The right superior vena cava, draining at the right atrium, was also present (yellow arrow in panel A).
- Using the same axial view, a significantly enlarged pulmonary artery was identified (asterisk in panel A), as a reflection of the aforementioned pulmonary hypertension. Importantly, the probable etiology of the exertional dyspnea was also identified, by the detection of a discrete subaortic membrane (yellow arrow in panel B) causing a fixed subaortic stenosis (yellow arrow in panel C; also detected using a left ventricular outflow tract view in panel E) as well as mild aortic regurgitation (asterisk in panel B).
- In addition, moderate tricuspid regurgitation was identified (asterisk in panel D).
- Three-dimensional volume rendering MR angiography showed normal pulmonary vein return (yellow arrows in panel H).
- After valvular aortic stenosis, subaortic aortic stenosis is the second more common form of aortic stenosis and is frequently related to other defects (more frequently ventricular septal defect, bicuspid aortic valve, aortic coarctation, and patent ductus arteriosus).
- These patients, according to the presence of symptoms and evidence for progression of the left ventricular outflow tract gradient, generally require surgical resection.

Further Reading

Qureshi A, Awuor S, Martinez M. Adult presentation of subaortic stenosis: another great hypertrophic cardiomyopathy mimic. Heart Lung Circ. 2015;24:e7-10.

Case 119

Peripheral Pulmonary Stenosis

Clinical History

- Seventeen-year-old female with Alagille syndrome.
- She underwent cardiac magnetic resonance (CMR) to rule out pulmonary artery stenosis.

Images

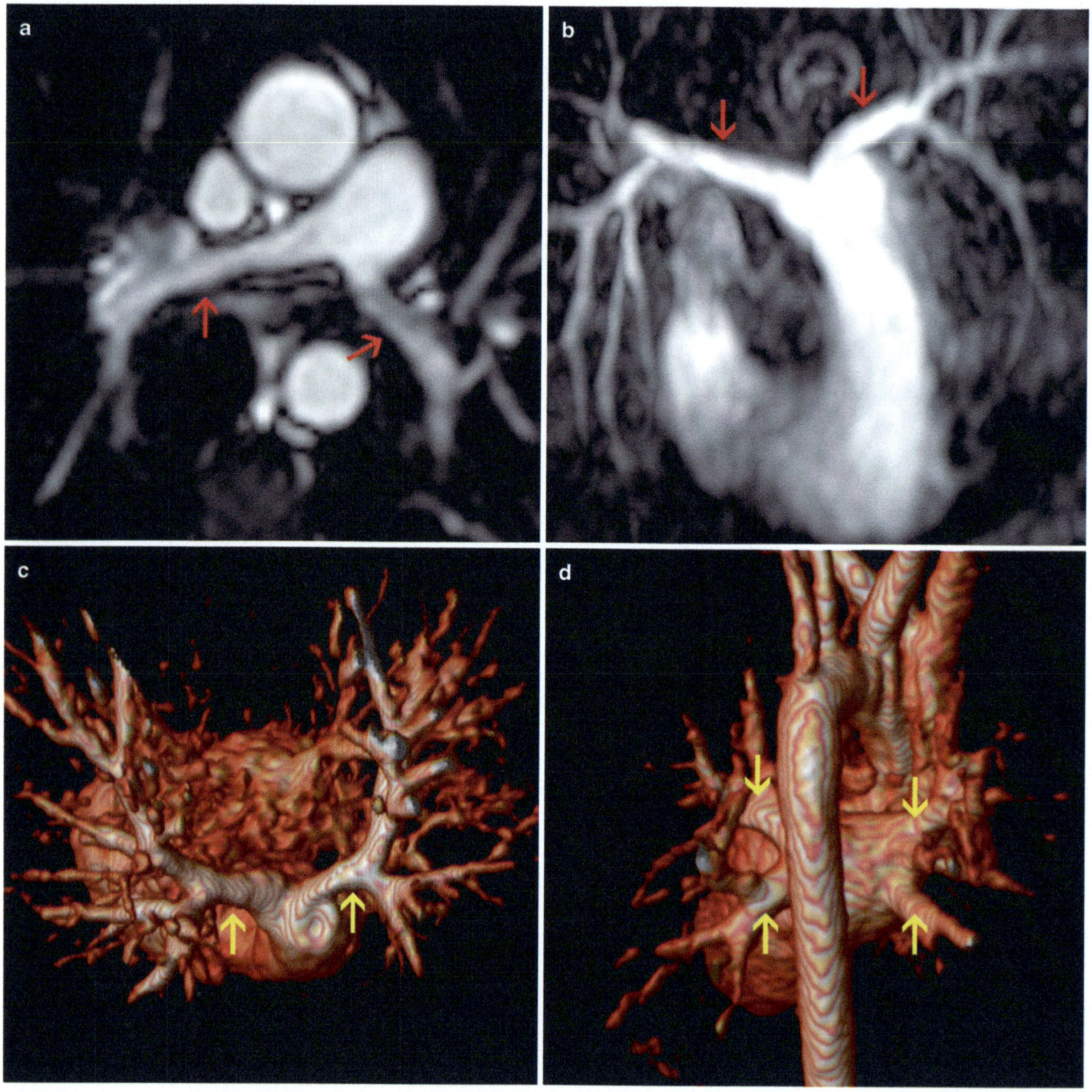

Findings and Interpretation

- Cine axial views at the level of the pulmonary artery bifurcation show a normal pulmonary artery trunk and diffuse narrowing of both pulmonary artery branches (red arrows in panel A).
- Contrast-enhanced MR angiogram using maximum intensity projection (panel B) and volume rendering (panel C) reconstructions demonstrates similar findings, with patent yet diffusely narrowed pulmonary artery branches.
- The patient had no additional cardiac or aortic defects, and both systemic and pulmonary vein returns (arrows in panel D) were normal.
- Alagille syndrome is a genetic disorder with an autosomal dominant inheritance that affects mostly the bile ducts but also affects the heart and other organs. Peripheral pulmonary stenosis is particularly common in these individuals.

Further Reading

Saleh M, Kamath BM, Chitayat D. Alagille syndrome: clinical perspectives. Appl Clin Genet. 2016;9:75–82.

Case 120

Pulmonary Atresia

Clinical History

- Twenty-eight-year-old female.
- Patient with a history of cyanotic congenital heart disease with surgery (central shunt with 4 mm goretex between right pulmonary branch and aorta).
- Currently with dyspnea New York Heart Association functional class II of 2 months duration associated with cough and expectoration. The patient is admitted for respiratory insufficiency and polyglobulia with a saturation of 72% with 21% with fraction of inspired oxygen (FiO2) that corrects 85% with 100% FiO2. Continuous murmur in pulmonary area. No fever. No edema.
- ECG: sinus rhythm, extreme right axis deviation, incomplete right bundle branch block, and poor progression of R waves in precordial leads.
- Transthoracic echocardiography with poor acoustic window revealed pulmonary atresia with intact septum and non-confluent pulmonary branches, the left fed by a large persistent ductus arteriosus and the right one hard to assess. Also tricuspid atresia with eccentric left ventricular hypertrophy and global hypokinesia with mild systolic dysfunction was observed. Indirect signs of pulmonary hypertension. No central shunt was observed.
- Referred to thoracic and cardiac computed tomography (CT) angiography for further cardiac and pulmonary evaluation.

Images

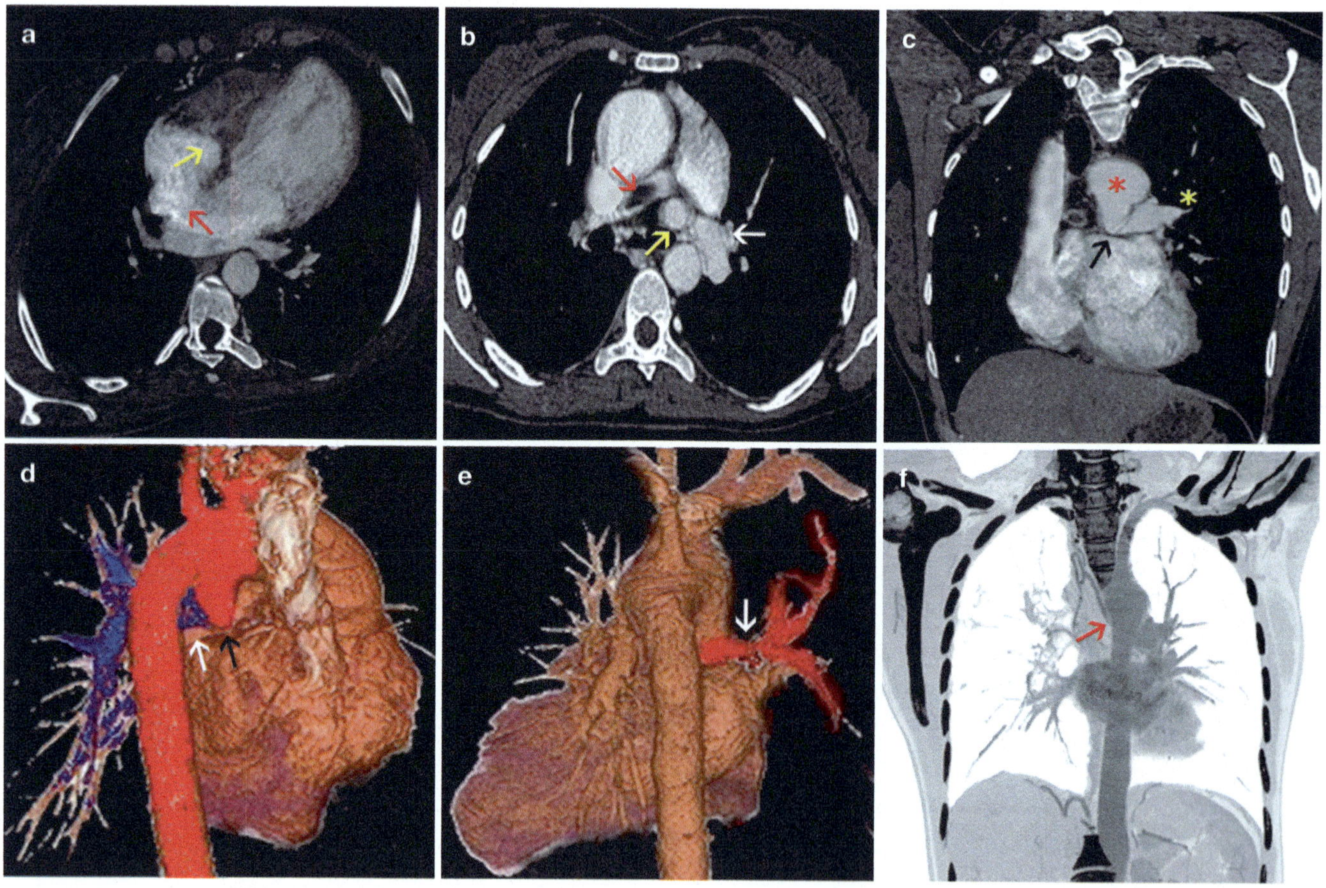

Findings and Interpretation

- Sequential segmental analysis was performed defining situs solitus, levocardia.
- Atrioventricular connection: univentricular with tricuspid atresia with rudimentary right ventricle (yellow arrow in panel A).
- Ventriculoarterial connection: pulmonary atresia with intact septum. The left branch of the pulmonary artery (white arrow in panel B, yellow asterisk in panel C, and white arrow in 3D reconstruction in panel D) is fed by a large ductus (yellow arrow in panel B, black arrows in panel C and in 3D reconstruction in panel D) as the sole

source of pulmonary flow, whereas in the right branch (white arrow in 3D reconstruction in panel E), an intraluminal thrombus is detected (red arrow in panel B).
- Development of collateral circulation from enlarged bronchial (red arrow in panel F) and right internal mammary arteries. There is thinning of segmental vessels in the right lung.
- The aorta is dilated with maximum diameter at the level of the aortic root.
- The described findings allowed to diagnose chronic pulmonary thromboembolism as probable cause of pulmonary hypertension associated to the base cardiopathy. Next steps might be perfusion ventilation scintigraphy and/or right cardiac catheterization.

Further Reading

Chikkabyrappa SM, Loomba RS, Tretter JT. Pulmonary atresia with an intact ventricular septum: preoperative physiology, imaging, and management. Semin Cardiothorac Vasc Anesth. 2018;22:245–55.

Galiè N, Humbert M, Vachiery JL, Gibbs S, Lang I, Torbicki A, et al. Guidelines on diagnosis and treatment of pulmonary hypertension.ESC clinical practice guidelines. Eur Heart J. 2016:37;67–119.

Case 121

Tetralogy of Fallot

Clinical History

- Fifty-one-year-old male.
- He has a history of tetralogy of Fallot, with surgical repair at the age of 6.
- Asymptomatic, 1 year ago he underwent catheter ablation due to arrhythmia (non-specified).
- Echocardiography revealed right ventricular (RV) dilatation with preserved systolic function and moderate tricuspid regurgitation (pulmonary artery systolic pressure of 38 mmHg); moderate aortic regurgitation with normal left ventricular (LV) size and preserved systolic function.
- Cardiac magnetic resonance (MR) was requested for further assessment.

Images

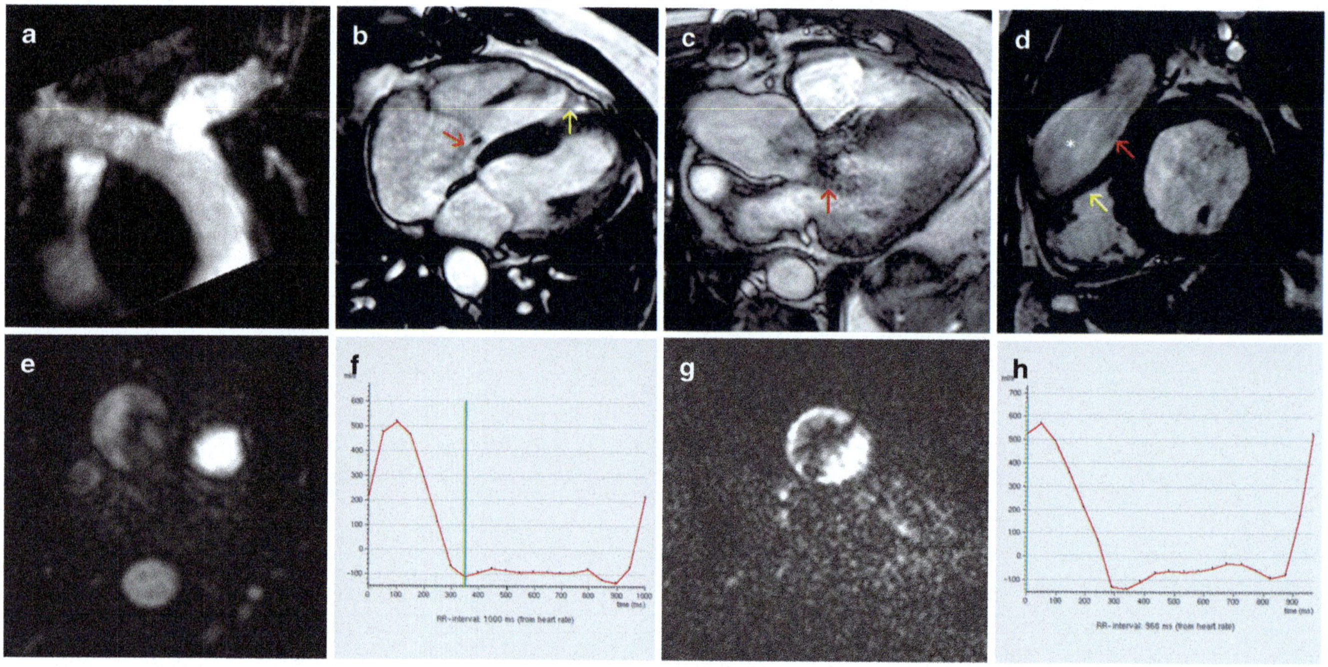

Findings and Interpretation

- Maximum intensity reconstruction of MR angiography (panel A) demonstrates normal pulmonary artery, both the pulmonary trunk and main branches.
- End-systolic cine four-chamber view (panel B) shows moderate tricuspid regurgitation (red arrow), with mildly dilated RV (end diastolic volume 97 ml/m^2) and ejection fraction of 40%, and hypertrophy of the moderator band (yellow arrows in panels B and D). The LV is mildly dilated (end-diastolic volume 103 ml/m^2), with mild systolic dysfunction (LV ejection fraction 45%).
- End-diastolic LV outflow tract view (panel C) shows a dilated aortic root and moderate to severe aortic regurgitation (red arrow).
- There is no residual ventricular septal defect, as shown in panels B and C.
- End-diastolic RV outflow tract view (panel D) shows moderate to severe pulmonary regurgitation (red arrow), with RV dilatation (asterisk) and hypertrophy of the moderator band (yellow arrow).
- Phase-encoding sequences in orthogonal planes at the pulmonary trunk (panels E–F) and the ascending aorta (panels G–H) established the following regurgitation fractions: pulmonary, 44%, and aortic, 39%.
- This case depicts the ability of cardiac MR to evaluate patients with tetralogy of Fallot. Pulmonary valve replacement among these patients is indicated when the RV dilatation reaches 140 ml/m^2.

Further Reading

Bokma JP, de Wilde KC, Vliegen HW, et al. Value of cardiovascular magnetic resonance imaging in noninvasive risk stratification in tetralogy of Fallot. JAMA Cardiol. 2017;2(6):678–83.

Case 122

Tetralogy of Fallot

Clinical History

- Fifty-six-year-old male.
- He has a history of tetralogy of Fallot, with surgical repair at the age of 13.
- Dyspnea functional class II. Holter monitoring revealed frequent ventricular premature beats, with duplets and bigeminy.
- Doppler echocardiography showed left ventricular (LV) dilatation with incremented LV filling pressures (E/e´15), a dilated aortic root, pulmonary hypertension (60 mmHg), mild mitral and aortic valve regurgitation, and a closed ventricular septal defect (VSD).
- Pulmonary branches could not be evaluated; therefore a cardiac magnetic resonance (MR) was requested for further assessment.

Images

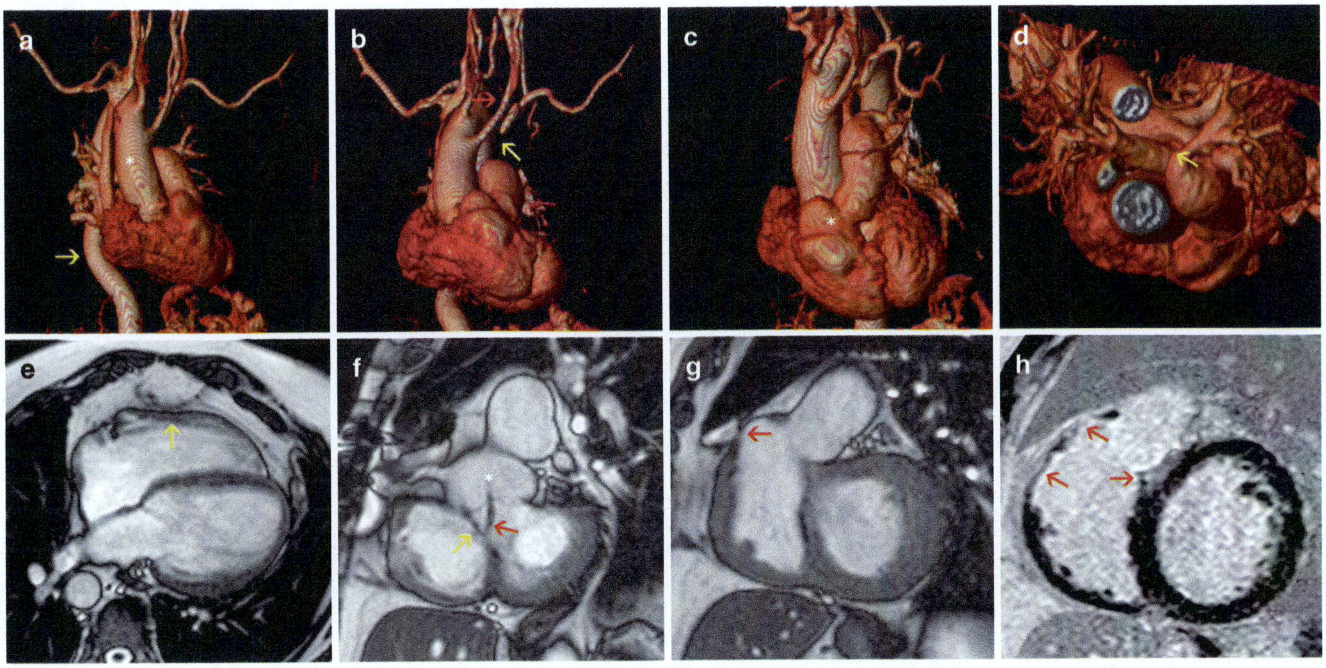

Findings and Interpretation

- Three-dimensional volume rendering reconstructions of MR angiography (panels A–D) demonstrate the presence of a dilated ascending aorta (asterisk in panel A) with a right aortic arch (yellow arrow in panel A), an independent and early origin of the left common carotid artery (red arrow in panel B). The left subclavian artery is occluded at the proximal segment (yellow arrow in panel B), with preserved distal flow provided by collateral circulation. A mild infundibular pulmonary stenosis is also detected (asterisk in panel C). When the ascending aorta is sculpted off, a significant stenosis of the left pulmonary artery is revealed (yellow arrow in panel D).
- As shown with an end-diastolic four-chamber view, both the left (end-diastolic volume 114 ml/m^2) and right (end-diastolic volume 95 ml/m^2) ventricles were dilated (panel E), and right ventricular hypertrophy was also noted (yellow arrow).
- Using a basal cine short-axis view at diastole (panel F) and systole (panel G), dilatation of the ascending aorta (asterisk in panel F) and mild to moderate aortic regurgitation (red arrow in panel F) were identified, and the full ventricular septal defect patch (yellow arrow in panel F) without shunt was depicted. The right ventricular outflow tract showed a thinned wall (red arrow in panel G), possibly related to the surgical procedure.
- Global left and right ventricular systolic function was normal, with ejection fraction of 51% for both.
- At inversion-recovery images, late gadolinium enhancement was detected at the right ventricular outflow tract (red arrows in panel H).

- The presence of significant left pulmonary artery stenosis might demand surgical or percutaneous repair in this patient.
- This case nicely depicts the ability of cardiac MR to evaluate patients with tetralogy of Fallot.

Further Reading

Bokma JP, de Wilde KC, Vliegen HW, et al. Value of cardiovascular magnetic resonance imaging in noninvasive risk stratification in tetralogy of Fallot. JAMA Cardiol. 2017;2:678–83.

Case 123

Tetralogy of Fallot

Clinical History

- Twenty-five-year-old female.
- Tetralogy of Fallot operated at 2 years old, in good clinical condition.
- Surveillance echocardiogram revealed a dilated right ventricle with increased volume, associated with severe pulmonary regurgitation.
- Cardiac computed tomography (CT) was performed to evaluate pulmonary arteries and pulmonary valve annulus.

Images

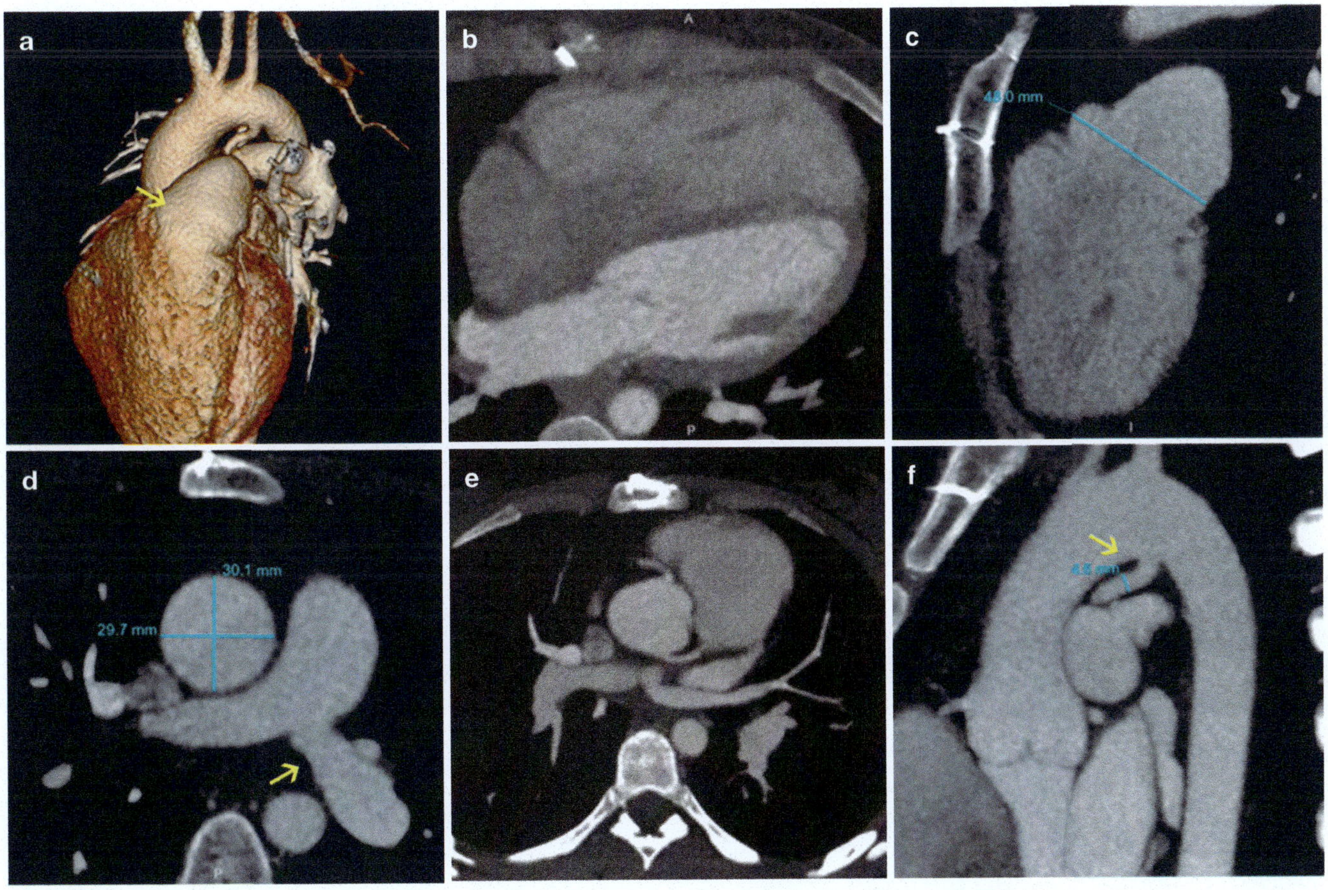

Findings and Interpretation

- Three-dimensional volume rendering reconstruction showing a dilated right ventricular (RV) outflow tract (arrow in panel A).
- Axial CT view showed a dilated RV with normal size of the other cardiac chambers (panel B).
- Dilated RV outflow tract in sagittal multiplanar reconstruction (panel C).
- Axial CT image demonstrating non-dilated pulmonary artery branches, with minimal stenosis in origin of left branch (arrow in panel D).
- Axial CT image showing normal origin of the coronary arteries (panel E).
- Sagittal multiplanar reconstruction showing a partially patent ductus arteriosus, interrupted before the anastomosis with the pulmonary artery (panel F).

- Pulmonary regurgitation is the most common complication following repair of tetralogy of Fallot, leading to progressive RV dilatation and systolic dysfunction.

Further Reading

Ahmed S, Johnson PT, Fishman EK, Zimmerman SL. Role of multidetector CT in assessment of repaired tetralogy of Fallot. Radiographics. 2013;33:1023–36.

Han BK, Lesser JR. CT imaging in congenital heart disease: an approach to imaging and interpreting complex lesions after surgical intervention for tetralogy of Fallot, transposition of the great arteries, and single ventricle heart disease. J Cardiovasc Comput Tomogr. 2013;7: 338–53.

Valente AM, Cook S, Festa P, et al. Multimodality imaging guidelines for patients with repaired tetralogy of Fallot: a report from the American Society of Echocardiography: developed in collaboration with the Society for Cardiovascular Magnetic Resonance and the Society for Pediatric Radiology. J Am Soc Echocardiogr. 2014;27:111–41.

Case 124

Tetralogy of Fallot

- Ten-month-old female.
- History of cyanosis since birth.
- Dyspnea on exertion.
- Referred for thoracic computed tomography (CT) angiography.

Images

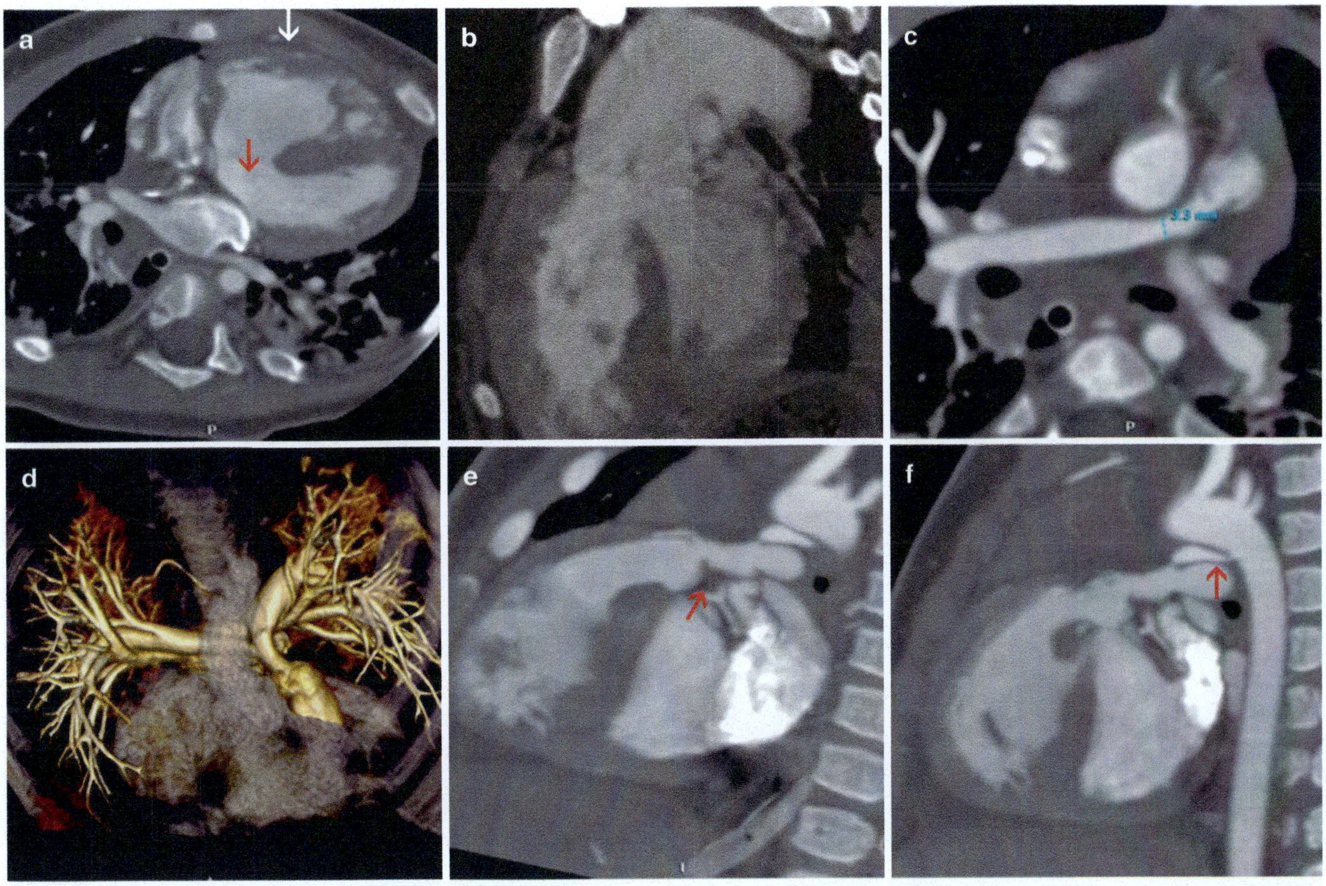

Findings and Interpretation

- Oblique CT image (panel A) shows a large ventricular septal defect (red arrow) and right ventricular hypertrophy (white arrow).
- Overriding of the aorta, positioned directly over the septal defect (panel B).
- CT axial (panel C) and volume rendering (panel D) views showing main pulmonary artery hypoplasia. Sagittal oblique CT image at the level of the main pulmonary artery bifurcation (panel E) shows a pulmonary infundibular stenosis (red arrow) associated with hypoplasia of the main pulmonary artery.
- Maximum intensity projection reconstruction (panel F) demonstrating an associated patent ductus arteriosus (red arrow).
- Several other abnormalities may occur in association with tetralogy of Fallot, including right aortic arch, atrial septal defect, and coronary artery anomalies.

Further Reading

Leschka S, Oechslin E, Husmann L, Desbiolles L, Marincek B, Genoni M, et al. Pre- and postoperative evaluation of congenital heart disease in children and adults with 64-Section CT. Radiographics. 2007 27:829–46.

Villafañe J, Feinstein JA, Jenkins KJ, Vincent RN, Walsh EP, Dubin AM, et al. Hot topics in tetralogy of Fallot. J Am Coll Cardiol. 2013;62:2155–66.

Case 125

Tetralogy of Fallot

Clinical History

- Thirty-nine-year-old male.
- Fallot tetralogy operated in three times.
- Pacemaker placed because of a complete atrioventricular block.
- Echocardiography revealed a dilated right ventricle and a calcified pulmonary homograph with severe pulmonary stenosis and regurgitation but was unable to evaluate the pulmonary branches.
- Cardiac computed tomography (CT) was performed to evaluate the pulmonary arteries.

Images

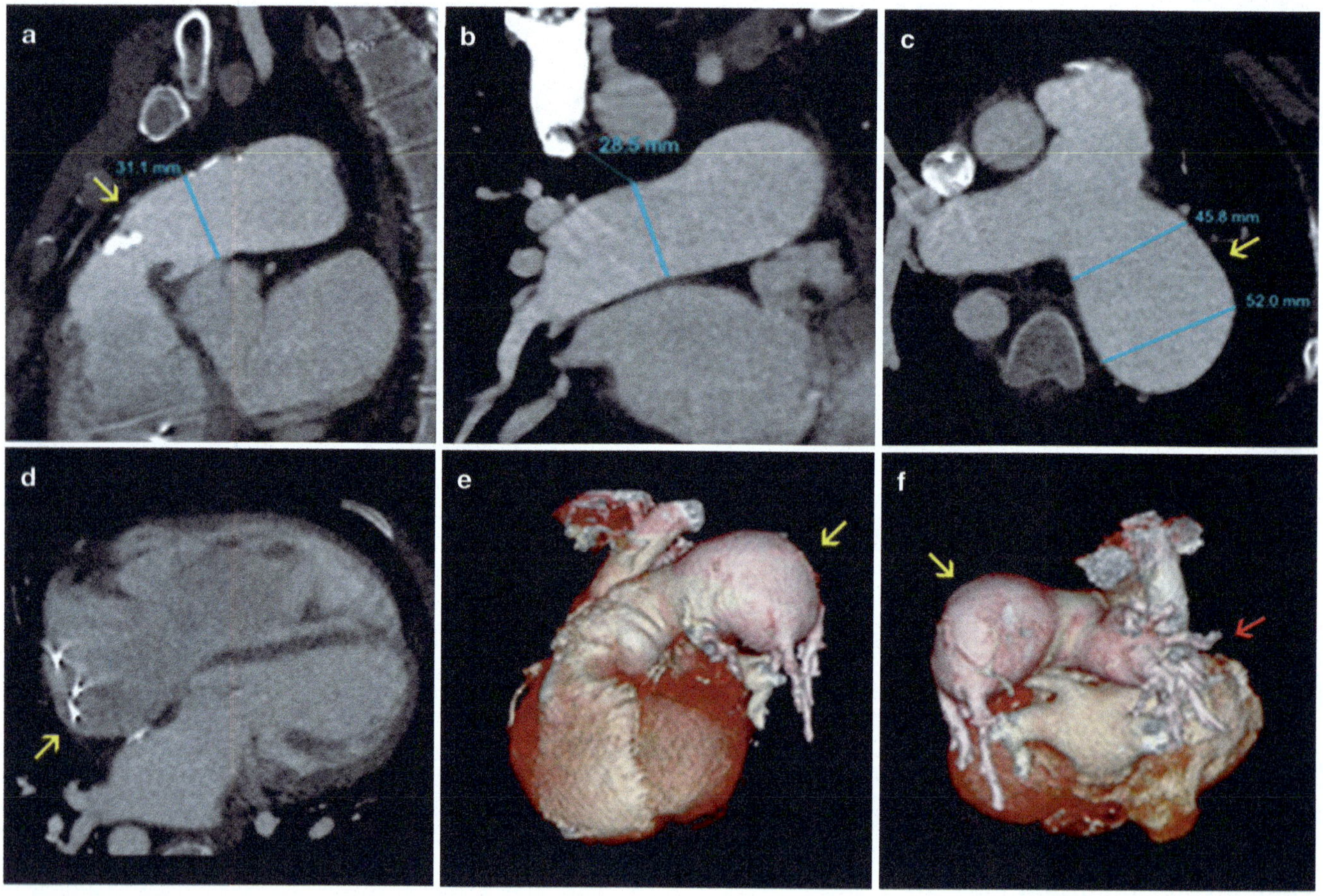

Findings and Interpretation

- Sagittal reformat showing calcified homograph at the annulus level (arrow in panel A).
- Coronal (panel B) and axial (panel C) views are illustrating severely dilated pulmonary arteries with aneurysm of left pulmonary branch.
- Four-chamber view (panel D) demonstrating a dilated right ventricle and permanent pacemaker (arrow).
- Three-dimensional volume rendering reconstructions of the heart and great vessels in anterior (panel E) and posterior (panel F) views showing a dilated right pulmonary artery (red arrow in panel F) and an aneurysmatic left pulmonary artery (yellow arrows).
- Pulmonary regurgitation is one of the most common surgical repair complications of tetralogy of Fallot. In general, pulmonary valve replacement is indicated when the right ventricular dilatation reaches 140 ml/m^2.

Further Reading

Ahmed S, Johnson PT, Fishman EK, Zimmerman SL. Role of multidetector CT in assessment of repaired tetralogy of Fallot. Radiographics. 2013;33:1023–36.

Han BK, Lesser JR. CT imaging in congenital heart disease: an approach to imaging and interpreting complex lesions after surgical intervention for tetralogy of Fallot, transposition of the great arteries, and single ventricle heart disease. J Cardiovasc Comput Tomogr. 2013;7:338–53.

Valente AM, Cook S, Festa P, et al. Multimodality imaging guidelines for patients with repaired tetralogy of Fallot: a report from the American Society of Echocardiography: developed in collaboration with the Society for Cardiovascular Magnetic Resonance and the Society for Pediatric Radiology. J Am Soc Echocardiogr. 2014;27:111–41.

Case 126

Pulmonary Atresia with Ventricular Septal Defect (VSD) and Major Aortic Pulmonary Collateral Arteries (MAPCAs)

Clinical History

- Ten-day-old newborn.
- Presented with cyanosis, hypoxia, and systolic murmur.
- Transthoracic echocardiogram showed pulmonary atresia with ventricular septal defect (VSD) and major aortic pulmonary collateral arteries (MAPCAs).
- A cardiac computed tomography (CT) scan was indicated to evaluate anatomy and guide surgical management.

Images

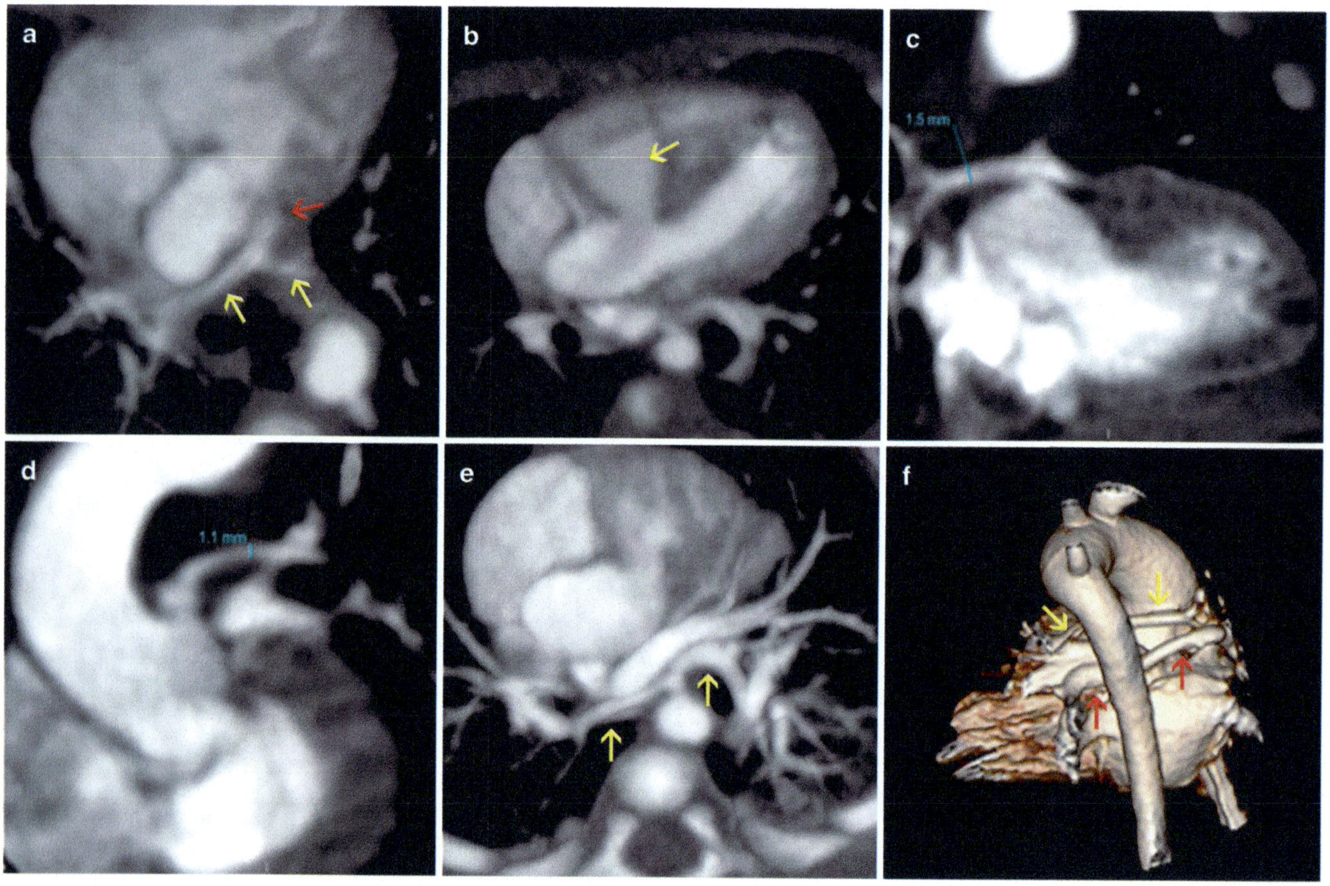

Findings and Interpretation

- Using an oblique axial view (panel A), atresia of the pulmonary trunk (red arrow) and pulmonary arteries (yellow arrows) are shown.
- Oblique three-chamber view (panel B) showing a large ventricular septal defect (arrow).
- Long-axis view showing the atretic right pulmonary artery (panel C).
- A basal short-axis view demonstrates the atretic left pulmonary artery (panel D).
- Major aortic pulmonary collateral arteries (MAPCAs) are exhibited (arrows in panel E).
- Three-dimensional volume rendering reconstruction (panel C) showing the pulmonary arteries (yellow arrows) and MAPCAs (red arrows).
- This is a very rare case of complex congenital heart disease that in a certain way can be considered the most severe form of tetralogy of Fallot. Until surgery, survival in these patients depends on the development of collateral circulation (MAPCAs).

Further Reading

Meinel FG, Huda W, Schoepf UJ, Rao AG, et al. Diagnostic accuracy of CT angiography in infants with tetralogy of Fallot with pulmonary atresia and major aortopulmonary collateral arteries. J Cardiovasc Comput Tomogr. 2013;7:367–75.

Presnell LB, Blankenship A, Cheatham SL, Owens GE, Staveski SL. Overview of pulmonary atresia and major aortopulmonary collateral arteries. World J Pediatr Congenit Heart Surg. 2015;6:630–9.

Qianjun Jia, Jianzheng Cen, Jinglei Li, et al. Anatomy of the retro-esophageal major aortopulmonary collateral arteries in patients with pulmonary atresia with ventricular septal defect: results from preoperative CTA. Eur Radiol. 2018;28:3066–74.

Case 127

Partial Anomalous Pulmonary Venous Return Caused by Malposition of Septum Primum

Clinical History

- Twenty-one-year-old female.
- No family history of congenital heart disease.
- Symptomatic. Dyspnea New York Heart Association functional class II–III during recent pregnancy. Systolic heart murmur in tricuspid and pulmonary areas.
- The ECG revealed right axis deviation and incomplete right bundle branch block.
- Transthoracic echocardiography confirmed right ventricular (RV) volume overload, with a RV systolic pressure of 62 mm Hg. A membrane was identified within the left atrium, interpreted as cor triatriatum. The pulmonary venous return could not be defined.
- Referred for cardiac computed tomography (CT) to define pulmonary venous connections.

Images

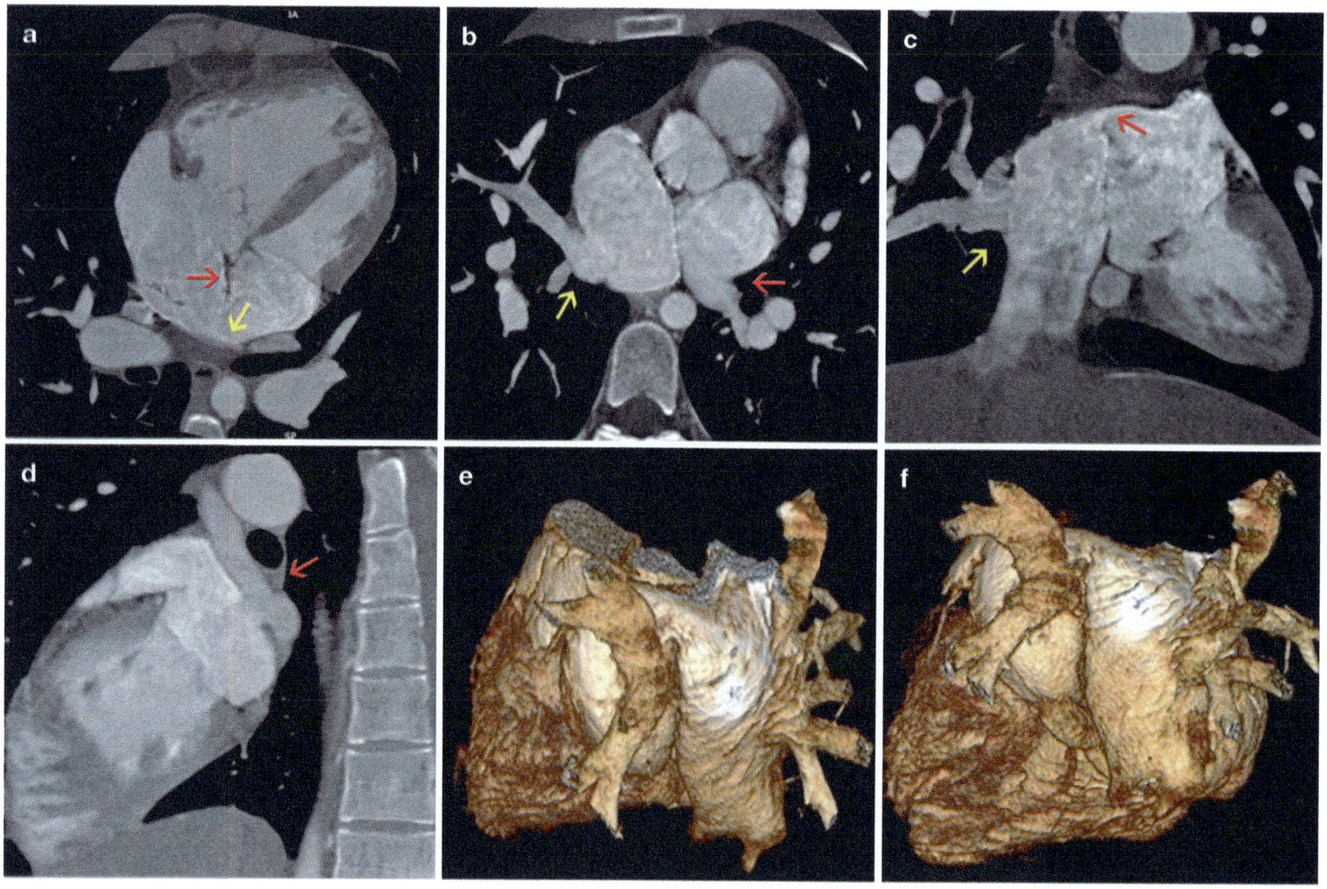

Findings and Interpretation

- Axial CT image (panel A) showing enlarged right atrium (RA) and RV. The left atrium (LA) shows a membrane as a result of the displacement of the septum primum, dividing the atrium into two cavities (red arrow).
- The right pulmonary veins drain to the right side of the membrane, within the RA (yellow arrow in panels B and C), whereas the left veins drain to the left side of the membrane within the LA (red arrow in panels B and D), leading to a partial anomaly of the pulmonary venous return. An atrial septal defect is observed between the septum primum and the posterior wall of the atrium (yellow arrow in panel A and red arrow in panel C).
- Three-dimensional volume rendering reconstructions (posterior views, panels E and F) demonstrate concordant pulmonary venous return. Partial anomaly of the venous return is produced by deviation of the septum primum. Left pulmonary veins enter the LA through a common trunk. Right pulmonary veins enter the RA through two independent trunks.

- The findings of malposition of the septum primum produced the partial anomaly of the pulmonary venous return, which caused dilatation of right cavities and signs of pulmonary hypertension.
- Corrective surgery was performed by closing the interatrial communication with an autologous pericardium patch, correcting the malposition of the septum primum and redirecting the right veins to the LA.

Further Reading

Cuttone F, Hadeed K, Lacour-Gayet F, Lucron H, Hascoet S, Acar P, et al. Isolated severe leftward displacement of the septum primum: anatomic and 3D echocardiographic findings and surgical repair. Interact Cardiovasc Thorac Surg. 2017;24:772–7.

Silvestri LM, Scarabotti A, Marino B. Leftward displacement of septum primum in children with congenital heart disease. Pediatr Cardiol. 2014;35:185.

Van Praagh S, Carrera ME, Sanders S, Mayer JE Jr., Van Praagh R. Partial or total direct pulmonary venous drainage to right atrium due to malposition of septum primum. Anatomic and echocardiographic findings and surgical treatment: a study based on 36 cases. Chest 1995;107:1488–98.

Case 128

Anomalous Pulmonary Vein Return

Clinical History

- Forty-nine-year-old female.
- She has known partial anomalous pulmonary venous return. Doppler echocardiogram revealed a pulmonary-to-systemic flow ratio (Qp/Qs) of 1.8:1, a systolic pulmonary pressure of 40 mmHg, and an abnormal interatrial septal flow not clearly defined.
- Referred for aortic computed tomography (CT) angiography for further evaluation of the venous return anatomy and to evaluate the interatrial septum.

Images

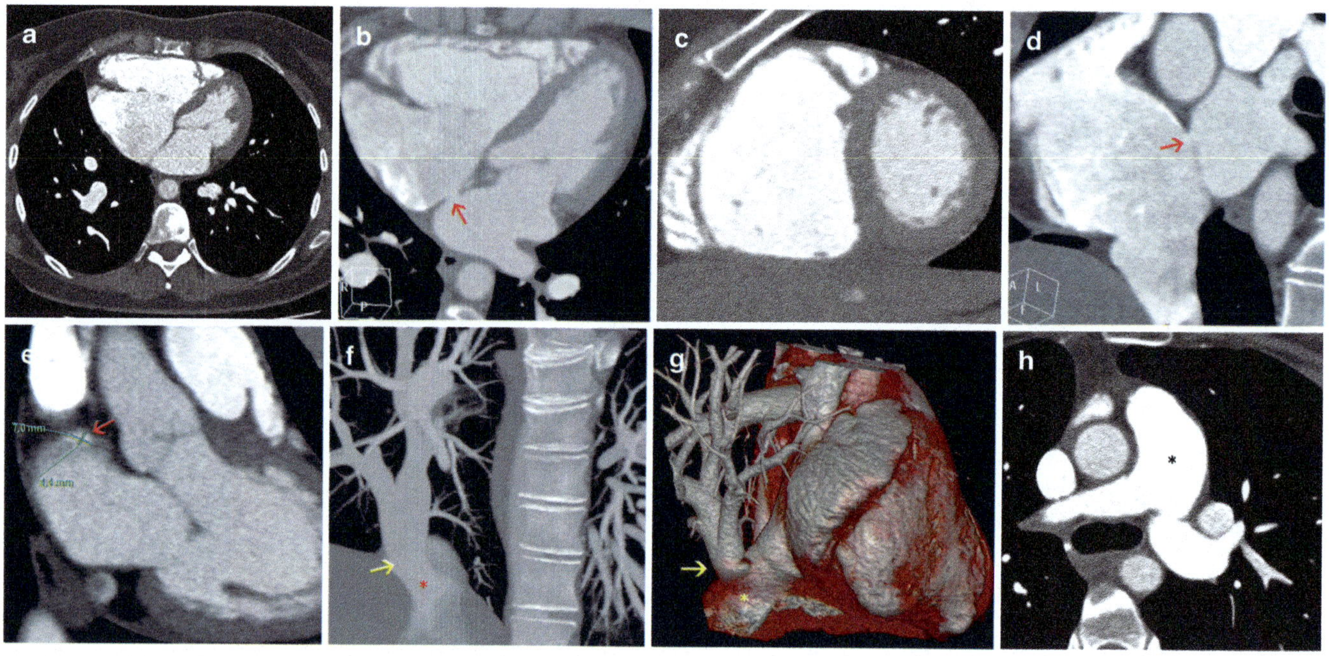

Findings and Interpretation

- Cardiac structures are displaced to the right hemithorax, and the right-sided chambers are dilated (panel A, axial view; panel B, four-chamber view; and panel C, basal short-axis view).
- A small, high, ostium secundum-type atrial septal defect (ASD) is detected (red arrow in panels B, D, and E). Panel D is a short axis at the atrial level, and panel E is an oblique sagittal plane passing through the interatrial septum.
- CT angiography allows accurate measurement of the ASD (4.4 mm × 7.0 mm, in panel E) and evaluates the relationship between the boundaries of the ASD and surrounding structures (panel E) relevant to eventual percutaneous closure, such as the superior vena cava and the aortic root.
- The right pulmonary veins have an anomalous drainage into the supradiaphragmatic inferior vena cava (yellow arrows in panels F and G).
- The inferior vena cava is dilated (*, in panels D, F, and G).
- The presence of a dilated pulmonary artery (*, in panel H) reflects the presence of pulmonary hypertension.
- This patient has an anomalous pulmonary venous return to the inferior vena cava, with moderate dilatation of the right cardiac chambers and signs of pulmonary hypertension.
- The ASD has a very small size and does not seem to add much to the left-to-right shunt.

Further Reading

Vida VL, Guariento A, Milanesi O, et al. The natural history and surgical outcome of patients with scimitar syndrome: a multi-centre European study. Eur Heart J. 2018;39:1002–11.

Case 129

Anomalous Pulmonary Vein Return

Clinical History

- Ten-year-old male.
- He has known right lung hypoplasia, associated with partial anomalous pulmonary venous return, with "scimitar" vein to the inferior vena cava.
- Referred for cardiac magnetic resonance (CMR) for further evaluation.

Images

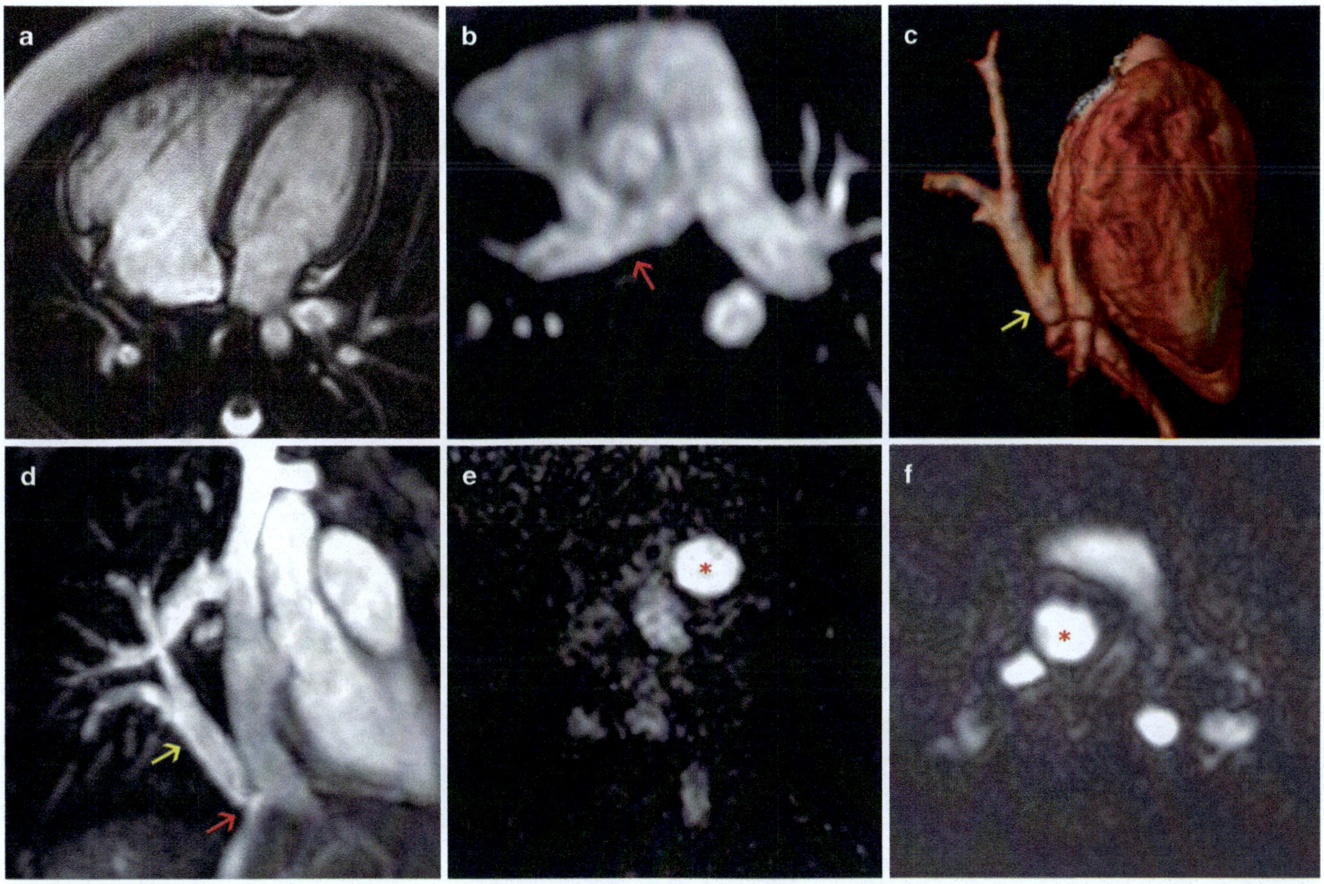

Findings and Interpretation

- There is a displacement of the cardiac structures to the right hemithorax, related to right lung hypoplasia (panel A).
- The right-sided chambers are mildly dilated (panel A), with preserved ventricular systolic function.
- Contrast-enhanced magnetic resonance angiography was performed (panels B–D). The right pulmonary artery is patent and hypoplastic (red arrow in panel B).
- The right pulmonary veins have an anomalous drainage into the supradiaphragmatic inferior vena cava (yellow arrows in panels C and D) and have a moderate stenosis at the scimitar drainage (red arrow in panel D).
- Phase-encoding gradient echo sequences performed perpendicular to the pulmonary artery (*, in panel E) and to the ascending aorta (*, in panel F) demonstrate a significant left-to-right shunt, with a pulmonary-to-systemic flow ratio (Qp/Qs) of 1.78:1.
- This is a typical case of scimitar syndrome, name given to the resemblance with the Middle East sword and comprising right lung hypoplasia, anomalous pulmonary venous return to the inferior vena cava, dextroposition of the heart, and occasionally anomalous systemic arterial supply to the right lung.
- These patients usually have high rates of survival, although this patient would probably benefit from surgical treatment.

Further Reading

Vida VL, Guariento A, Milanesi O, et al. The natural history and surgical outcome of patients with scimitar syndrome: a multi-centre European study. Eur Heart J. 2018;39:1002–11.

Case 130

Anomalous Vein Return

Clinical History

- Seventeen-year-old male.
- Dilated right ventricle and coronary sinus.
- Transthoracic echocardiogram revealed an anomalous pulmonary and systemic vein return and an atrial septal defect.
- Patient was referred for cardiac computed tomography (CT) to evaluate pulmonary and systemic vein return.

Images

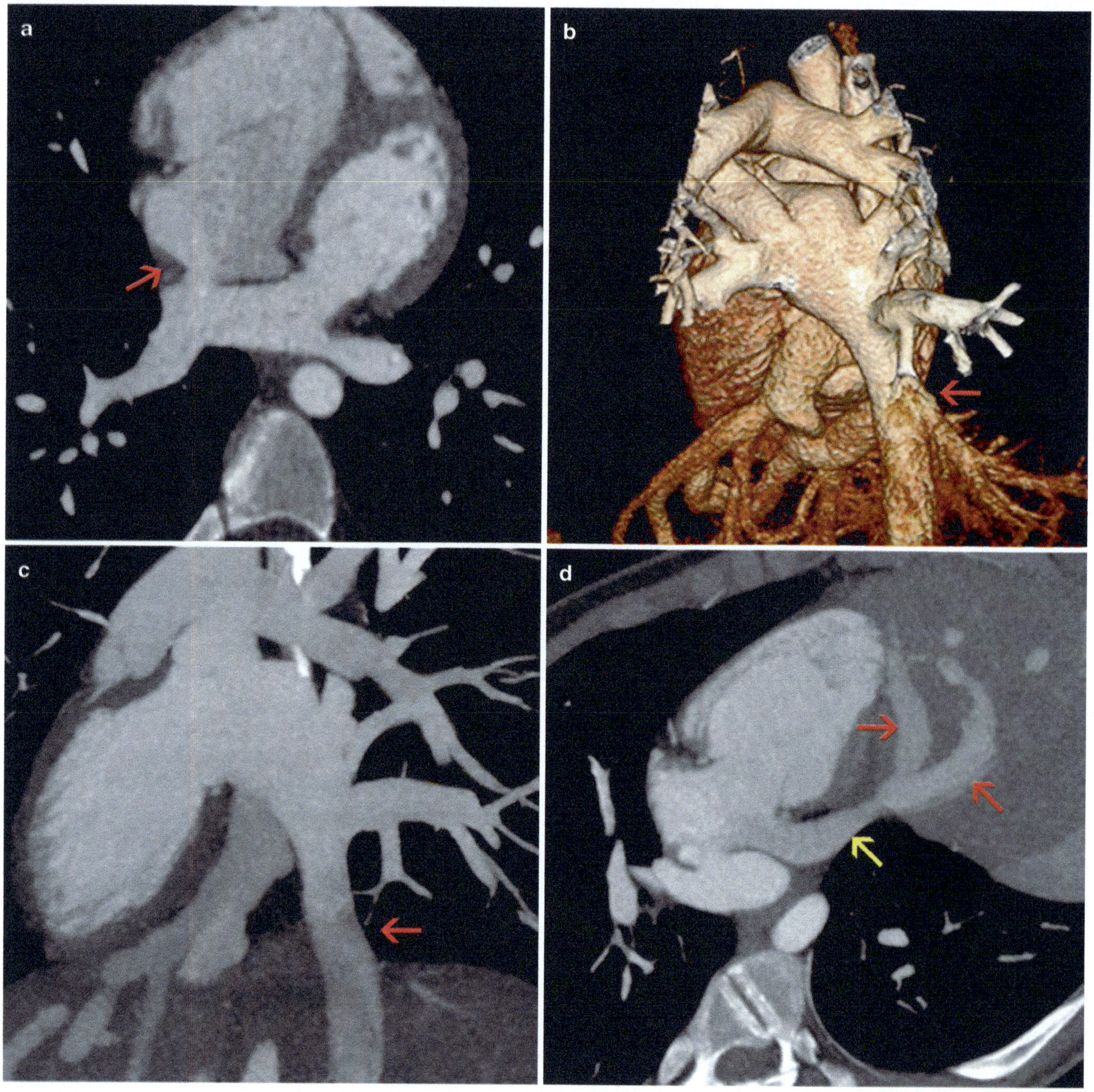

Findings and Interpretation

- A sinus venosus atrial septal defect (ASD, arrow) is detected using a low four-chamber view (panel A). Right ventricular dilatation is also present.
- The inferior vena cava is draining in the left atrium (arrows in panels B and C).
- Suprahepatic veins (red arrows in panel D) are draining into the coronary sinus (yellow arrow in panel D).
- This rare case of anomalous systemic and pulmonary vein return associated with ASD shows the usefulness of cardiac CT as preoperative anatomical assessment of patients with congenital heart disease.

Further Reading

Kivisto S, Hanninen H, Holmstrom M. Partial anomalous pulmonary venous return and atrial septal defect in adult patients detected with 128-slice multidetector computed tomography. J Cardiothorac Surg. 2011;6:126.

Case 131

Anomalous Vein Return

Clinical History

- Twenty-two-year-old male.
- History of left ventricular non-compaction and ventricular arrhythmia. Referred for evaluation in the cardiac transplant service.
- Transthoracic echocardiogram showed mild left ventricular dysfunction and a dilated coronary sinus.
- Cardiac computed tomography (CT) was performed to assess anatomy as pre-operatory evaluation before cardiac transplant surgery.

Images

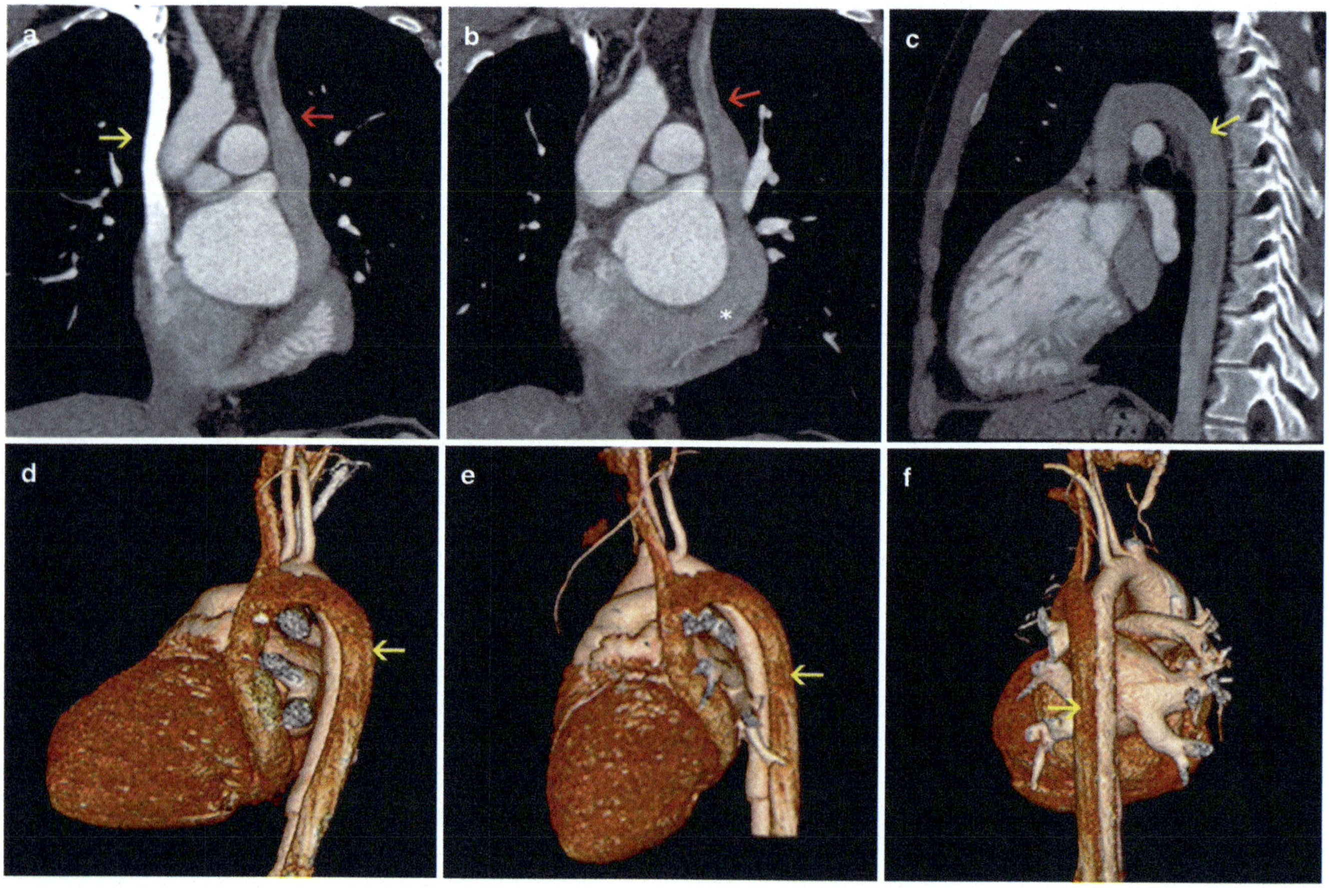

Findings and Interpretation

- Coronal multiplanar reconstructions (MPR) (panels A and B) show a double superior vena cava system with superior right vena cava (yellow arrow in panel A) and persistent superior left vena cava (red arrows). The left persistent superior vena cava drains to a dilated coronary sinus (asterisk in panel B).
- Given the absence of the intrahepatic portion of the vena cava, a dilated azygos system runs through the left side of the chest and makes an arch over the left pulmonary artery. MPR sagittal (panel C) and three-dimensional volume rendering reconstructions (panels D–F) show the dilated azygos system draining into the persistent superior left vena cava (yellow arrows).
- According to this finding, patient was refused for cardiac transplant at this time.

Further Reading

Tyrak KW, Holda J, Holda MK, Koziej M, Piatek K, Klimek-Piotrowska W. Persistent left superior vena cava. Cardiovasc J Afr. 2017;28:e1–4.

Case 132

Ebstein's Anomaly

Clinical History

- Fifty-seven-year-old female.
- Known Ebstein's anomaly with atrial septal defect.
- Right heart failure. Progressive severe desaturation.
- Transthoracic echocardiogram showed severe right ventricular dysfunction, severe tricuspid regurgitation, and an ostium secundum atrial septal defect.
- Referred for evaluation in the cardiac transplant service.
- Cardiac computed tomography (CT) scan was performed as preoperative evaluation of cardiac anatomy.

Images

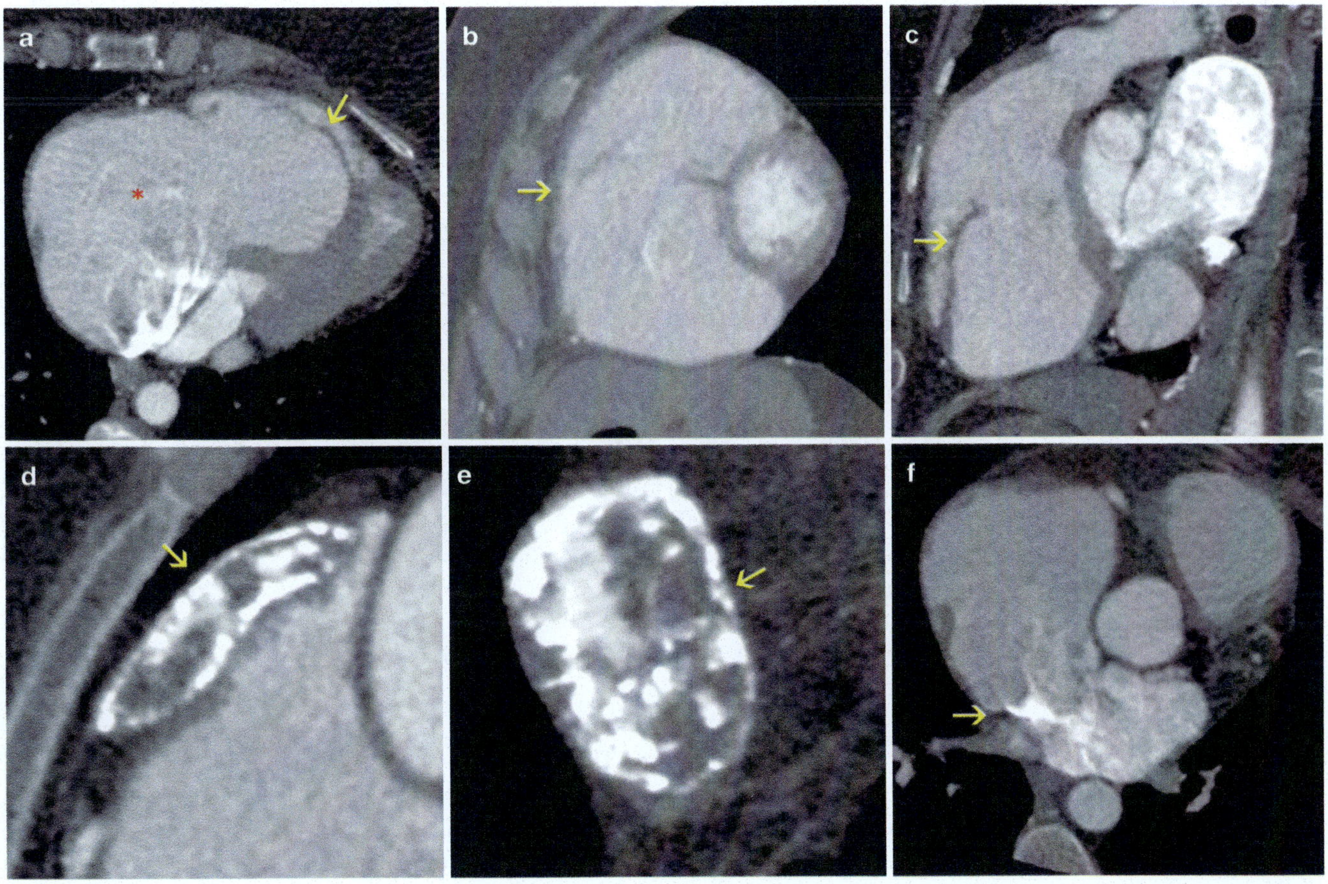

Findings and Interpretation

- A low axial view (panel A) showed severely dilated right atrium (asterisk) with apical displacement of the septal tricuspid valve leaflet (arrow), leading to atrialization of the right ventricle.
- Oblique coronal (panel B) and sagittal (panel C) views showing the displacement of the tricuspid valve (arrows).
- Calcified right atrial appendage (arrow, in panels D and E).
- Axial view illustrating a large ostium secundum atrial septal defect (panel F).
- Ebstein's anomaly is a very rare congenital heart defect, usually associated with other anomalies such as atrial and ventricular septal defects. Furthermore, patients with Ebstein's anomaly might have concomitant Wolff-Parkinson-White syndrome. Given the presence of heart failure, surgery is indicated in this patient.

Further Reading

Gaurav Aggarwala, MD, Brad Thompson, MD, Edwin van Beek, et al. Multislice computed tomography angiography of Ebstein anomaly and anomalous coronary artery. J Cardiovasc Comp Tomogr. 2007;1:168–9.

Joseph F. Zikria, MD, Evan H. Dillon, MD, et al. Common CTA features of Ebstein anomaly in a middle-aged woman with a heart murmur and dyspnea on exertion. J Cardiovasc Comput Tomogr. 2012;6:431–2.

Case 133

Transposition of the Great Arteries (D-TGA)

Clinical History

- Seventeen-year-old male.
- History of transposition of the great arteries (D-TGA) repaired at 11 months of age with atrial switch procedure.
- Currently asymptomatic.
- Given a suboptimal echocardiographic window, cardiac magnetic resonance (MR) was indicated for assessment.

Images

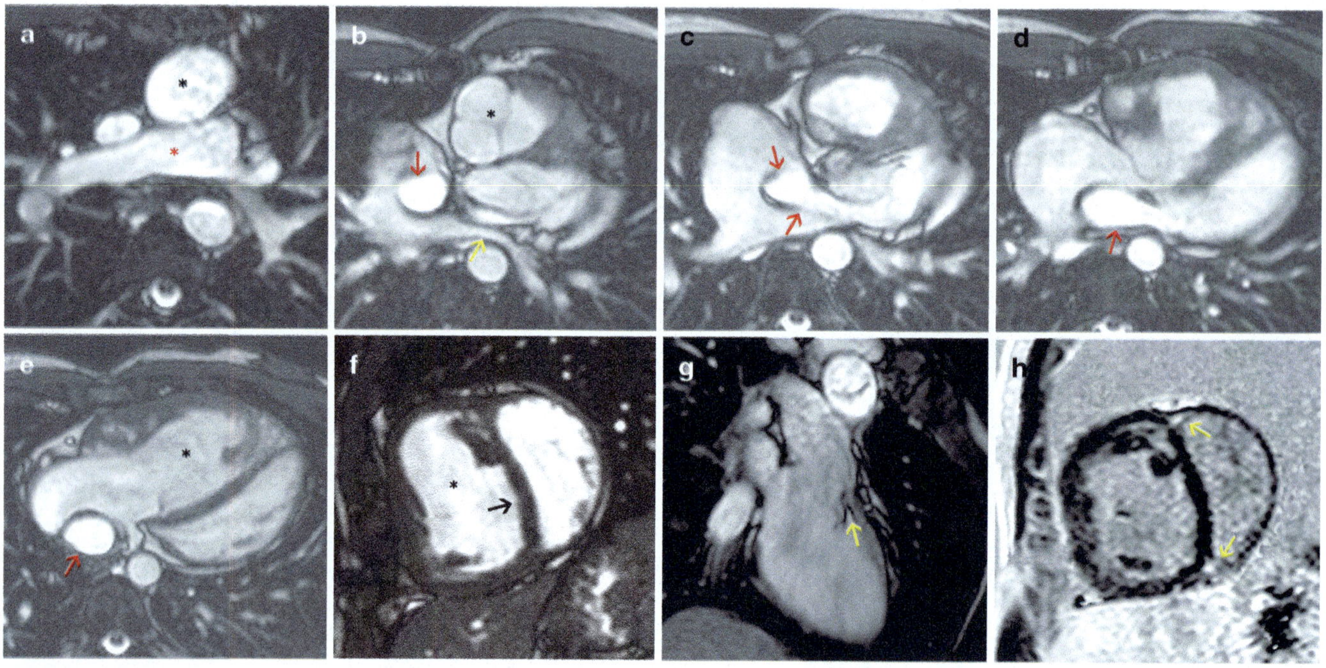

Findings and Interpretation

- Cine MR axial imaging views from the aortic arch to the diaphragm (panels A–D) are useful in patients with complex congenital heart disease.
- The ascending aorta has an anterior position (black asterisk in panels A and B), and the pulmonary artery is located in a posterior position (red asterisk in panel A).
- In the atrial switch procedure (Mustard/Senning), a baffle or intra-atrial conducts/tunnels are used to redirect caval flow (deoxygenated blood) to the left atrium and left ventricle, which in D-TGA is connected to the pulmonary artery. Therefore, it allows correction of D-TGA.
- The intra-atrial baffle connecting the superior vena cava toward the mitral valve is clearly depicted (red arrows in panels B–D) and is patent with no obstructions. Note that the inferior vena cava (red arrow in panel E) is not connected to the right atrium.
- There is no interatrial septum (excised); therefore the pulmonary veins (yellow arrow in panel B) drain the oxygenated blood to the tricuspid valve and right ventricle, which in D-TGA is connected to the aorta.
- The systemic ventricle (right ventricle) is dilated and hypertrophic (asterisk in panels E and F), with rightward displacement (black arrow in panel F), leading to dynamic obstruction of the subpulmonary outflow tract (yellow arrow in panel G) associated to the significant septal shift.
- Inversion-recovery images (panel H) show focal intramural areas of late gadolinium enhancement at the insertion sites of the systemic ventricle over the interventricular septum (yellow arrows in panel H), reflecting pressure overload.

Further Reading

ECG guidelines for the management of grown-up congenital disease (new version 2010): the Task Force on the management of grown-up congenital disease of the European Society of Cardiology (ESC). Eur Heart J. 2010;31:2915–57.

Case 134

Double Aortic Arch

Clinical History

- Twelve-year-old female.
- Trisomy 21. History of hypothyroidism, celiac disease, gastroesophageal reflux, and asthma.
- ECG and transthoracic echocardiography without abnormalities.
- Referred to thoracic computed tomography (CT) angiography to assess pulmonary parenchyma and great vessels.

Images

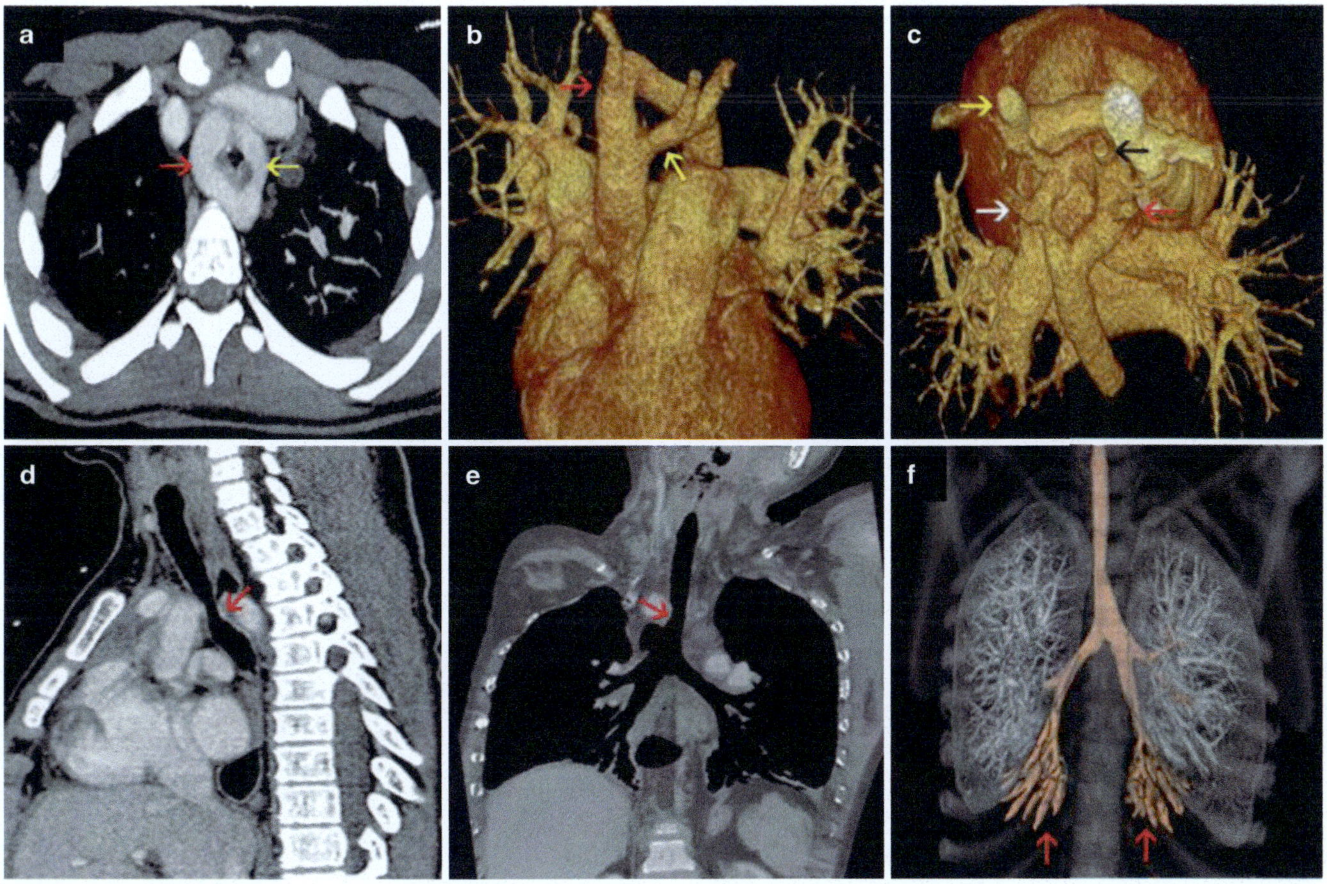

Findings and Interpretation

- Axial CT image (panel A) and volume rendering reconstruction, anterior view (panel B), demonstrated the presence of a double aortic arch with a dominant right arch (red arrow) and a left arch of smaller size (yellow arrow).
- From each of the arches emerged the primitive carotid arteries (yellow and black arrows in panel C) and subclavian arteries, respectively (white and red arrows in panel C).
- Compression of the airway and the esophagus by the double aortic arch is present (arrows in panels D and E). There was also the presence of bilateral saccular bronchiectasis (arrows in panel F).
- A double aortic arch occurs when the distal portion of the right dorsal aorta fails to regress. The two arches form a complete ring, encircling the trachea and esophagus. The right arch is dominant in the majority of cases, followed by left dominant, with codominant arches being the least common. The left and right carotid and subclavian arteries generally arise from their respective arches. Symptoms are frequently present during childhood that could be confused with asthma. Affected children may have cough, stridor, dyspnea, and upper respiratory tract infections.
- The CT angiography allowed us to perform the diagnosis and plan the corrective surgery.

Further Reading

Backer CL, Mongé MC, Popescu AR, et al. Vascular rings. Semin Pediatr Surg. 2016;25:165–75.

Muller CO, Derycke L, Kheniche A, et al. Routine multi detector computed tomography evaluation of tracheal impairment compared to laryngo-tracheal endoscopy in children with vascular ring. Pediatr Surg Int. 2018;34:879–84.

Zhang Q, Fu Z, Dai J, Geng G, Fu W, Tian D. Recurrent wheezing and cough caused by double aortic arch, not asthma. Case Rep Cardiol. 2017;2017:8079851.

Case 135

Congenitally Corrected Transposition of the Great Arteries (L-TGA)

Clinical History

- Thirty-eight-year-old male.
- Asymptomatic, under surveillance of congenitally corrected transposition of the great arteries (L-TGA).
- Referred to cardiac magnetic resonance (CMR) for further evaluation.

Images

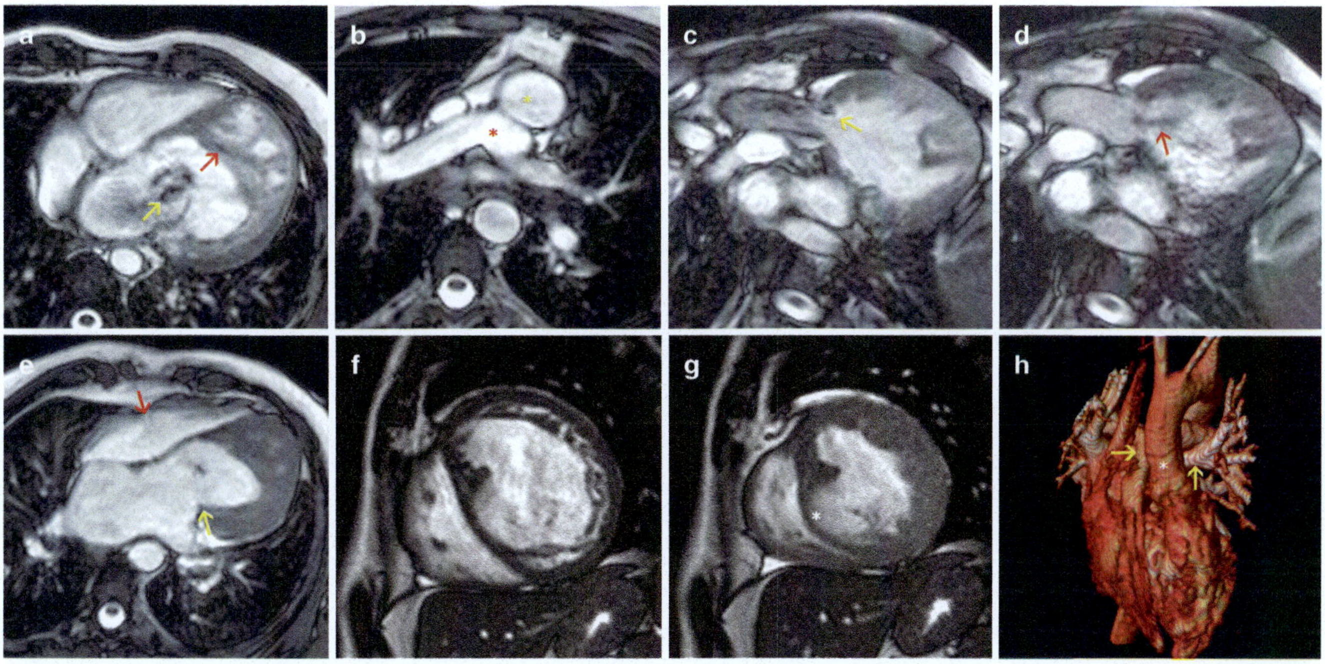

Findings and Interpretation

- L-TGA has a very low prevalence (<1% of all congenital heart disease). In L-TGA, there is both atrioventricular and ventriculoarterial discordance, leading to great vessels in a parallel position. In other words, the ventricles are inverted: the aorta arises from the right ventricle (which is in the left side) in an anterior position; and the pulmonary artery arises from the left ventricle (which is in the right side). Associated lesions can be frequently identified among these patients, being ventricular septal defects the most common.
- Cine images using axial planes at a low ventricular level (panel A) and at the level of the great vessels (panel B) depict the L-TGA, with right ventricle (RV) in a left position (panel A), clearly recognized by the identification of an hypertrophic moderator band (red arrow). In panels C and D, there is confirmation of the aorta rising from the morphologically RV (systemic ventricle). Note the presence of mild subaortic stenosis, likely related to focal subvalvular thickening (yellow arrow in panel C), and moderate aortic regurgitation (red arrow in panel D).
- The four-chamber view (panel E) nicely depicts that the systemic atrioventricular valve (yellow arrow) has a more apical location compared to the pulmonary atrioventricular valve (red arrow). This configuration is in opposition to the normal positioning, with the tricuspid valve in a more apical position.
- Moderate to severe mitral regurgitation is also observed (yellow arrow in panel A).
- End-diastolic (panel F) and end-systolic (panel G) views show a dilated systemic ventricle, with dyskinetic motion of basal septal wall (asterisk in panel G).
- Three-dimensional MR angiography volume rendering reconstruction (panel H) portrays the anterior position of the aorta (asterisk) and the posterior pulmonary artery (arrows).

- Axial views can be extremely useful among patients with complex congenital heart disease.
- Patients with isolated L-TGA often remain asymptomatic until adulthood and might even be misinterpreted as a dilated cardiomyopathy.
- Complications in these patients are generally related to heart failure due to a morphologically right ventricle supporting systemic pressures, as well as to conduction abnormalities.

Further Reading

ECG guidelines for the management of grown-up congenital disease (new version 2010): the Task Force on the management of grown-up congenital disease of the European Society of Cardiology (ESC). Eur Heart J. 2010;31:2915–57.

Case 136

Pulmonary Atresia with Ventricular Septal Defect

Clinical History

- Fifteen-day-old female.
- Breathing and feeding difficulty.
- Developing cyanosis.
- Referred for thoracic computed tomography (CT) angiography for evaluation of the great vessels.

Images

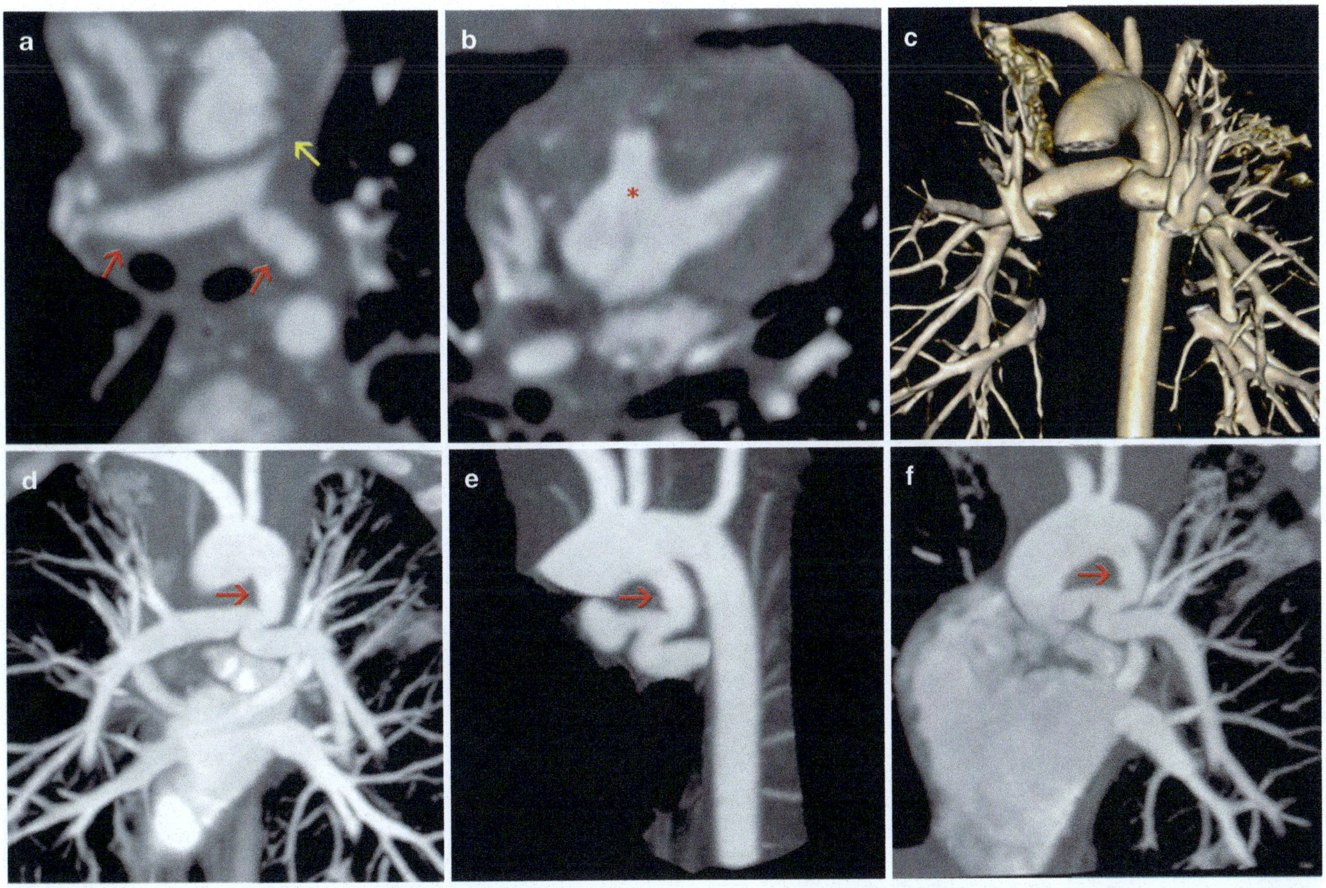

Findings and Interpretation

- Axial CT image (panel A) shows atresia of the main pulmonary artery (arrow). The right and left pulmonary arteries (red arrows) are not connected with the right ventricle.
- Axial CT image (panel B) demonstrates a ventricular septal defect (*).
- Three-dimensional volume rendering reconstruction (panel C) and maximum intensity projection image in coronal plane (panel D) show normal-sized confluent pulmonary arteries supplied by a large patent ductus arteriosus (arrows in panels D–F) without major aortopulmonary collateral arteries.
- Pulmonary atresia with ventricular septal defect represents the extreme form of the tetralogy of Fallot. It can be an isolated lesion or associated with a genetic syndrome. It has been demonstrated that tetralogy of Fallot with pulmonary atresia belongs to a spectrum of cone-truncated cardiac malformations that can be associated with 22q11 monosomies.

Further Reading

Rajeshkannan R, Moorthy S, Sreekumar KP, Ramachandran PV, Kumar RK, Remadevi KS. Role of 64-MDCT in evaluation of pulmonary atresia with ventricular septal defect. AJR Am J Roentgenol. 2010;194:110–8.

Case 137

Hemitruncus Arteriosus

Clinical History

- Full-term male newborn, of 2390 grams.
- At 3 days of age begins with tachypnea, with respiratory rate >50 bpm, and tachycardia. Oxygen therapy was required because his arterial oxygen saturation was 75–80% in room air.
- Chest X-ray showed increased pulmonary vascularization in both lung fields.
- Cardiac examination: grade 3/6 systolic regurgitation murmur. ECG with signs of right pressure overload with presence of positive T waves in V1. Transthoracic echocardiography revealed signs of severe (suprasystemic) pulmonary hypertension, right aortic arch, and emergence of the left branch of the pulmonary artery from the ascending aorta with turbulence at its origin. The right branch of the pulmonary artery originated from the main pulmonary artery.
- Referred to thoracic computed tomography (CT) angiography to define the anatomy of the pulmonary artery and aorta and confirm the clinical and echocardiographic suspicion of hemitruncus.

Images

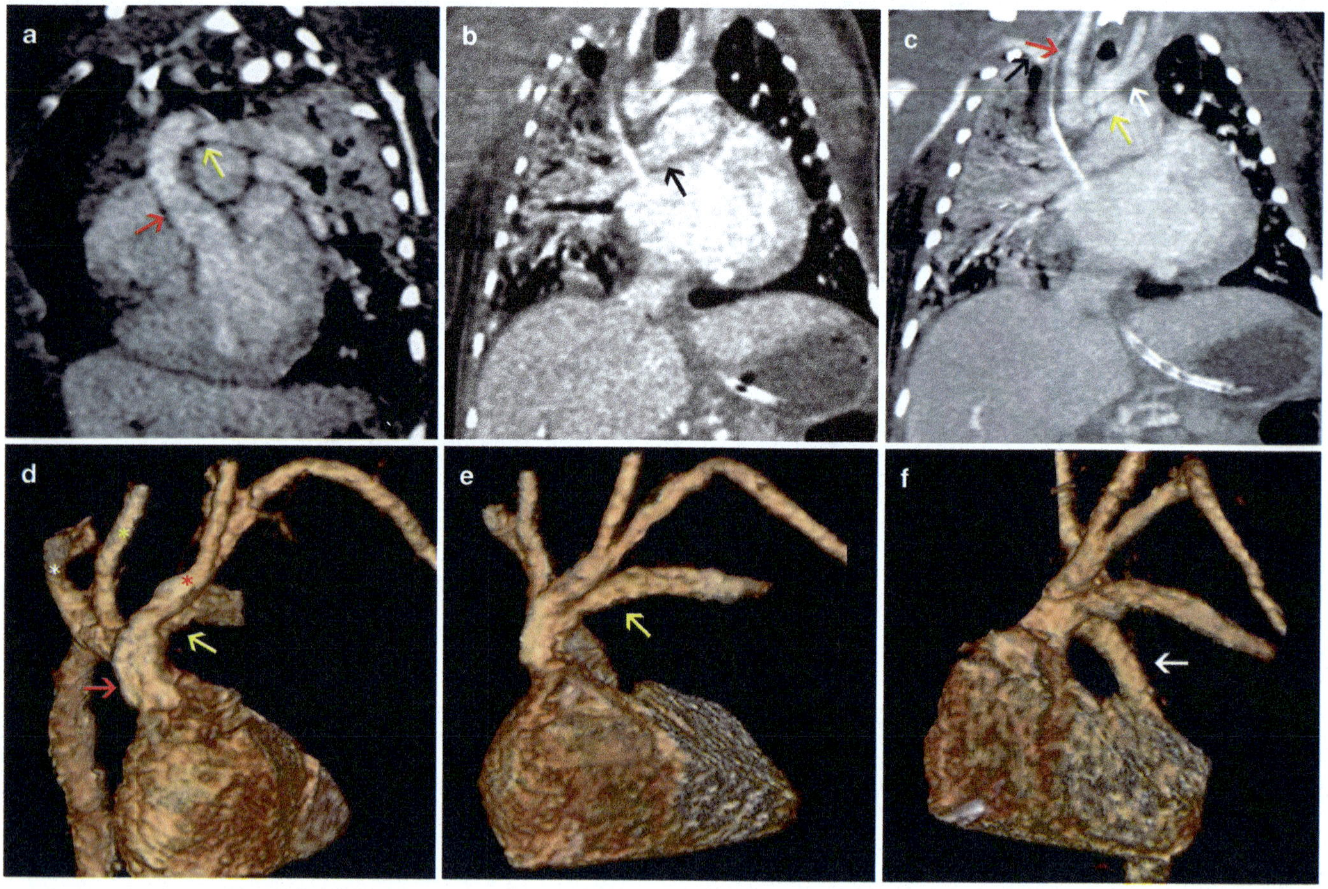

Findings and Interpretation

- Multiplanar reconstructions (panels A–C) and three-dimensional volume rendering reconstructions (panels D–F) showing an anomalous origin of the left branch of the pulmonary artery (yellow arrow in panels A, C–E) from the ascending aorta (red arrow in panel A and D) are identified, with stenosis at its origin (hemitruncus).
- The right branch (black arrow in panel B) emerges from the main pulmonary artery. Right aortic arch (white arrow in panel F) with the first branch being the left brachiocephalic arterial trunk (white arrow in panel C and red asterisk in panel D), then the right primitive carotid artery (red arrow in panel C and yellow asterisk in panel D), and finally the right subclavian artery (black arrow in panel C and white asterisk in panel D).
- CT angiography aided the confirmation of the diagnosis and guidance of the corrective surgery by reinserting the left branch of the pulmonary artery into the main pulmonary artery, with subsequent improvement in pulmonary hypertension.
- If it is not diagnosed, early development of pulmonary hypertension and irreversible pulmonary vascular changes occur inevitably when the affected lung is exposed to unrestricted aortic flow and systemic pressure, while the contralateral lung receives the entire right ventricular output.

Further Reading

Bi W, Ren W, Song G, Shang C, Pan F, Xu M. Anomalous origin of one pulmonary artery from the ascending aorta (hemitruncus) in a premature infant: a case report and literature review. J Clin Ultrasound. 2014;42:367–70.

Haywood LJ, Chakryan Y, Kim D, Boltzer T, Rivas G, Shavelle D. Abnormal origin of the right pulmonary artery from ascending aorta (Hemitruncus Arteriosus). J Investig Med High Impact Case Rep. 2014;2:2324709614536139.

Nathan M, Rimmer D, Piercey G, del Nido PJ, Mayer JE, Bacha EA, et al. Early repair of hemitruncus: excellent early and late outcomes. J Thorac Cardiovasc Surg. 2007;133:1329–35.

Prifti E, Bonacchi M, Murzi B, Crucean A, Leacche M, Bernabei M, et al. Anomalous origin of the right pulmonary artery from the ascending aorta.J Card Surg. 2004;19:103–12.

Case 138

Common Arterial Trunk (Truncus Arteriosus)

Clinical History

- Twenty-four-day-old male with cyanosis.
- Evolves with progressive signs of congestive heart failure.
- Drop in pulmonary vascular resistance.
- Referred for cardiac computed tomography (CT) for further assessment.

Images

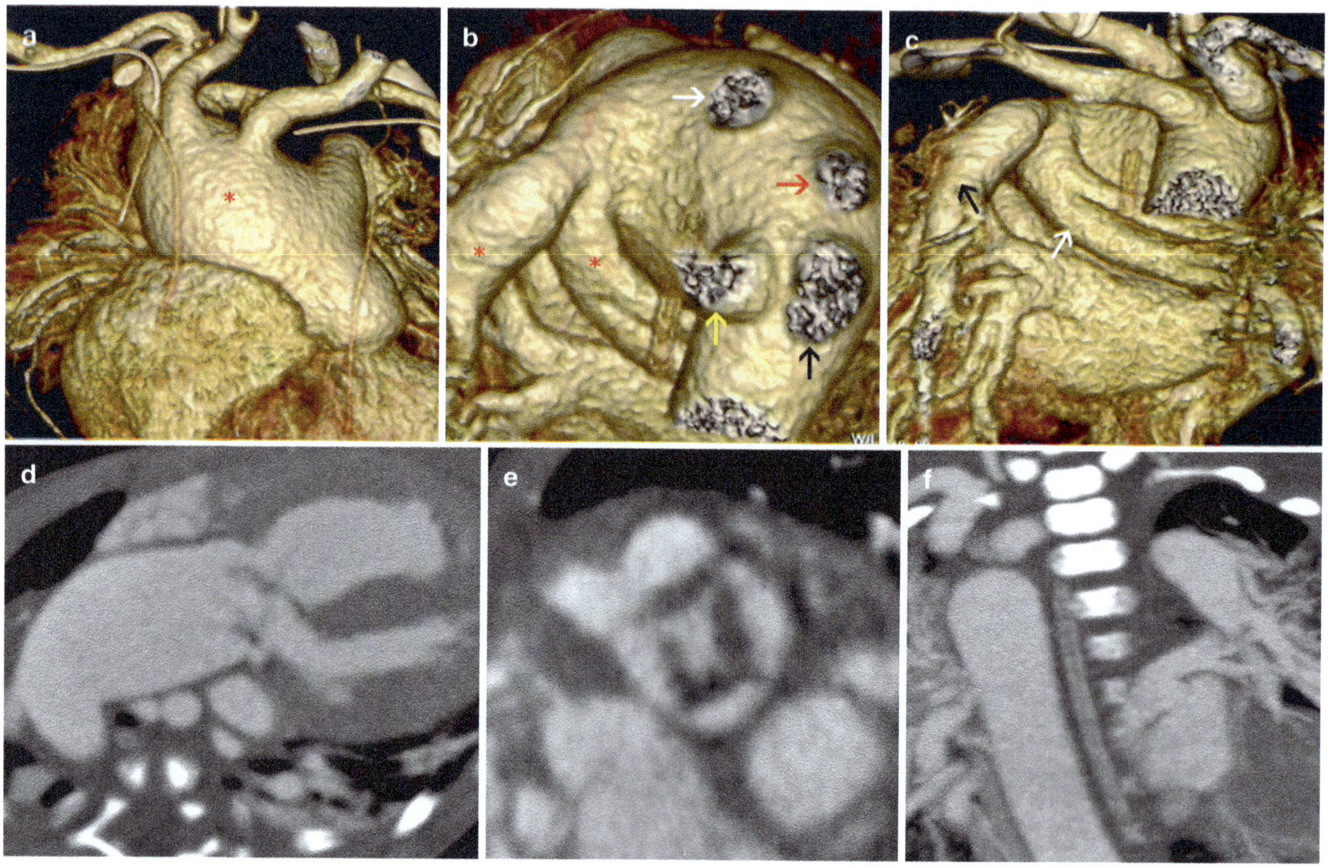

Findings and Interpretation

- Volume rendering reconstruction (anterior view) acquired using ECG-gated CT (panel A) shows a single large artery (truncus) (*), originating from the base of the heart and giving rise to the systemic supraaortic and pulmonary vessels.
- Volume rendering reconstruction (superior view, panel B) shows the truncus giving rise to the two main pulmonary arteries (asterisks). Ostium of left carotid artery (white arrow), right carotid artery (red arrow), aberrant left subclavian artery (yellow arrow), and right subclavian artery (black arrow).
- Volume rendering reconstruction (posterior view, panel C) demonstrates the left (black arrow) and right (white arrow) pulmonary arteries originated from the posterior side of the truncus. The descending aorta was visually sectioned for a better understanding of the anatomy.
- The common artery trunk receives the output of both ventricles (panel D).
- Double oblique plane at the level of the truncal valve (panel E) shows a single dysplastic valve with four leaflets. This may cause regurgitation, stenosis, or both.
- Coronal plane (panel F) showing a right descending aorta.
- Truncus arteriosus is usually an isolated finding, though it can occasionally be associated with DiGeorge syndrome, right aortic arch with mirror-image branching, and CATCH-22 deletion.

Further Reading

Leschka S, Oechslin E, Husmann L, Desbiolles L, Marincek B, Genoni M, et al. Pre- and postoperative evaluation of congenital heart disease in children and adults with 64-Section CT. Radiographics 2007;27:829–46.

Paul JF, Serraf A. Truncus arteriosus and double aortic arch. Circulation. 2002;105:e170.

Case 139

Total Anomalous Pulmonary Venous Return

Clinical History

- Four-week-old male
- Severe developing cyanosis followed by symptoms of congestive heart failure
- Referred for thoracic computed tomography (CT) angiography

Images

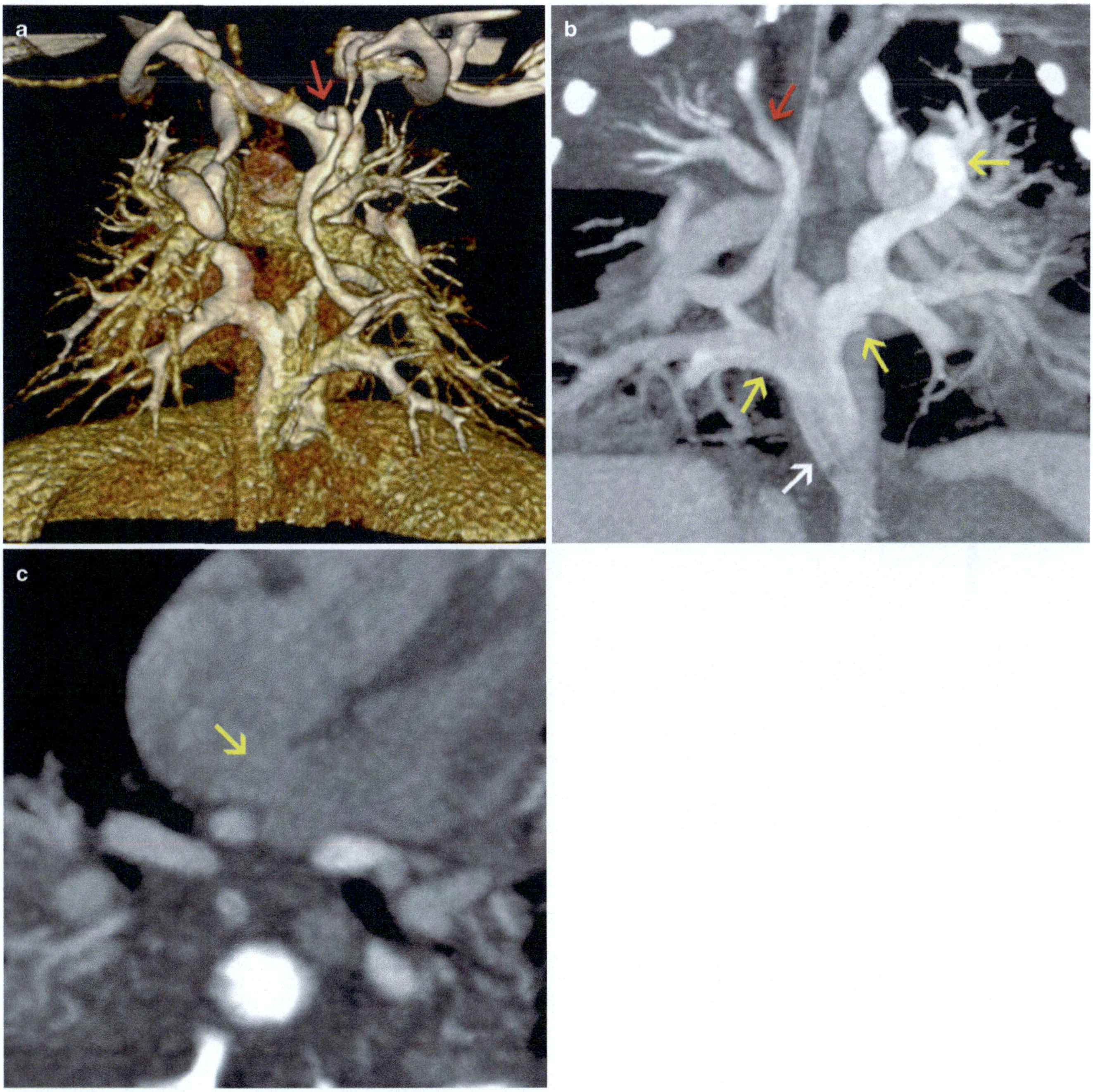

Findings and Interpretation

- Three-dimensional CT volume rendering reconstruction (panel A) and maximum intensity projection (MIP) posterior view (panel B) demonstrate the anomalous pulmonary vein return (yellow arrows). Two pulmonary veins on the right side and one inferior pulmonary vein on the left side form a confluence behind the right atrium. The pulmonary venous confluence drains into a tortuous abnormal vein or collector (white arrow) that drains into the inferior vena cava. Pulmonary veins from the superior left lung drain into the left superior brachiocephalic vein (red arrow in panels A and B) through a vertical vein.
- Axial MIP view (panel C) showing a large atrial septal defect (yellow arrow) allowing patient survival.
- Total anomalous pulmonary venous return is a very rare congenital malformation (2.5 per 100,000 live births) characterized by the disconnection of all 4 of the pulmonary veins from the left atrium and the redirection of oxygenated blood to the right atrium either directly or indirectly via the superior or the inferior vena cava.

Further Reading

Dyer KT, Hlavacek AM, Meinel FG, De Cecco CN, McQuiston AD, Schoepf UJ, et al. Imaging in congenital pulmonary vein anomalies: the role of computed tomography. Pediatr Radiol. 2014;44:1158–68.

Leschka S, Oechslin E, Husmann L, Desbiolles L, Marincek B, Genoni M, et al. Pre- and postoperative evaluation of congenital heart disease in children and adults with 64-section CT. RadioGraphics. 2007;27:829–46.

Rajiah P, Kanne JP. Computed tomography of pulmonary venous variants and anomalies. J Cardiovasc Comput Tomogr. 2010;4:155–63.

Case 140

Univentricular Heart: Fontan Circulation

Clinical History

- Twenty-six-year-old female.
- She has known double outlet right ventricle with Fontan surgery in childhood.
- Cardiac magnetic resonance (MR) was requested for further assessment.

Images

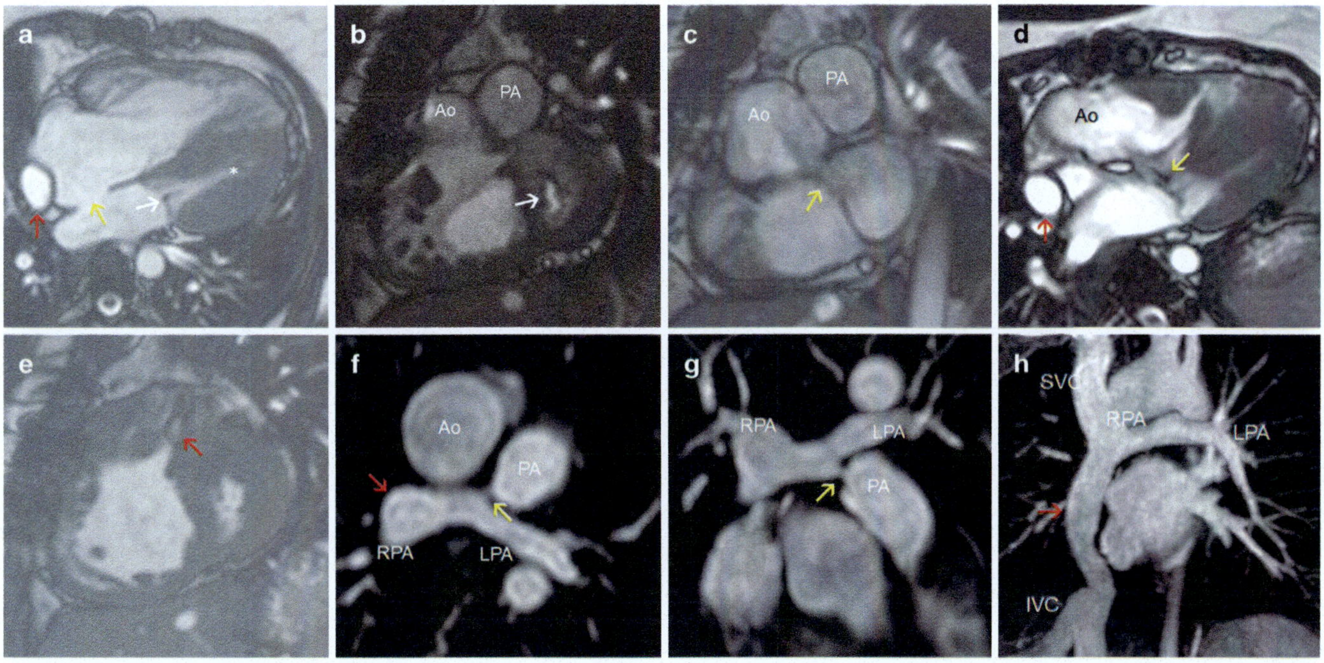

Findings and Interpretation

- End-diastolic cine axial view (panel A) shows the presence of an extracardiac conduit (red arrow, also shown in panels D, F, and H). The right ventricle (RV), dilated and hypertrophic, is the single functional ventricle (double outlet RV), whereas the left ventricle (LV) is hypoplastic and hypertrophic (asterisk in panel A).
- A large nonrestrictive atrial defect is also identified (yellow arrow in panel A), as well as severe mitral stenosis (white arrows in panels A and B), and a restrictive subaortic ventricular septal defect (yellow arrows in panels C and D).
- The aorta (Ao) and the pulmonary artery (PA) arise from the RV (panel B).
- Using basal short-axis views (panels B, C, and E) and a LV outflow tract view (panel D), no stenosis of the aortic valve or LV outflow tract is identified, whereas marked signal void at the right ventricular outflow tract is displayed (red arrow in panel E).
- Maximum intensity reconstructions of MR angiography (panels F to H) demonstrate interruption of the PA with minimum anterograde passage before the bifurcation (yellow arrow in panels F and G) and preserved right (RPA) and left (LPA) pulmonary arteries provided by the cavopulmonary anastomosis by the fenestrated extracardiac conduit (red arrows in panels F and H). SVC and IVC refer to superior and inferior vena cava.
- Double outlet RV is one type of single ventricle congenital heart diseases. Superior cavopulmonary anastomosis (bidirectional Glenn procedure), with later redirection also of the inferior vena cava to the PA by an extracardiac conduit (Fontan-Kreutzer procedure), allows to bypass the RV and therefore to avoid volume overload, with passive blood flow to the lungs.
- Among these patients, the presence of a large (nonrestrictive) atrial septal defect allows nonrestricted flow of pulmonary vein blood to the single ventricle.
- Given this successful surgical procedure and improved postsurgical care, many patients with this complex congenital disease reach the adulthood with much better prognosis than in the past.

Further Reading

Kreutzer C, Kreutzer J, Kreutzer GO. Reflections on five decades of the fontan kreutzer procedure. Front Pediatr. 2013;1:45.

Kreutzer GO, Schlichter AJ, Kreutzer C. The Fontan/Kreutzer procedure at 40: an operation for the correction of tricuspid atresia. Semin Thorac Cardiovasc Surg Pediatr Card Surg Annu. 2010;13:84–90.

Case 141

Univentricular Heart: Glenn Procedure

Clinical History

- Twenty-two-year-old male.
- He has known single ventricle congenital heart disease with pulmonary atresia and with Glenn surgery plus tricuspid ligation during childhood.
- Cardiac magnetic resonance (MR) was requested for further assessment.

Images

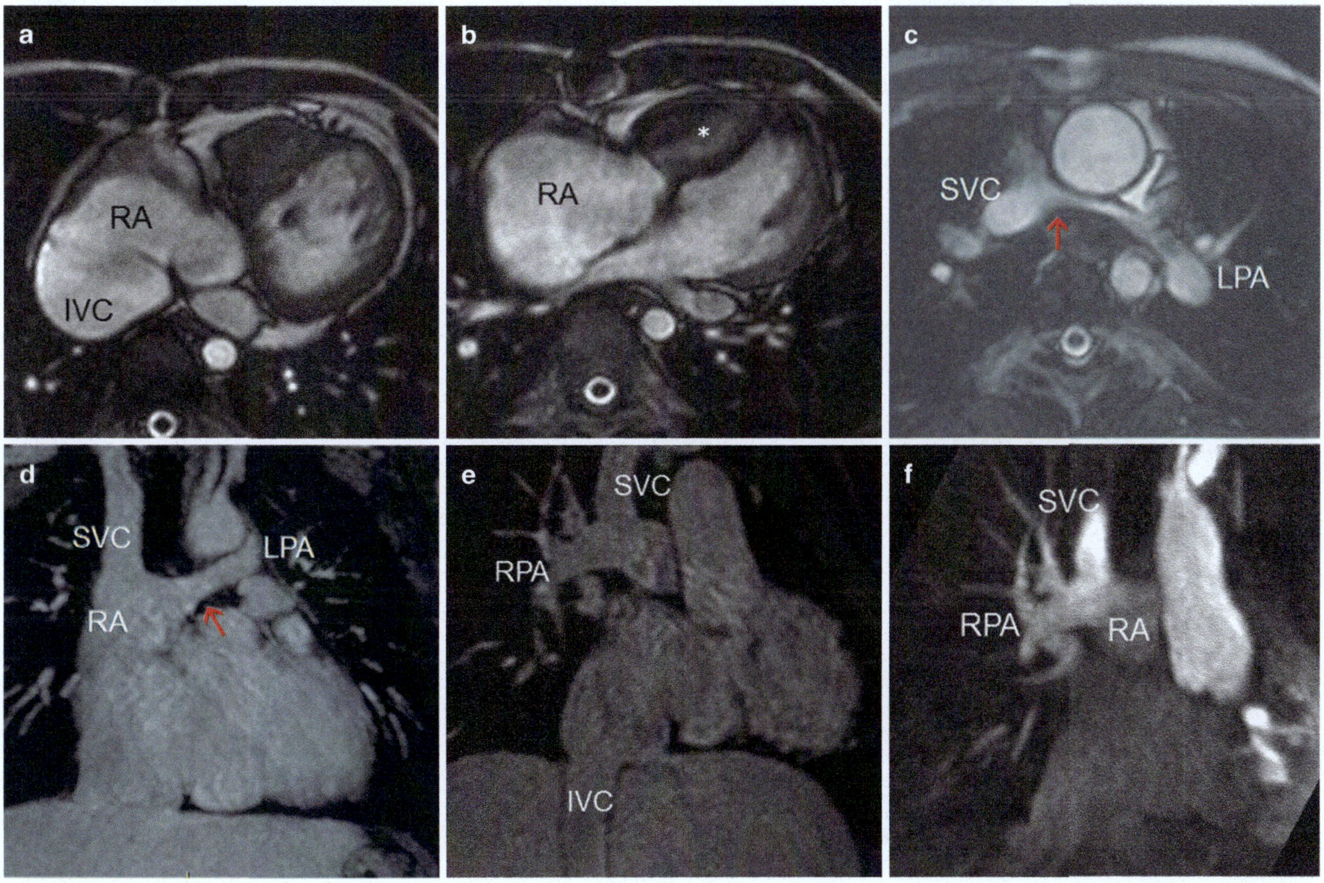

Findings and Interpretation

- Cine axial views (panels A and D) show a rudimentary right ventricle (asterisk in panel B), intact interventicular septum, and a dilated inferior vena cava (IVC), draining at a dilated right atrium (RA).
- An upper axial view (panel C) portrays the superior vena cava (SVC) connected to the right pulmonary artery (RPA, arrow in panel C). All vessels are patent. Same findings are observed in panels D to F using MR angiogram reconstructions. LPA refers to left pulmonary artery.
- Superior cavopulmonary anastomosis (bidirectional Glenn procedure) allows to bypass the atretic right ventricle and therefore to avoid volume overload, with passive blood flow from the upper body to the lungs. Nonetheless, vein return from the lower body though the IVC drains at the RA, therefore both structures are greatly dilated.

Further Reading

Gupta SK, Juneja R, Anderson RH, Gulati GS, Devagorou V. Clarifying the anatomy and physiology of totally anomalous systemic venous connection. Ann Pediatr Cardiol. 2017;10:269–77.

Case 142

Univentricular Heart: Double Left Ventricular Inlet with Coarctation of the Aorta

Clinical History

- Two-day-old female
- Cyanosis
- Signs of congestive heart failure
- Referred for thoracic computed tomography (CT) angiography

Images

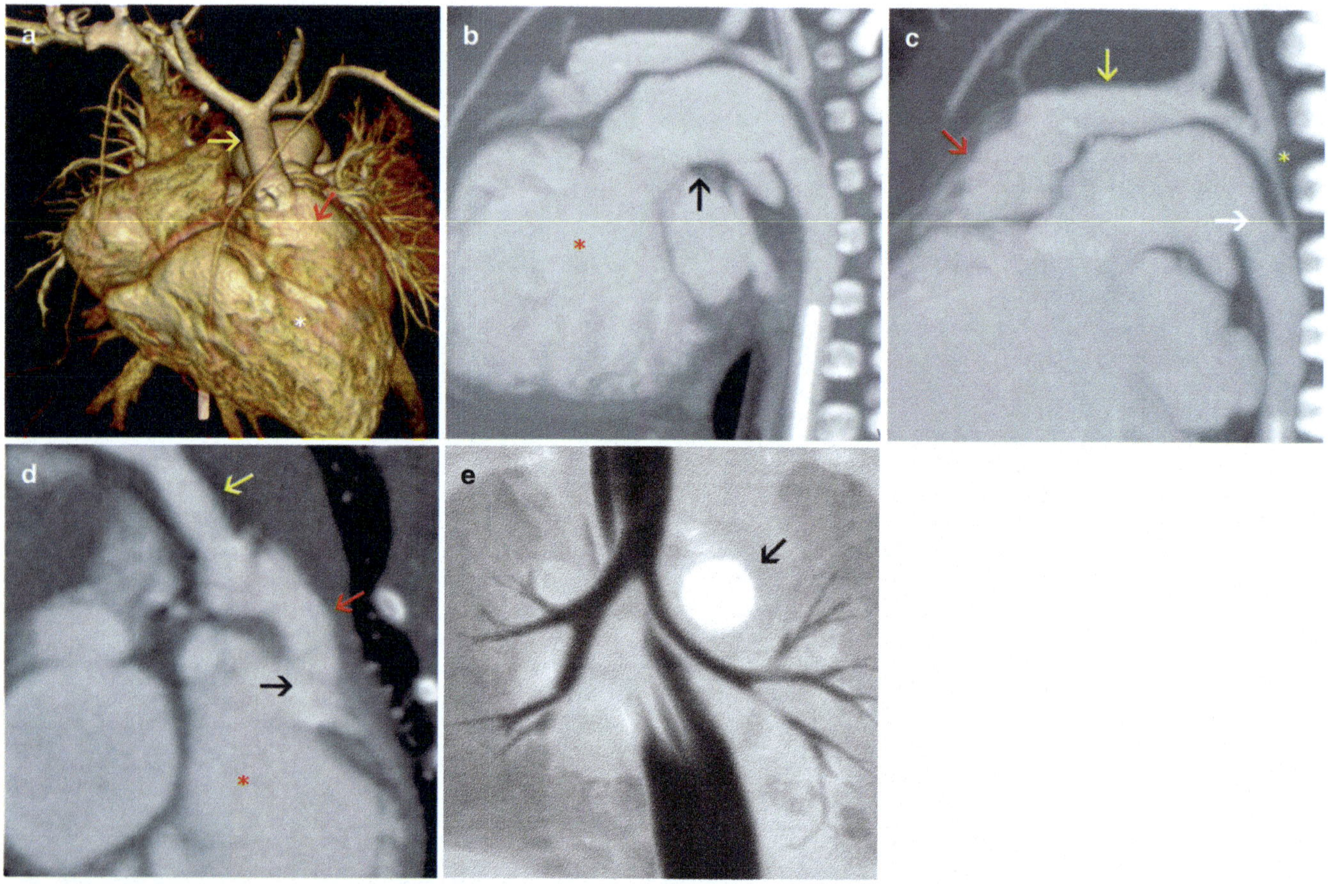

Findings and Interpretation

- Volume-rendered three-dimensional CT reconstruction at an anterior view (panel A) shows a single common ventricle (asterisk) which is morphologically left, with a single atrioventricular connection with both atria emptying into it (double left ventricular inlet). There is a small subaortic outlet chamber (incomplete or rudimentary ventricle) (red arrow). The aorta (yellow arrow) arises in a left anterior position.
- Maximum intensity projection (MIP) sagittal planes (panels B and C) show a dilated common pulmonary artery (black arrow) arising from the dominant ventricle (asterisk in panel B). Note that the great arteries are in a parallel and transposed position. The aorta (yellow arrow in panel C) arises from the rudimentary chamber (red arrow) in an anterior position. There is a patent ductus arteriosus (white arrow) connecting the pulmonary artery and the descending aorta. Note the severe hypoplasia of the aortic arch constituting an aortic coarctation (yellow asterisk in panel C).
- Thin section oblique coronal plane (panel D) demonstrates the subaortic outlet chamber connected via a bulboventricular foramen (black arrow) to the sub-pulmonary dominant ventricle (asterisk). There is no atrioventricular connection to the subaortic outlet chamber.
- Minimum-intensity projection coronal plane (panel E) shows the dilated pulmonary artery (black arrow) compressing the left main bronchus.

Further Reading

Leschka S, Oechslin E, Husmann L, Desbiolles L, Marincek B, Genoni M, et al. Pre- and postoperative evaluation of congenital heart disease in children and adults with 64-Section CT. Radiographics. 2007;27:829–46.

Case 143

Univentricular Heart

Clinical History

- Forty-year-old female.
- Non-operated univentricular heart.
- Progressive dyspnea.
- Transthoracic echocardiogram revealed a single left ventricle with rudimentary nonfunctional right ventricle. Anterior position of the aorta and severe pulmonary stenosis were also detected, with inadequate visualization of the pulmonary branches.
- Cardiac computed tomography (CT) scan was required to evaluate the pulmonary arteries.

Images

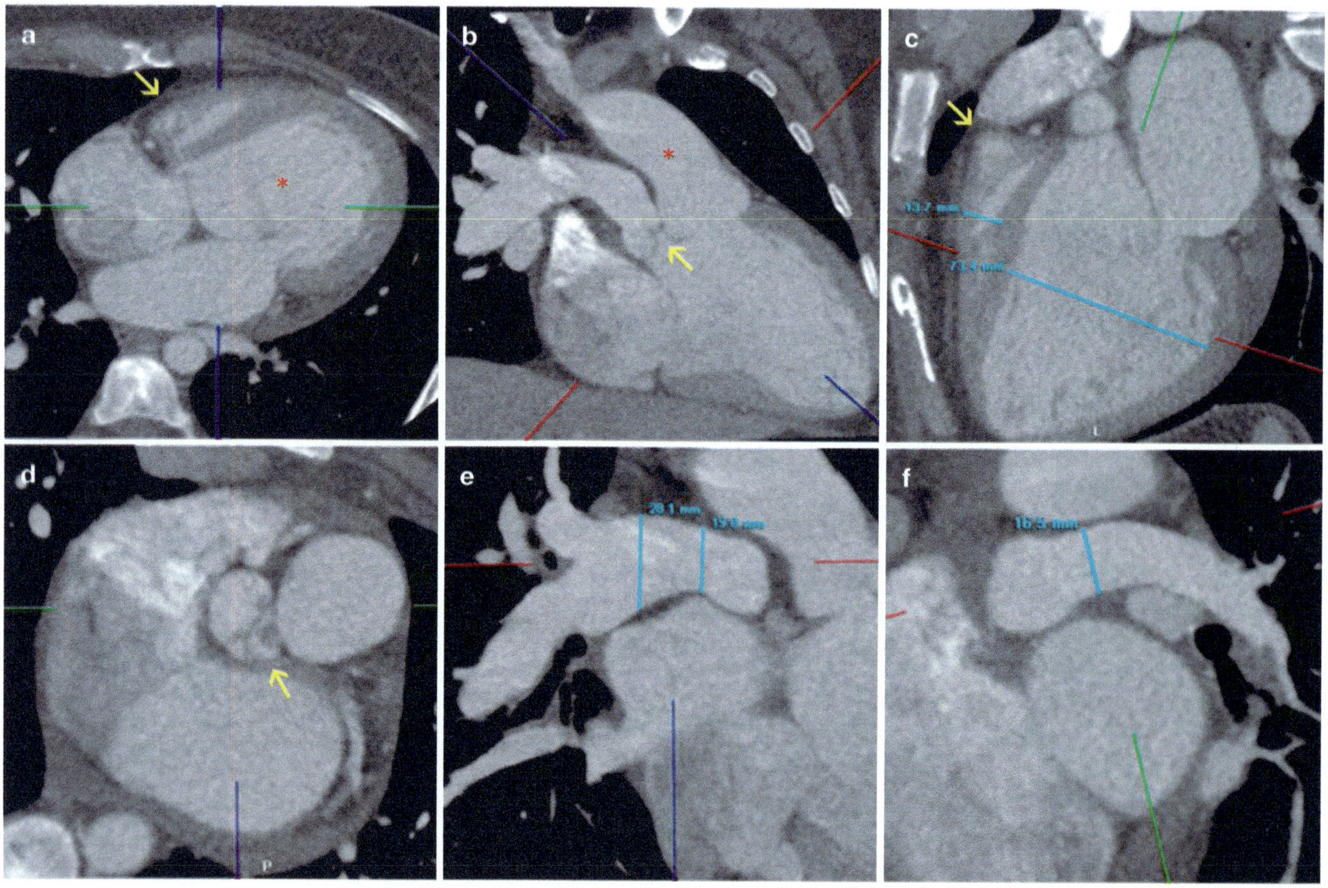

Findings and Interpretation

- Axial and oblique CT views (panels A–C) show a dilated single ventricle (asterisk) and a rudimentary right ventricle (arrows).
- Anterior aorta (asterisk in panel B) and posterior and thickened pulmonary valve (yellow arrows in panels B and D) arise from the single ventricle. Pulmonary branches are dilated (panels E and F).
- Univentricular heart with double inlet is a very rare congenital cardiac anomaly. A large portion of these patients have associated pulmonary stenosis, as is in this case.

Further Reading

Dillman JR, Hernandez RJ. Role of CT in the evaluation of congenital cardiovascular disease in children. AJR Am J Roentgenol. 2009;192:1219–31.

Menon SC, Hagler DJ. Double-outlet left ventricle: diagnosis and management. Curr Treat Options Cardiovasc Med. 2008;10:448–52.

Prakash A, Powell AJ, Geva T. Multimodality noninvasive imaging for assessment of congenital heart disease. Circ Cardiovasc Imaging. 2010;3:112–25.

Case 144

Lung Sequestration

Clinical History

- Twenty-seven-year-old male.
- Non-smoker, 3-year history of persistent dry cough, occasionally pleuritic chest pain at the right lung lower zone.
- Physical examination was remarkable for decrease breath sounds on the right lower lung field, in the paravertebral region.
- Past clinical history of several hospital admissions since young adulthood because of recurrent pneumonias in the right lung. Previous evaluations which included chest X-ray demonstrated a persistent consolidation in the right lower lobe that failed to resolve after antibiotic treatments.
- Referred for thoracic computed tomography (CT) angiography with the presumptive diagnosis of lung sequestration.

Images

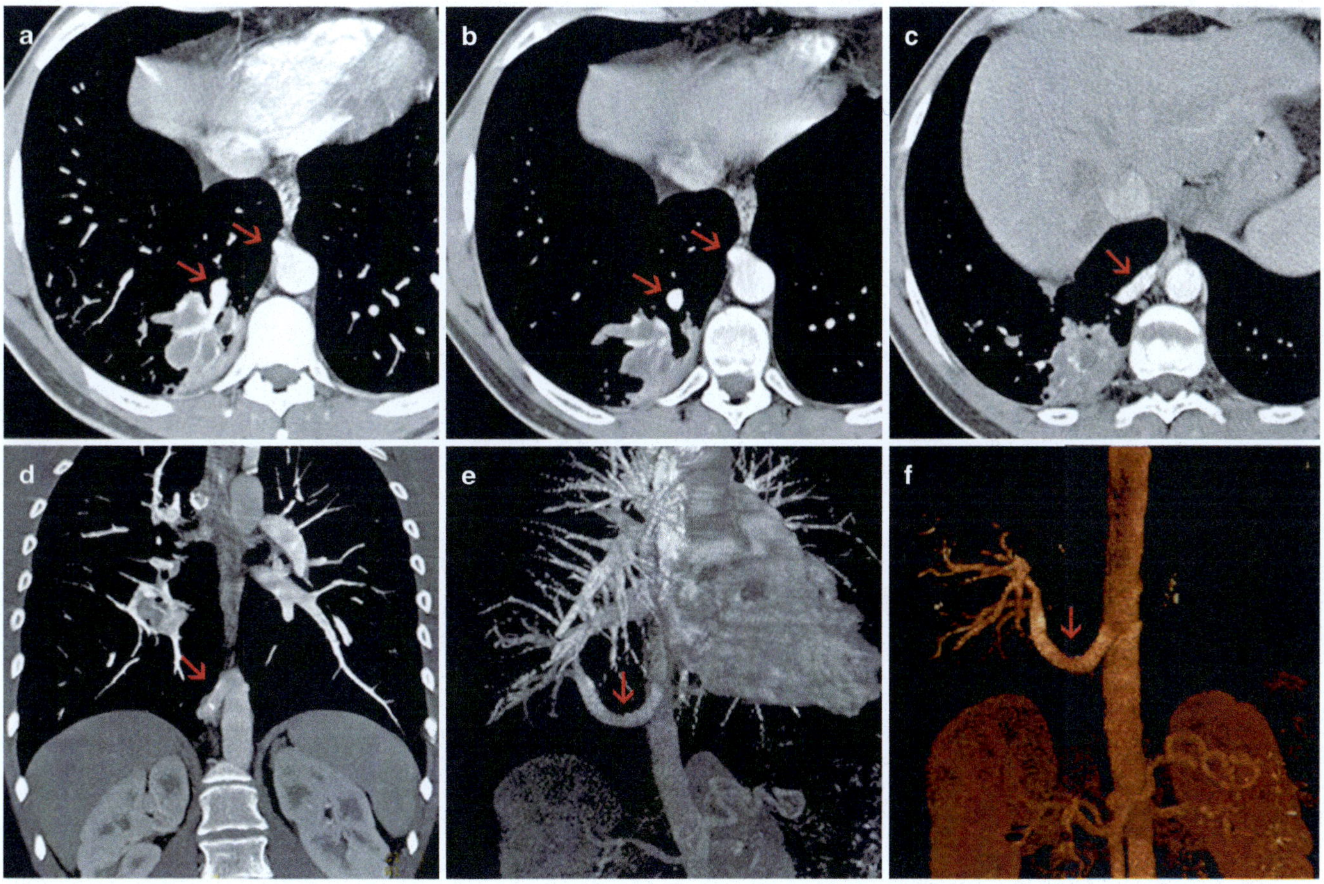

Findings and Interpretation

- Axial CT images with soft tissue window (panels A–C) show a focal consolidation at the posterior basal segment of the right lower lobe. There is an anomalous artery arising from the antero-right aspect of the descending thoracic aorta (arrow) that supplies the consolidated lung.
- Coronal MPR (panel D), MIP (panel E), and volume rendering (panel F) images demonstrate the aberrant artery arising for the right aspect of the descending thoracic aorta (arrow) above the level of the diaphragm.
- The location of the lung lesion, its persistence over time, and the identification of a systemic feeding vessel suggest the diagnosis of intralobar pulmonary sequestration.
- Pulmonary sequestration represents a bronchopulmonary foregut airway malformation. First described by Rektorzik in 1861, it characterizes for dysplastic lung tissue without identifiable communication to the tracheobronchial tree that receives its blood supply from an anomalous systemic artery, usually from the aorta.

- On CT, it typically manifests as a focal opacity, located most frequently in the posterior basal segment of the left lower lobe. The second most common location is the posterior basal segment of the right lower lobe. These two locations represents the 98% of the cases. Bilateral involvement is uncommon.
- Intralobar sequestration is usually diagnosed later than extralobar sequestration, being usually diagnosed in adult life after repetitive pulmonary infections.
- Chest CT angiography allows identification of the abnormal feeding vessel originating from descending thoracic aorta, providing a comprehensive vascular and thoracic anatomical assessment.

Further Reading

Berrocal T, Madrid C, Novo S, Gutiérrez J, Arjonilla A, Gómez-León N. Congenital anomalies of the tracheobronchial tree, lung, and mediastinum: embryology, radiology, and pathology. Radiographics. 2004;24(1):e17.

Frazier AA, Rosado de Christenson ML, Stocker JT, Templeton PA. Intralobar sequestration: radiologic-pathologic correlation. RadioGraphics. 1997; 17:725–45.

Zylak CJ, Eyler WR, Spizarny DL, Stone CH. Developmental lung anomalies in the adult: radiologic-pathologic correlation. Radiographics. 2002;22 Spec No:S25–43.

Case 145

Lung Sequestration

Clinical History

- Eight-year-old girl.
- Normal physical examination, with absence of respiratory symptoms.
- Chest auscultation was remarkable for decreased breath sounds on the left lower lung field, without rhonchi or rales sounds. A non-enhanced chest CT scan showed a focal, round hyperlucency area of lung parenchyma at the posterior basal segment of the left lower lobe, in association with anomalous enlarged vessels.
- No previous clinical history of lower respiratory infections.
- Referred for thoracic computed tomography (CT) angiography with the presumptive diagnosis of bronchopulmonary foregut airway malformation.

Images

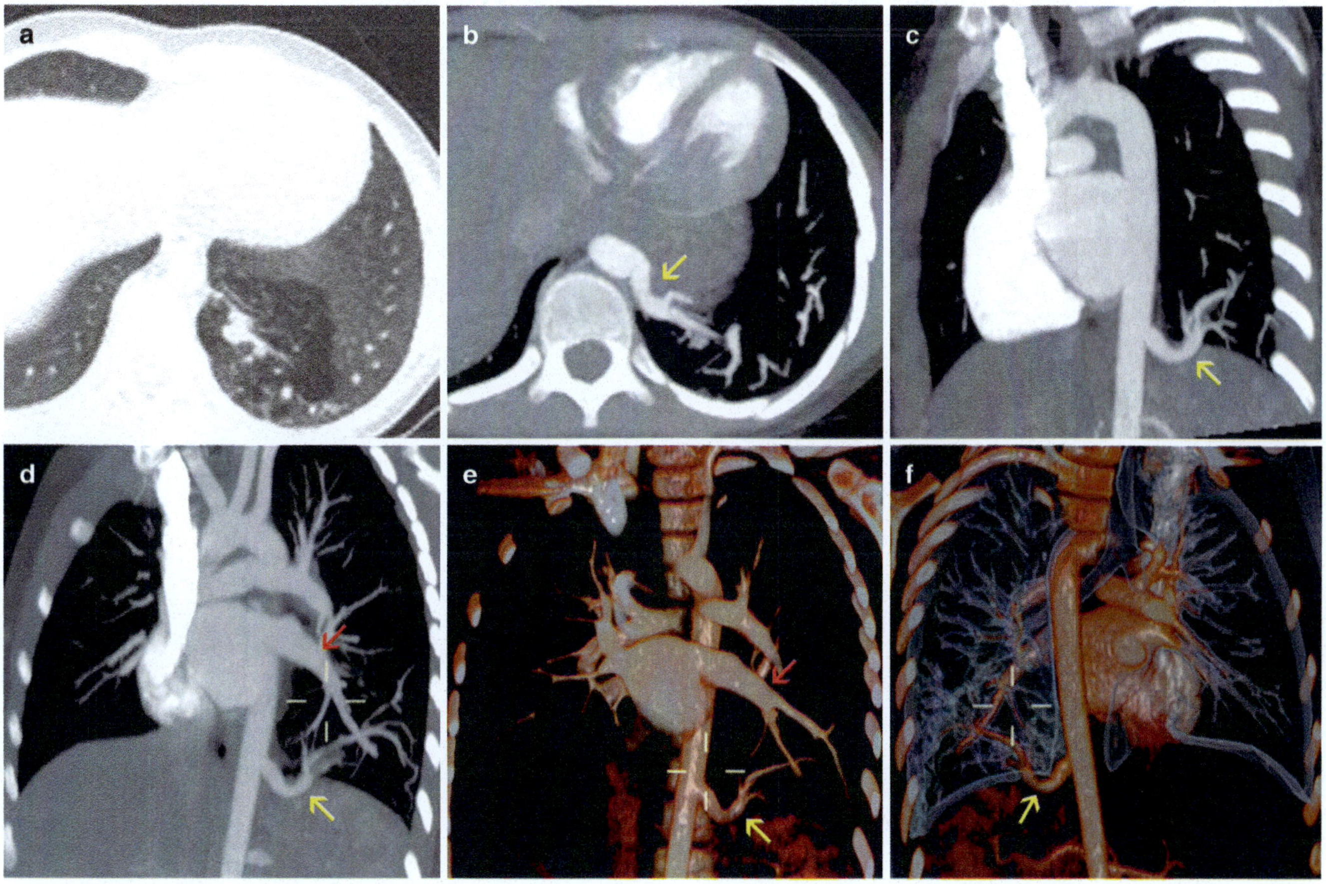

Findings and Interpretation

- Axial CT image with lung window (panel A) shows a focal, well-delimitated hypoattenuated area of lung parenchyma at the posterior basal segment of the left lower lobe, in association with anomalous enlarged vessels.
- Axial maximum intensity projection (MIP, panel B) and coronal oblique (panel C) CT angiography images demonstrate an aberrant artery arising for the left aspect of the descending aorta (yellow arrow) at the level of the diaphragm feeding the abnormal lung parenchyma.
- Coronal MIP image (panel D) and volume rendering images, anterior (panel E) and posterior (panel F) views, depict the feeding artery (yellow arrow) and a normal venous drainage via the pulmonary circulation to the left atrium.
- Image findings are consistent with the diagnosis of intralobar pulmonary sequestration.
- Pulmonary sequestration represents a bronchopulmonary foregut airway malformation. It refers to a segment of lung parenchyma without connection with the tracheobronchial tree that receives its blood supply from a systemic artery, usually from the aorta.

- They can be classified as extralobar or intralobar sequestration, according to its relationship with the pleural investment. Intralobar sequestration accounts for 75% of all cases. The abnormal lung tissue lies within normal pulmonary visceral pleura, and the venous drainage commonly occurs via the pulmonary veins. In cases of extralobar sequestration, the abnormal lung parenchyma has its own pleural investment, and venous drainage most commonly occurs via systemic veins into the right atrium.
- Lesions are preferentially located in the lower lobes, being left-sided lesions more common. Intralobar sequestration is usually diagnosed later than extralobar sequestration, being usually found in childhood or adulthood after repetitive pulmonary infections. Associated diseases, such as congenital heart disease, diaphragmatic hernia, or hypogenetic lung syndrome, are more common findings with the extralobar type (60%).
- The abnormal feeding artery may also arise below the diaphragm from the celiac or splenic artery or from an intercostal artery.
- CT angiography allows detailed anatomical assessment with excellent spatial and temporal resolution, giving a comprehensive vascular and thoracic anatomical assessment.

Further Reading

Alivizatos P, Cheatle T, de Leval M, Stark J. Pulmonary sequestration complicated by anomalies of pulmonary venous return. J Pediatr Surg. 1985;20(1):76–9.

Berrocal T, Madrid C, Novo S, Gutiérrez J, Arjonilla A, Gómez-León N. Congenital anomalies of the tracheobronchial tree, lung, and mediastinum: embryology, radiology, and pathology. Radiographics. 2004;24(1):e17.

Zylak CJ, Eyler WR, Spizarny DL, Stone CH. Developmental lung anomalies in the adult: radiologic-pathologic correlation. Radiographics. 2002;22 Spec No:S25–43.

Case 146

Pulmonary Arteriovenous Malformation

Clinical History

- Fifty-seven-year-old female.
- With brain and liver metastasis from breast primary cancer treated with systemic chemotherapy.
- Currently, the patient has prolonged febrile syndrome and chills. Infective endocarditis was suspected. Transthoracic echocardiography identified a small 2.5 mm "vegetation-like" lesion on the aortic valve. The differential diagnosis with papillary fibroelastoma of the aortic valve was considered.
- History of right breast cancer treated with breast-conserving surgery, chemotherapy, and radiotherapy. Brain and liver metastasis developed.
- Referred for contrast-enhanced cardiac and thoracic computed tomography (CT) scans.

Images

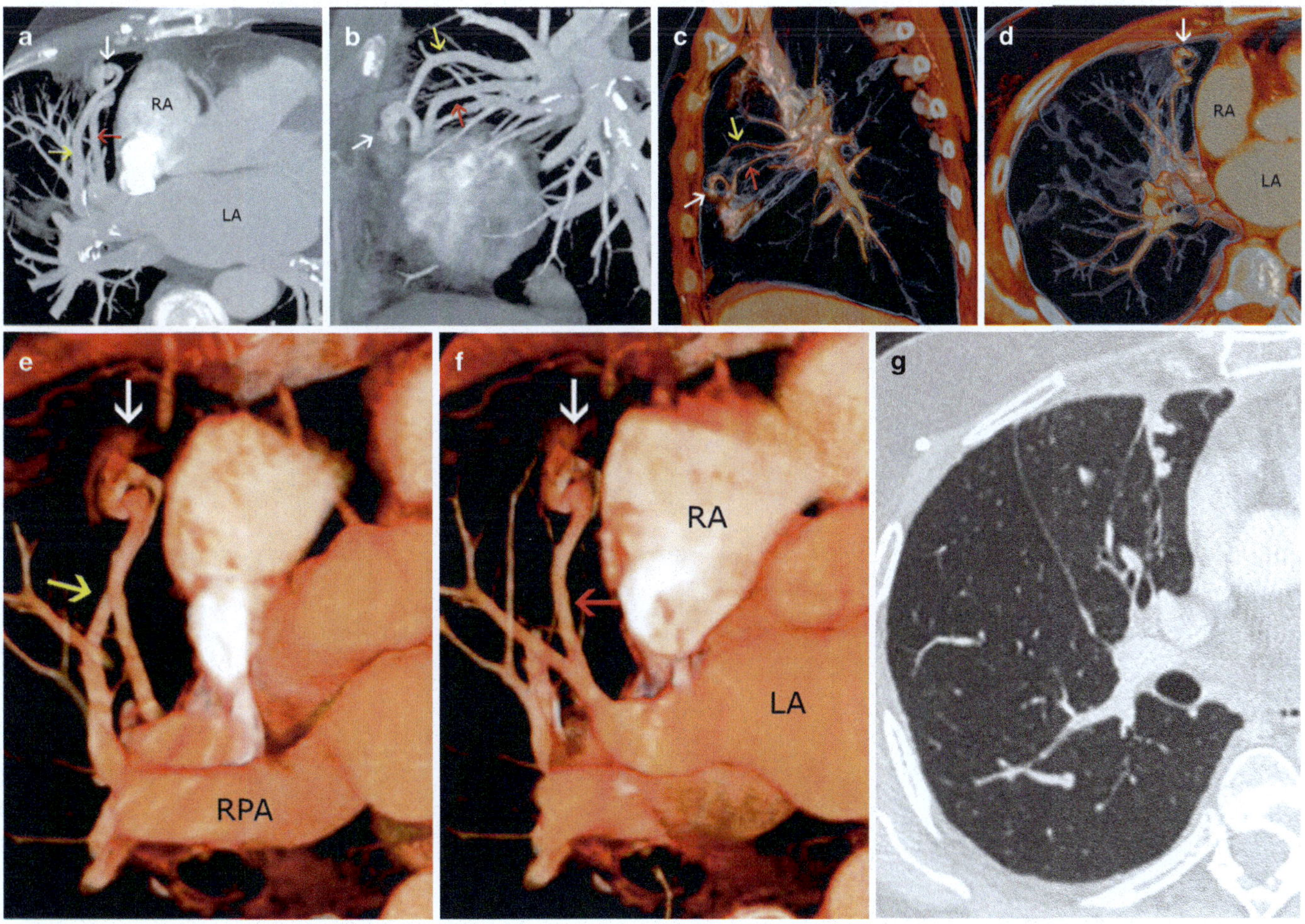

Findings and Interpretation

- Non-calcified round opacity connected with anomalous serpiginous dilated vascular structures projecting into the medial segment of the right middle lobe. Findings are consistent with the diagnosis of a simple pulmonary arteriovenous malformation (PAVM).
- Axial (panel A) and sagittal (panel B) maximum intensity projection images and sagittal (panel C) and superior three-dimensional views (panels D–F) demonstrate an anomalous enlarged right middle lobe pulmonary artery (feeding artery, yellow arrow), a round opacity consistent with the nidus or aneurysmal part of the PAVM (white arrow), and the draining vein (red arrow) draining directly into the right superior pulmonary vein. RA, right atrium; LA, left atrium, RPA, right pulmonary artery. Axial CT image, lung window (panel G) shows a partial collapse of the right middle lobe secondary to fibrotic changes, adjacent to the dilated vascular structures.

- PAVM consists of abnormal communications between the pulmonary artery and pulmonary veins, providing a right-to-left shunt (high-flow, low-resistance vascular malformation). Usually congenital, they can be secondary to pulmonary infections, trauma, or metastatic disease among other causes.
- Based on the angioarchitecture, they can be classified as simple PAVM (80% of cases), characterized by the presence of a single feeding segmental artery and a single draining pulmonary vein, and as complex PAVM (20% of cases), with the identification of two or more feeding arteries or draining veins.
- Simple PAVM are usually asymptomatic and diagnosed incidentally in the investigation of another issues. Complex PAVM with severe right-to-left shunt can manifest with cyanosis, hemoptysis, or respiratory distress syndrome.
- Contrast-enhanced chest CT and pulmonary CT angiography allow detailed anatomical assessment of both lung and vascular structures, with excellent spatial and temporal resolution, giving a comprehensive vascular and thoracic anatomical assessment. CT evaluation includes size, angioarchitecture, location, and timing of enhancement of the lesion.

Further Reading

Coulier B. Detection of pulmonary arteriovenous malformations by multislice spiral CT angiography. JBR-BTR. 2003;86:28.

Hashemzadeh S, Daryani A. Pulmonary arteriovenous malformation. J Cardiovasc Thorac Res 2009;1:37–40.

Papagiannis J, Apostolopoulou S, Sarris G, Rammos S. Diagnosis and management of pulmonary arteriovenous malformations. Images Paediatr Cardiol. 2002;4:33–49.

Case 147

Pulmonary Hypertension

Clinical History

- Thirty-year-old female.
- History of pulmonary hypertension.
- She underwent cardiac magnetic resonance (CMR) to rule out specific etiologies including left-sided heart disease, cardiac shunt, patent ductus arteriosus (PDA), and chronic thromboembolism.

Images

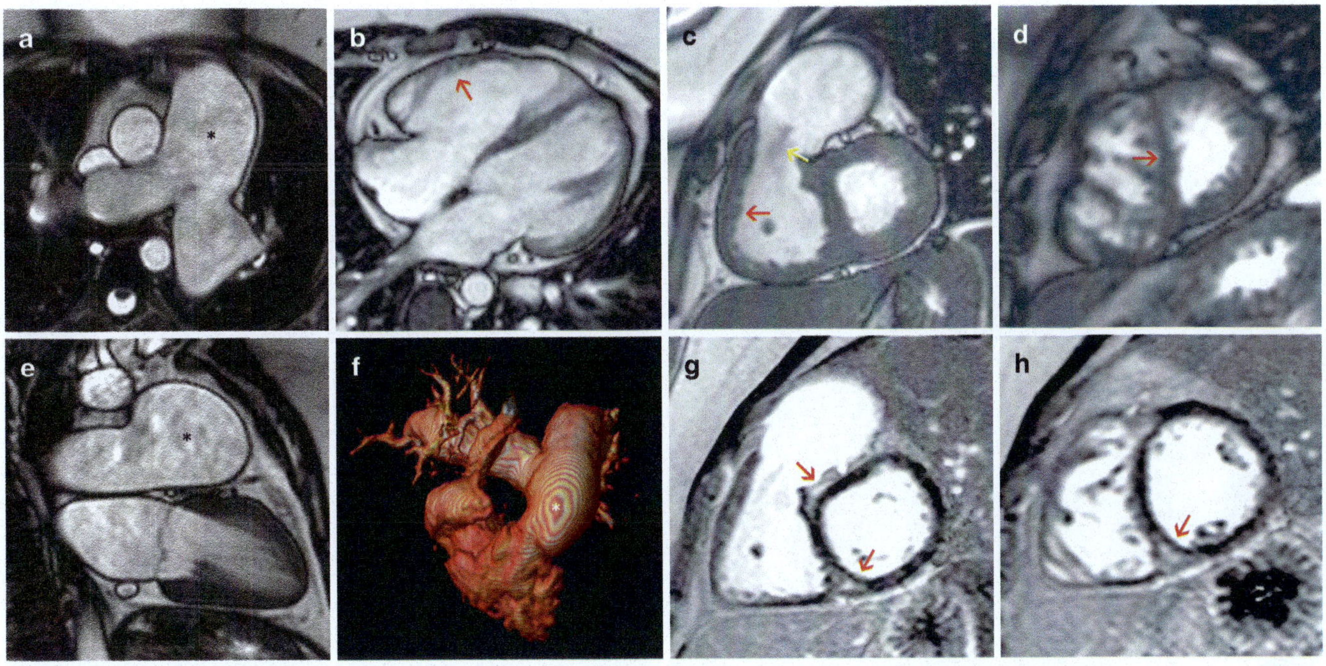

Findings and Interpretation

- Cine axial views from the aortic arch to the diaphragm are very useful among these patients to exclude PDA and atrial septal defect. In addition, pulmonary artery size and patency can be assessed accurately. In this case, the pulmonary artery trunk (asterisk in panel A) is markedly enlarged (48 mm), as well as the main pulmonary branches.
- Right ventricular (RV) hypertrophy is documented using a four-chamber view (red arrow in panel B) and a basal short-axis view (red arrow in panel C). Mild pulmonary regurgitation is also detected (yellow arrow in panel C).
- RV pressure overload leads to a significant leftward septal shift (red arrow in panel D).
- The severe pulmonary artery dilatation is clearly observed using a two-chamber view.
- Contrast-enhanced magnetic resonance angiography was performed (panel F), showing large and patent main and segmentary pulmonary branches.
- At inversion-recovery imaging, intramural/subepicardial late gadolinium enhancement at the insertion sites upon the septum is a hallmark of RV pressure overload.
- This case nicely depicts the ability of CMR to evaluate patients with pulmonary hypertension.
- Primary pulmonary hypertension is a very rare disease, generally idiopathic, although some reports suggest a familial form with autosomal dominant inheritance, enabling a higher susceptibility to vasoconstrictors. The prognosis is poor, and no definite treatment has been established though several strategies are available.

Further Reading

McLaughlin VV, Hoeper MM, Channick RN, Chin KM, Delcroix M, Gaine S, et al. Pulmonary arterial hypertension-related morbidity is prognostic for mortality. J Am Coll Cardiol. 2018;71:752–63.

Swift AJ, Rajaram S, Campbell MJ, Hurdman J, Thomas S, Capener D, et al. Prognostic value of cardiovascular magnetic resonance imaging measurements corrected for age and sex in idiopathic pulmonary arterial hypertension. Circ Cardiovasc Imaging. 2014;7:100–6.

Case 148

Left Ventricle Dual Chamber

Clinical History

- Forty-four-year old male.
- Asymptomatic.
- As part of a medical check-up, a transthoracic echocardiogram was done showing a dual-chamber left ventricle.
- A cardiac magnetic resonance (CMR) was requested to verify the diagnosis.

Images

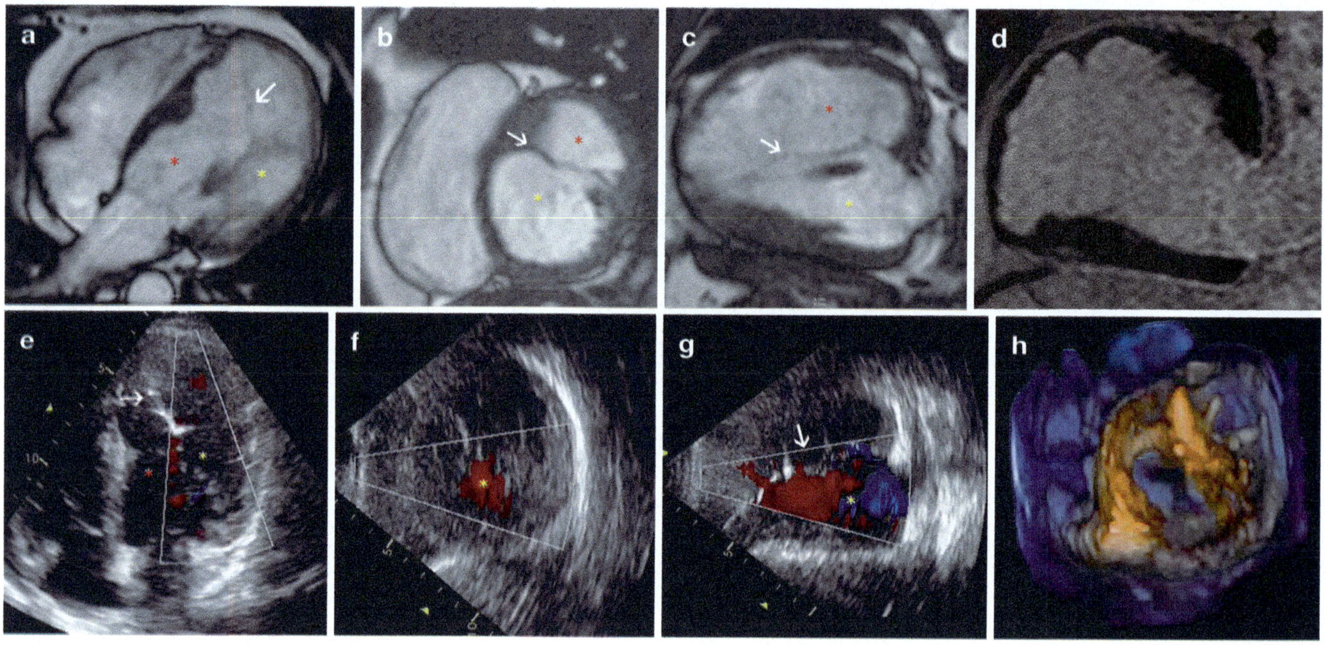

Findings and Interpretation

- Four-chamber (panel A), short-axis (panel B), and two-chamber (panel C) cine images showing a left ventricle (LV) with dual chamber. A thin soft tissue band (arrow) is dividing the LV into two chambers, one accessory (red asterisk) and another the main chamber (yellow asterisk). The main chamber is the one that has the papillary muscles and the mitral valve.
- Late enhancement image (panel D) shows normal myocardial signal intensity.
- Transthoracic echocardiogram in four-chamber (panel E), short-axis (panel F), and two-chamber (panel G) views showing similar findings than CMR with the two LV chambers divided by a fibrous band.
- Double-chambered LV (DCLV) is a congenital rare disease characterized by the presence of two ventricular cavities divided by a septum or abnormal muscular band.
- It is usually diagnosed at neonatal or pediatric age.
- Differential diagnosis include:
  - Diverticulum: there is narrow neck connecting the ventricular cavity with a normal morphological and functional wall. It is associated with middle line congenital abnormalities that affect the diaphragm, abdominal wall, and pericardium (Cantrell syndrome).
  - Aneurysm: fibrotic sac with dyskinetic movement.
- CMR can accurately evaluate and perform a precise diagnosis among these different pathologies.

Further Reading

Gufler H, Anderson RH, Annette M, Voigtlaender T. Double-chambered left ventricle in a patient with chest pain. Clin Res Cardiol. 2018;107(12):1180–82.

Vijayvergiya R, Goel R, Patel R. Double chamber right ventricle and left ventricle: a rare association. Indian Heart J. 2015;67:489–90.

Case 149

Left Persistent Isolated Superior Vena Cava

Clinical History

- Forty-year old male.
- Familiar history of dilated cardiomyopathy.
- A transthoracic eco was done and a left persistent vena cava was identified.
- A computed tomography coronary angiography (CTCA) was requested for further evaluation.

Images

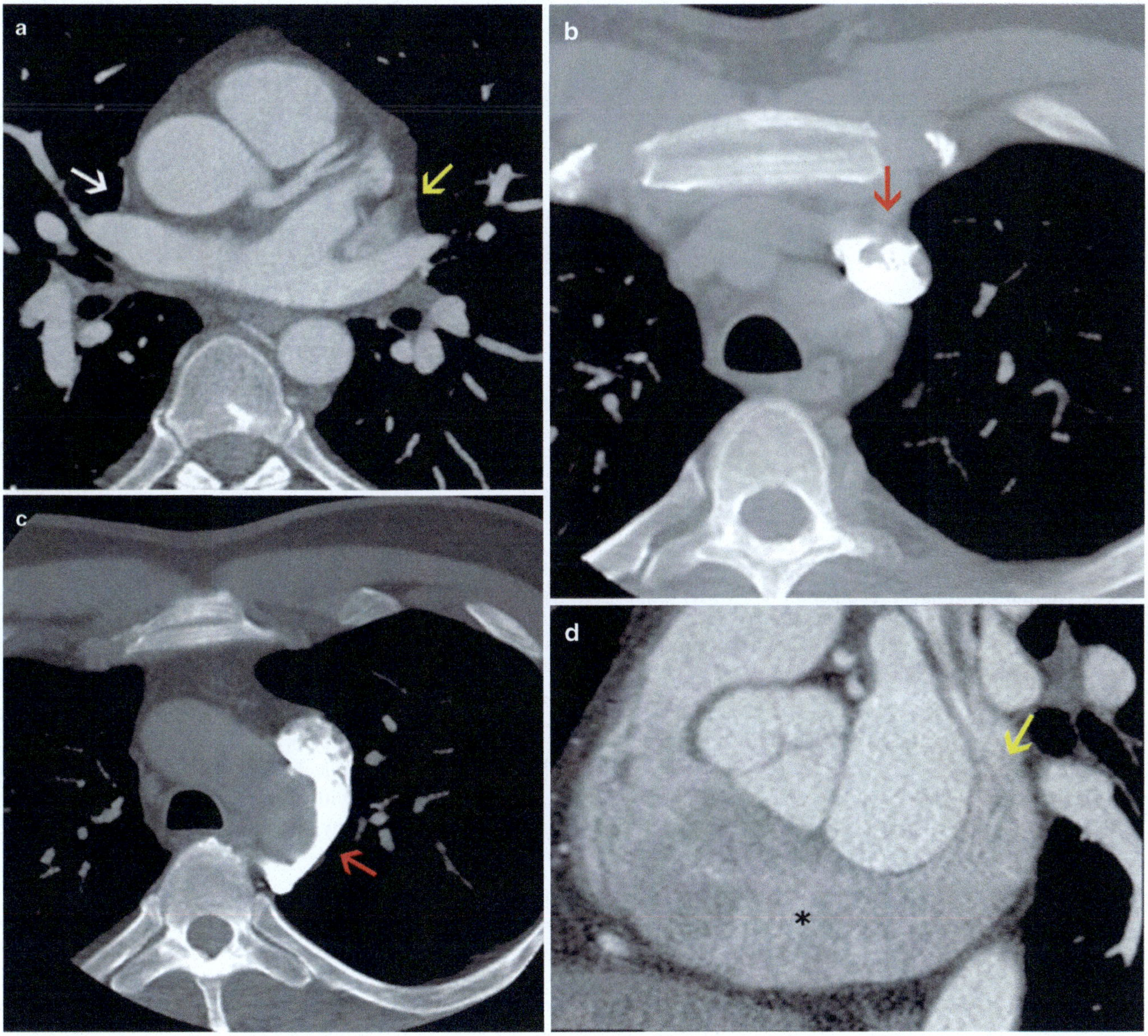

(continued)

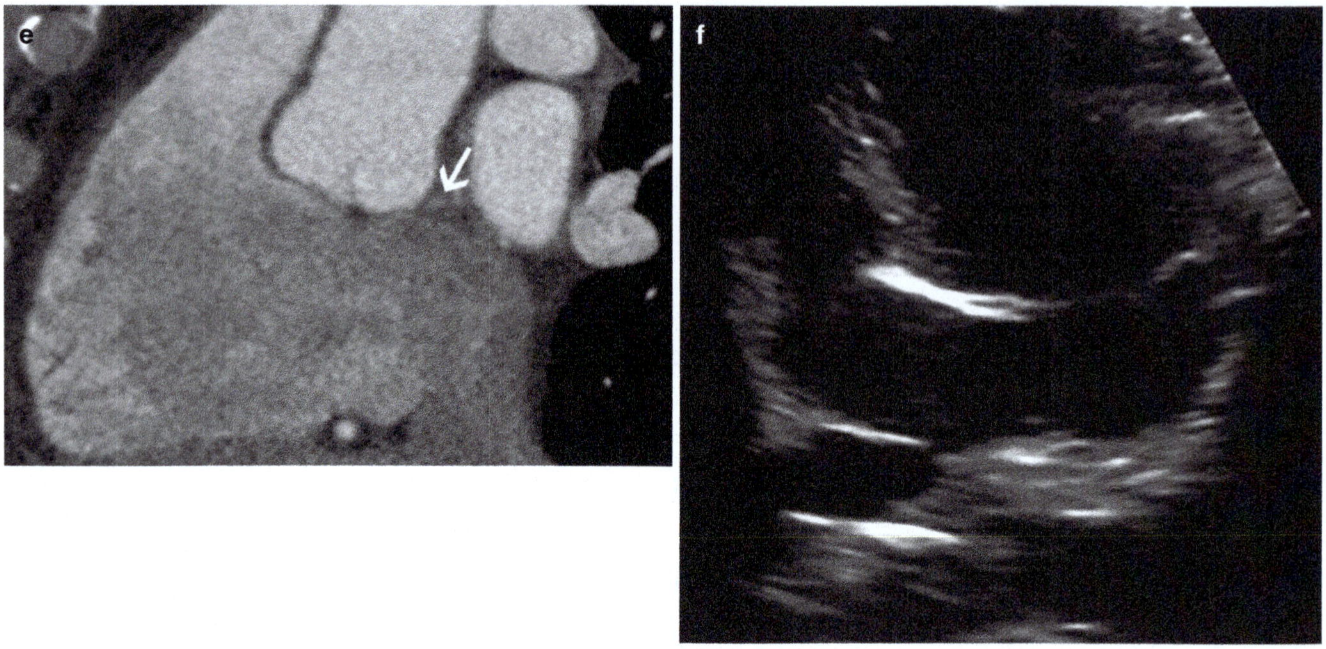

Findings and Interpretation

- Axial CT image (panel A) showing the absence of superior vena cava (SVC) (white arrow) with persistent left superior vena cava (LPSVC) (yellow arrow) (panel A).
- Axial CT images (panels B and C) with soft tissue window showing the brachiocephalic venous trunk draining into the LPSVC (arrows).
- Left sagittal multiplanar reconstruction (MPR) (panel D) showing the LPSVC (arrow) arriving to the coronary sinus (asterisk).
- Right sagittal MPR (panel E) showing the absence of SCV (arrow).
- Transthoracic echocardiogram (panel F) showing similar findings.
- Left persistent isolated superior vena cava with absence of right superior vena cava is a rare condition with a frequency of 0.07–0.13%.
- It is usually asymptomatic, but it can pose difficulties with central venous access, pacemaker implantation, and cardiothoracic surgery. This condition is also associated with an increased incidence of congenital heart disease, arrhythmias, and conduction disturbances.

Further Reading

Conti S, Khaykin Y. Pacemaker implantation in a challenging anatomy: isolated persistent left superior vena cava and azygos continuation of interrupted inferior vena cava. Clin Case Rep. 2018;6(4):709–11.

Uçar O, Paşaoğlu L, Ciçekçioğlu H, et al. Persistent left superior vena cava with absent right superior vena cava: a case report and review of the literature. Cardiovasc J Afr. 2010;21:164–6.

Case 150

Cor Triatriatum

Clinical History

- Sixty-three-year-old male.
- He underwent a primary percutaneous angioplasty due to an ST-elevation acute myocardial infarction.
- During hospitalization a transthoracic echocardiogram revealed cor triatriatum.
- Cardiac magnetic resonance (CMR) was indicated for further assessment.

Images

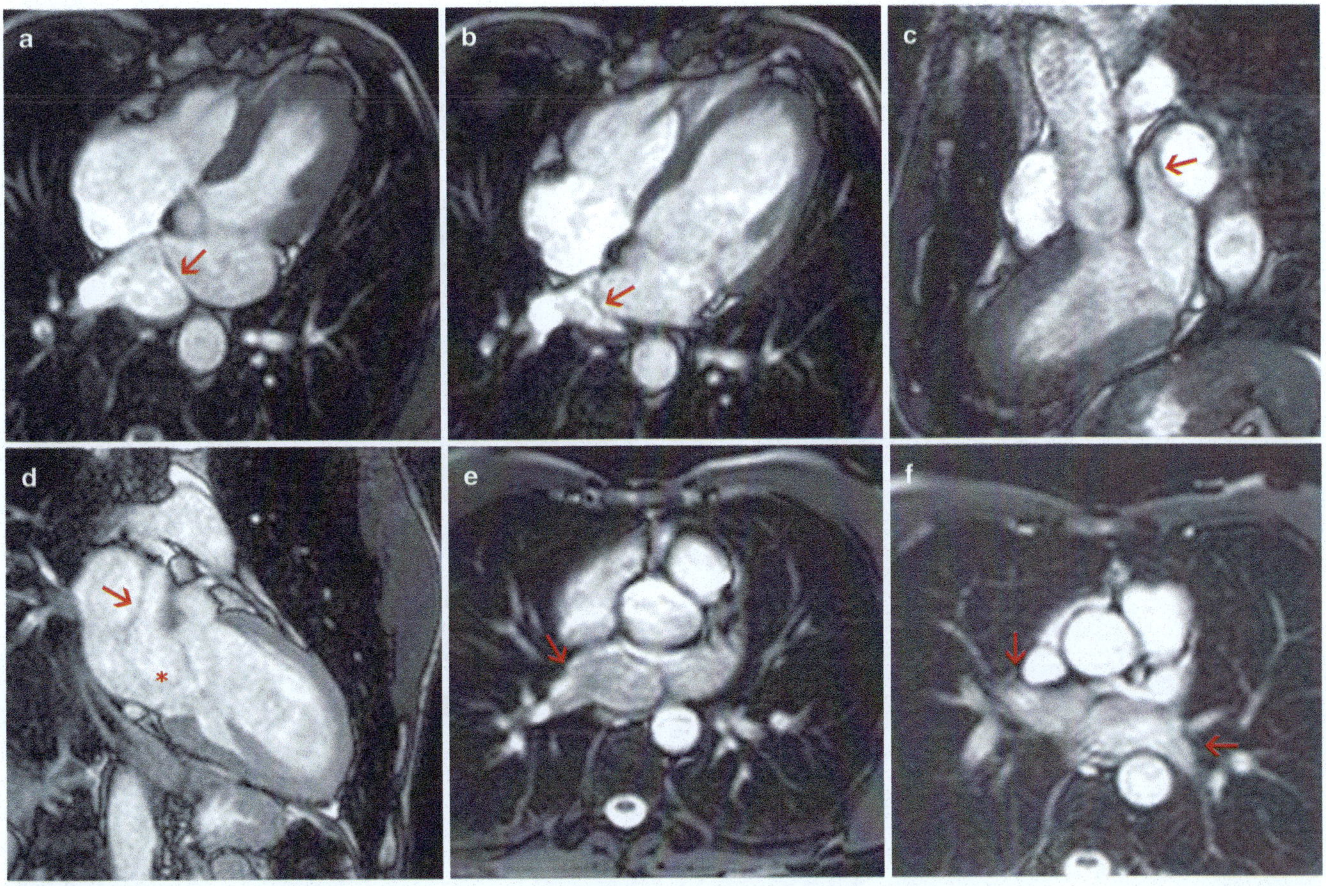

Findings and Interpretation

- At cine images in four-chamber (panels A and B), three-chamber (panel C), and two-chamber (panel D) views, a fibromuscular membrane dividing the left atrium was observed (arrows), without evidence of flow obstruction (asterisk).
- At axial scout views (panels E and F), normal pulmonary veins draining into the pulmonary venous chamber are observed (arrows).
- Cor triatriatum is a rare congenital heart defect where the left atrium (cor triatriatum sinistrum) or right atrium (cor triatriatum dextrum) is divided by a thin membrane. In the case of cor triatriatum sinistrum, the membrane divides the left atrium into two well-differentiated chambers: one is proximal, posterior, and related to the pulmonary veins (pulmonary venous chamber); and the other is distal, anterior, and adjacent to the mitral valve orifice and in which the left atrial appendage is located (true left atrium). It is associated with other malformations such as pulmonary vein stenosis and atrial septal defect.
- CMR allows defining accurately the anatomy of the membrane and the atria. In addition, it simultaneously enables the evaluation of associated pathologies.

Further Reading

Anderson RH, Baker EJ, Redington A, Rigby ML, Penny D, Wernovsky G. Paediatric cardiology. 3rd ed. Philadelphia: Elsevier.

Case 151

Bicuspid Aortic Valve

Clinical History

- Seventy-seven-year-old female.
- During a routine stress echocardiogram (hypercholesterolemia), an ascending aorta dilatation and a bicuspid aortic valve are detected, with absence of regurgitation and mild stenosis (effective orifice area of 1.7 cm^2 and peak gradient of 18 mmHg).
- Referred to non-contrast cardiac magnetic resonance (CMR) for further evaluation of thoracic aorta dimensions.

Images

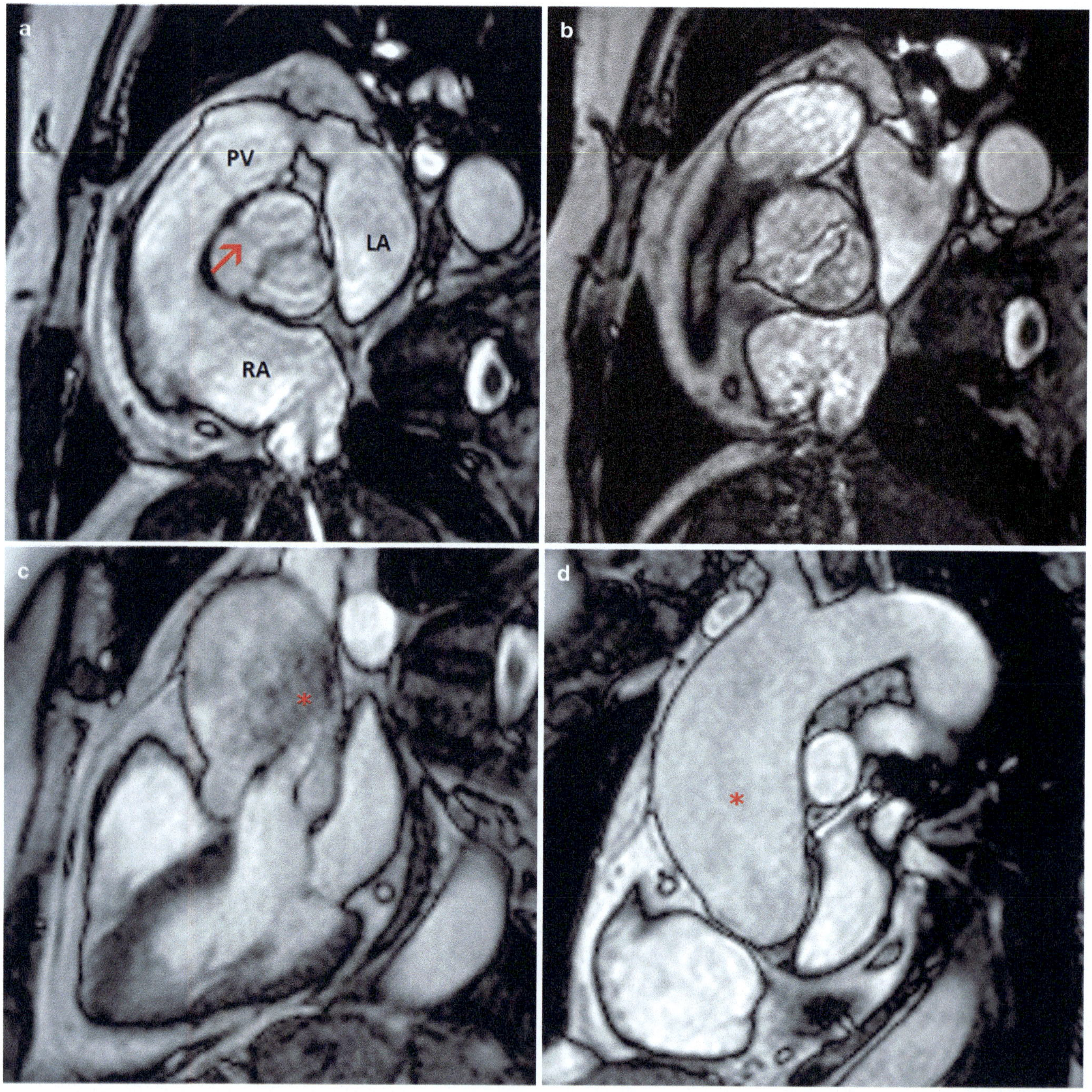

Findings and Interpretation

- Diastolic (panel A) and systolic (panel B) cine images at the aortic valve plane demonstrate a type 1 bicuspid aortic valve, with an anterior raphe (arrow) at 11 o'clock.
- Manual planimetry revealed a mild stenosis (effective valve area of 1.76 cm^2), and no regurgitation was detected.
- A dome-shaped opening is observed at a left ventricular outflow tract view (panel C), with mild acceleration (*) of the systolic transvalvular flow.
- Using cine images and oblique sagittal views, accurate measurements of the thoracic aorta can be obtained without the need of contrast.
- In this case, the aortic diameters were of 40 mm at the sinus portion and of 49 mm at the tubular portion.
- Bicuspid aortic valve is the most frequent congenital cardiac anomaly (1–2% of the general population) and can variably impact valve function, from none to severe aortic regurgitation and/or stenosis. The most common classification of bicuspid aortic valve is based on the number of raphes (type 0, without raphe; type 1, with 1 raphe; and type 2, with 2 raphes). Most patients with bicuspid aortic valve have a dilated ascending aorta and are therefore at a higher risk of aortic dissection. This case nicely depicts that a very accurate assessment of the aortic valve and of the thoracic aorta dimensions can be performed without the need of contrast.

Further Reading

Michałowska IM, Kruk M, Kwiatek P, et al. Aortic pathology in patients with bicuspid aortic valve assessed with computed tomography angiography. J Thorac Imaging. 2014;29:113–7.

Nistri S, Sorbo MD, Marin M, et al. Aortic root dilatation in young men with normally functioning bicuspid aortic valves. Heart. 1999;82:19–22.

Sievers HH, Schmidtke C. A classification system for the bicuspid aortic valve from 304 surgical specimens. J Thorac Cardiovasc Surg;133:1226–33.

Case 152

Ebstein's Anomaly

Clinical History

- Seventeen-year-old female.
- She has known Ebstein's anomaly.
- Referred to delayed-enhancement cardiac magnetic resonance (DE-CMR) for further evaluation.

Images

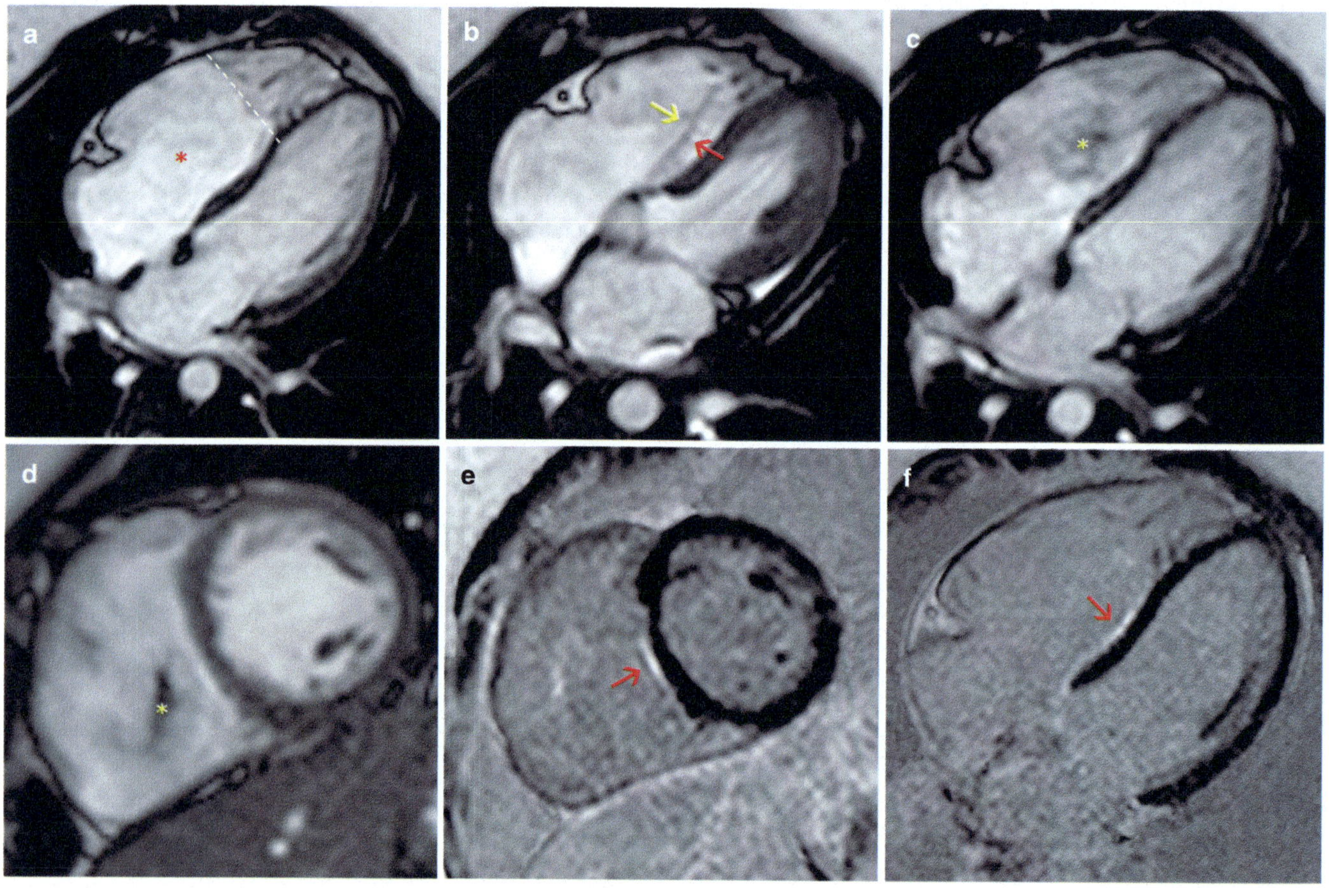

Findings and Interpretation

- A marked apical (downward) displacement of the tricuspid valve is clearly observed using four-chamber views (panels A–C).
- Instead of the normal position at the atrioventricular groove, the tricuspid valve is apically displaced (dashed lined in panel A). Particularly, the septal leaftlet is displaced (red arrow in panel B) and less frequently the posterior tricuspid leaflet (yellow arrow in panel B). These leads to an atrialized right ventricle (asterisk in panel A). Also, the underlying tricuspid valve dysplasia usually leads to different degrees of tricuspid regurgitation, whose regurgitating jet is obviously apically displaced (asterisk in panel C).
- A systolic short-axis view at the mid-ventricular level shows the abnormally low regurgitating jet (asterisk in panel D).
- At inversion-recovery images, the right ventricular aspect of the mid- and basal interventricular septum shows thin subendocardial enhancement (fibrosis).
- Ebstein's anomaly (EA) is a very rare congenital heart defect, accounting for less than 1% of all congenital heart defects. As a genetic cardiomyopathy, EA can also be associated with other disorders such as atrial and ventricular septal defects, patent foramen ovale, hypertrophic and dilated cardiomyopathy, and left ventricular non-compaction, among others. Also, a large number of patients with EA have concomitant Wolff-Parkinson-

White syndrome, related to the atrialized right ventricular tissue. Among these patients, surgery is only indicated in the presence of significant and progressive right heart dilatation or systolic failure.

Further Reading

Yuan SM. Ebstein's anomaly: genetics, clinical manifestations, and management pediatrics and neonatology 2017;58:211–5.

Case 153

Scimitar Syndrome

Clinical History

- Forty-four-year-old male.
- Symptoms of increasing fatigue and dyspnea with a history of poor exercise tolerance.
- Posteroanterior chest X-ray showed an anomalous vascular shadow in the right lower lung field, associated with a small right lung and dextrocardia.
- Referred for thoracic computed tomography (CT) angiography.

Images

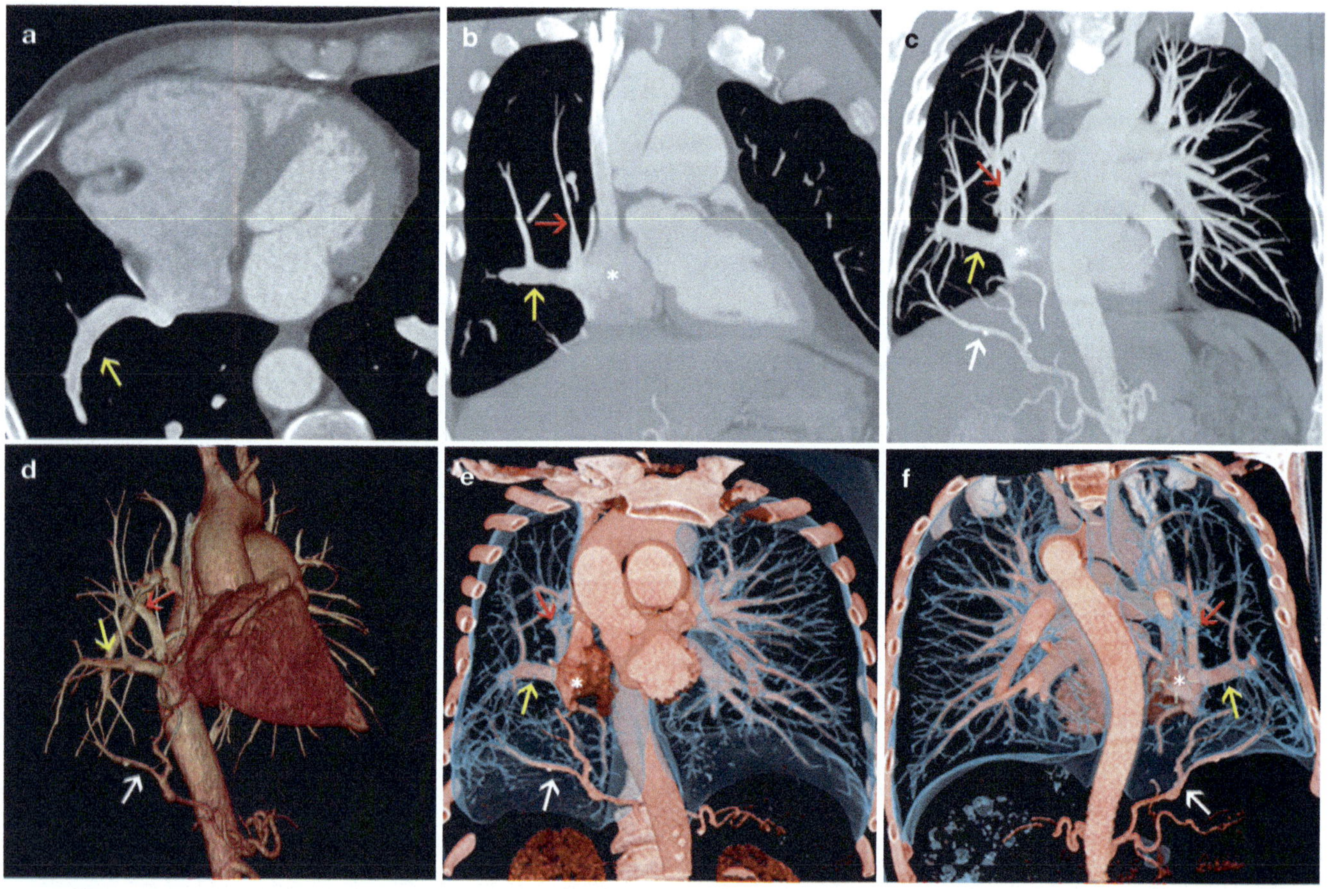

Findings and Interpretation

- The right lung is small in size, the left lung is hyperinflated, and the mediastinum shifted to the affected side, with dextrocardia.
- Axial CT image (panel A) and coronal multiplanar reconstruction (panel B) demonstrate an anomalous enlarged inferior lobe pulmonary vein (yellow arrow) and a superior lobe pulmonary vein (red arrow) draining into the right atrium (asterisk). The superior vena cava is normal. The right ventricle as well as the pulmonary arterial trunk are enlarged.
- Coronal maximum intensity reconstruction (panel C), three-dimensional coronal oblique (panel D), anterior (panel E), and posterior (panel F) views, show the presence of a systemic arterial supply from an aberrant artery (white arrow) arising from the infradiaphragmatic aorta. The scimitar syndrome consists in a combined lung and vascular anomalies, with an abnormal development of the lung (hypogenetic lung, almost always on the right side), associated with a systemic arterial supply and anomalous venous return to the systemic venous system, usually into the inferior vena cava or right atrium. It results in a left-to-right shunt as pulmonary venous blood flows directly into the right side of the heart or systemic veins. Accompanying cardiovascular anomalies are frequent.
- CT angiography allows detailed anatomical assessment with excellent spatial and temporal resolution, giving a comprehensive vascular and thoracic anatomical assessment.

Further Reading

Alivizatos P, Cheatle T, de Leval M, Stark J. Pulmonary sequestration complicated by anomalies of pulmonary venous return. J Pediatr Surg. 1985;20(1):76–9.

Berrocal T, Madrid C, Novo S, Gutiérrez J, Arjonilla A, Gómez-León N. Congenital anomalies of the tracheobronchial tree, lung, and mediastinum: embryology, radiology, and pathology. Radiographics. 2004;24(1):e17.

Zylak CJ, Eyler WR, Spizarny DL, Stone CH. Developmental lung anomalies in the adult: radiologic-pathologic correlation. Radiographics. 2002;22 Spec No:S25–43.

Case 154

Kawasaki Disease

Clinical History

- Seven-month-old male.
- Episode of high-grade fever (40 °C/104 °F) that did not respond to antipyretic medication. No other associate symptoms were present.
- Chest X-ray was within normal limits. Transthoracic echocardiography showed dilatation of the mid-segment of the right coronary artery (RCA).
- Referred for computed tomography coronary angiography (CTCA) for further evaluation.

Images

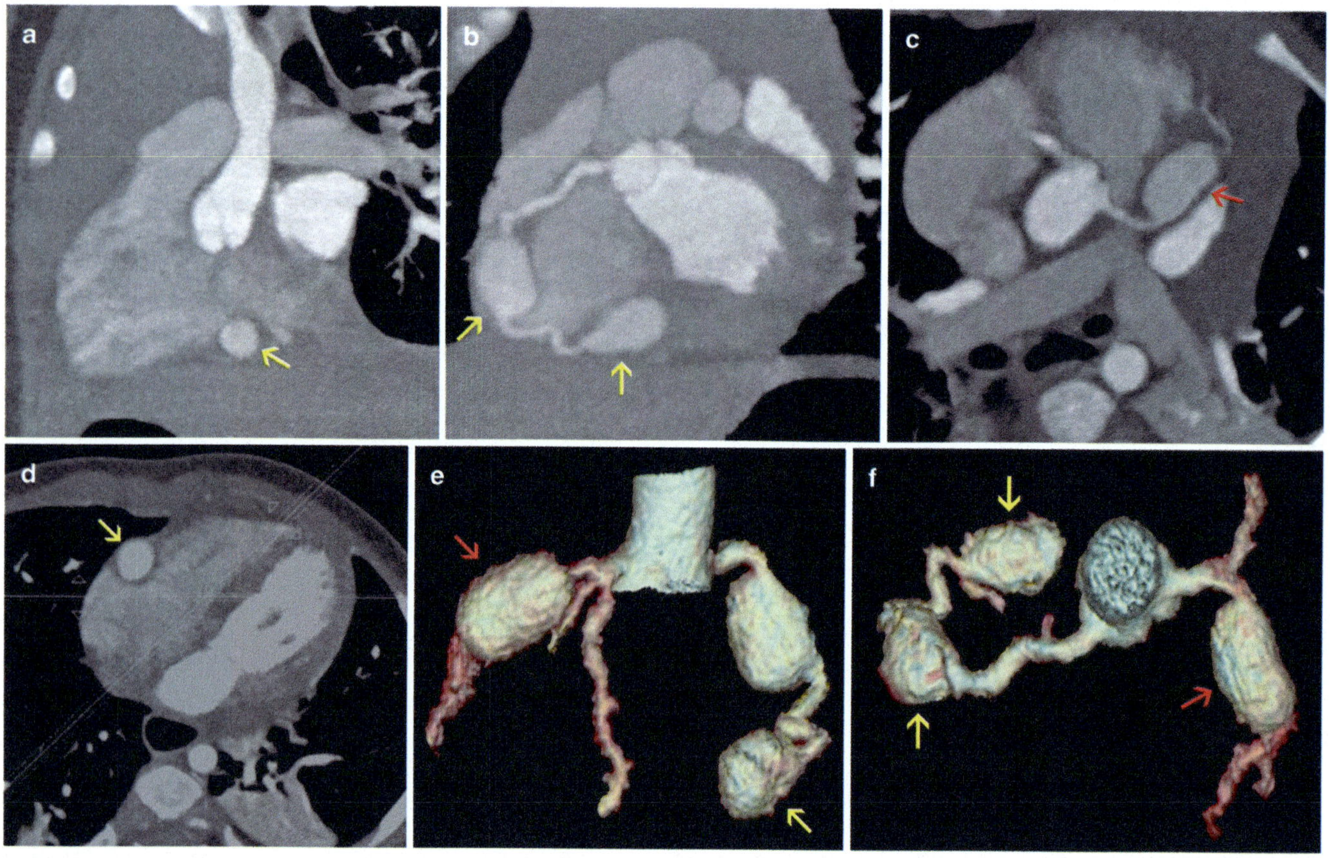

Findings and Interpretation

- CTCA demonstrates multiple coronary artery aneurysms in the right coronary artery (RCA) (yellow arrows) and left anterior descendending artery (LAD) (red arrows).
- Sagittal (panel A), coronal (panel B), and axial (panel D) CT images illustrating two aneurysms in the RCA (panel C).
- Axial CT image showing an aneurysm in the mid segment of the LAD (panel C). Volume rendering images in coronal posterior view (panel E) and superior projection (panel F) showing the coronary aneurysms.
- Kawasaki disease (KD) is an acute idiopathic vasculitis that affects infants and children. Coronary artery abnormalities develop in 15–25% of untreated patients.
- Although transthoracic echocardiography is the modality of choice for evaluation of children with this pathology, in many cases distal vessels cannot be well assessed, and other imaging modalities are required. Invasive coronary angiography is an alternative, but its invasive nature precludes its use for follow-up imaging. Also it is limited to detect coronary wall changes.
- CTCA is a noninvasive technique that permits identification of coronary anomalies and evaluation of the lumen and vessel wall. Additionally, current cardiac CT studies can be performed with acceptable radiation exposure, making CT a good imaging technique to diagnose and follow up these patients.

- With early diagnosis and adequate management, there has been a significant decrease in the appearance of coronary abnormalities. Nevertheless, around 3–5% of treated patients will still develop vessel damage that include stenotic lesions (segmental or localized) and occlusions. Segmental stenosis can be found in 15% of patients, most frequently compromising the RCA. In cases of severe stenosis, the most common location is the proximal segment of the LAD.
- Coronary abnormalities may regress. Nonetheless, in half of the patients, vessel remodeling may occur within the following years. The majority of these children may progress with severe residual disease and complications during the adulthood.
- CTCA is a good imaging modality for evaluation of children with KD in acute and chronic phase of the disease. Current CT studies can be performed with very low radiation doses.

Further Reading

Duan Y, Wang X, Cheng Z, Wu D, Wu L. Application of prospective ECG-triggered dual-source CT coronary angiography for infants and children with coronary artery aneurysms due to Kawasaki disease. Br J Radiol. 2012;85:e1190–7.

Kim JW, Goo HW. Coronary artery abnormalities in Kawasaki disease: comparison between CT and MR coronary. Acta Radiol. 2013;54:156–63.

Peng Y, Zeng J, Du Z, et al. Usefulness of 64-slice MDCT for follow-up of young children with coronary artery aneurysm due to Kawasaki disease: initial experience. Eur J Radiol. 2009;69:500–9.

Yu Y, Sun K, Wang R, et al. Comparison study of echocardiography and dual-source CT in diagnosis of coronary artery aneurysm due to Kawasaki disease: coronary artery disease. Echocardiography. 2011;28:1025–34.

Cardiac Masses and Tumors

7

Patricia M. Carrascosa, Gastón A. Rodríguez-Granillo, Alejandro Deviggiano, Diego Perez de Arenaza, and Macarena C. De Zan

Background

Cardiac masses are frequently detected and evaluated with echocardiography. However, in many cases further diagnosis is required with higher resolution techniques such as cardiac magnetic resonance (CMR).

Aside from lacking acoustic window limitations, CMR has additional advantages over echocardiography such as greater field of view, superior tissue contrast, and improved tissue discrimination allowing a better assessment of the components of cardiac masses (such as fat, water, vascularization, fibrosis, necrosis).

CMR enables a detailed assessment of the relationship with adjacent structures, aiding the planification of the potential surgical strategies. It also allows accurate surveillance of mass progression or regression after treatment.

Cardiac tumors are very rare (0.06% of all primary tumors), but when they are present, they can evolve to severe complications including thromboembolic events, compressive symptoms, and fatal arrhythmias.

Discrimination Between Tumors and Pseudotumors

Cardiac masses can be classified as pseudotumors (nonneoplastic structures/lesions that may simulate cardiac tumors) and tumors. During routine clinical practice, the most frequent cause of misdiagnosis of a cardiac tumor is thrombus, being the most common location the left ventricular apex and less frequently the left atrium. By means of accurate tissue characterization (Table 7.1), CMR allows a precise discrimination between thrombus and cardiac tumors. Other nonneoplastic structures that can simulate tumors at echocardiography involve caseous calcification of the mitral valve, prominent crista terminalis, giant coronary aneurysm, elongated Chiari network and/or prominent Eustachian valve, large hiatal hernia, and prominent pericardial fat among others.

Cardiac tumors are initially classified as primary and secondary. Primary tumors are further classified as benign or malignant tumors. The prevalence of each subtype has regional- and age-related variations. Overall, cardiac myxoma is the most frequent benign cardiac tumor (approximately 50% of all benign cardiac tumors), commonly affecting the left atrium, with implantation at the fossa ovalis. Fibroelastoma is the second benign cardiac tumor in prevalence (and the most common if valves are involved, representing 75% of valvular tumors). Among children, rhabdomyoma is the most common cardiac tumor. These tumors are usually multiple and can regress spontaneously.

P. M. Carrascosa (✉)
Departments of CT, MR, and Research, Department of Cardiovascular Imaging, Diagnostico Maipu, Buenos Aires, Argentina

University of Buenos Aires, Buenos Aires, Argentina

Latin American Committee of the Society of Cardiovascular Computed Tomography, Buenos Aires, Argentina
e-mail: patriciacarrascosa@diagnosticomaipu.com.ar

G. A. Rodríguez-Granillo
Department of Cardiovascular Imaging, Department of Research, Diagnostico Maipu, Buenos Aires, Argentina

National Council of Scientific and Technical Investigations (CONICET), Buenos Aires, Argentina

A. Deviggiano
Department of Cardiovascular Imaging, Diagnostico Maipu, Buenos Aires, Argentina

Cardiac CT and MRI Council of the Argentinian Society of Cardiology, Buenos Aires, Argentina

D. P. de Arenaza
Cardiovascular Imaging Section, Department of Cardiology, Hospital Italiano de Buenos Aires, Buenos Aires, Argentina

M. C. De Zan
Cardiovascular CT and MR, CEMIC and Fundación Centro Diagnostico Nuclear, Buenos Aires, Argentina

P. M. Carrascosa et al. (eds.), *Clinical Atlas of Cardiac and Aortic CT and MRI*, https://doi.org/10.1007/978-3-030-03682-9_7

Table 7.1 General magnetic resonance characteristics of most common cardiac masses and tumors

Cardiac mass	T1-weighted	T2-weighted	First-pass perfusion	LGE
Pseudotumors				
Thrombus	Hypo	Hypo	–	–
Crista terminalis	Iso	Iso	–	–
Caseous calcification	Hypo	Hypo	–	+ (homogeneous, with peripheral rim)
Tumors				
Benign:				
Myxoma	Iso	Hyper	– (or minimal)	+ (heterogeneous)
Lipoma	Hyper	Intermediate	–	–
Fibroelastoma	Hypo	Iso/hyper	–	+
Fibroma	Iso	Hypo	–	++ (homogeneous)
Hemangioma	Iso	+	+	+
Rhabdomyoma	Iso	Iso/hyper	–	Minimum
Malignant:				
Angiosarcoma	Heterogenous	Heterogenous	+	+ (heterogenous, mostly peripheral)
Rhabdomyosarcoma	Iso	Hyper	+	+
Undifferentiated sarcoma	Iso	Hyper	+	+ (heterogeneous)
Lymphoma	Iso	Intermediate	–	–/mild
Metastasis	Hypo	Hyper	+	+ (heterogeneous)

LGE late gadolinium enhancement

The most frequent malignant primary cardiac tumor is angiosarcoma, usually with right atrium localization. Cardiac metastases (secondary cardiac tumors) are far more frequent than primary tumors, found in approximately 10% of autopsies of patients dying from cancer. The most frequent cancer with cardiac metastasis is melanoma, followed by lung, breast, and renal cancer.

CMR is a very useful technique to evaluate cardiac tumors and pseudotumors. Applying all the available sequences and views, tumor and tissue characterization can be done that may help to determine the presence of malignancy indicators (Table 7.2).

Table 7.2 Cardiac magnetic resonance (CMR) findings suggestive of malignancy

CMR indicators of tumor malignancy	
Tumor characteristics	Tissue characteristics
Large size > 5 cm	Tissue heterogeneity
Irregular borders	T1/T2 mass hemorrhage and necrosis
Direct invasion/infiltration	Hemorrhagic pericardial effusion
Right heart involvement	Contrast enhancement
Pericardial/pleural involvement	
Growth through a major vessel	
Effusion and nodular masses	
Involvement of >1 chamber	

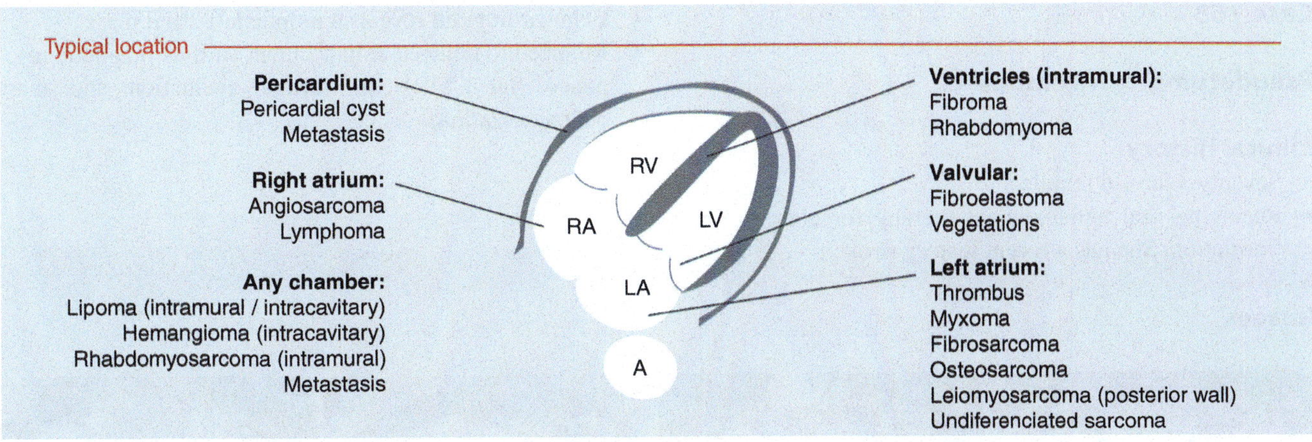

Fig. 7.1 Most common cardiac masses and tumors according to the localization

Cardiac masses (pseudotumors and tumors) have different behavior in T1-weighted, T2-weighted, first-pass perfusion, and late gadolinium enhancement (LGE) summarized in Table 7.1 and also have, in most cases, distinctive localization (Fig. 7.1). Cardiac computed tomography is also a valuable tool for the assessment of cardiac masses and tumors, particularly to visualize the relationship with surrounding adjacent structures, thus facilitating the guidance of surgical strategies.

Further Reading

Chan AT, Plodkowski AJ, Pun SC, Lakhman Y, Halpenny DF, Kim J, et al. Prognostic utility of differential tissue characterization of cardiac neoplasm and thrombus via late gadolinium enhancement cardiovascular magnetic resonance among patients with advanced systemic cancer. J Cardiovasc Magn Reson. 2017; 19(1):76.

Klatt EC, Heitz DR. Cardiac metastasis. Cancer. 1990;65(6):1456–9.

Maybrook RJ, Afzal MR, Parashar S, Deibert B, Chivington M, Walker JY, et al. Intrinsic and extrinsic cardiac Pseudotumors: echocardiographic evaluation and review of the literature. Echocardiography. 2016;33(1):117–32.

Paraskevaidis IA, Michalakeas CA, Papadopoulos CH, Anastasiou-Nana M. Cardiac tumors. ISRN Oncol. 2011;2011:208929.

Patel R, Lim RP, Saric M, Nayar A, Babb J, Ettel M, et al. Diagnostic performance of cardiac magnetic resonance imaging and echocardiography in evaluation of cardiac and Paracardiac masses. Am J Cardiol. 2016;117(1):135–40.

Pazos-López P, Pozo E, Siqueira ME, García-Lunar I, Cham M, Jacobi A, et al. Value of CMR for the differential diagnosis of cardiac masses. JACC Cardiovasc Imaging. 2014;7(9):896–905.

Rajiah P, Kanne JP, Kalahasti V, Schoenhagen P. Computed tomography of cardiac and pericardiac masses. J Cardiovasc Comput Tomogr. 2011;5(1):16–29.

Randhawa K, Ganeshan A, Hoey ET. Magnetic resonance imaging of cardiac tumors: part 1, sequences, protocols, and benign tumors. Curr Probl Diagn Radiol. 2011;40(4):158–68.

Case 155

Pseudotumors: Thrombus

Clinical History

- Seventy-year-old female.
- Receiving oral anticoagulant therapy for chronic atrial fibrillation. She has a recent history stroke.
- Echocardiogram reveals a mobile left atrial mass.
- Referred to delayed enhancement cardiac magnetic resonance (DE-CMR) for further evaluation and mass characterization.

Images

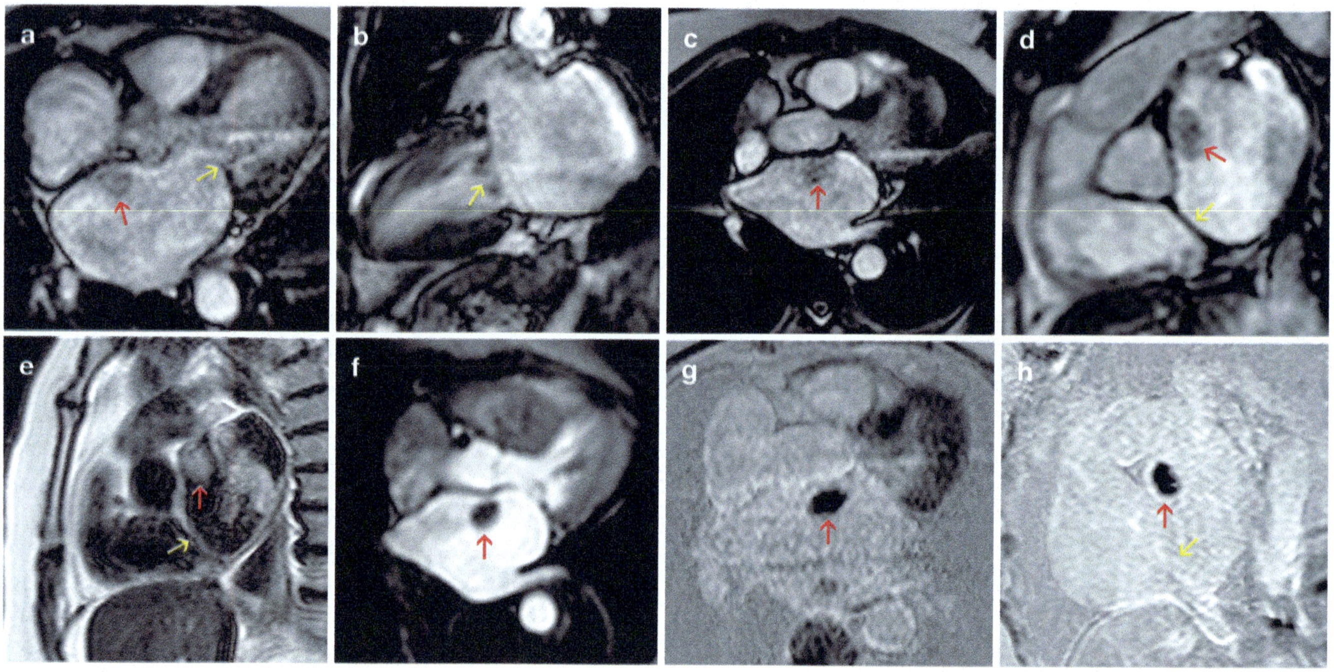

Findings and Interpretation

- Image quality is affected due to cardiac arrhythmia (atrial fibrillation).
- The left ventricle has a normal size (end diastolic volume 51 ml/m^2) and has a normal systolic function (ejection fraction 61%).
- There is moderate to severe dilatation of the left atrium (panels A and B), and this seems to be related in part to a moderate mitral stenosis (yellow arrows in panels A and B).
- At the left atrial's roof, there is a homogeneous, well-defined, mobile mass (red arrows in panels A, C, and D), with a mid-signal intensity (isointense) in T2-weighted images (panel E).
- Panels C, F, and G correspond to high horizontal long axis views and panels D, E, and H to short-axis views at the atrial level.
- Panels D, E, and H demonstrate that the interatrial septum and the fossa ovalis are not affected by the mass.
- First-pass perfusion images (panel F) show lack of vascularization of the atrial mass.
- At inversion-recovery images (panels G and H), the mass does not show any late gadolinium enhancement.
- This is a case of left atrial thrombi in a patient with mitral stenosis and chronic atrial fibrillation. Atrial thrombi, when adhered or located next to interatrial septum, can resemble a cardiac myxoma. As shown, DE-CMR is very useful to define the etiology in these cases.

Further Reading

Lu HT, Nordin R, Othman N, et al. Biatrial thrombi resembling myxoma regressed after prolonged anticoagulation in a patient with mitral stenosis: a case report. J Med Case Rep. 2016;10:221.

Case 156

Pseudotumors: Crista Terminalis

Clinical History

- Fifty-five-year-old male.
- Asymptomatic, without unremarkable clinical history.
- A routine echocardiogram identified a slightly mobile mass adhered to the posterior right atrium wall.
- Referred to cardiac magnetic resonance (CMR) for further evaluation.

Images

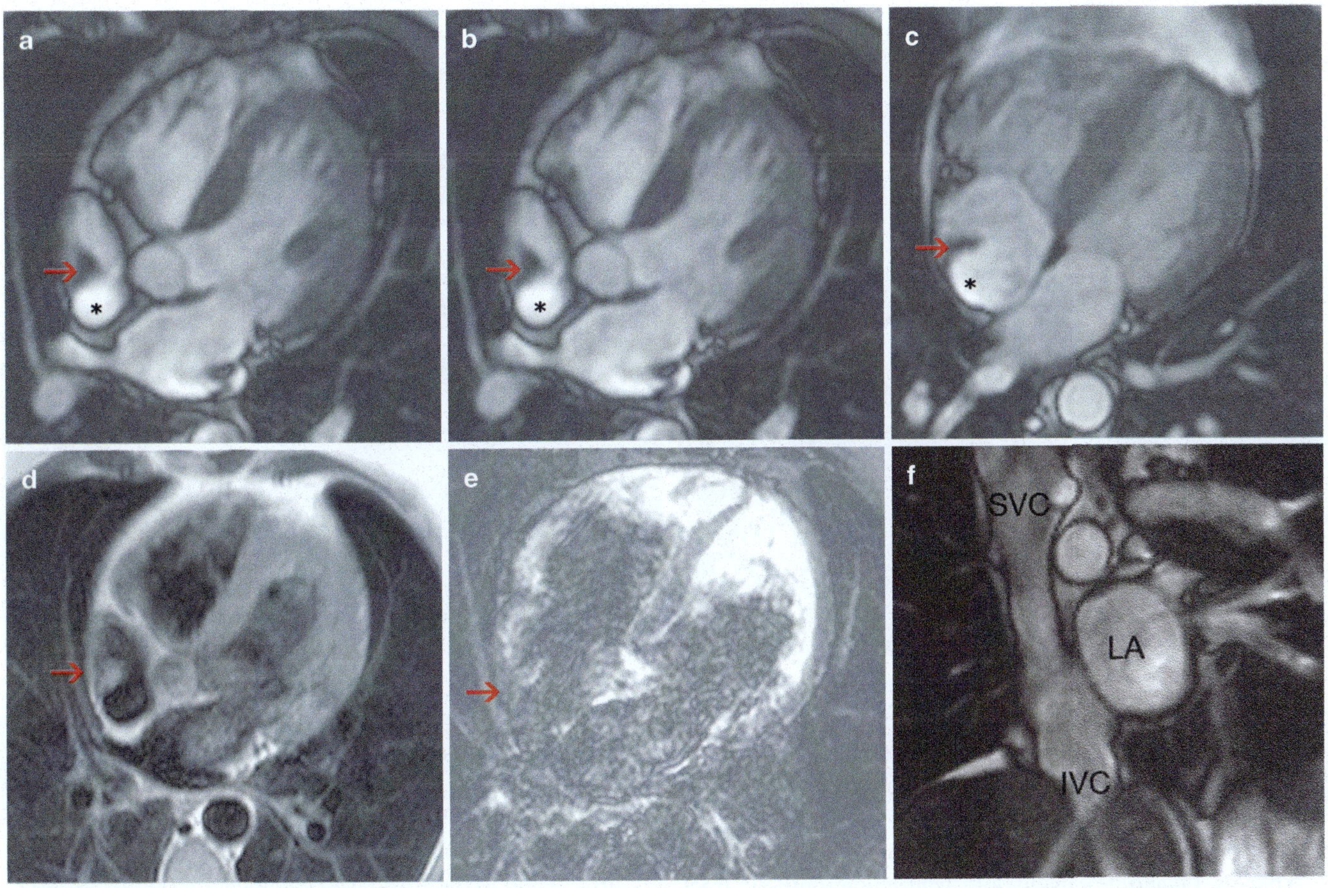

Findings and Interpretation

- Axial cine views (panels A to C) are very useful among patients with suspected cardiac masses.
- A non-infiltrating, well-circumscribed, slightly mobile mass (red arrows in panels A to E) extending from the superior vena cava (asterisk in panel A) to the inferior vena cava (asterisk in panel C).
- The structure has the same signal intensity compared to the myocardium in T1-weighted (panel D) and T2-weighted (panel E) images.
- A basal short-axis view at the level of both caval veins demonstrated that all adjacent structures are normal. SVC refers to superior vena cava, IVC to inferior vena cava, and LA to left atrium.
- A prominent crista terminalis is a relatively common cause of suspected masses at the posterior wall of the right atrium. This structure is a fibromuscular ridge formed by the junction of the sinus venosus and primitive right atrium, and in some cases it can be particularly large and mimic a cardiac mass.

Further Reading

Gaudio C, Di Michele S, Cera M, Nguyen BL, Pannarale G, Alessandri N. Prominent crista terminalis mimicking a right atrial mixoma: cardiac magnetic resonance aspects. Eur Rev Med Pharmacol Sci. 2004;8:165–8.

Case 157

Pseudotumors: Caseous Calcification of the Mitral Valve

Clinical History

- Seventy-eight-year-old female.
- Echocardiogram with an incidental cardiac mass at the mitral valve.
- Referred to delayed enhancement cardiac magnetic resonance (DE-CMR) for further evaluation and mass characterization.

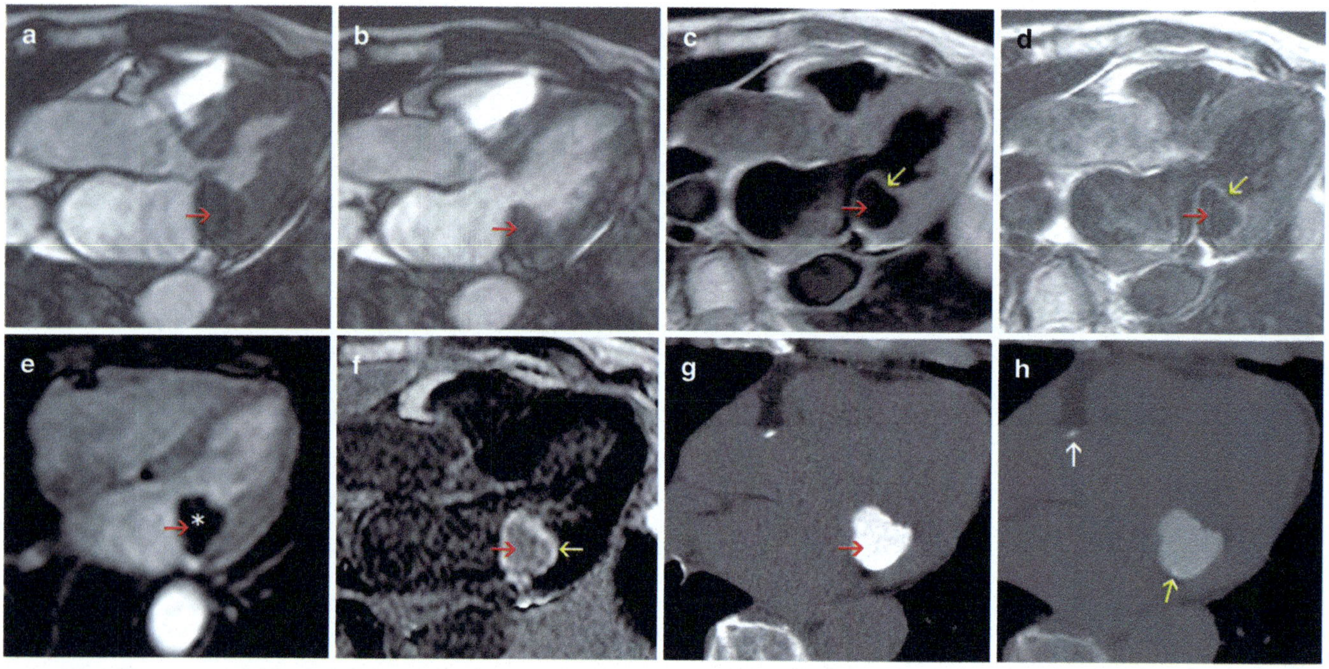

Findings and Interpretation

- The left ventricle has a normal size (end diastolic volume 59 ml/m^2) and normal systolic function (ejection fraction 74%).
- CMR images (panels A–F) and CT non-contrast images (panels G and H) using left ventricular outflow tract views.
- The mitral valve has a normal function, without regurgitation or stenosis (panels A and B).
- The posterior mitral valve annulus shows a well-circumscribed, homogeneous non-infiltrative mass (red arrows).
- The mass has low signal intensity at T1- and T2-weighted images (panels C and D), with a thin overlying cap (yellow arrows).
- First-pass perfusion images show lack of vascularization of the mass (*, in panel E).
- At inversion-recovery images (panel F), the mass shows homogeneous late enhancement, of higher intensity at the overlying cap (yellow arrow in F).
- Non-enhanced CT shows a high-attenuation (~450 Hounsfield units) mass at the posterior mitral valve annulus. By adjusting window and width levels (panel H), it becomes clear that the core of the mass has much lower density levels compared to the overlying calcified cap (red arrow) and to the aortic wall calcification (white arrow).
- Caseous calcification of the mitral valve is a benign condition that usually requires no medical or surgical intervention. It usually involves old patients and is commonly misdiagnosed as a tumor or even as an abscess.
  - Histopathology analyses have found that it involves amorphous eosinophilic acellular material, surrounded by inflammatory cells and a periphery rim of calcifications and necrosis.

Further Reading

Elgendy IY, Conti CR. Caseous calcification of the mitral annulus: a review. Clin Cardiol. 2013;36:E27–31.

Case 158

Myxoma

Clinical History

- Seventy-seven-year-old male.
- Asymptomatic. He has an incidental left atrial mass identified in a routine echocardiogram.
- Given the patient's age, he was referred to cardiac CT angiography (CTA) instead of magnetic resonance as pre-operatory evaluation of the interatrial septum and the coronary artery tree.

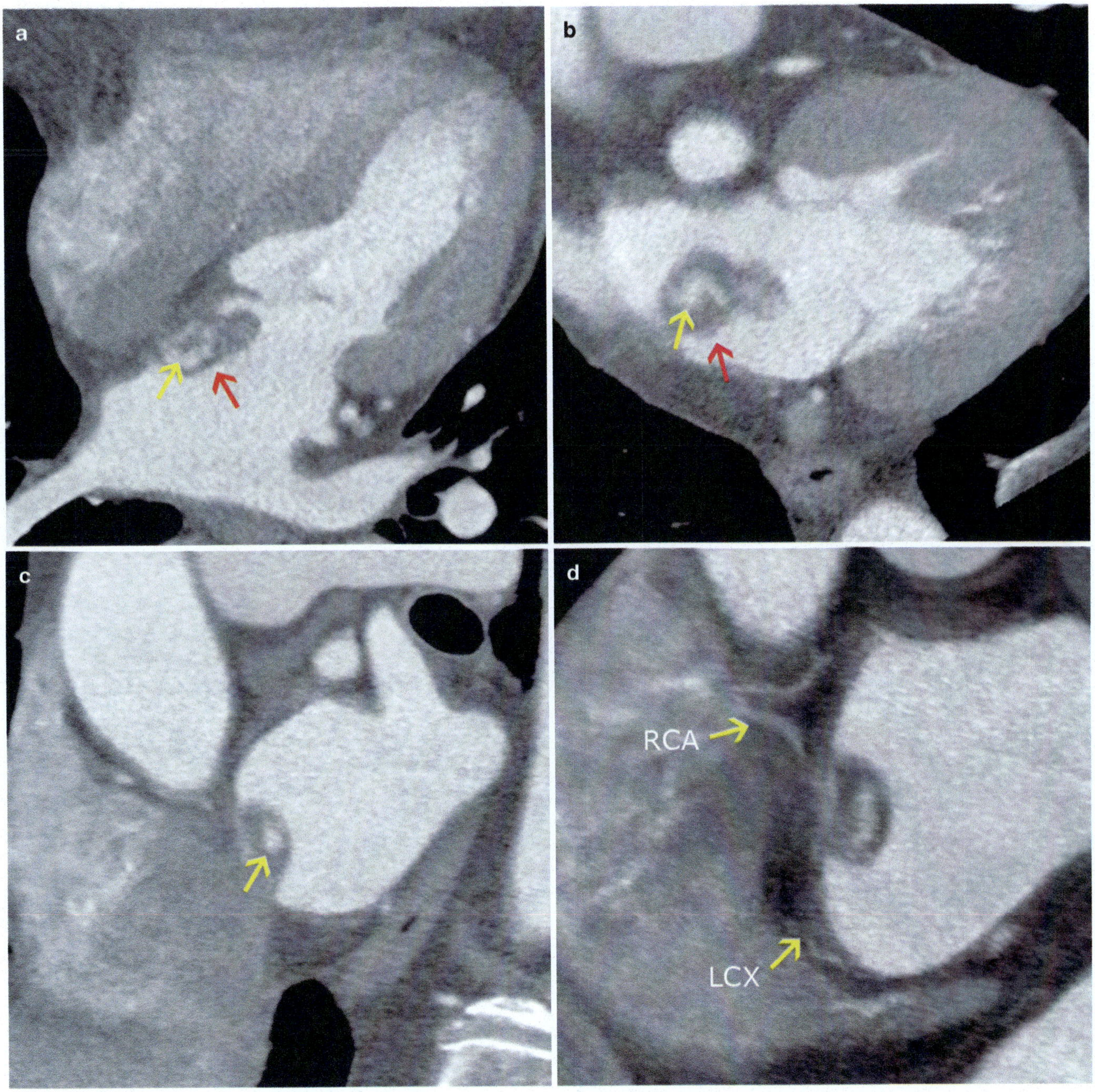

Findings and Interpretation

- At the fossa ovalis, the interatrial septum shows a polypoid, mildly irregular, heterogeneous, non-infiltrating mass (red arrows in panels A and B). The mass has a core of serpiginous high-attenuation areas and absence of calcifications (yellow arrow in panels A, B, and C).
- There is also neovascularization from the left circumflex and right coronary arteries (panel D).
- According to the tissue characteristics and to the location possibly corresponds to a left atrial myxoma.
- Cardiac myxomas are the most common benign primary cardiac tumor in adults.
- Of note, this case shows high-attenuation areas suggestive of sinusoidal vascular channels, as well as neovascularization/feeding vessels.
- Surgical excision is generally the treatment of choice, particularly in the presence of large masses with high likelihood of thromboembolic events.
- In the presence of neovascularization such as in this case, care must be taken to avoid coronary artery to left atrium fistulas as a surgical complication.

Further Reading

Burns AC, Osula S, Harley A, et al. Left circumflex coronary artery to left atrial fistula in a patient with mitral regurgitation after excision of a left atrial myxoma. Ann Thorac Surg. 2001;72:1732–3.

Kim TJ, Seol SH, Kim JK, et al. Multiple feeding vessels from left circumflex artery and right coronary artery to myxoma in left atrium. J Thorac Dis. 2013;5:E236–9.

Case 159

Myxoma

Clinical History

- Forty-two-year-old female.
- She presents with atypical chest pain.
- An echocardiography was performed as initial diagnostic test which shows a mobile round mass placed in the left atrium (LA). Due to its characteristics, a LA myxoma was diagnosed.
- A cardiac magnetic resonance (CMR) was requested for a better assessment of the lesion size, site of insertion, and to confirm the diagnosis.

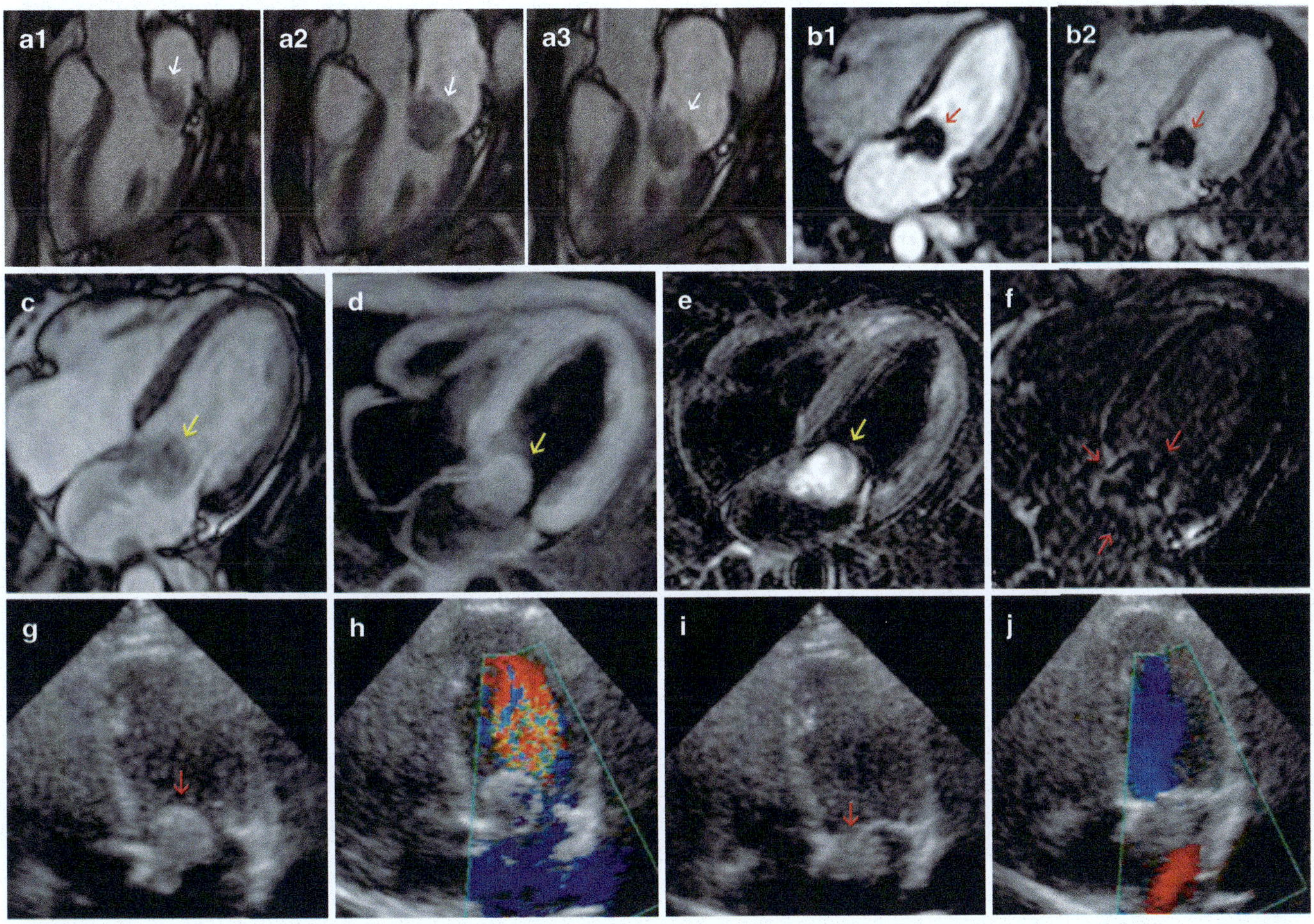

Findings and Interpretation

- Three-chamber cine view at different cardiac phases (panel A) showing a round isointense mass in the LA that is mobile and protruding through the mitral valve (arrow).
- Perfusion imaging at early and late times at four-chamber views illustrates hardly no gadolinium uptake by the mass (panel B).
- Four-chamber cine image showing the isointense mass passing through the mitral valve from the LA to the left ventricle (arrow in panel C).
- Black blood T1-weighted with fat suppression image (panel D) is showing no fat component in the isointense lesion (arrow). Four-chamber black blood T2-weighted (panel E) demonstrating the rounded hyperintense mass (arrow).
- Late-enhancement inversion recovery (IR) at four-chamber view showing minimal peripheral enhancement of the mass (arrow in panel F) due to fibrosis with no central enhancement (necrosis).
- Echocardiographic four-chamber view (panels G and I) and Doppler imaging (panels H and J) showing the round lesion in the LA protruding through the mitral valve.
- Cardiac myxoma is the most frequent primary cardiac tumor. It is an intracavitary neoplasm that can occur anywhere in the heart. The majority (75%) are placed in the LA (75% have a pedunculated attachment to the atrial

septum near the fossa ovalis), 20% in the right atrium, 5% in either the right or the left ventricle.

- Middle-aged woman are more frequently affected. They can be asymptomatic or present with vague complaints such as atypical chest pain, palpitations, or intermittent shortness of breath.
- Depending on their size and mobility, myxomas can promote obstruction of ventricular filling, with subsequent dyspnea, recurrent pulmonary edema, and right-sided heart failure mitral or tricuspid valve stenosis. Also embolism can occur in 30–40% of the patients especially when they are placed in the LA. Calcification can be present in these tumors but is rare. When present, the lesion is commonly located in the right atrium.
- Myxomas may show homogeneous or heterogeneous enhancement in late IR sequences according to the histological characteristics of the tumor. The areas of enhancement represent inflammation, whereas the non-enhanced regions correspond to necrosis.

Further Reading

Fuchs J, Leszczyszyn D, Mathew D. Cardiac myxoma causing acute ischemic stroke in a pediatric patient and a review of literature. Pediatr Neurol. 2014;50:525–9.

Giménez Roca C, Felipe Villalobos A, Cambra Lasaosa FJ, et al. Fever, asthenia, myalgia and murmur due to cardiac myxoma]. An Pediatr (Barc). 2013;79:257–60.

Ise H, Ishikawa N. Nakanishi S, et al. Giant left atrial myxoma causing acute ischemic stroke in a child. Surg Case Rep. 2018;4:6.

Case 160

Myxoma

Clinical History

- Forty-seven year-old male.
- In sinus rhythm.
- Admitted with a ischemic stroke with hemorrhagic conversion, comprising the lenticulocapsular region.
- Echocardiogram revealed a left atrial mass adhered to the interatrial septum and with diastolic prolapse to the left ventricular inflow tract.
- A delayed enhancement cardiac magnetic resonance (DE-CMR) was performed to characterize the mass.

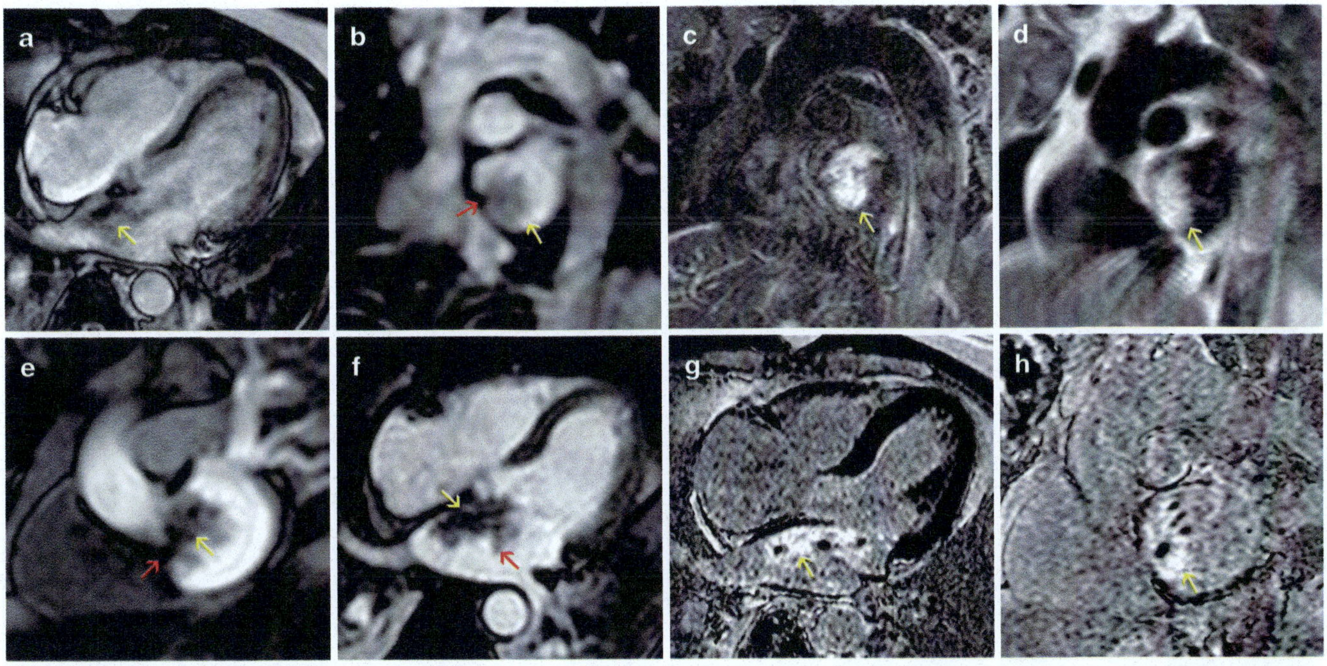

Findings and Interpretation

- DE-CMR was performed with general anesthesia; therefore, free-breathing images were obtained.
- Free-breathing cine images (panel A, four-chamber view; panel B, short-axis at the atrial level) show a non-infiltrating, polypoid, irregular, heterogeneous, mobile mass (approximately 40 mm × 53 mm) anchored at the interatrial septum fossa ovalis (red arrow in panel B) and reaching the inflow tract during diastole.
- The mass is markedly hyperintense at T2-weighted images (panel C) and mildly hyperintense at T1-weighted images (panel D).
- At first-pass perfusion imaging (panels E and F), the mass does not show significant vascularization. These images also depict the pedicle at the fossa ovalis (red arrow in panel E) and a distinctive small mobile area suggestive of adhered thrombotic material (red arrow in panel F).
- Inversion-recovery images (panels G and H) show diffuse late enhancement, with spared focal non-enhanced areas.
- Given the topography and tissue characteristics, this seems to correspond to a left atrial myxoma.
- As depicted in this case, though benign, between 25% and 50% of these tumors can lead to thromboembolic events, posing a major risk of morbidity and mortality. Surgical excision is indicated.

Further Reading

Keeling IM, Oberwalder P, Anelli-Monti M, et al. Cardiac myxomas: 24 years of experience in 49 patients. Eur J Cardiothorac Surg. 2002;22:971–7.

Percell RL Jr, Henning RJ, Siddique Patel M. Atrial myxoma: case report and a review of the literature. Heart Dis. 2003;5:224–30.

Case 161

Papillary Fibroelastoma

Clinical History

- Fifty-year-old female.
- Asymptomatic.
- A routine echocardiography identified a 9 mm mobile mass attached to the aortic valve. Differential diagnosis between valve vegetation and cardiac valve tumor was considered.
- Referred for cardiac magnetic resonance imaging (CMR) for better characterization of the mass.

Images

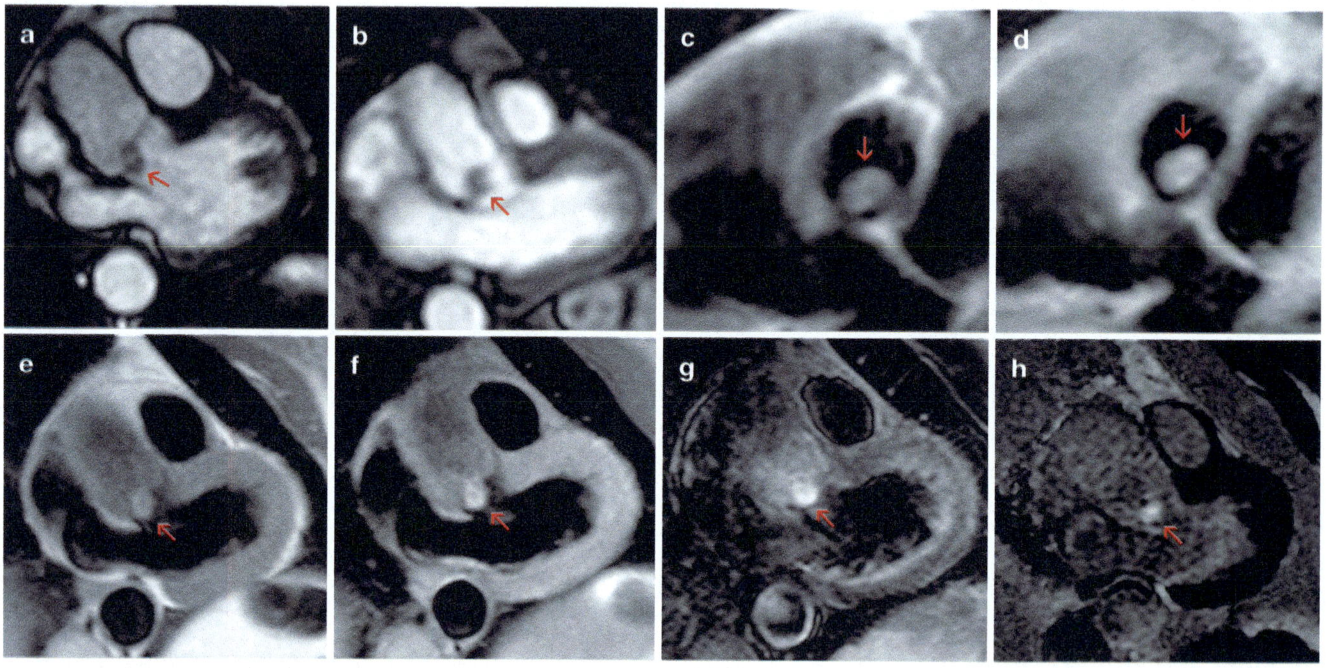

Findings and Interpretation

- CMR images demonstrate a pedunculated 7 × 9 mm mass attached to the ventricular aspect of the non-coronary aortic leaflet (red arrows).
- Three-chamber cine image (panel A) shows the small hypointense lesion at the aortic valve. There is absence of contrast enhancement during the perfusion imaging (panel B). Orthogonal views (panels C and D) and three-chamber views (panels E and F) black blood T1-weighted images without and with fat suppression, respectively, show the lesion hanging from the non-coronary aortic leaflet and projecting to the left ventricle cavity.
- The lesion is hyperintense on T2-weighted images, as shown on this three-chamber T2-weighted black blood image (panel G), and it has homogeneous late gadolinium enhancement on inversion-recovery images.
- Papillary fibroelastoma is the second most common type of cardiac tumors in adults (less than 10%), being the most common valvular tumor. Most of them occur as solitary lesions on the left side of the heart and are ≤15 mm in diameter.
- The clinical presentation varies from asymptomatic patients to severe cases most likely due to embolic complications such as cerebral embolic events and chest pain. In cases of tumor prolapse into coronary ostia, patients can suffer myocardial infarction or even sudden death.
- Differential diagnosis between thrombus in transit, valve vegetation, and cardiac valve tumor should be considered.
- The management of asymptomatic patients is controversial. In many cases, especially in elderly patients, long-term oral anticoagulation is an option. However, due to the high possibility of embolization, symptomatic lesions should undergo surgery. Surgical treatment is considered curative and safe.

Further Reading

Abu Saleh WK, Al Jabbari O, Ramlawi B, et al. Cardiac papillary fibroelastoma: single-institution experience with 14 surgical patients. Tex Heart Inst J. 2016;43:148–51.

Carino D, Nicolini F, Molardi A, et al. Unusual locations for cardiac papillary Fibroelastomas. J Heart Valve Dis. 2017;26:226–230.

Pinheiro Santos J, Banazol N, Cruz Tomás A, Varela-Afonso D, Fragata J. Cardiac fibroelastoma: 10-year experience. Rev Port Cir Cardiotorac Vasc. 2017;24:161.

Val-Bernal JF, Mayorga M, Garijo MF, et al. Cardiac papillary fibroelastoma: retrospective clinicopathologic study of 17 tumors with resection at a single institution and literature review. Pathol Res Pract. 2013;209:208–14.

Case 162

Lipoma

Clinical History

- Forty-seven-year-old male.
- Asymptomatic.
- In a routine cardiologic checkup, echocardiography revealed a mass in the septal wall with characteristics of lipoma.
- A cardiac magnetic resonance (CMR) was requested for a better determination of the extension of the mass and to confirm the diagnosis.

Images

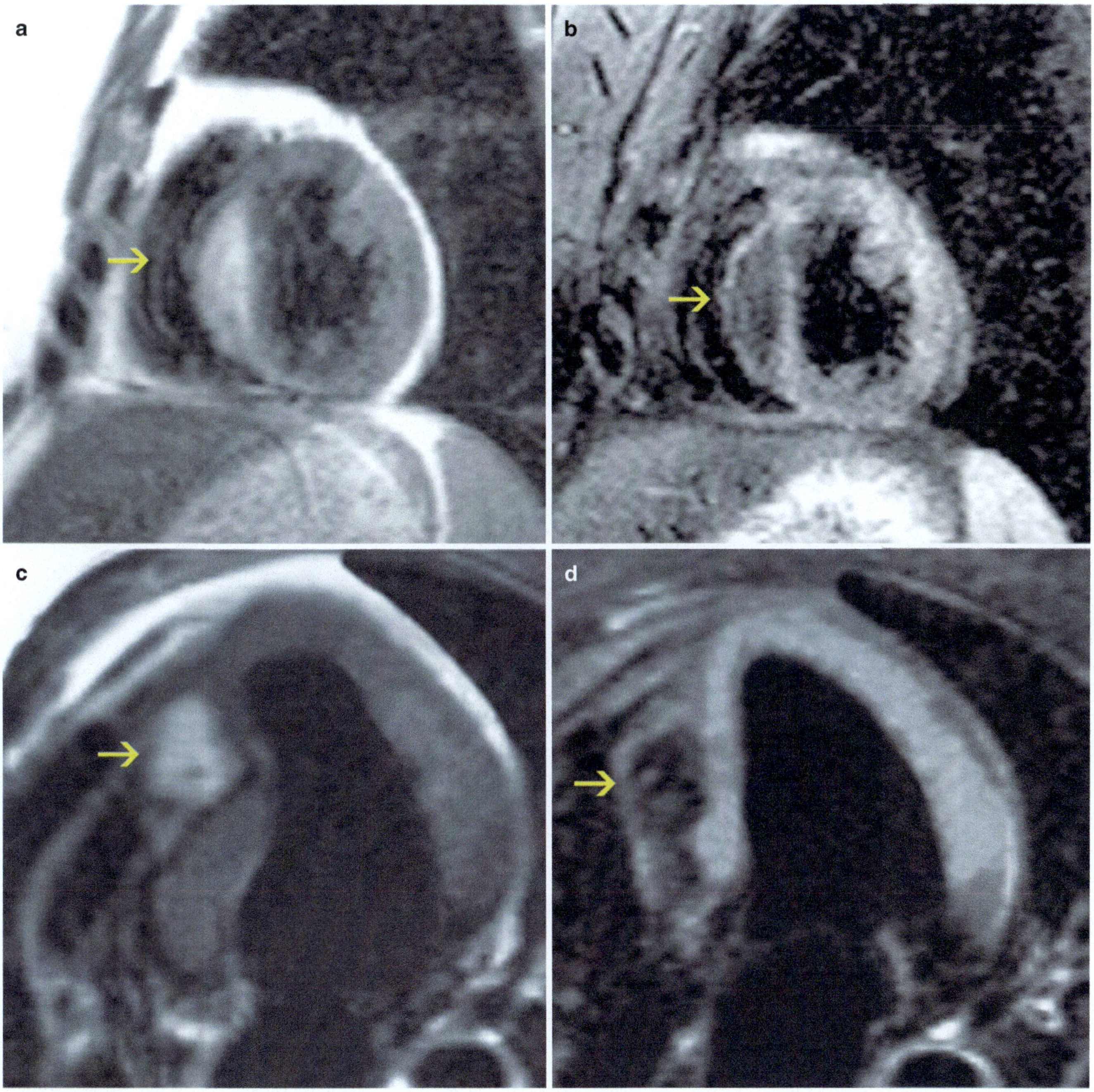

Findings and Interpretation

- Short-axis black blood T1-weighted showing a hyperintense mass in the septal wall (arrow, panel A). Short-axis black blood T1-weighted with fat suppression is showing the hypointense mass (arrow, panel B) compatible with lipoma.
- Four-chamber black blood T1-weighted without and with fat suppression (panels C and D) is illustrating the same lesion hyperintense and hypointense, respectively.
- Cardiac lipomas are rare benign tumors of the heart. They are frequently asymptomatic, for that reason they are usually diagnosed incidentally.
- Typical locations are endocardium of the right atrium and the left ventricle wall.
- They may cause life-threatening complications by rapid growth. Surgical excision is the main therapeutic intervention, which is always performed in cases of symptomatic lipoma or when malignancy is suspected.
- Multimodality imaging would be of great help in the diagnosis of cardiac lipoma. However, diagnostic modality of choice is CMR, and echocardiography is a convenient method for follow-up.

Further Reading

D'Souza J, Shah R, Abbass A, Burt JR, Goud A, Dahagam C. Invasive cardiac lipoma: a case report and review of literature. BMC Cardiovasc Disord. 2017;17:28.

Fang L, He L, Chen Y, Xie M, Wang J. Infiltrating lipoma of the right ventricle involving the interventricular septum and tricuspid valve: report of a rare case and literature review. Medicine (Baltimore). 2016;95:e2561.

Wu S, Teng P, Zhou Y, Ni Y. A rare case report of giant epicardial lipoma compressing the right atrium with septal enhancement. J Cardiothorac Surg. 2015;10:150.

Case 163

Hemangioma

Clinical History

- Twenty-year-old male.
- As part of a routine examination prior to starting physical activity, he underwent an echocardiogram that revealed a well-delineated mass in the lateral wall of the left ventricle suggestive of hemangioma.
- A cardiac magnetic resonance (CMR) imaging was requested for further characterization.

Images

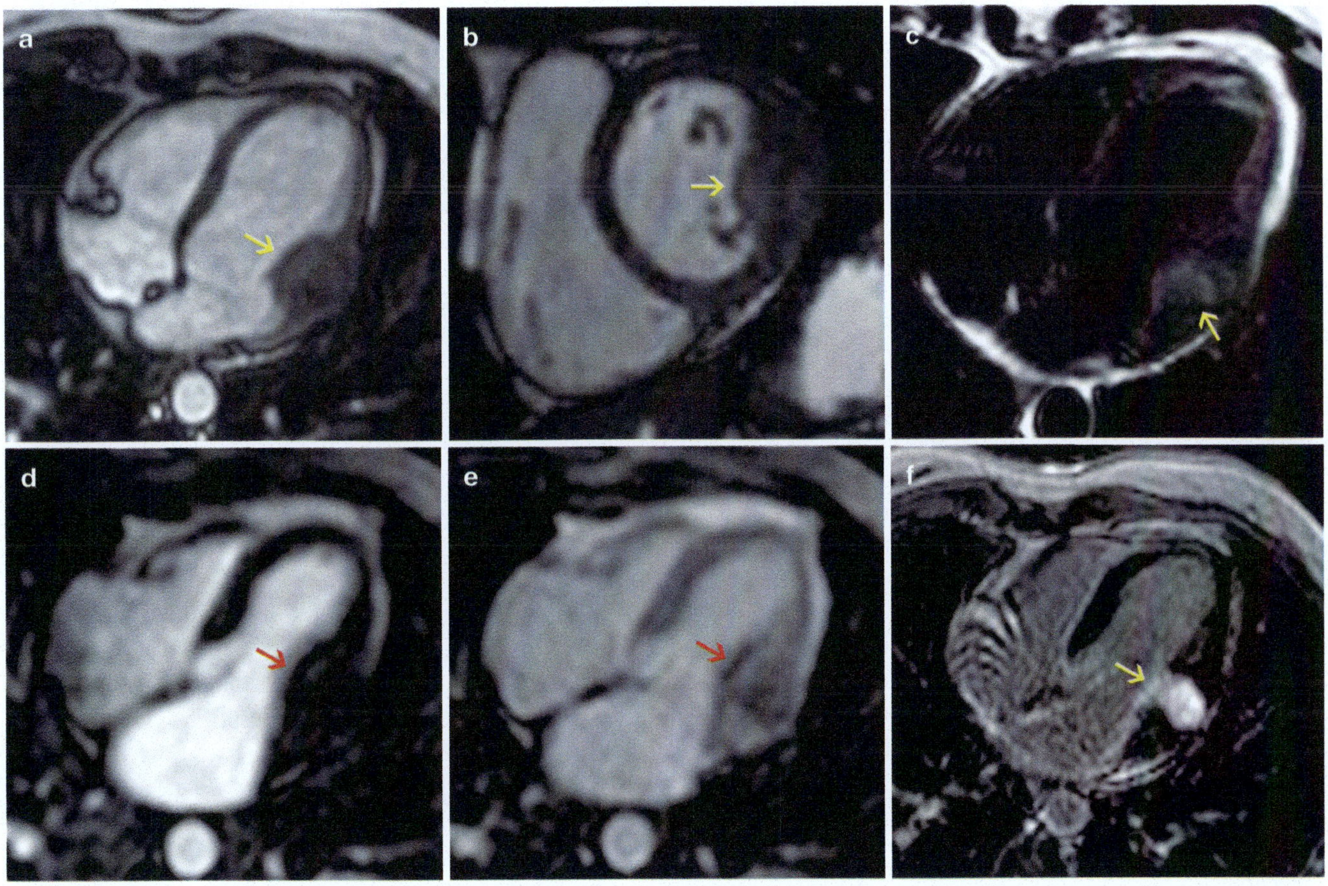

Findings and Interpretation

- Four-chamber cine image (panel A) and short-axis cine image at basal plane (panel B) showing a focal enlargement of the lateral wall (arrows) at the posterobasal segment, isointense with the myocardial wall, and with focal central areas slightly hypointense.
- Short-axis T2-weighted image (panel C) showing the area of wall enlargement hyperintense (arrow).
- Early and late perfusion four-chamber images (panels D and E) showing the perfusion of the posterobasal lateral wall (arrow). The mass stains slightly at early stages, starting from the periphery to the central area.
- Four-chamber late-enhancement inversion-recovery image (panel F) showing a focal, round, well-bounded hyper-enhanced mass (arrow).
- Cardiac hemangiomas are quite rare benign tumors of vascular origin often detected incidentally during routine examinations.

- Hemangiomas are composed of blood vessels (capillaries, capillary hemangioma, or large cavernous vascular channels, cavernous hemangioma).
- In general they are solitary, mainly located in the lateral wall of the left ventricle, the anterior wall of the right ventricle, and the septum. Notwithstanding, in 30% of the cases, they are multiple. Half of these tumors grow intramural; the other half are intracavitary.
- In CMR they appear as mass with intermediate signal intensity on T1-weighted images and a high signal intensity on T2-weighted images. After contrast administration, the increase in signal intensity is related on the blood flow through the tumor. High-flow hemangiomas demonstrate a much lower increase in signal intensity than low-flow hemangiomas.

Further Reading

Jiang WJ, Li JH, Dai J, et al. Cardiac hemangioma at the apex of the right ventricle: a case report and literature review. J Thorac Cardiovasc Surg. 2014;147:e18–21.
Li W, Teng P, Xu H, et al. Cardiac hemangioma: a comprehensive analysis of 200 cases. Ann Thorac Surg. 2015;99:2246–52.
Vacirca SR, Nardi P, Ferlosio A, et al. Multifocal cardiac hemangioma. J Card Surg. 2018;33:310–2.
Zhang B, Xu Z, Tang H, et al. Intermuscular hemangioma of the left ventricle. J Card Surg. 2012;27:572–5.

Case 164

Hemangioma

Clinical History

- Thirty-nine-year-old female.
- Asymptomatic.
- During a health control, a transthoracic echocardiogram revealed a mass in the right atrium, most likely a myxoma.
- Cardiac magnetic resonance (CMR) was indicated for further assessment.

Images

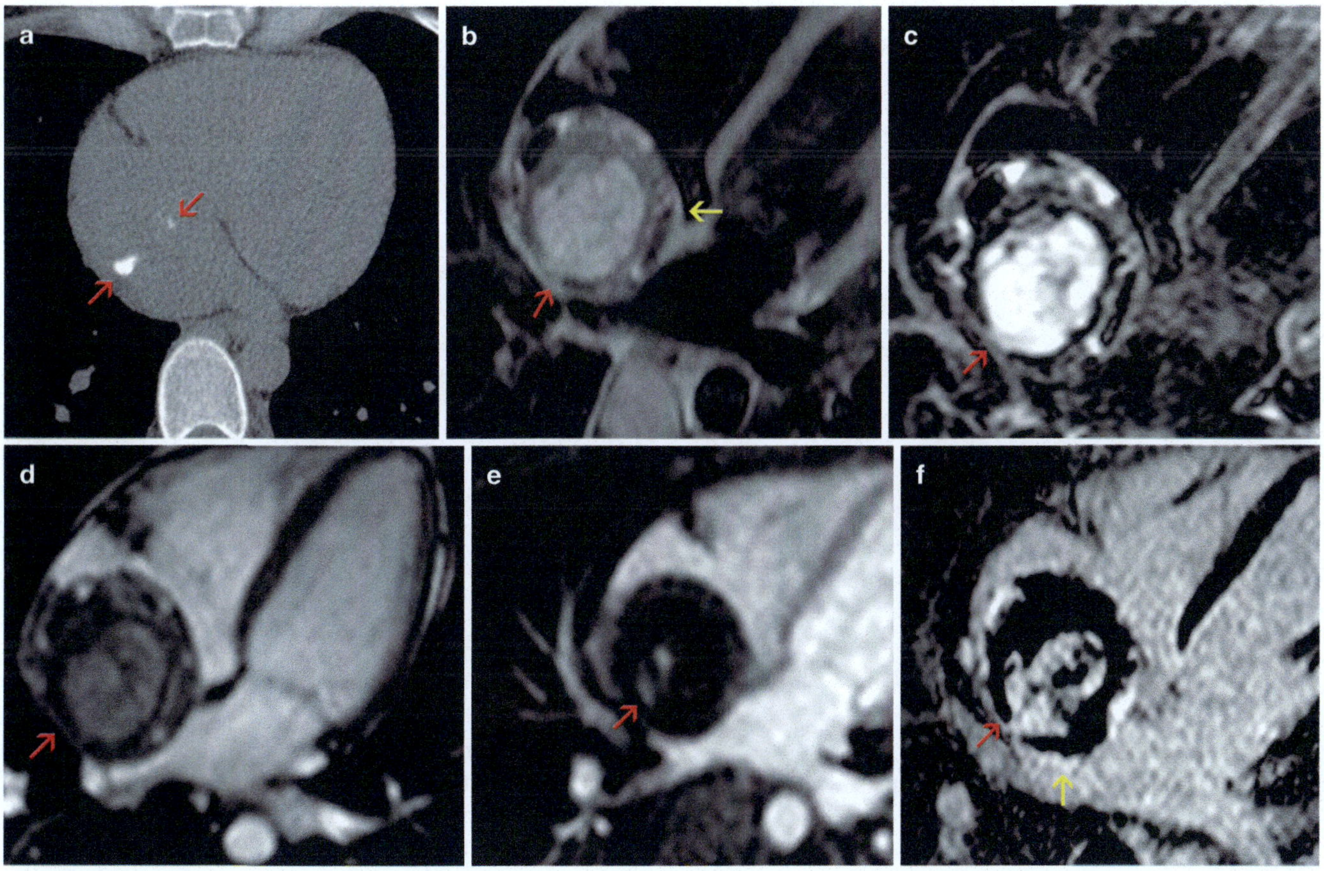

Findings and Interpretation

- At axial views, non-enhanced computed tomography (CT) identified a calcified intracavitary mass adjacent to the interatrial septum (red arrows in panel A).
- CMR using T1-weighted with fat saturation (panel B), T2-weighted (panel C), cine images (panel D), first-pass perfusion (panel E), and late-enhancement (panel D) images demonstrated a 5 × 6 cm mass adhered to the posterior wall of the right atrium. The mass is well-circumscribed, heterogeneous, and non-pedunculated, with a central core [markedly high signal intensity in T2-weighted, slightly high in T1-weighted, and with late gadolinium enhancement (arrows)] and a peripheral low signal intensity areas in T1 and T2 with focal interspersed high-intensity areas. The mass is covered by a structure (capsule?) (yellow arrows) slightly hyperintense in T1. The core exhibits uptake of contrast at first-pass perfusion images (arrow in panel E). There is heterogeneous and diffuse late gadolinium enhancement in the core as well as in the periphery/capsule (yellow arrow in panel F).
- Hemangioma is an extremely rare primary benign cardiac tumor. Blood vessel tumors can be located in any part of the heart, including endocardium, myocardium, and epicardium. It can be classified into capillary, cavernous, epithelioid, and arteriovenous type. At CMR, they are heterogeneous, iso- or hypointense in T1 and hyperintense in T2, with a typical heterogeneous late enhancement. CT allows demonstration of calcifications.

Further Reading

Templin C. Difficult differential diagnosis of a right atrial intracardiac mass. Int J Cardiol. 2008;125:e19–20.

Case 165

Hydatidosis

Clinical History

- Sixty-year-old male.
- Referred for multiples cysts on the heart and thoracic cavities. The patient had a history of pericarditis that required hospitalization at young age and had onset of atypical chest pain 3 months prior to the hospital referral.
- The physical exam was unremarkable.
- Echocardiography showed a large intracardiac cyst on the right atrium.
- Cardiac magnetic resonance (CMR) was performed for further assessment.

Images

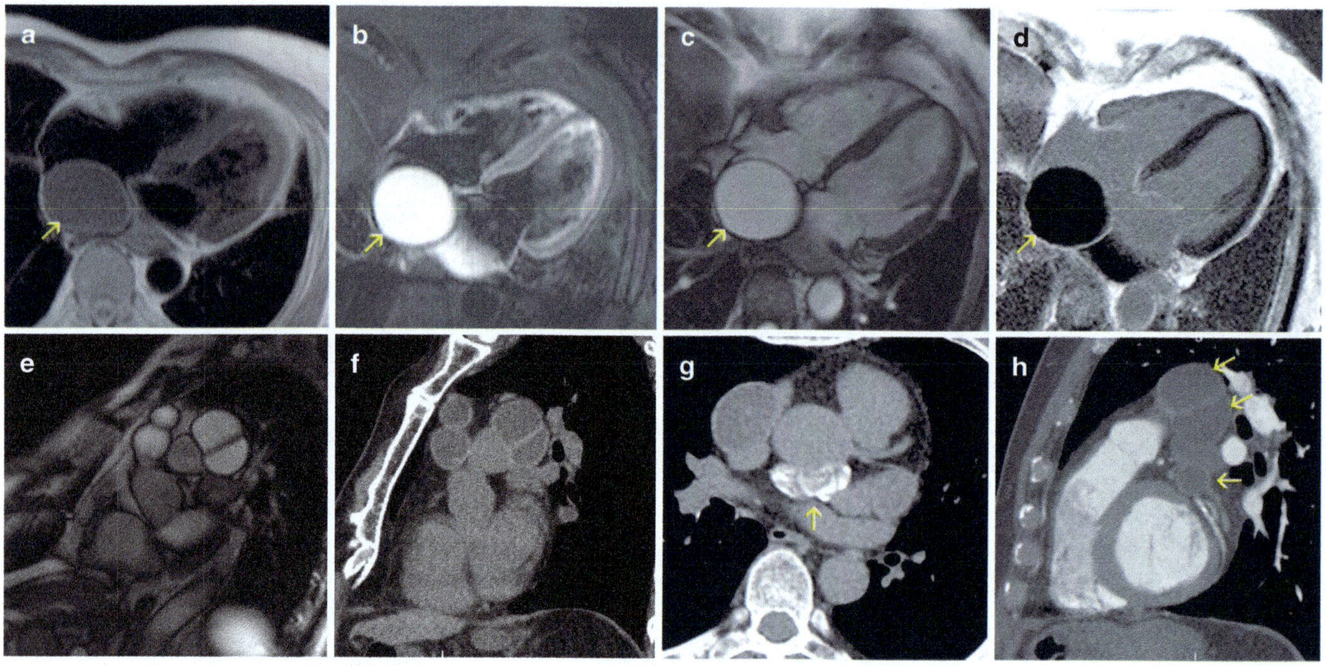

Findings and Interpretation

- CMR was performed showing multiples cysts in relation with the heart and great vessels. In total, seven cysts were identified with a largest cyst of 6.6 cm of diameter located in relationship with the posterior wall of the right atrium (arrow in panels A to D). The cysts had low signal in T1-weighted images (panel A), high signal in cine images (panels C and E), very high signal in fat-saturation T2-weighted images (panel B), and very low signal in phase-sensitive late gadolinium enhancement (LGE) images (panel D).
- Computed tomography (CT) displayed the cysts with low attenuation density and well-defined capsule and identified a semisolid cyst with calcifications (arrow) behind the aortic root (panels F–H). A latex agglutination test for echinococcosis was positive. The patient underwent successful surgical removal of cardiac and thoracic cystic and pericardiectomy. One month before and after the surgery, the patient received orally albendazole.
- Cardiac echinococcosis is an infrequently encountered entity, but with clinical suspicion and early diagnosis, it can be successfully managed with good outcomes.
- Hydatidosis should be included in the differential diagnosis of a solid, echogenic, cardiac nodule. CMR and CT help in the detection, characterization, and extension of these lesions expanding findings of transthoracic echocardiography. The treatment for cardiopulmonary hydatid cysts is surgical, followed by anthelmintics.

Further Reading

Kahlfuß S, Flieger RR, Kai T, Yilmaz K. Diagnosis and treatment of cardiac echinococcosis. Heart. 2016;102:1348–53.

Stojkovic M, Rosenberger K, Kauczor HU, Junghanss T, Hosch W. Diagnosing and staging of cystic echinococcosis: how do CT and MRI perform in comparison to ultrasound? PLoS Negl Trop Dis. 2012;6:e1880.

Case 166

Extramedullar Location of Multiple Myeloma (Cardiac Plasmocytoma)

Clinical History

- Fifty-four-year-old male.
- Hospitalized in intensive care unit for cough, dyspnea, fever, and pericardial effusion on a background of a 1-year history of multiple myeloma under treatment with oral corticosteroid and thalidomide.
- The cardiovascular examination showed jugular vein distension and sinus tachycardia but was otherwise unremarkable.
- Chest radiograph showed an increased cardiothoracic index with globular cardiac silhouette and bilateral pulmonary infiltrates.
- Echocardiography showed a large pericardial effusion with a right atrial mass. Initial clinical management included pericardiocentesis and antibiotics for pneumonia.
- Cardiac magnetic resonance (CMR) was performed for further assessment.

Images

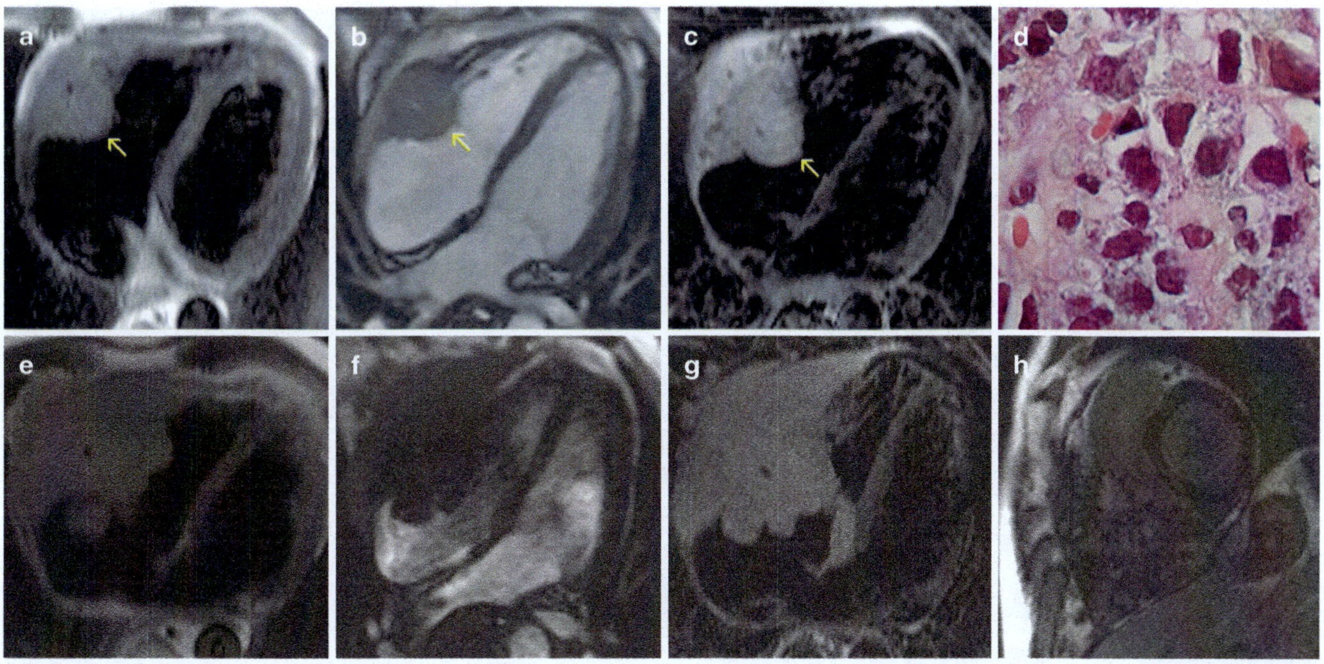

Findings and Interpretation

- CMR demonstrated a pericardial 11 cm mass attached to the right atrium groove extending to right atrium and basal free wall of right ventricle and apparently breaching tissue planes and track around the pericardium. The tumor was isointense on T1-weighted image (arrow in panel A).
- Cine imaging showed a hypointense mass compared to the myocardium (arrow in panel B), whereas T2-weighted fat-saturation imaging displayed a high signal intensity mass (arrow in panel C), suggesting high water content compared to myocardium.
- After gadolinium, the mass was very heterogeneous with areas suggestive of avascularity and/or necrosis. The cytological analysis of the pericardial effusion showed the presence of plasmocytoid cells (panel D).
- The patient underwent systemic chemotherapy with bortezomib. After 2 months, the patient was rehospitalized for fever and dyspnea.
- Follow-up CMR (panels E–H) showed a large increase in tumor size with extrapericardium extension. Imaging characteristics were similar on T1-weighted (panel E) and T2-weighted (panel G) but with a higher enhancement after gadolinium administration (panel H). The patient died by sepsis.
- Primary malignant cardiac tumors are very rare. Among these tumors, cardiac plasmocytoma is extremely rare and is the subject of few case reports. Multiple imaging methods, including echocardiography, CMR, and positron-emission tomography/computed tomography, are valuable and complementary to each other in these patients for diagnosis and optimal management.

Further Reading

Vigo F, Ciammella P, Valli R, Cagni E, Iotti C. Extraskeletal multiple myeloma presenting with an atrial mass: a case report and a review of the literature. J Med Case Rep. 2012;6:236.

Case 167

Leiomyosarcoma Metastasis

Clinical History

- Sixty-four year old female.
- Presented progressive dyspnea.
- A plain X-ray film showed an enlarged right hilum; chest computed tomography (CT) was complemented.
- Chest CT illustrated a 5 cm mass in the right hilum in contact with the cardiac silhouette that enhanced significantly after intravenous contrast administration. Additionally, two pulmonary nodules of 8 mm and 5 mm were detected in the mid right lobe and superior left lobe, respectively.
- A transthoracic ultrasound showed a huge mass in the right thorax that entered the left atrium, mobile, that protruded to the left ventricle in diastole through the mitral valve. For that reason it produced obstruction of the ventricular filling and moderate increment of pulmonary pressures. Mild pericardial fluid was also observed.
- A cardiac magnetic resonance (CMR) was requested to complete the evaluation.

Images

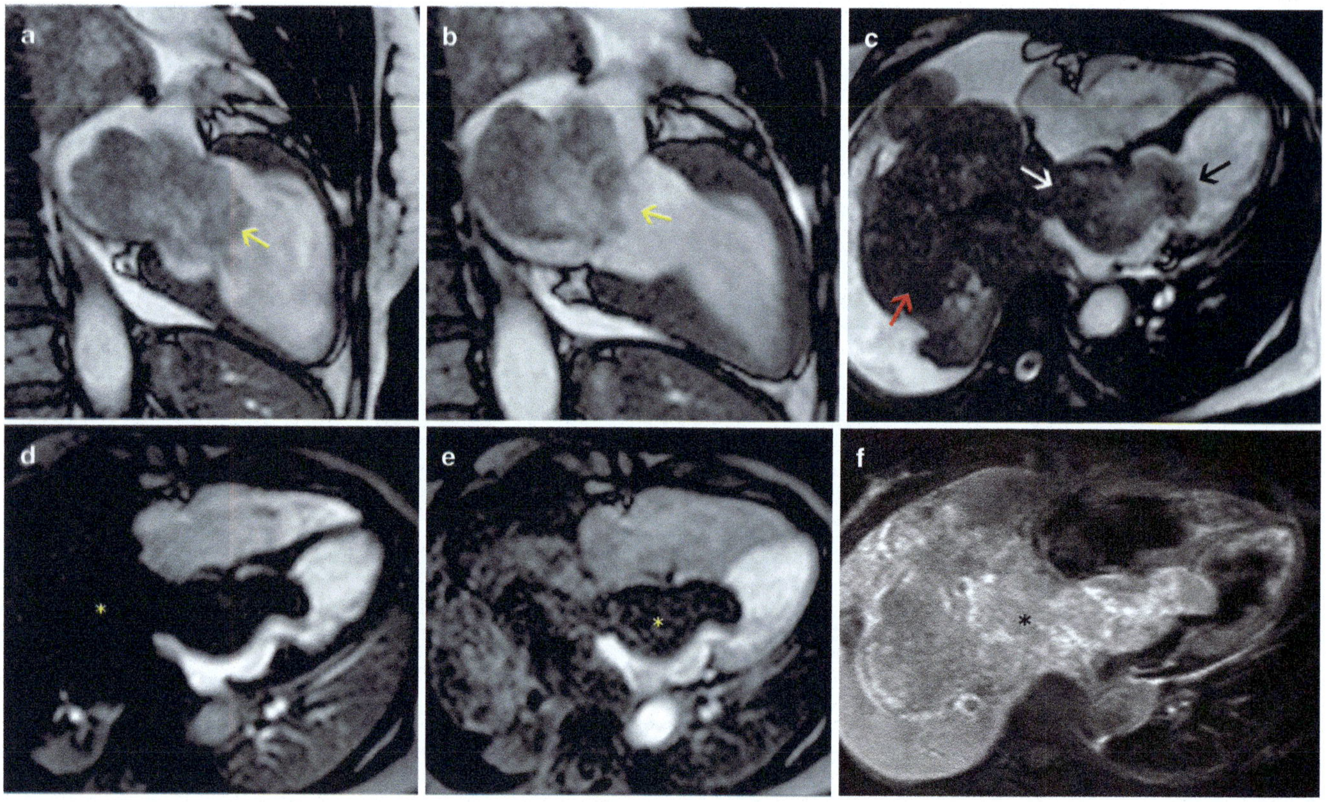

Findings and Interpretation

- Two-chamber cine images in diastole (panel A) and systole (panel B) show a mobile huge mass located in the left atrium (yellow arrow) that extends through the mitral valve to the left ventricle (panel A).
- Four-chamber cine images show that the mass origin is placed in the right hemithorax (red arrow) and extends through the pulmonary vein (white arrow) to the left atrium (panel C).
- Perfusion images (panels D and E) show the perfusion of the mass over time (asterisk in panel E).
- Late-enhancement sequence (panel F) shows that the mass is highly enhanced (asterisk).
- Uterine leiomyosarcomas (ULMS) are rare tumors, with an incidence of 0.64 cases per 100,000 women. The common sites of metastases are the lung, peritoneum, and bone. Cardiac metastases are very rare. In general they involve the right heart and associated structures.
- In general, these tumors may spread to the heart and pericardium by one of four pathways: (1) retrograde lymphatic extension, (2) hematogenous spread, (3) direct contiguous extension, and (4) transvenous extension.
- Early diagnosis of cardiac metastases may be difficult. Signs and symptoms are nonspecific and highly variable, related to the localization, size, and composition of the cardiac mass. Due to its low cost, portability, widespread

availability, and lack of ionizing radiation, transthoracic ultrasound remains the first-line imaging modality for the evaluation of a patient with a suspected cardiac mass. It allows identification of the mass and evaluation of other cardiac structures and function.

- However, CMR is used in many cases due to better anatomic delineation, tissue characterization, and tumor extension. CMR helps delineate the surface and margins of the mass, as well as the potential myocardial invasion (important information that will help in the decision of the surgical technique). Also perfusion sequences can help assessing the presence and extent of vascularization of the mass.
- In patients with extrauterine disease spread, additional surgical resection of metastatic disease or systemic chemotherapy is recommended, depending on the staging of the disease. ULMS is biologically aggressive.

Further Reading

Katayama K, Takahashi S, Sueda T. Rupture of a metastatic uterine leiomyosarcoma invading the right atrium causing cardiac tamponade. Ann Thorac Surg. 2017;104(1):e83.

Peng YJ,Hueng GG, LeeHS. Acute heart failure as manifestation of metastatic uterine leiomyosarcoma to the heart and lung. Heart Lung. 2004;33:46–9.

Sripariwuth A, Xu B, Shih-Lin HS, et al. Multimodality Cardiac Imaging Assessment of a Large Metastatic Pericardial Leiomyosarcoma. CASE (Phila). 2018;2:156–162.

8 Pericardial Disease

Patricia M. Carrascosa, Alejandro Deviggiano,
and Gastón A. Rodríguez-Granillo

Background

Different noninvasive diagnosis modalities are available to evaluate suspected or established pericardial disease. Echocardiography is the most used method due to its safety, availability, and low cost. Nonetheless, it has limited value in discriminating pericardial thickness, and in differentiation between constrictive pericarditis and restrictive cardiomyopathy, with similar clinical presentation and hemodynamic characteristics. Computed tomography (CT) is the method of choice to detect the presence of pericardial calcium, especially in chronic or constrictive pericarditis. Although it is unable to identify calcium, cardiac magnetic resonance (CMR) provides superior tissue discrimination and determines the hemodynamic significance of pericardial disease. In contrast to echocardiography, both techniques can differentiate paracardiac structures from the pericardium and epicardial fat.

The pericardium is a relatively inelastic sac that surrounds the heart and the origin of the great vessels. It is constituted by a visceral and a parietal layer. The visceral pericardium is a thin layer of mesothelial cells that covers the epicardium, epicardial fat, and coronary arteries. The parietal pericardium is thicker and composed of fibrous tissue. Between both layers, there is a virtual space containing 25–50 mL of serous fluid that provides lubrication. The pericardium measures approximately 1.2 mm in diastole and 1.7 mm in systole and presents several recesses that make up the transverse sinus (superior) and oblique sinus (behind the left atrium).

In CMR, the normal pericardium is best visualized over the right ventricular free wall and the cardiac apex. In cine sequences, the pericardium is observed as a hypointense line with underlying hyperintensity areas in case of pericardial fluid. In black blood sequences (T1 and T2), the pericardium constitutes a hypointense line between epicardial and mediastinal fat.

Congenital Absence of the Pericardium

Congenital absence of the pericardium is a rare anomaly. Absence of the pericardium can be either complete or partial, occurring more often on the left than the right side. Left-sided complete absence of pericardium is the most common form. CT scan through the great vessels shows interposition of the lung between the ascending aorta and main pulmonary artery and excessive levoposition and levorotation of the cardiac structures (Fig. 8.1).

Pericardial Cyst

Pericardial cysts are congenital encapsulated cysts implanted on the pericardium that are not connected with the pericardial cavity. They typically occur in the cardiophrenic sulcus (90%), most often right-sided (70%). They appear as non-enhanced, well-defined mass, adjacent to the pericardium, with low intensity on T1-weighted and high intensity on T2-weighted images, and hypodense in CT (Fig. 8.2).

P. M. Carrascosa (✉)
Departments of CT, MR, and Research, Department of Cardiovascular Imaging, Diagnostico Maipu, Buenos Aires, Argentina

University of Buenos Aires, Buenos Aires, Argentina

Latin American Committee of the Society of Cardiovascular Computed Tomography, Buenos Aires, Argentina
e-mail: patriciacarrascosa@diagnosticomaipu.com.ar

A. Deviggiano
Department of Cardiovascular Imaging, Diagnostico Maipu, Buenos Aires, Argentina

Cardiac CT and MRI Council of the Argentinian Society of Cardiology, Buenos Aires, Argentina

G. A. Rodríguez-Granillo
Department of Cardiovascular Imaging, Department of Research, Diagnostico Maipu, Buenos Aires, Argentina

National Council of Scientific and Technical Investigations (CONICET), Buenos Aires, Argentina

P. M. Carrascosa et al. (eds.), *Clinical Atlas of Cardiac and Aortic CT and MRI*, https://doi.org/10.1007/978-3-030-03682-9_8

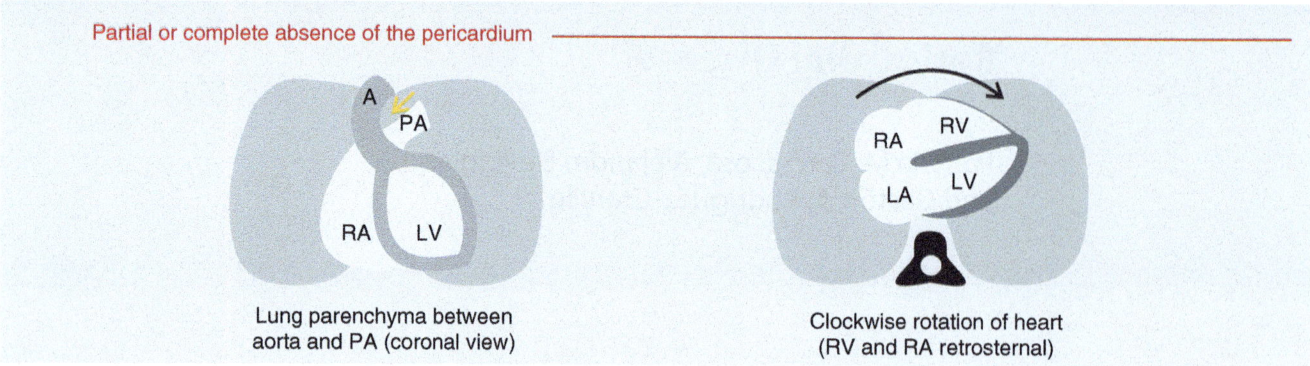

Fig. 8.1 Schematic representation of congenital absence of the pericardium

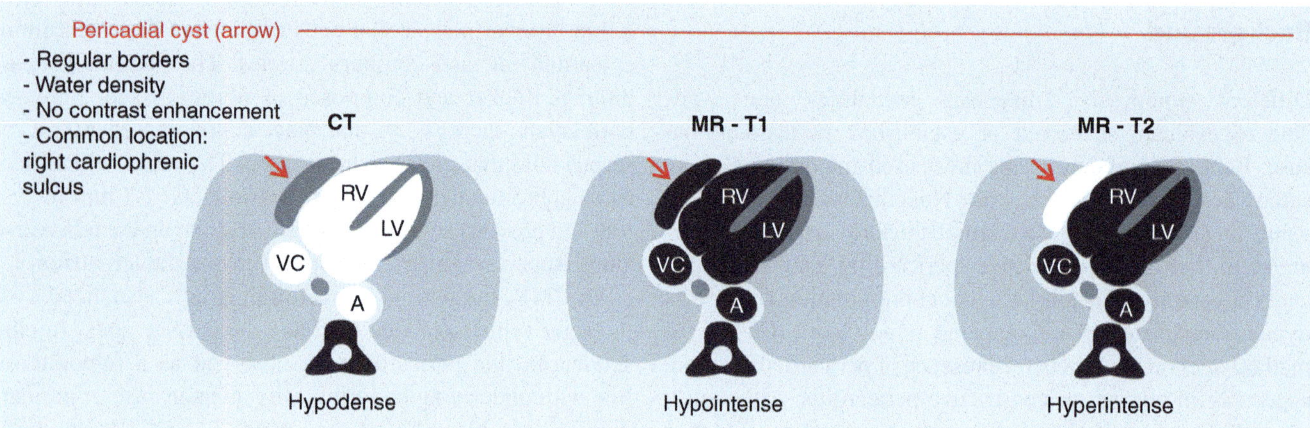

Fig. 8.2 Schematic representation of pericardial cyst

Pericardial Effusion

Pericardial effusion is the presence of an abnormal amount of fluid and/or an abnormal character of fluid in the pericardial space. It can be caused by a variety of local and systemic disorders, or it may be idiopathic. CMR detects small-volume effusions, septations, and pericardial thickening and differentiates liquid from fat with higher sensitivity than echocardiography. In addition, it allows determining the distribution of the pericardial fluid that tends to accumulate adjacent to the posterolateral left ventricle region.

In cine sequences, the pericardial effusion is hyperintense and can be correctly quantified in a similar manner to the calculation of ventricular volumes, delineating the contour of the pericardial sac in contiguous sections in the short-axis plane throughout the entire heart. In the black blood T1- and T2-weighted sequences, pericardial effusion is hypointense and hyperintense, respectively, and does not enhance with intravenous contrast. In the presence of hemorrhage or infection, the pericardial effusion becomes inhomogeneous with regions of different intensities depending on the elapsed time (Fig. 8.3). In CT, pericardial effusion has low density values in case of transudates. CT attenuation values (Hounsfield units) are significantly related to the albumin content of the pericardial fluid; therefore higher density values reflect an exudative process (Table 8.1).

Pericardial Inflammation

Acute pericarditis is an inflammatory process of the pericardium of sudden onset. It usually has viral etiology, although it can be caused by various systemic diseases such as systemic lupus erythematosus or as a complication of acute myocardial infarction. It is usually accompanied by pericardial effusion. The diagnosis is usually clinical without requiring complementary methods of high complexity. CMR may show spillover and pericardial thickening and/or demonstrate areas of inflammation through late enhancement. In the black blood T1 and T2 sequences, the pericardium is hypointense and hyperintense, respectively, and may present delayed enhancement (Fig. 8.4).

Chronic pericarditis is defined by a progressive sclerosing pericarditis with fibroblasts, collagen, and fibrin deposition. It may progress toward an end-stage, chronic fibrosing

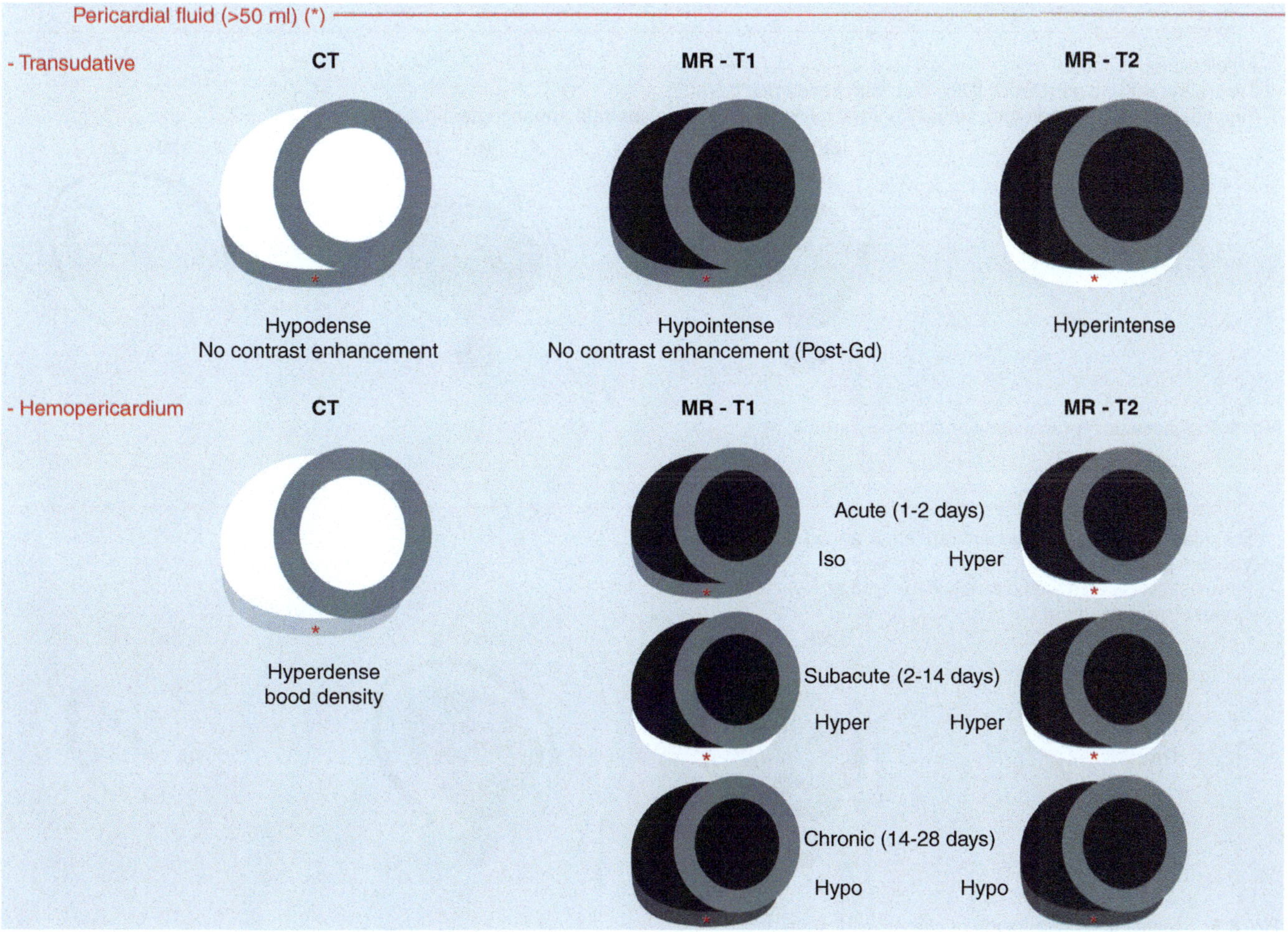

Fig. 8.3 Schematic representation of pericardial effusion

Table 8.1 Approximate probability of different types of pericardial effusion according to the CT attenuation values

	Transudative effusion	Exudative effusion	Hemopericardium
Hounsfield units	<5 HU	>5 HU	>20 HU

pericarditis. The pericardium tends to be thickened, with irregular contours. The key feature of this end-stage is a stiff pericardium with constriction of the heart (Fig. 8.5).

Constrictive Pericarditis

Constrictive pericarditis is defined as biventricular diastolic dysfunction due to cardiac constriction related to a thickened, fibrotic, and/or calcified pericardium. In most cases it is of viral or tuberculous etiology, but it may be due to connective tissue diseases, neoplasms, and traumatism. With a lower frequency, it can be a complication of chronic dialysis, radiation, and cardiac surgery.

As mentioned previously, its differentiation from restrictive cardiomyopathy is fundamental and difficult to attain using echocardiography.

The main morphological alterations in the CMR are the following (Fig. 8.6):

- Pericardial thickening: pericardial thickness equal or greater than 4 mm, irregular margins, and hypointense signal in black blood sequences T1 and T2 due to the presence of calcium and/or fibrosis.
- Tubular aspect of both ventricles with predominance of the right ventricle.
- Signs of systemic venous hypertension: dilatation of the vena cava and suprahepatic veins.
- Delayed pericardial enhancement: in cases of associated inflammation.

Occasionally, pericardial thickening is not generalized but is confined to regions that generate functional compromise such as the atrioventricular groove, with the rest of the pericardium showing normal appearance. That is why it is

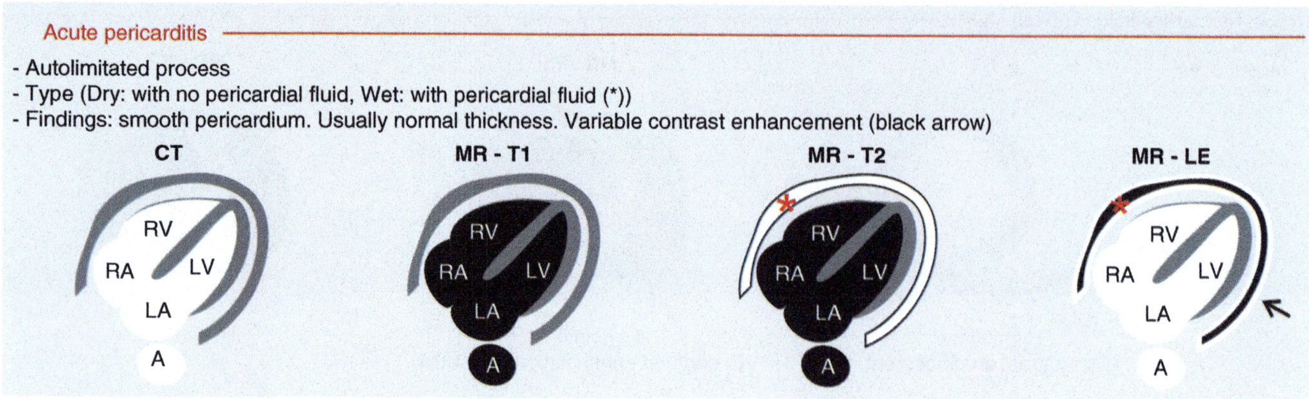

Fig. 8.4 Schematic representation of acute pericarditis

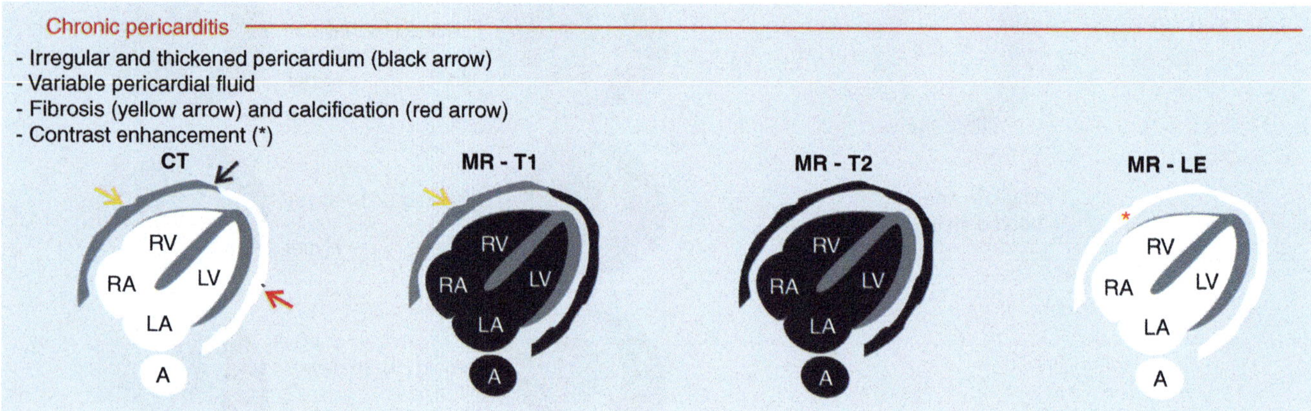

Fig. 8.5 Schematic representation of chronic pericarditis

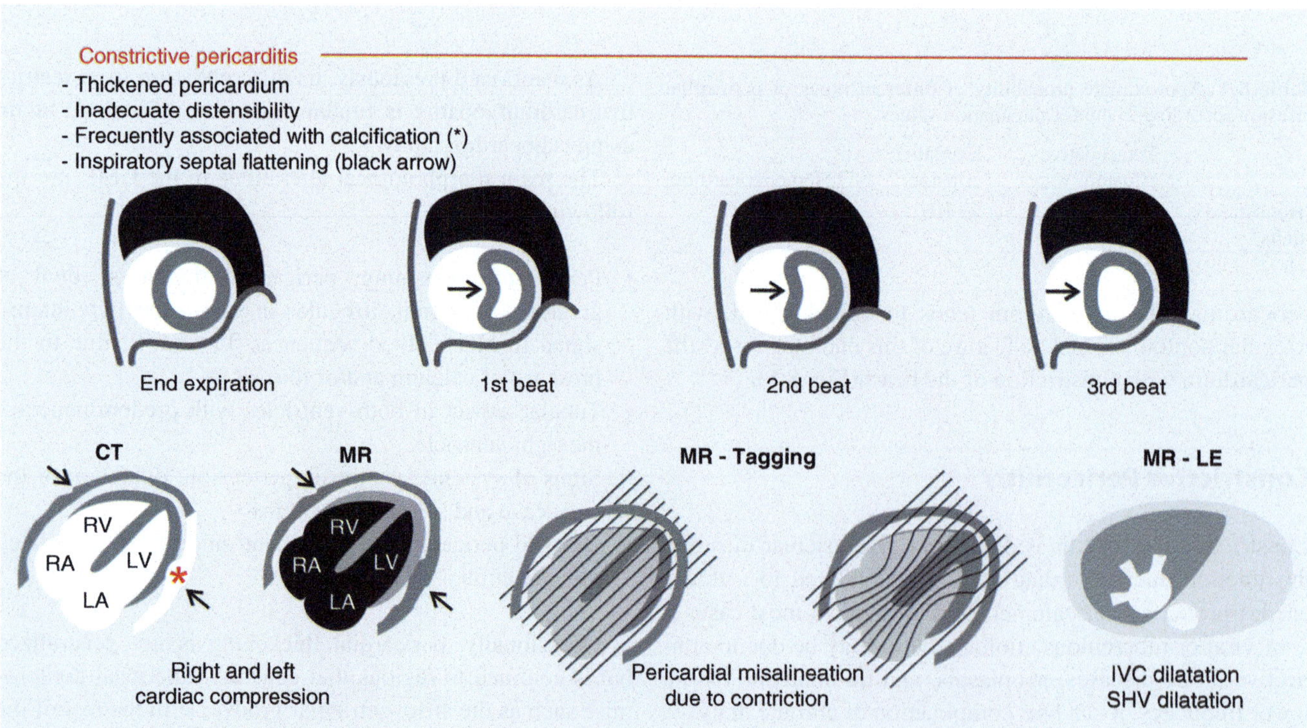

Fig. 8.6 Schematic representation of constrictive pericarditis. IVC refers to inferior vena cava, and SHV to suprahepatic veins

advisable to make acquisitions in multiple planes and with different sequences.

In cine images it is possible to demonstrate an incremented interventricular dependence characteristic of this entity. To better understand the images, it is necessary to know the respiratory influence on cardiac filling. During inspiration, the intrathoracic pressure is reduced, and there is an increase in venous return to the right cavities, decreasing, on the contrary, the filling of the left cavities by the accumulation of blood in the pulmonary veins. Due to the thinness of the RV free wall, the increase in ventricular filling during inspiration in the presence of a rigid pericardium limits its expansion, and the displacement of the interventricular septum toward the left ventricular cavity generates a characteristic septal bounce and flattening. To evaluate this phenomenon, free-breathing cine images are obtained. In this way, the protodiastolic flattening of the interventricular septum during the first three beats subsequent to the inspiratory excursion can be identified (Fig. 8.6).

Tagging CMR-tagging images can detect fibrotic adhesions of pericardial layers. The acquisition must be carried out on the four-chamber view with linear tags. In constrictive pericarditis, the loss of continuity of the tag is not evident as in normal physiology (Fig. 8.6).

Further Reading

Çetin MS, Özcan Çetin EH, Özdemir M, Topaloğlu S, Aras D, Temizhan A, et al. Effectiveness of computed tomography attenuation values in characterization of pericardial effusion. Anatol J Cardiol. 2017;17(4):322–7.

Francone M, Dymarkowski S, Kalantzi M, Rademakers FE, Bogaert J. Assessment of ventricular coupling with real-time cine MRI and its value to differentiate constrictive pericarditis from restrictive cardiomyopathy. Eur Radiol. 2006;16:944–51.

Misselt AJ, Harris SR, Glockner J, Feng D, Syed IS, Araoz PA. MR imaging of the pericardium. Magn Res Imaging Clin N Am. 2008;16:185–99.

Taylor AM, Dymarkowski S, Verbeken EK, Bogaert J. Detection of pericardial inflammation with late-enhancement cardiac magnetic resonance imaging: initial results. Eur Radiol. 2006;16:569–74.

Case 168

Pericardial Effusion

Clinical History

- Fourteen-year-old male.
- He has diagnosis of pectus excavatum under evaluation for surgical candidacy (Nuss procedure, minimally invasive placement of a stainless steel bar behind the sternum).
- Referred for cardiac magnetic resonance (CMR) for the assessment of the presence and extent of cardiac compression.

Images

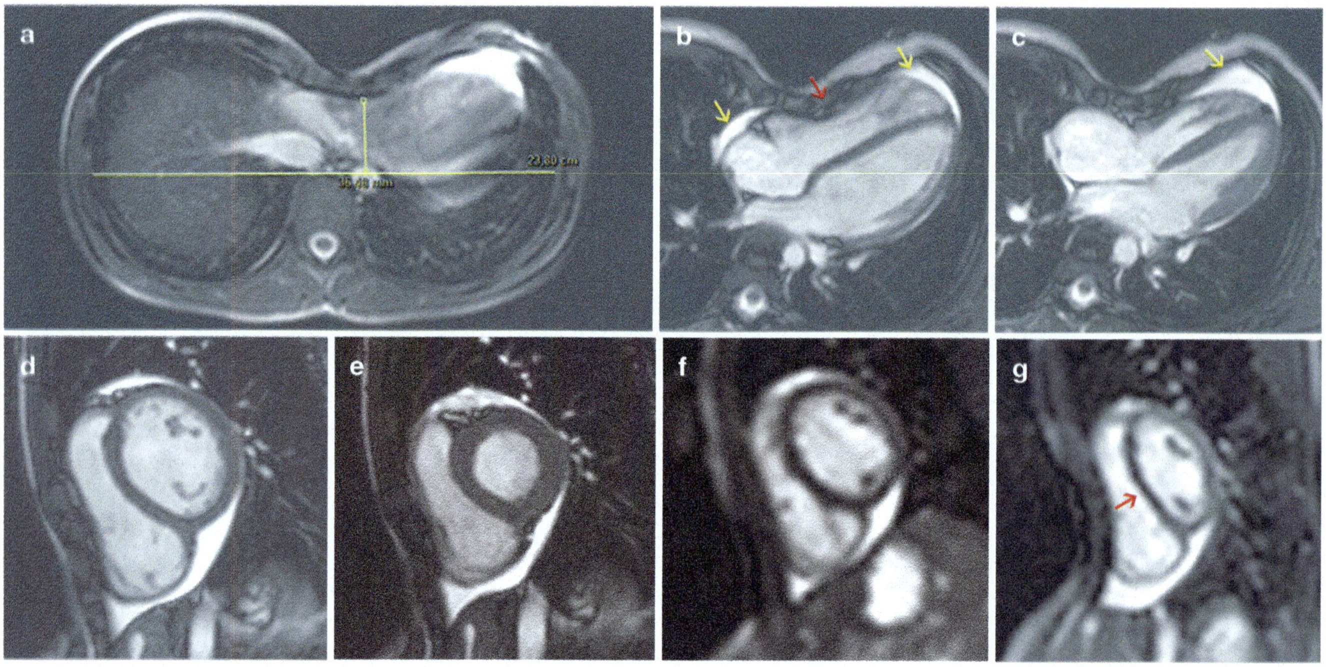

Findings and Interpretation

- Scout views at the diaphragmatic level (panel A) revealed a significant sternal depression (pectus excavatum), with a Haller index (transverse/posterior-anterior ratio) of 6.5.
- Diastolic (panel B) and systolic (panel C) four-chamber views demonstrated external compression of the right ventricular free wall by the sternum (red arrow in panel B) and pericardial effusion (yellow arrows in panels B and C).
- Diastolic (panel D) and systolic (panel E) short-axis views show mild to moderate pericardial effusion and preserved systolic function.
- Using real-time cine images (panels F and G), a significant increment in ventricular eccentricity index during inspiration related to septal shift (red arrow in panel G) was identified.
- Pectus excavatum, originally deemed only a cosmetic issue that can occasionally have a psychosocial impact, has been recently related to several cardiac and pulmonary adverse morphological and functional findings. In this case, aside from mild to moderate pericardial effusion, we detected an exaggerated interventricular dependence (identified as a significant septal shift and associated to a less distensible right ventricle).

Further Reading

Deviggiano A, Vallejos J, Vina N, Martinez-Ferro M, Bellia-Munzon G, Carrascosa P, et al. Exaggerated interventricular dependence among patients with pectus excavatum: combined assessment with cardiac MRI and chest CT. AJR Am J Roentgenol. 2017;208:854–61.

Case 169

Pericardial Effusion

Clinical History

- Forty-three-year-old female with cough and palpitations.
- Doppler echocardiography revealed moderate pericardial effusion without signs of hemodynamic compromise and a high systolic pulmonary artery pressure (34 mmHg).
- A cardiac magnetic resonance was requested for further assessment.

Images

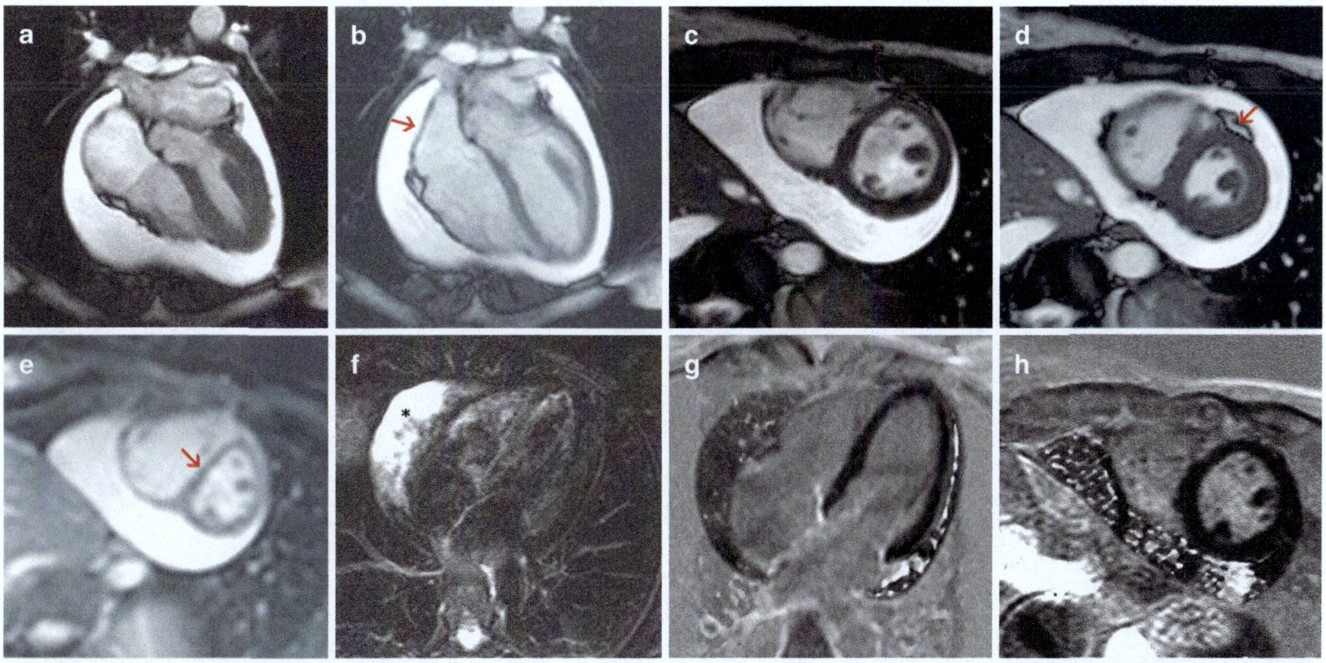

Findings and Interpretation

- Moderate to severe pericardial effusion (calculated volume of 290 mL), with normal pericardial thickness. End-systolic (panel A) and end-diastolic (panel B) four-chamber cine views show large pericardial effusion, with incipient telediastolic collapse (arrow in panel B). Atrial and ventricular dimensions as well as systolic function are preserved.
- End-diastolic (panel C) and end-systolic (panel D) short-axis views highlight the presence of a marked sisto-diastolic displacement of the heart during the cardiac cycle within the enlarged pericardial sac, reflecting the so-called "swinging heart" motion, that is responsible for the beat-to-beat variation of the electrocardiographic cardiac axis, amplitude, and even morphology.
- Septal flattening during inspiration (panel E) further reflects incremented filling pressures.
- At T2-weighed imaging, there is no evidence of myocardial or pericardial edema, with high-intensity signal of the pericardial fluid (asterisk in panel F).
- Likewise, inversion-recovery imaging (panels G and H) did not show evidence of late gadolinium enhancement.
- Identification of the underlying cause of pericardial effusion can be troublesome since a large number of possible etiologies might be involved (idiopathic, infections, traumatic, neoplasic, radiation-induced, autoimmune, myocardial infarction, end-stage renal failure, hypothyroidism).
- Pericardial drainage is only indicated with clinical tamponade, which was not the case in this patient.

Further Reading

Bogaert J, Francone M. Cardiovascular magnetic resonance in pericardial diseases. J Cardiovasc Magn Res. 2009;11:14.

Sagrista-Sauleda J, Sarrias Merce A, Soler-Soler J. Diagnosis and management of pericardial effusion. World J Cardiol. 2011;3:135–43.

Case 170

Acute Pericarditis

Clinical History

- A 27-year-old female.
- Hospitalized for acute chest pain that increased in deep inspiration.
- Non-specific ECG changes.
- Negative cardiac enzymes.
- Normal echocardiogram.
- A cardiac magnetic resonance (CMR) was requested for further evaluation.

Images

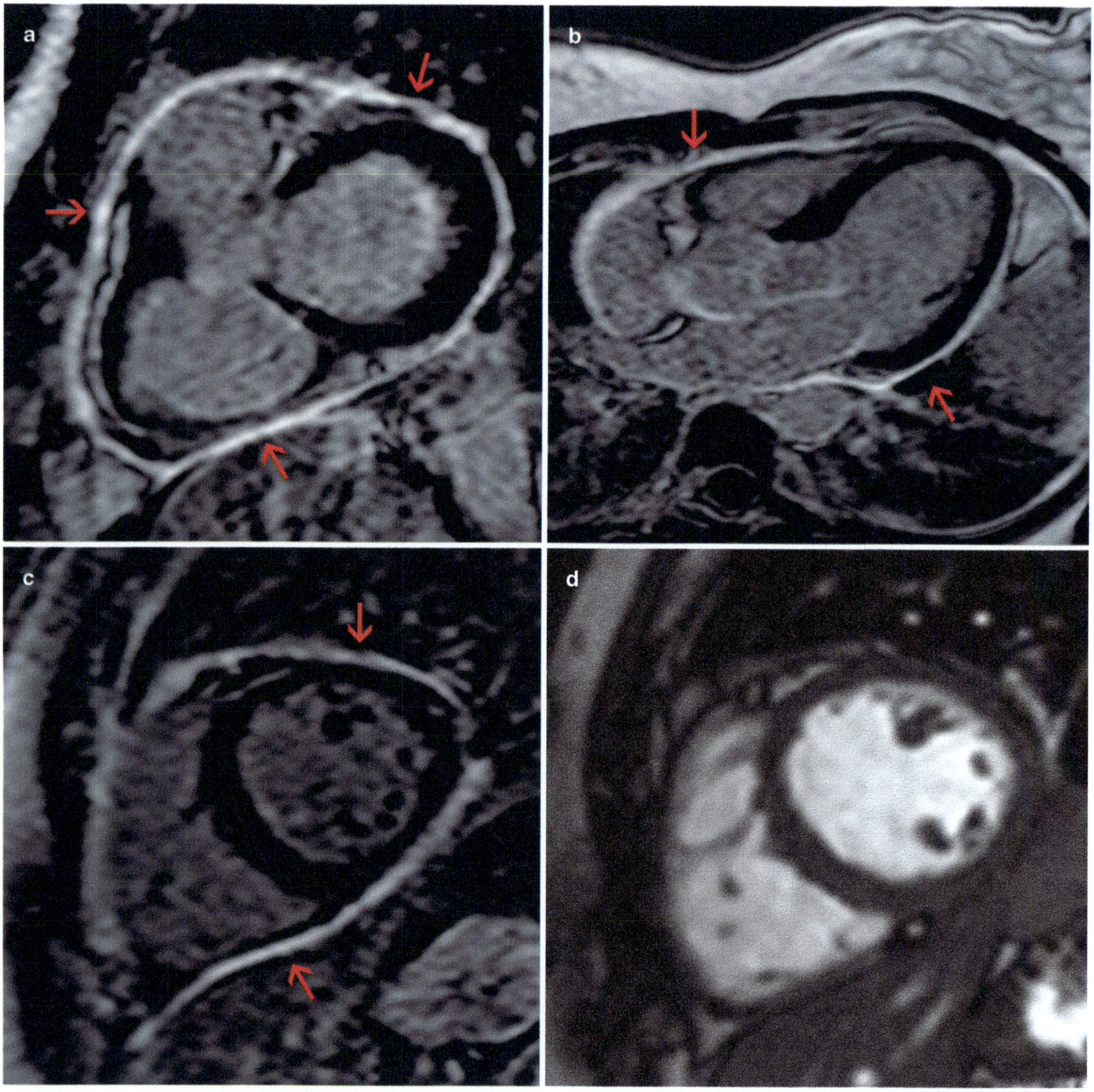

Findings and Interpretation

- Delayed enhancement inversion-recovery images (panels A–C) showed diffuse abnormal pericardial uptake of gadolinium (red arrows). Note the absence of pericardial effusion (panel D).
- Acute pericarditis is defined as an inflammatory pericardial syndrome with or without pericardial effusion. CMR late enhancement can be used to visualize pericardial inflammation in patients with clinical suspicion of pericardial disease.

Further Reading

Bogaert J, Francone M. Cardiovascular magnetic resonance in pericardial diseases. J Cardiovasc Magn Reson. 2009;11:14.

Taylor AM, Dymarkowski S, Verbeken E, Bogaert J. Detection of pericardial inflammation with late-enhancement cardiac magnetic resonance imaging: initial results. Eur Radiol. 2006;16:569–74.

Case 171

Pericarditis

Clinical History

- Thirty-five-year-old male.
- Coronary risk factors: none.
- Forty-five days ago he was admitted with respiratory symptoms and pericarditis that required pericardiocentesis.
- Referred for delayed enhancement cardiac magnetic resonance (DE-CMR) due to persisting symptoms.

Images

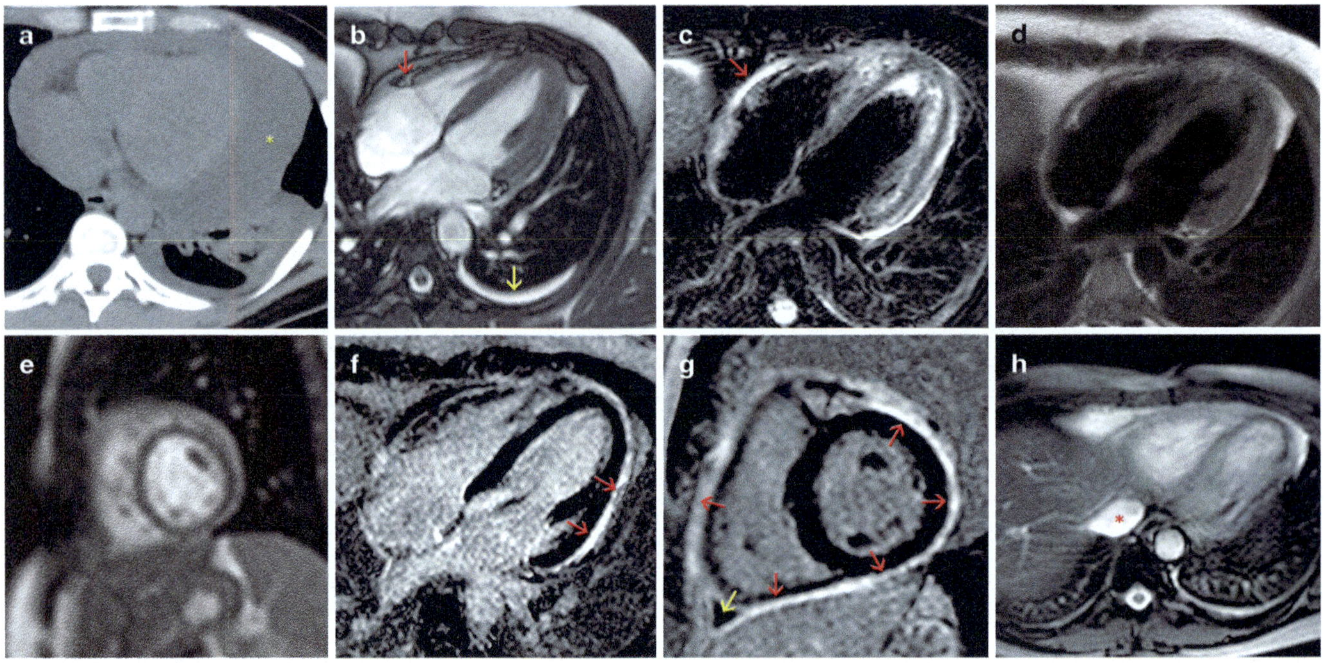

Findings and Interpretation

- Left ventricular (LV) dimensions were normal (end-diastolic volume 81 mL/m^2), with normal systolic function (ejection fraction 53%).
- Non-contrast chest computed tomography performed 45 days before CMR revealed severe pericardial effusion (*, in panel A) that required pericardiocentesis.
- Systolic four-chamber cine image (panel B) showed normal systolic function and minimal pericardial (red arrow) and pleural (yellow arrow) effusions.
- Confrontation of T2-weighted (panel C) and T1-weighted (panel D) images allow discrimination between pericardial effusion (panel C) and pericardial thickening.
- The absence of septal motion changes (particularly of significant leftward excursion) during inspiration (panel E) reveals the lack of ventricular filling impairment that can be found in constrictive pericarditis. Supporting this, the inferior vena cava has a normal size (*, in panel H)
- Inversion-recovery images (four-chamber view, panel F; and short-axis view, panel G) show extensive pericardial late gadolinium enhancement (LGE, red arrows). Note the presence of minimal pericardial fluid (yellow arrow) and the absence of myocardial LGE.
- It is important to define the etiology of pericarditis (viral vs. non-viral, tuberculosis, radiation or drug-induced, connective tissue disorders, among others), commonly non-discernable with CMR.
- As in myocarditis, one of the most effective therapeutic strategies is to restrict physical activity at least for 3 months. Aspirin or nonsteroidal anti-inflammatory drugs (NSAIDs) are the backbone of myocarditis and pericarditis therapy.
- In cases such as this one with extensive LGE, adjuvant therapy with low-dose colchicine might be recommended to prevent recurrences and progression to constrictive disease. Also, moderate doses of corticosteroids might be a second option among non-responders to aspirin or NSAIDs.

Further Reading

Adler Y, Charron P, Imazio M, et al. 2015 ESC Guidelines for the diagnosis and management of pericardial diseases the task force for the diagnosis and management of pericardial diseases of the European society of cardiology (ESC). Eur Heart J. 2015;36:2921–64.

Case 172

Myopericarditis

Clinical History

- Sixty-four-year-old male.
- Coronary risk factors: hypertension.
- One month ago he was hospitalized due to acute chest pain and non-specific ST-T changes. He underwent a negative chest pain unit including invasive coronary angiography and stress echocardiography with absence of ischemia.
- Referred for delayed enhancement cardiac magnetic resonance (DE-CMR) due to heart failure symptoms.

Images

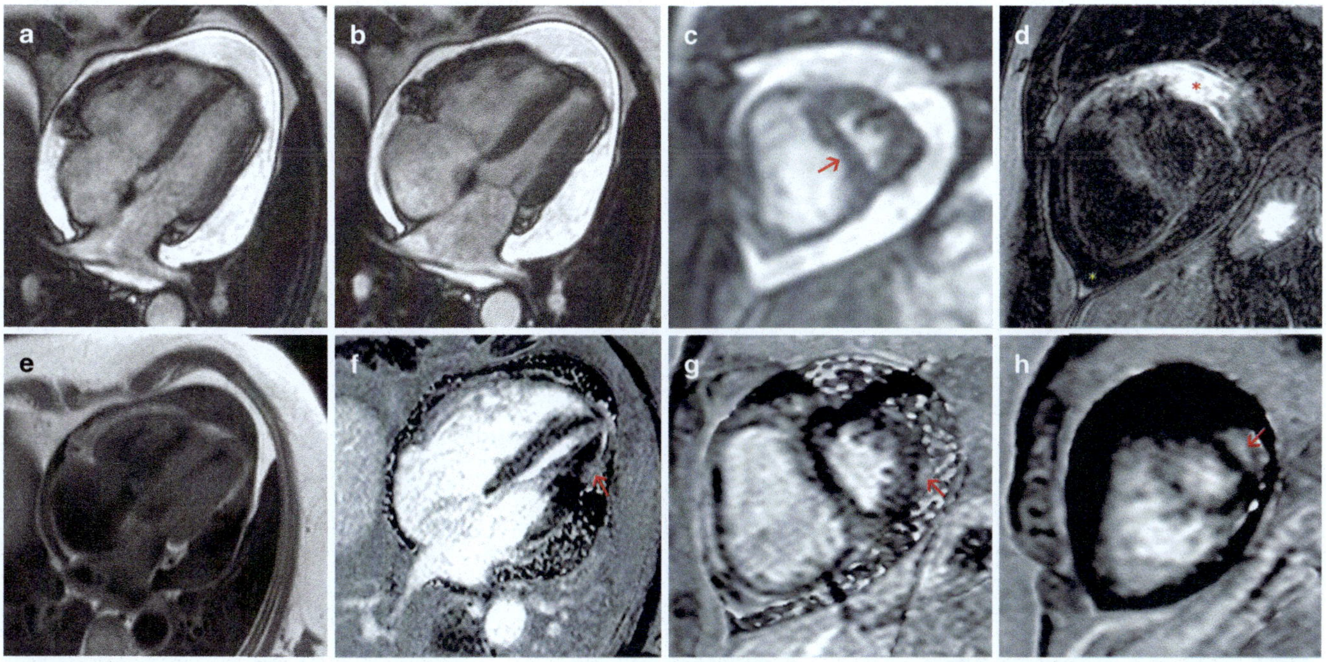

Findings and Interpretation

- Left ventricle (LV) was small (end-diastolic volume 33 mL/m^2), with a tubular shape, and biventricular systolic function was normal (LV ejection fraction 62%).
- Four-chamber cine views (diastolic, panel A; systolic, panel B) show severe pericardial effusion (442 mL), with very subtle increment in pericardial thickness (but <2 mm).
- Using free-breathing real-time cine images (panel C), an exaggerated interventricular dependence is demonstrated by the presence of significant septal excursion to the left (red arrow) during inspiration.
- T2-weighted images (panel D) do not show evidence of any significant myocardial edema. Of note, pericardial effusion in heterogeneous (high and low intensity, *), suggestive of exudative fluid.
- T1-weighted images (panel E) show that pericardial thickness, though very mildly incremented, is within the upper normal range.
- Inversion-recovery images (four-chamber view, panel F; short-axis views, panels G and H) show patchy areas of subepicardial late gadolinium enhancement (red arrows), whereas the pericardium is not involved.
- This is a case of myopericarditis, with severe pericardial effusion and evidence of impaired ventricular filling. While viral infections are the most common cause, eosinophilic myocarditis, connective tissue disorders, inflammatory bowel disease, and drug-induced/radiation-induced etiologies should be excluded.

Further Reading

Adler Y, Charron P, Imazio M, et al. 2015 ESC Guidelines for the diagnosis and management of pericardial diseases the task force for the diagnosis and management of pericardial diseases of the European society of cardiology (ESC). Eur Heart J. 2015;36:2921–64.

Case 173

Constrictive Pericarditis

Clinical History

- Eighty-year-old male.
- Coronary risk factors: hypertension.
- Admitted with cough, dyspnea, and unremarkable ECG findings. Chest x-ray revealed a large consolidation/ pleural effusion of the basal right lung field.
- Non-contrast chest computed tomography (CT) showed large right pleural effusion and a thickened pericardium.
- Doppler echocardiography reported a preserved systolic function with a restrictive left ventricular (LV) filling pattern.
- Cardiac magnetic resonance was requested to confirm constrictive pericarditis.

Images

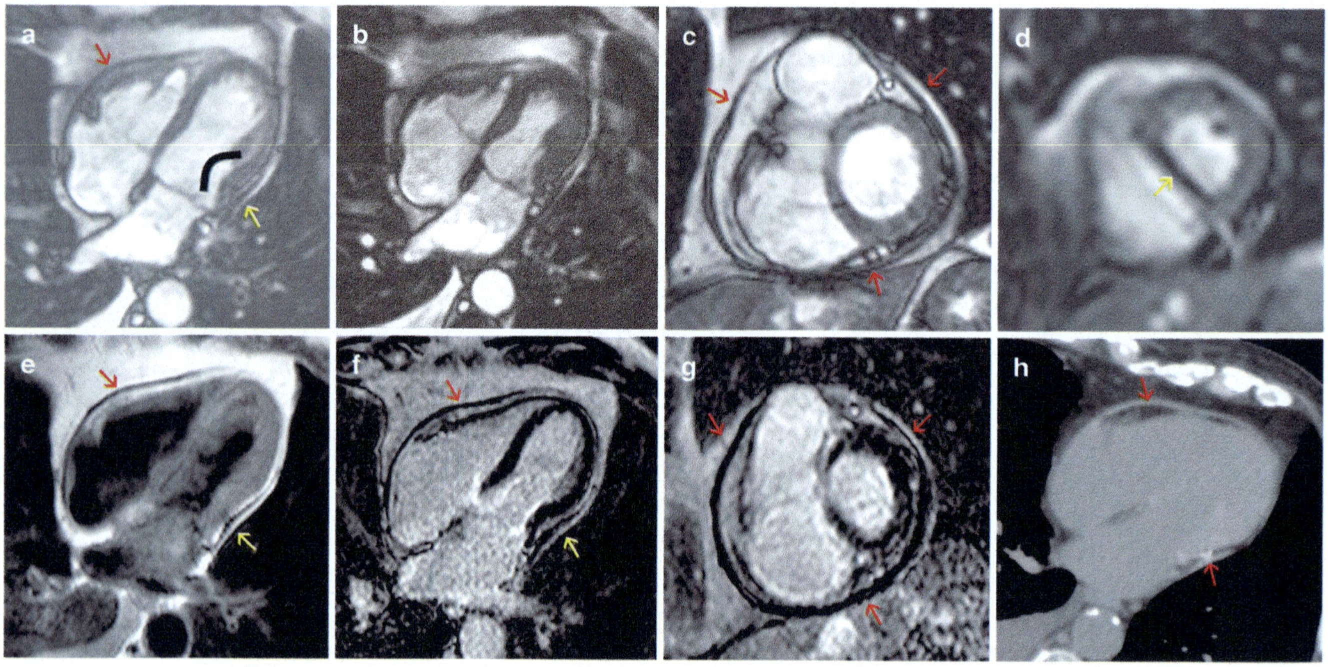

Findings and Interpretation

- End-diastolic four-chamber view (panel A) showed normal chamber dimensions and a thickened pericardium over the right ventricle (red arrow in panel A) and over the basal lateral LV wall (yellow arrow). Of note, the basal lateral wall has an abnormal inward convexity (curved line in panel A), commonly observed in the presence of constrictive pericarditis. Such segmental inward displacement, reflecting cardiac compression by the overlying thickened pericardium, is also observed in T1-weighted images (panel E), in inversion-recovery images (panel F) and in CT images (panel H).
- Systolic function was preserved (panel B).
- A basal short-axis view (panel C) depicts the diffuse circumferential pericardial thickening (maximum thickness 4.5 mm).
- Short-axis free-breathing images demonstrate septal flattening during inspiration (yellow arrow in panel F), reflecting the presence an incremented interventricular dependence due to a non-distensible pericardium that leads to impaired ventricular filling.
- Four-chamber T1-weighted images (panel E) can be used to measure the thickened pericardium.
- Inversion-recovery images (panels F and G) show lack of late gadolinium enhancement.
- Axial CT shows a thickened, yet non-calcified pericardium (arrows in panel H). Note that the minimal calcification underlying the basal lateral wall corresponds to the left circumflex artery.
- Constrictive pericarditis is a very rare cause of heart failure, commonly related to right-sided symptoms. The etiology is widely diverse, including idiopathic, postsurgical,

post-viral, tuberculous, and radiation-induced, among others. Of note, contrary to the general belief, atrial dilatation might be absent, as well as pericardial calcification.

- Although anti-inflammatory medical treatment might lead to reversion in some cases, surgical pericardiectomy is generally indicated.

Further Reading

Aldweib N, Farah V, Biederman RWW. Clinical utility of cardiac magnetic resonance imaging in pericardial diseases. Curr Cardiol Rev. 2018;14:200–12.

Bogaert J, Francone M. Pericardial disease: value of CT and MR imaging. Radiology. 2013;267:340–56.

Case 174

Constrictive Pericarditis

Clinical History

- Thirty-six-year-old female.
- Positive serology for Chagas disease.
- History of pulmonary tuberculosis and ascites.
- Dyspnea, New York Heart Association functional class II–III.
- Doppler echocardiogram showed increased pericardial thickness, abnormal septal motion (septal shudder and bounce), and tubular-shaped appearance of the right ventricle.
- Cardiac magnetic resonance (CMR) and computed tomography (CT) were required as pre-surgical studies.

Images

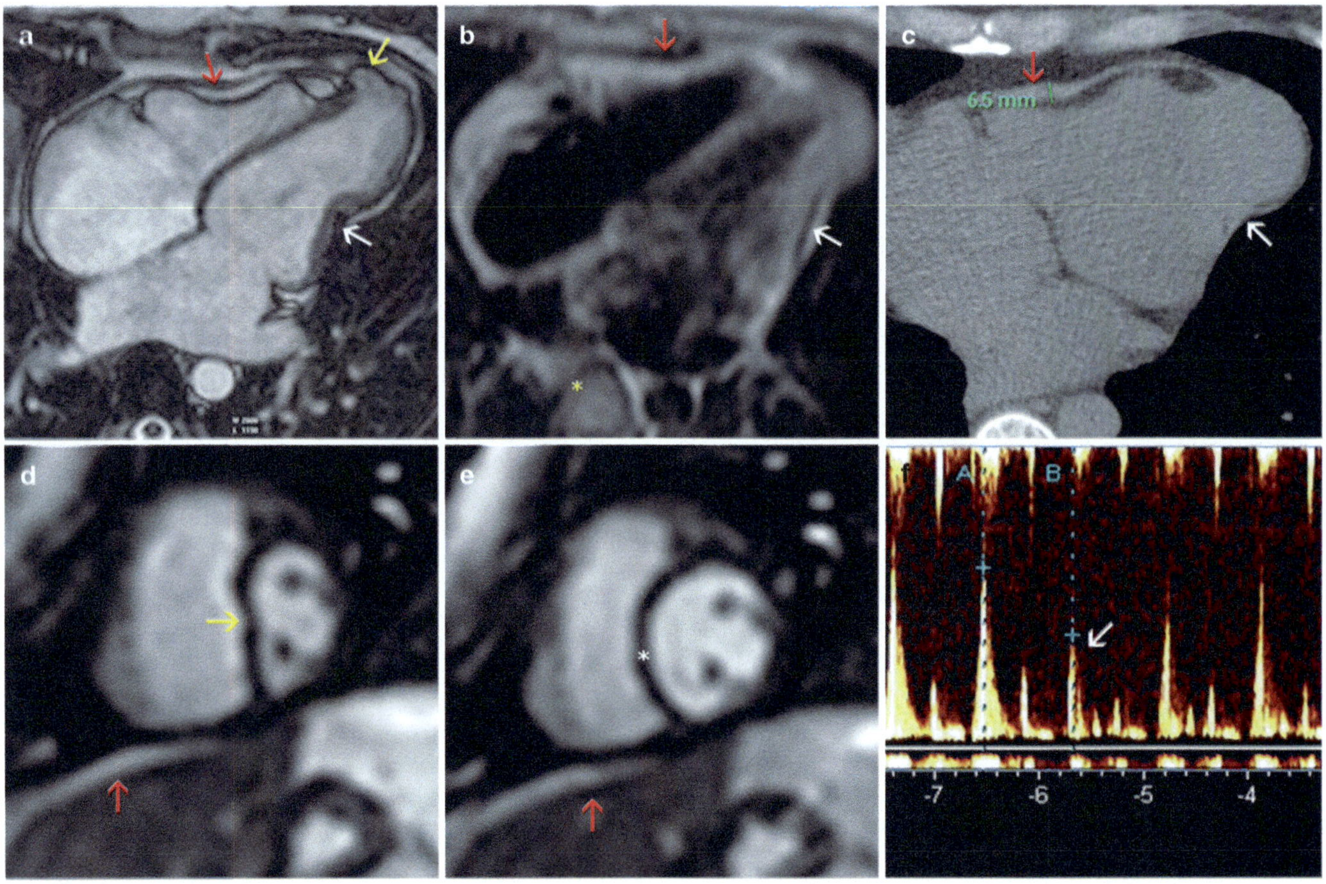

Findings and Interpretation

- Diastolic four-chamber view depicted at cine CMR (panel A) and T1-weighted image without fat suppression (panel B). Diffuse hypointense pericardial thickening is found on the basal and medial portions of the right ventricle (red arrows) and midportion of the left ventricle (white arrow). The thickened areas are compressing the adjacent cardiac cavities. Apical left ventricle aneurysm was observed (yellow arrow in panel A). A non-contrast CT (panel C) showed a non-calcified pericardial thickening with a maximum pericardial thickness of 6.5 mm.
- Short-axis free-breathing (real-time) cine images at onset of inspiration (panel D) and at onset of expiration (panel E) freezed at early ventricular filling. Septal inversion (significant septal leftward excursion) occurs at inspiration (yellow arrow), with normalization at expiration (asterisk), leading to an abnormal respiratory septal shift. This finding is related with an increased interventricular dependence. The red arrow indicates the position of the left hemidiaphragm, which is used to define the phase of the respiratory cycle.

- Doppler echocardiogram (panel F) exhibited a >25% reduction in E wave velocity (white arrow) during inspiration.
- These findings are characteristic of the constrictive pericarditis, a progressive condition characterized by pericardial fibrosis, with or without calcification, which results in chronic refractory congestive heart failure and for which pericardiectomy is often required. CMR and/or CT are usually requested as pre-surgical evaluation to determine the anatomical and functional compromise, as well as the presence of calcium at the pericardial level.

Further Reading

Bogaert J, Francone M. Pericardial disease: value of CT and MR imaging. Radiology. 2013;267:340–56.

Francone M, Dymarkowski S, Kalantzi M, Rademakers FE, Bogaert J. Assessment of ventricular coupling with real-time cine MRI and its value to differentiate constrictive pericarditis from restrictive cardiomyopathy. Eur Radiol. 2006;16:944–51.

Case 175

Pericardial Cyst

Clinical History

- Eighty-year-old female.
- Asymptomatic, without coronary risk factors.
- She has a known pericardial cyst.
- A cardiac magnetic resonance (CMR) was requested for further assessment.

Images

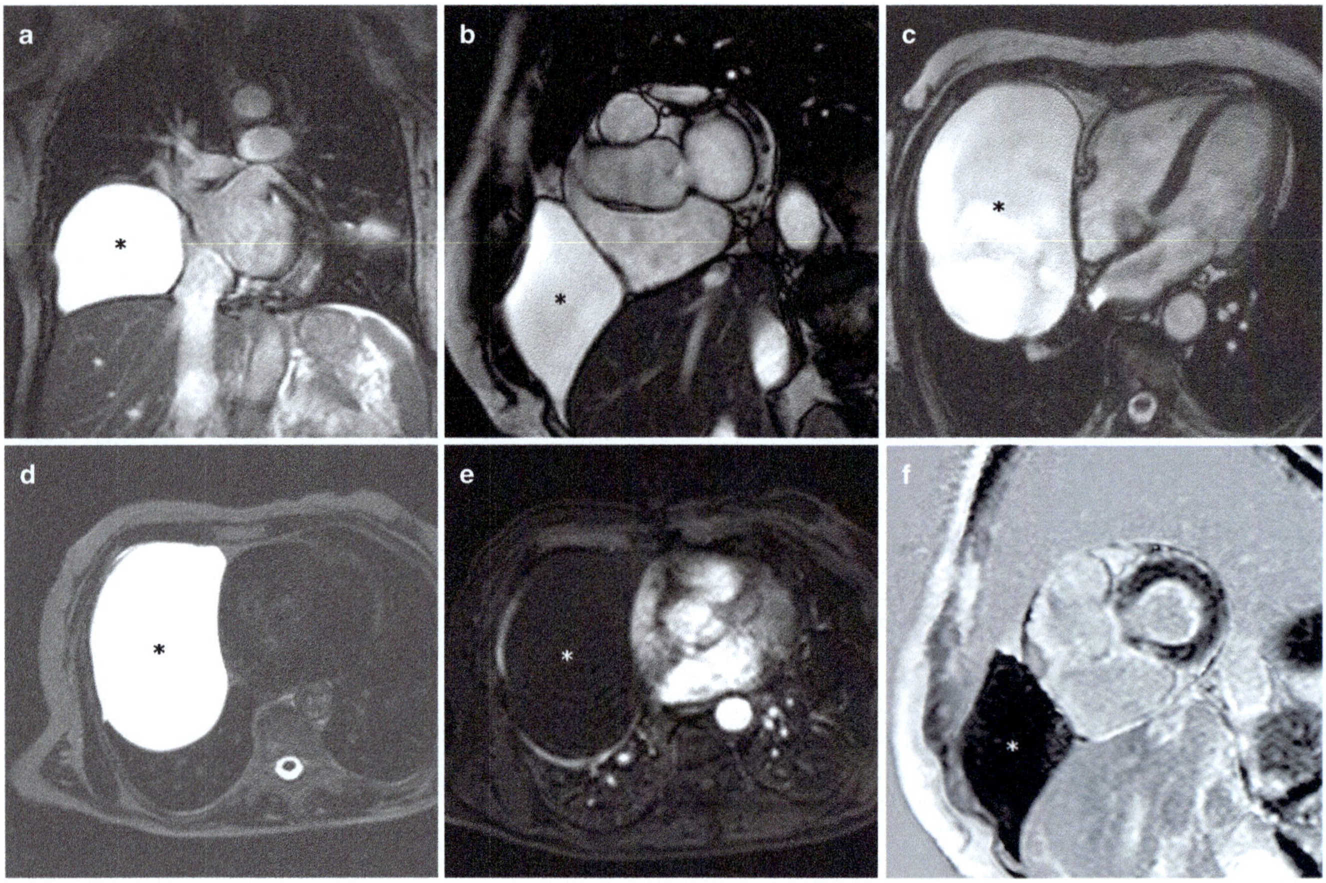

Findings and Interpretation

- A very large paracardiac mass is detected at the right cardiophrenic sulcus (asterisk in panels A–F).
- The mass is homogeneous, well circumscribed and encapsulated, with high signal intensity in T2-weighted images (panel D), and it does not infiltrate the adjacent structures.
- In addition, it has no early (panel E) or late (panel F) gadolinium uptake.
- Most pericardial cysts are located in the right cardiophrenic sulcus and less frequently left-sided. These congenital encapsulated cysts are benign and usually asymptomatic, unless they compress adjacent structures. Also, very rarely, complications such as inflammation, hemorrhage, or rupture have been reported.

Further Reading

Bogaert J, Francone M. Cardiovascular magnetic resonance in pericardial diseases. J Cardiovasc Magn Res. 2009;11:14.

Case 176

Congenital Absence of Pericardium

Clinical History

- Twenty-three-year-old male.
- History of chest pain.
- Normal physical examination.
- Normal echocardiogram.
- Chest X-ray showed marked levoposition of the cardiac silhouette; therefore a cardiac magnetic resonance (CMR) was indicated.

Images

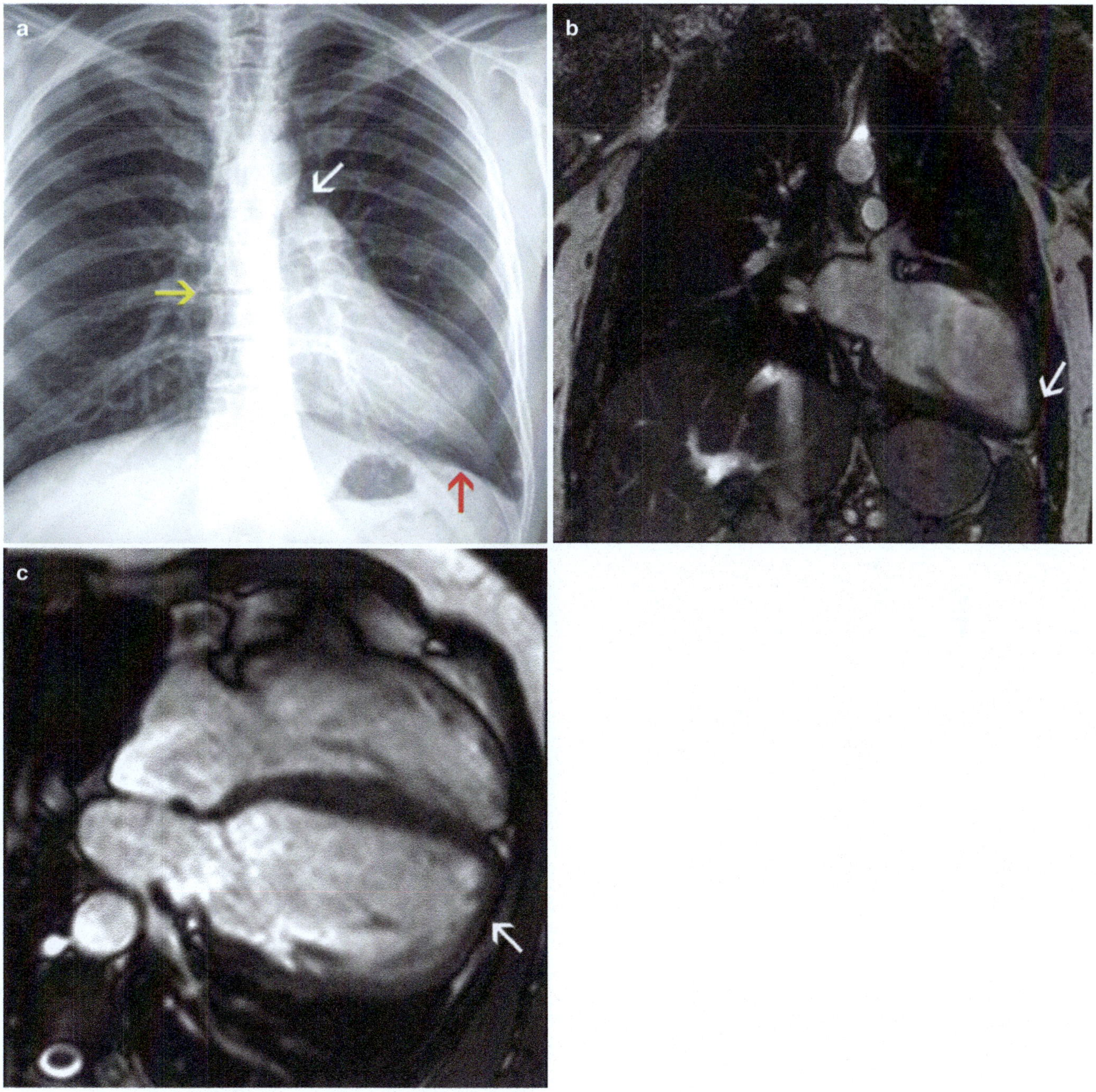

Findings and Interpretation

- Posterior-anterior chest X-ray showed marked levoposition of the cardiac silhouette without tracheal deviation, prominent main pulmonary artery, right heart border superimposed on the spine (yellow arrow), and interposition of lung parenchyma between the aortic arch and left pulmonary artery (white arrow) and between the cardiac base and the left hemidiaphragm (red arrow).
- Cine CMR image in coronal (panel B) and four-chamber (panel C) views confirm heart levoposition, with the apex in a lateral location (arrow). The pericardium cannot be visualized, making the diagnosis of congenital absence of left-sided pericardium.
- Congenital absence of the pericardium is rare and can be either complete or partial, occurring more often on the left than the right side. Left-sided complete absence of pericardium is the most common form.

Further Reading

Shah AB, Kronzon I. Congenital defects of the pericardium: a review. Eur Heart J Cardiovasc Imaging. 2015;16:821–7.

Aortic Disease

9

Carlos M. Capuñay, Jimena B. Carpio, Fernando Abramzon, Maria Jose Bosaleh, Gastón A. Rodríguez-Granillo, and Patricia M. Carrascosa

Background

The prevalence of aortic disease is in continuous growth due to the population aging and the ineffective control of the atherosclerosis process and prevention programs. Accurate assessment of aortic size plays an important role in the detection of pathology and in the management of the patients with cardiovascular disease.

Aortic size varies according to the anatomic location, and it has linear association with age and gender. In healthy average mid-aged patients, the aorta reaches ~30–35 mm in the ascending aorta, ~25 mm in the thoracic descending aorta, and ~20 mm in the abdominal aorta. The aortic wall consists of three layers: the innermost layer is the intima, the middle layer is the media (larger in comparison with other arteries), and the outer layer is the adventitia.

C. M. Capuñay
Departments of CT and MR, and Research, Department of Cardiovascular Imaging, Diagnostico Maipu, Buenos Aires, Argentina

J. B. Carpio
Department of CT and MR, Diagnóstico Maipú, Buenos Aires, Argentina

F. Abramzon
Cardiovascular Imaging, Department of Radiology, Hospital de Trauma y Emergencias "Dr. Federico Abete", University of Buenos Aires, Buenos Aires, Argentina

M. J. Bosaleh
Department of Pediatrics, Pediatric Cardiology Section, Department of Radiology, Section of CT and MR, Hospital Nacional Alejandro Posadas, Buenos Aires, Argentina

G. A. Rodríguez-Granillo
Department of Cardiovascular Imaging, Department of Research, Diagnostico Maipu, Buenos Aires, Argentina

National Council of Scientific and Technical Investigations (CONICET), Buenos Aires, Argentina

P. M. Carrascosa (✉)
Departments of CT, MR, and Research, Department of Cardiovascular Imaging, Diagnostico Maipu, Buenos Aires, Argentina

University of Buenos Aires, Buenos Aires, Argentina

Latin American Committee of the Society of Cardiovascular Computed Tomography, Buenos Aires, Argentina
e-mail: patriciacarrascosa@diagnosticomaipu.com.ar

Aortic Aneurysm

Aortic aneurysm (AA) has multifactorial etiologies, with secondary structural modifications of the arterial wall and dilatation of the vessel over 50% of its normal diameter. Most of the AAs are secondary to atherosclerotic disease. Nevertheless, the AA of the ascending aorta has a different origin not associated to atherosclerosis and more related to congenital or acquired degeneration of the vascular wall structures and the influence of hemodynamic stress forces. In general, the enlargement of the ascending aorta affects the right aortic wall, where the wall shear stress is greater than in other aortic locations. In particular cases such as in patients with Marfan disorders, the AA compromises the aortic root due to distorted systolic flow turbulences that can also be associated to bicuspid aortic valve. Computed tomography (CT) is undoubtedly the best imaging modality for the diagnosis, characterization, surveillance, guidance of percutaneous or surgical repair, and postsurgical follow-up of AA.

Imaging Protocol

Multidetector CT scanners with ≥16 rows are recommended. Current CT angiography (CTA) protocols consist on a contrast-enhanced ECG-gated scan in arterial phase. Thin slice thickness of 1–2 mm is recommended. In patients with previous history of surgical aortic repair or endovascular treatment, the CT scan protocol includes a pre-contrast CT image acquisition to facilitate identification of endovascular

P. M. Carrascosa et al. (eds.), *Clinical Atlas of Cardiac and Aortic CT and MRI*, https://doi.org/10.1007/978-3-030-03682-9_9

devices and postsurgical grafts and delayed post-contrast imaging during the venous phase for visualization of slow-flow endoleaks.

Aortic Measurements on Cross-Sectional Imaging

The thoracic aorta undergoes dynamic changes during the cardiac circle, leading to a variation in aortic size of up to 2.5–3 mm between systole and diastole, especially in the aortic root and ascending aorta. As a consequence, end-systolic gated acquisitions are preferred for most accurate measurements.

On CTA and magnetic resonance imaging (MRI), the aortic lumen should be measured including the vessel wall and at the site of maximal dilatation for each of the aortic segments. Measurements should be performed on truly orthogonal images with respect to the aortic lumen at the different segments of the aorta (Figs. 9.1 and 9.2).

Current guidelines state that asymptomatic ascending AAs greater or equal than 55 mm and that descending thoracic aorta aneurysm greater than or equal to 55–60 mm require surgical repair. Special recommendations include

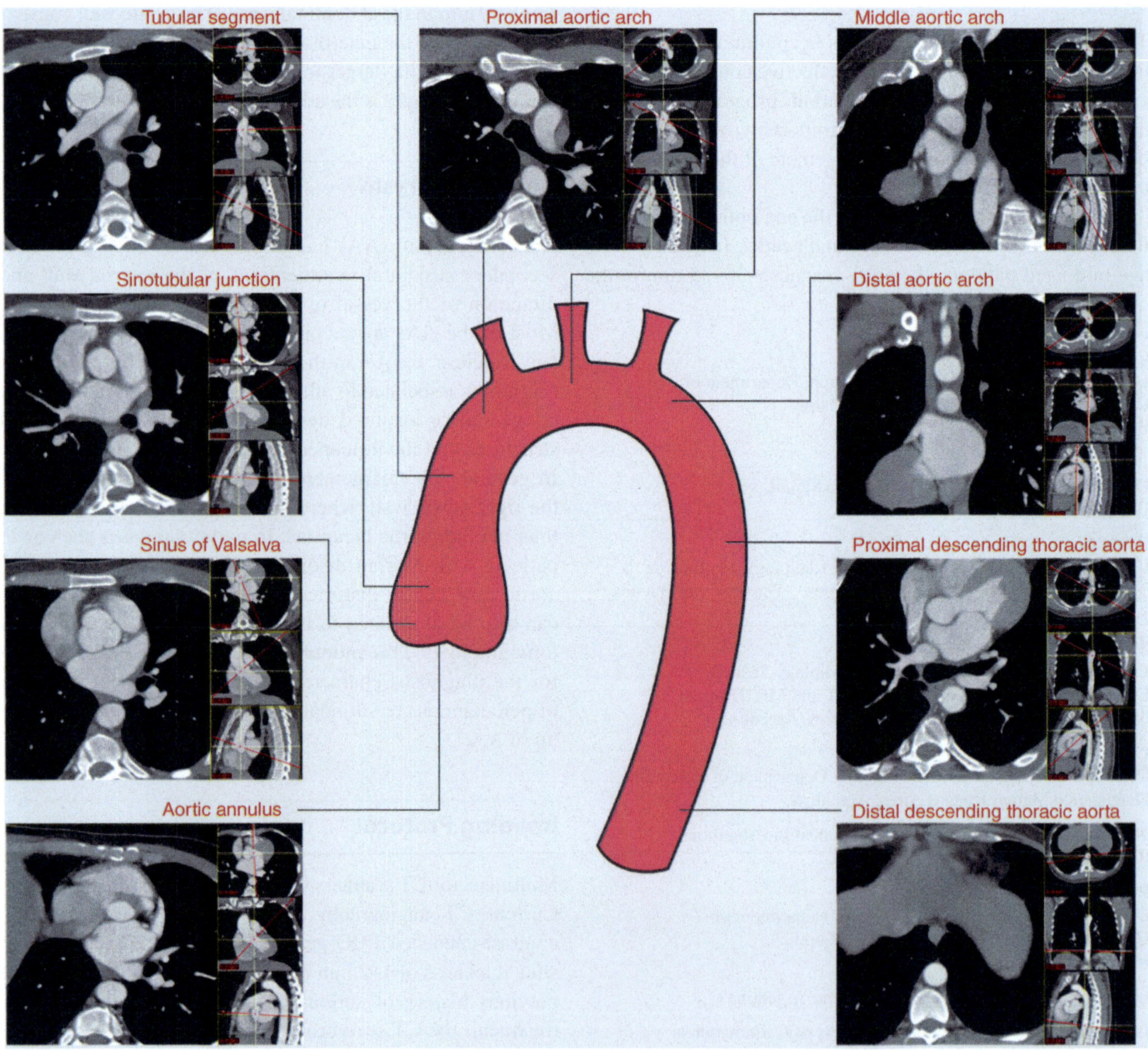

Fig. 9.1 Thoracic aorta segmentation and the corresponding true orthogonal images on computed tomography

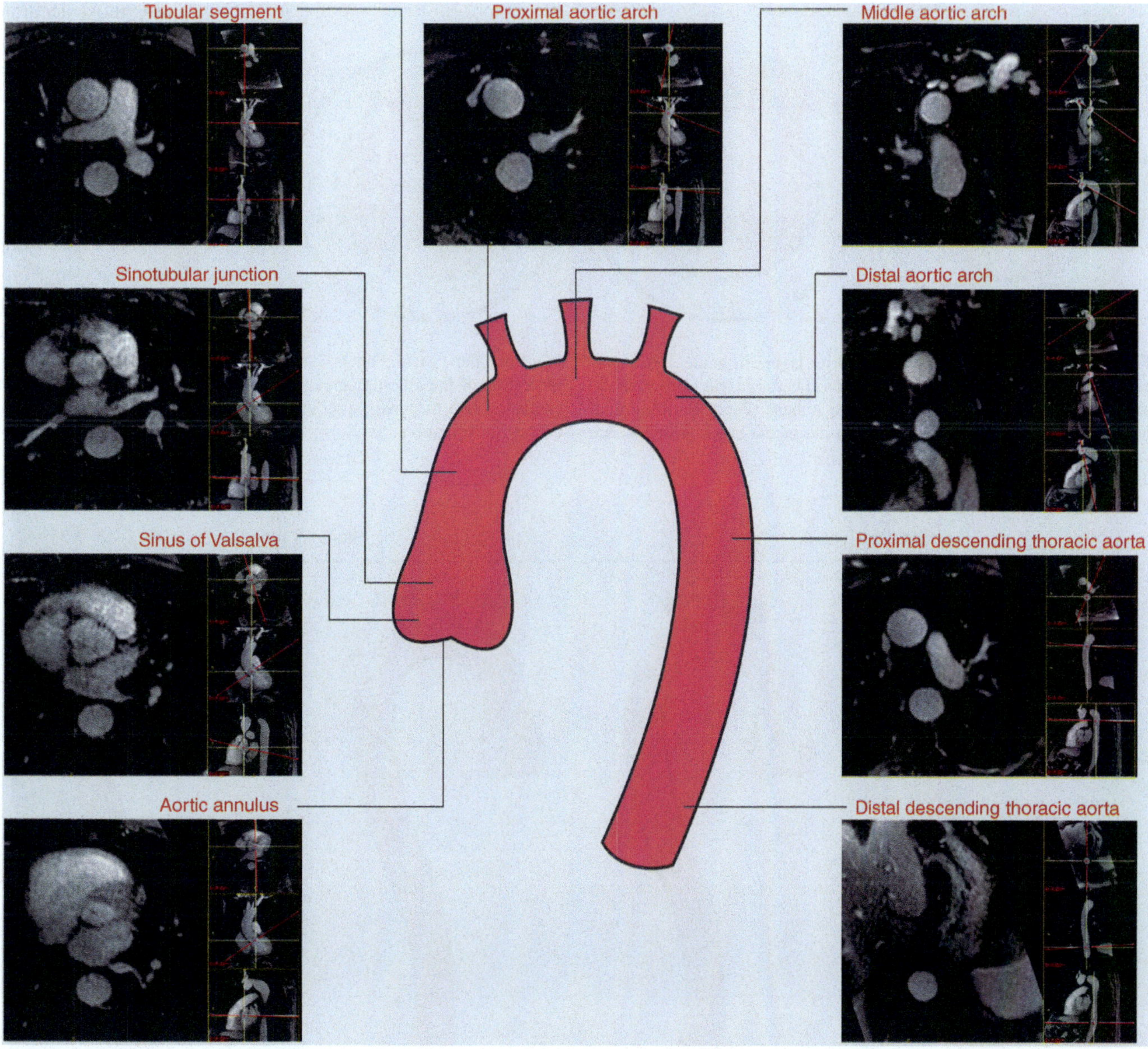

Fig. 9.2 Thoracic aorta segmentation and the corresponding true orthogonal images on magnetic resonance imaging

patients with Marfan disease [requiring ascending aorta surgery if ≥50 mm or ≥ 45 mm in the presence of risk factors such as rapid increase (>3 mm/year), family history of aortic dissection, and/or severe mitral or aortic regurgitation] and patients undergoing aortic valve replacement (>45 mm threshold).

Acute Aortic Syndromes

Acute aortic syndromes (AAS) describe three life-threatening vascular conditions of the thoracic aorta that include typical aortic dissection (AD), intramural hematoma (IMH), and penetrating atherosclerotic ulcer (PAU) (Fig. 9.3). These have many features in common and are clinically indistinguishable. Noninvasive imaging modalities have an important role in the diagnosis, management, and follow-up of these conditions. CTA is the preferred imaging modality in the acute clinical scenario, while CTA and MR angiography (MRA) are both useful in the chronic stage of the disease, being aware that these patients have lifelong medical treatment and will need a close surveillance with continuing imaging studies.

The cornerstone of the diagnosis of AAS is the correct identification of the location and extension of the aortic lesion, which defines the treatment options, prognosis, and life expectancy of the patient. The Stanford classification is currently in use and has replaced the DeBakey classification (Fig. 9.4).

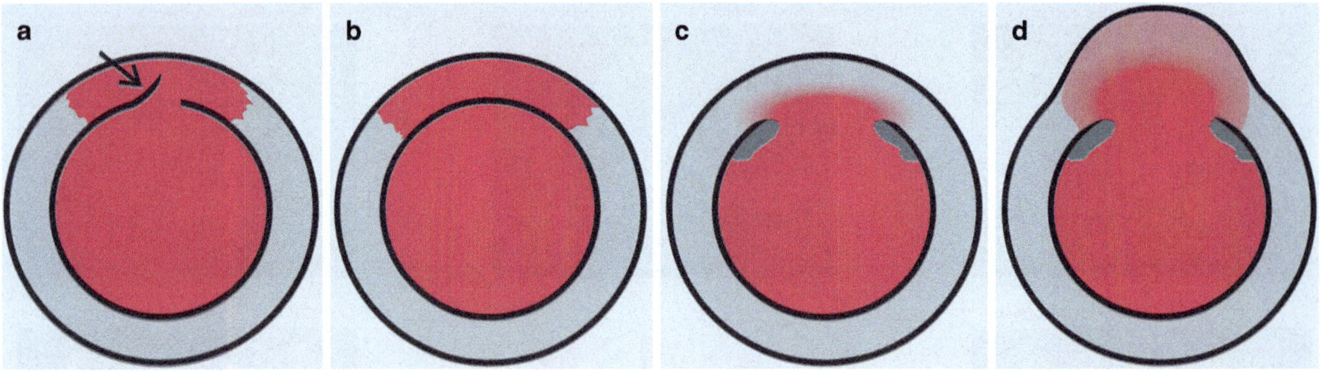

Fig. 9.3 Schematic changes of the aortic layers in acute aortic syndromes. Panel A. Typical aortic dissection. There is a tear (arrow) of the intima and the formation of two aortic lumens. Panel B. Intramural hematoma. There is hemorrhage within the media layer, with absence of intimal flap or tear. Panels C and D. Penetrating aortic ulcer. There is ulceration of the atheromatous plaque, with erosion of the intima and extension into the media producing a hematoma, with potential false aneurysm formation

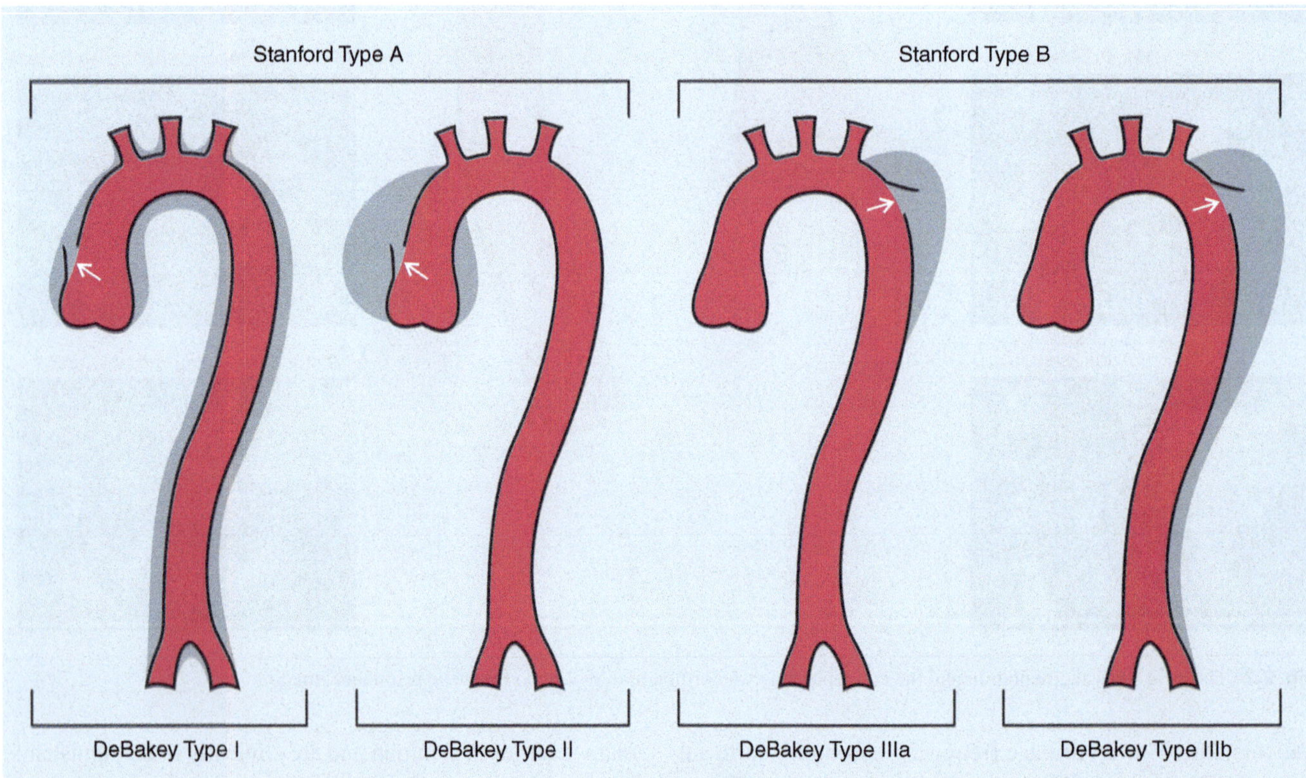

Fig. 9.4 Acute aortic syndrome classifications. The Stanford classification better correlates to patient's treatment options than the DeBakey classification, and it is widely used. Stanford Type A includes dissections involving the ascending aorta; the aortic arch and the descending aorta can also be involved. Stanford Type B includes lesions involving the descending aorta distal to the left subclavian artery (only thoracic or thoracoabdominal aorta). DeBakey type I dissections involve the ascending aorta, the aortic arch, and usually the descending aorta. DeBakey type II lesions only are confined to the ascending aorta. DeBakey type III lesions are confined to the descending aorta distal to the left subclavian artery; subtype "a" only the thoracic segment and subtype "b" the thoracoabdominal segment

Imaging Protocol

Multidetector CT scanners with ≥64 rows are recommended for the evaluation of patients with suspected AAS, providing isotropic image datasets that can be reconstructed in any plane. Current CT protocols must include an ECG-gated non-contrast acquisition of the thoracic aorta, followed by contrast-enhanced ECG-gated CTA in arterial phase from 3 cm above the aortic arch and to the pubis. ECG gating is essential to reduce cardiac motion artifacts, particularly in the aortic root. Thin slice thickness of 1–2 mm is recommended. If AD is diagnosed, a venous phase can be also performed for better characterization of the true and false lumen.

Aortic Dissection (AD)

AD is the most common entity of the AAS, accounting for 70–90% of the cases. It is categorized as acute or chronic in relation to the onset of symptoms (time frame of 14 days). Stanford type A AD has a high mortality rate (near 90% on non-treated patients) and is almost always surgically treated in the acute setting, while type B AD has in general a conservative (medical) treatment. For that reason, imaging modalities aimed at early diagnosis of AAS should allow an early recognition and characterization of AD as well as identification of the presence of any associated complications (Table 9.1).

Imaging findings on the non-enhanced CT scan include the internal displacement of intimal calcifications. The most important finding on contrast-enhanced CTA in this entity is the visualization of an intimal flap that separates the false lumen from the true lumen. The site of the intimal tear can be identified nearly always. Several imaging features are described for an appropriate differentiation between the two lumens (Fig. 9.5).

Table 9.1 Key findings in acute aortic syndromes

CT and MRI imaging findings in acute aortic syndromes
Visualization of an intimal flap (AD)
Identification of the true and false lumen (AD)
Localization of the intimal tear site and reentry (AD)
Integrity of aortic wall (IMH, PAU)
Involvement of arterial branches (AD, IMH)
Compromise of organ perfusion (AD, IMH)
Pericardial and/or pleural effusions (AD, IMH)
Compromise of periaortic tissue
Coexisting aortic lesions (aneurysms, atherosclerosis, valvular lesion)

CT computed tomography, *MRI* magnetic resonance imaging, *AD* aortic dissection, *IMH* intramural hematoma, *PAU* penetrating aortic ulcer

Intramural Hematoma (IMH)

IMH represents the 5–25% of all AAS. It is secondary to spontaneous hemorrhage in the medial layer of the aortic wall, due to rupture of the vasa vasorum. The evolution of IMH can be variable, ranging from resolving spontaneously to progression to typical aortic dissection, aneurysm formation, and/or rupture. Table 9.2 enumerates features to stratify and predict the progression and risk of death of patients with IMH.

Non-enhanced CT images are extremely useful for a prompt and accurate identification of IMH. It manifests as a crescent-shaped area of high attenuation (more than 40 Hounsfield units) in the aortic wall that remains unmodified after contrast administration. No dissection flap is present. The most common locations are the descending thoracic aorta (60–70%), the ascending aorta (30%), and the aortic arch (10%).

Table 9.2 High risk findings of intramural hematoma

Imaging features that represent a greater risk of life and progression of the intramural hematoma
Involvement of the ascending aorta
Intramural hematoma thickness greater than 10 mm
Diameter of the aorta greater than 50 mm
Association with penetrating atherosclerotic ulcer
Large/progressive pleural effusion
Large/progressive pericardial effusion
Enlargement of intramural hematoma on follow-up images

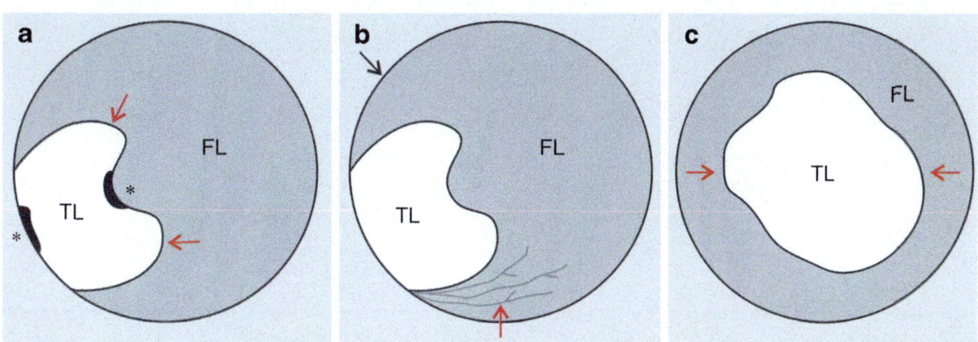

Fig. 9.5 Discrimination between the true and the false lumen with computed tomography angiography. In most cases, the true lumen (TL) has a greater contrast opacification than the false lumen (FL), where the blood flow is usually slower and more turbulent. Panel A: Cross-sectional scheme of the aorta, showing two aortic lumens separated by the presence of an intimal flap (arrow). The TL typically has a smaller cross-sectional area than the FL. Main features indicative of the TL include outer wall calcification and eccentric flap calcification (asterisks). Panel B: The cobweb sign (red arrow) consists on linear areas of low attenuation representing collagenous media remnants, only seen in the FL. The beak sign (black arrow) refers to the acute angle at the edge of the FL around the TL. Panel C: The wind sock sign represents an unusual type A aortic dissection in which there is a circumferential intimal tear (arrows) with intimo-intimal intussusception between the TL and the FL. The inner lumen is invariably the true one

Penetrating Atherosclerotic Ulcer (PAU)

PAU constitutes an ulceration of an atherosclerotic aortic lesion that erodes and penetrates the internal elastic intima of the aortic wall, with extension of blood into the media. The most common locations are the descending thoracic aorta (90%) and the aortic arch.

Classical imaging features in these patients are the presence of extensive atherosclerotic plaques and intimal calcifications, focal displacement of intimal calcifications (on non-enhanced CT images), and focal contrast filled outpouching of the aortic wall within the extensive aortic atheroma.

There is few evidence of the natural history of PAU. Described complications include development of saccular aneurysms, focal dissections, and aortic rupture. High-risk imaging features indicating endovascular/surgical treatment consist of aortic diameter greater than 55 mm, a >10 mm neck, and the presence of periaortic hematoma.

Further Reading

Carrascosa P, Capuñay C, Deviggiano A, Rodríguez-Granillo GA, Sagarduy MI, Cortines P, Carrascosa J, Parodi JC. Thoracic aorta cardiac-cycle related dynamic changes assessed with a 256-slice CT scanner. Cardiovasc Diagn Ther. 2013;3:125–8.

Erbel R, Aboyans V, Boileau C, Bossone E, Di Bartolomeo R, Eggebrecht H, et al. 2014 ESC guidelines on the diagnosis and treatment of aortic diseases: document covering acute and chronic aortic diseases of the thoracic and abdominal aorta of the adult. The task force for the diagnosis and treatment of aortic diseases of the European Society of Cardiology (ESC). Eur Heart J. 2014;35(41):2873–926.

Goldstein SA, Evangelista A, Abbara S, Arai A, Asch FM, Badano LP, et al. Multimodality imaging of diseases of the thoracic aorta in adults: from the American Society of Echocardiography and the European Association of Cardiovascular Imaging: endorsed by the Society of Cardiovascular Computed Tomography and Society for cardiovascular magnetic resonance. J Am Soc Echocardiogr. 2015;28(2):119–82.

Hallinan JT, Anil G. Multi-detector computed tomography in the diagnosis and management of acute aortic syndromes. World J Radiol. 2014;6:355–65.

Litmanovich D, Bankier AA, Cantin L, Raptopoulos V, Boiselle PM. CT and MRI in diseases of the aorta. Am J Roentgenol. 2009;193(4):928–40.

Case 177

Double Aortic Arch

Clinical History

- Two-year-old male.
- Patient started with inspiratory stridor worsening with feeding.
- Also referred apneic attacks, noisy breathing, and cough.
- Referred for thoracic computed tomography (CT) angiography to rule out vascular ring.

Images

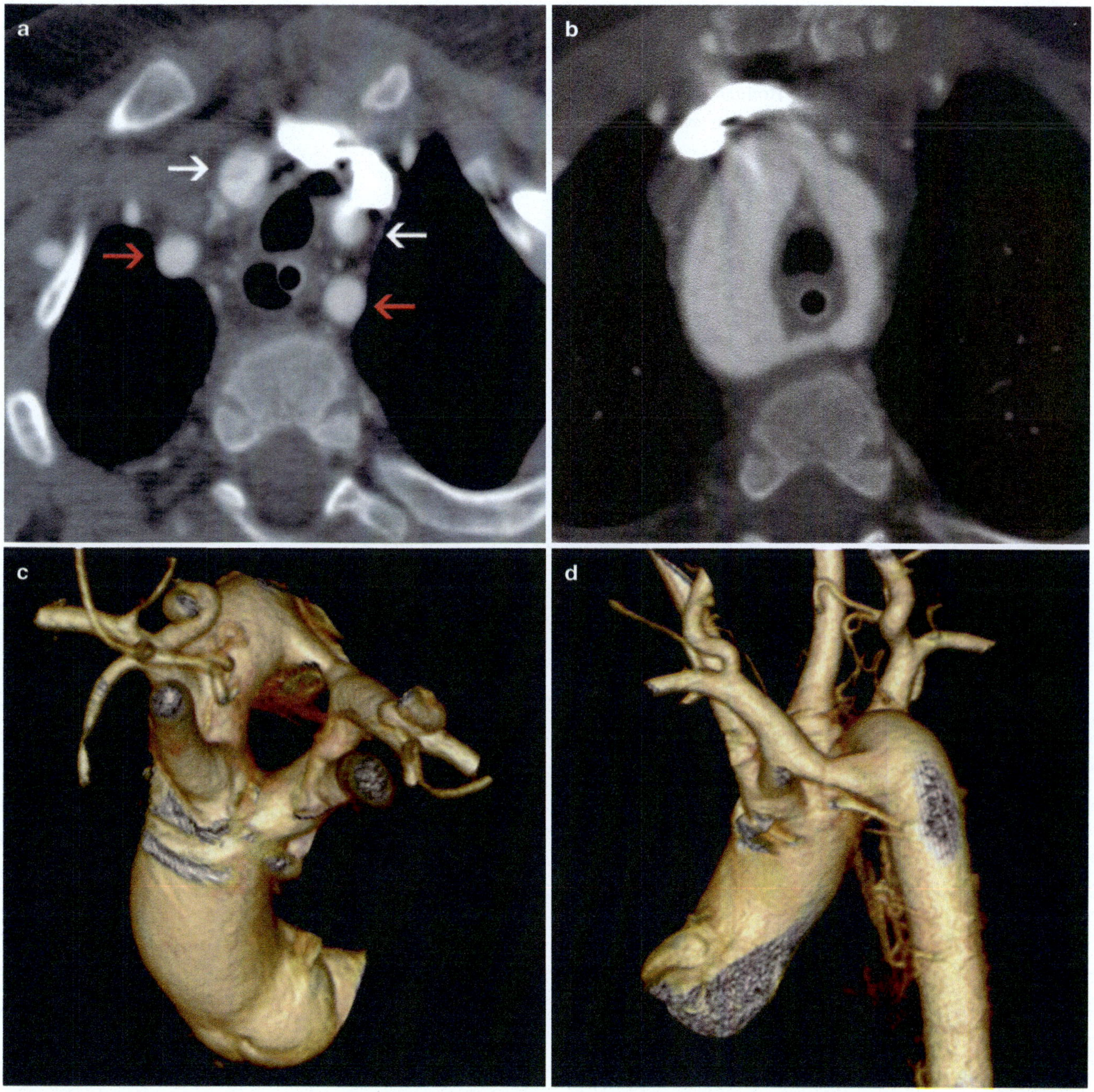

Findings and Interpretation

- Axial CT image (panel A) shows symmetric takeoff of four aortic branches at the thoracic inlet with two ventral carotid (white arrows) and two dorsal subclavian (red arrows) arteries. This sign is called "four-artery sign."
- Panel B shows two arches that surround the trachea and esophagus. The extremity of the right side is greater caliber than contralateral arch. Both archs are joined posterior generating a reduction of the esophageal lumen. Its patency is preserved due to a nasogastric tube.
- Volume rendering images from a cephalic view (panel C) and posterior oblique view (panel D) show a complete vascular ring formed by right and left aortic arches that arise from the ascending aorta. Both arches give rise to a common carotid artery and a subclavian artery.
- Double aortic arch is the most common cause of a vascular ring and is seldom associated with congenital heart disease. It results from persistence of both left and right 4th aortic arches that usually arise from the ascending aorta during development. The smaller arch may be partially atretic.

Further Reading

Maldonado JA, Henry T, Gutiérrez FR. Congenital thoracic vascular anomalies. Radiol Clin N Am. 2010;48:85–115.

Paul JF, Serraf A. Truncus arteriosus and double aortic arch. Circulation. 2002;105:e170.

Case 178

D-Transposition of the Great Arteries (D-TGA)

Clinical History

- Ten-year-old male.
- History of transposition of the great arteries (D-TGA) with corrective surgery with arterial switch performed at 10 days of life.
- Currently with chest pain and normal ECG.
- Transthoracic echocardiography with a poor echocardiographic window that impairs the assessment of the coronary arteries and the main pulmonary artery. Biventricular systolic and diastolic function are preserved.
- Exercise testing and Holter monitoring were normal.
- SPECT myocardial perfusion imaging with pharmacological stress showed evidence of mild ischemia in the left circumflex artery territory.
- Referred for cardiac computed tomography (CT) angiography to evaluate coronary and pulmonary artery anatomy.

Images

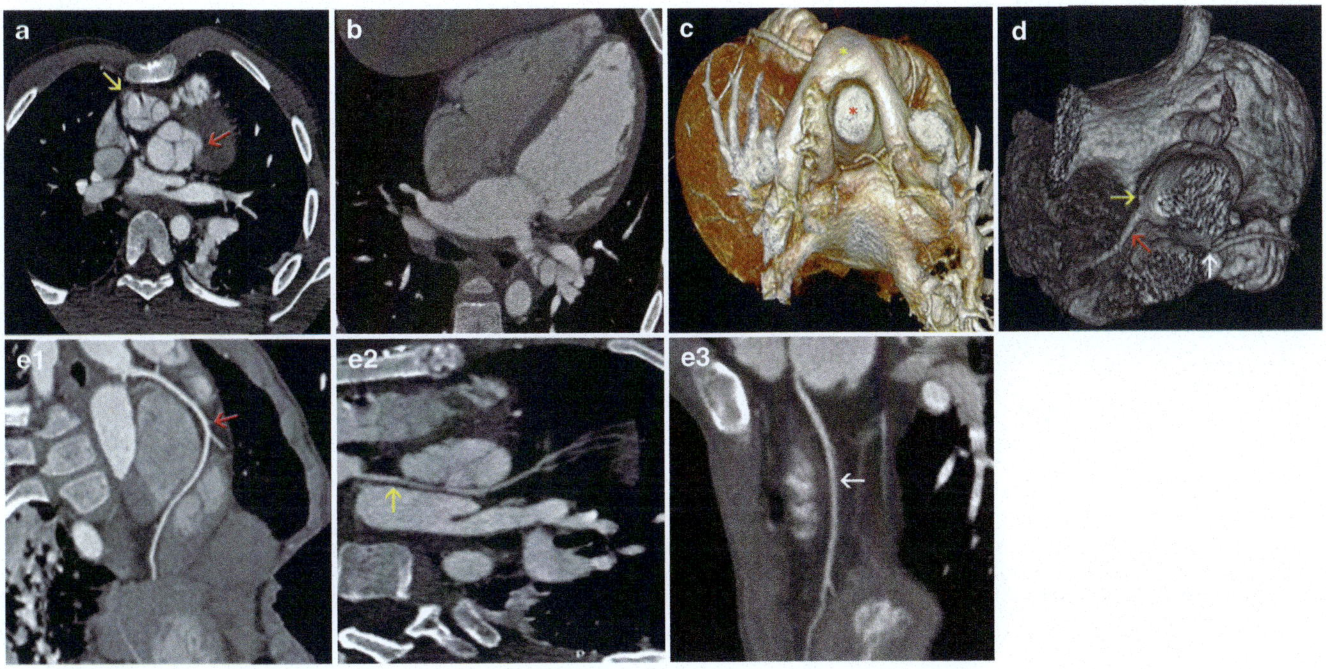

Findings and Interpretation

- CT angiography revealed the presence of atrioventricular (panel B) and ventriculoarterial concordance after corrective surgery with pulmonary artery (yellow asterisk in panels A and C) overlying the aorta (red arrow in panel A and red asterisk in panel C) (Lecompte maneuver).
- Coronary artery pattern observed after arterial switch: origin of the left anterior descending artery (white arrow in panel D) from the left coronary sinus, with a slight ostial narrowing (white arrow in panel D). The right coronary artery trunk gives origin to the right coronary artery (red arrow in panels D and E) and the left circumflex artery; the latter emerges in an acute angle and then follows a path between the aorta and the left atrium (yellow arrow in panels D and E).

- Cardiac CT allowed to assess the anatomy of the pulmonary branches and the outflow tracts of both ventricles, but most importantly the coronary anatomy.
- Transfer of the coronary arteries is a crucial step during the arterial switch operation for D-TGA in the case of abnormalities of origin or distribution of these arteries.
- Follow-up with ECG, exercise test, echocardiogram, and myocardial perfusion is important in these patients, and coronary artery angiography should be performed in case stenosis is suspected.

Further Reading

Legendre A, Losay J, Touchot-Koné A, Serraf A, Belli E, Piot JD, et al. Coronary events after arterial switch operation for transposition of the great arteries. Circulation. 2003;108 Suppl 1:II186–90.

Pasquali SK, Hasselblad V, Li JS, Kong DF, Sanders SP. Coronary artery pattern and outcome of arterial switch operation for transposition of the great arteries a meta-analysis. Circulation. 2002;106:2575–80.

Sithamparanathan S, Padley SP, Rubens MB, Gatzoulis MA, Ho SY, Nicol ED. Great vessel and coronary artery anatomy in transposition and other coronary anomalies: a universal descriptive and alphanumerical sequential classification. JACC Cardiovasc Imaging. 2013;6:624–30.

Case 179

Double Aortic Arch

Clinical History

- Six-year-old girl.
- With airway obstructive symptoms, such as inspiratory/expiratory laryngeal stridor and bronchospasm and cough.
- Past medical history indicates normal prenatal controls. Frequent episodes of respiratory tract infection and difficulty swallowing semisolid and solid foods (since the age of 3) were also documented.
- The presence of a vascular ring was suspected. Echocardiography suggested the presence of a double aortic arch. The patient was referred for thoracic computed tomography (CT) angiography to confirm the diagnosis.

Images

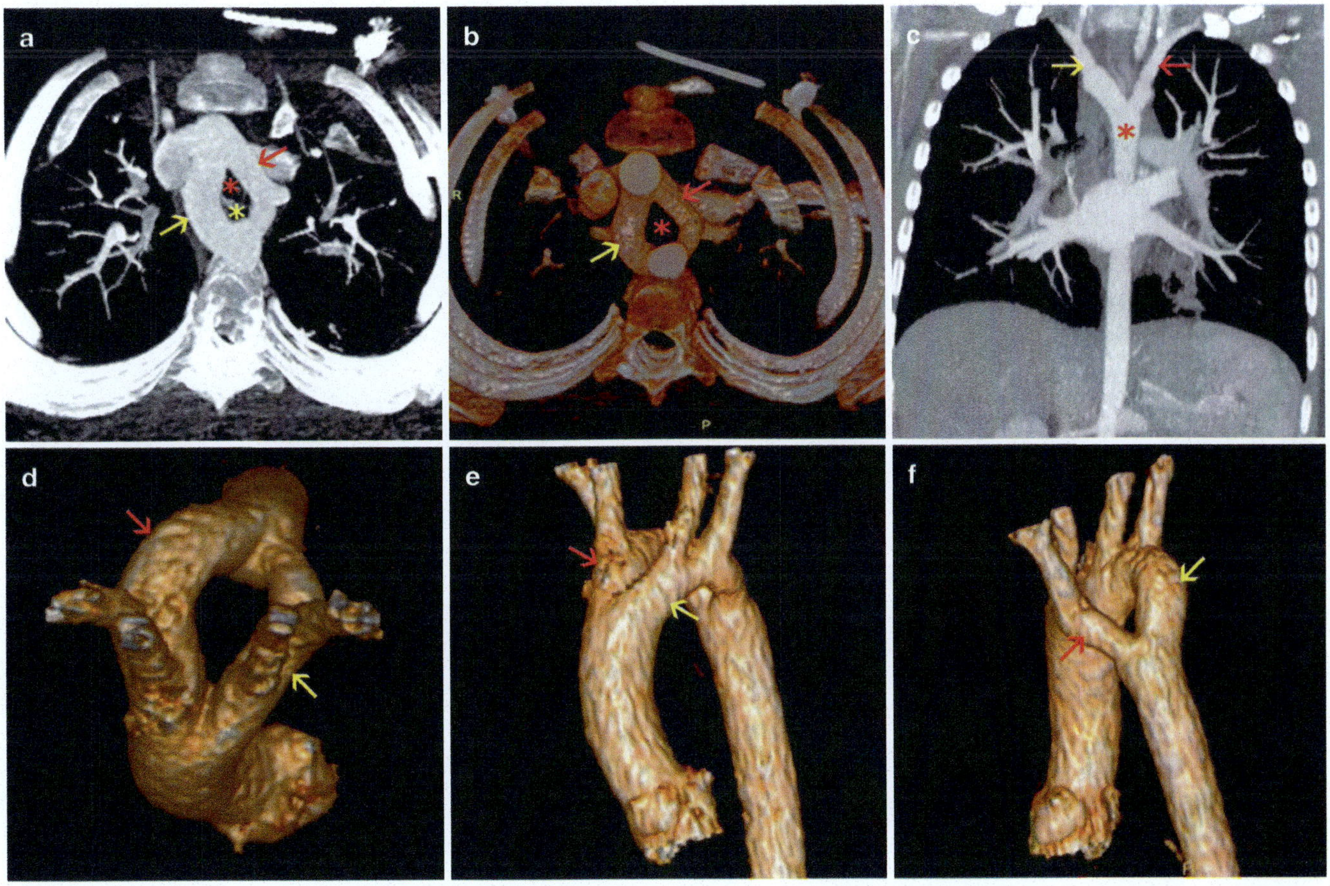

Findings and Interpretation

- CT angiography of the aorta shows a congenital anomaly of the aortic arch that constitutes a complete vascular ring. The right aortic arch (yellow arrow) and the left aortic arch (red arrow) join at the proximal segment of descending thoracic aorta.
- Axial maximum intensity projection image, superior view (panel A), and three-dimensional axial inferior view (panel B) show that the trachea (red asterisk) and esophagus (yellow asterisk) are surrounded and compressed by the double aortic arch. The coronal multiplanar reconstruction (panel C) demonstrates that the arches join at the proximal portion of a left-sided descending thoracic aorta (asterisk).
- Three-dimensional upper (panel D), left anterior (panel E), and posterior (panel F) views demonstrate a symmetrical double aortic arch, characterized by the right carotid and right subclavian arteries arising from the right arch and the left subclavian and left carotid arteries arising from the left arch, each separately.
- Vascular rings refer to congenital malformations of the aortic arch that encircle the esophagus and trachea, representing

less than 1% of all cardiovascular congenital malformations. They occur early in embryologic development due to the failure of the normal regression of the aortic arches. In cases of the double aortic arch, there is a failure in the regression of the distal right fourth arch. Both the fourth right and left arches persist and join the descending thoracic aorta, compressing the trachea and esophagus.

- Clinically, the onset and severity of symptoms depend on the tightness of the ring. Most patients present with laryngeal stridor, recurrent respiratory infections, or swallowing disorders within the first months/years of life. Association with congenital heart disease is rare. Surgical repair is indicated in symptomatic patients.
- CT angiography provides excellent image and accurate preoperative evaluation of the vascular anatomy and its relationship to the trachea and esophagus.

Further Reading

Fenández-Tena A, Martínez-González C. Double aortic arch diagnosed in a 44-year-old woman with recurring respiratory infections. Respir Med Case Rep. 2017;20:176–8.

Kanabuchi K, Noguchi N, Kondo T. Vascular tracheobronchial compression syndrome in adults: a review. Tokai J Exp Clin Med. 2011;36(4):106–11.

Park SC, Zuberbuhler JR. Vascular ring and pulmonary sling. In: Anderson RH, Baker EJ, Macartney RF, Rigby ML, Shinerbourne EA, Tynan M, editors. Paediatric cardiology. 2nd ed. London Harcourt Publishers; 2002. pp. 1559–1575.

Case 180

Right Aberrant Subclavian Artery and Related Kommerell Diverticulum

Clinical History

- Forty-year-old male.
- 3-year history of dysphagia lusoria.
- No respiratory or other gastrointestinal symptoms were present.
- The diagnosis of vascular ring is suggested on a barium esophagram.
- The patient was referred for thoracic magnetic resonance angiography (MRA) to confirm the diagnosis.

Images

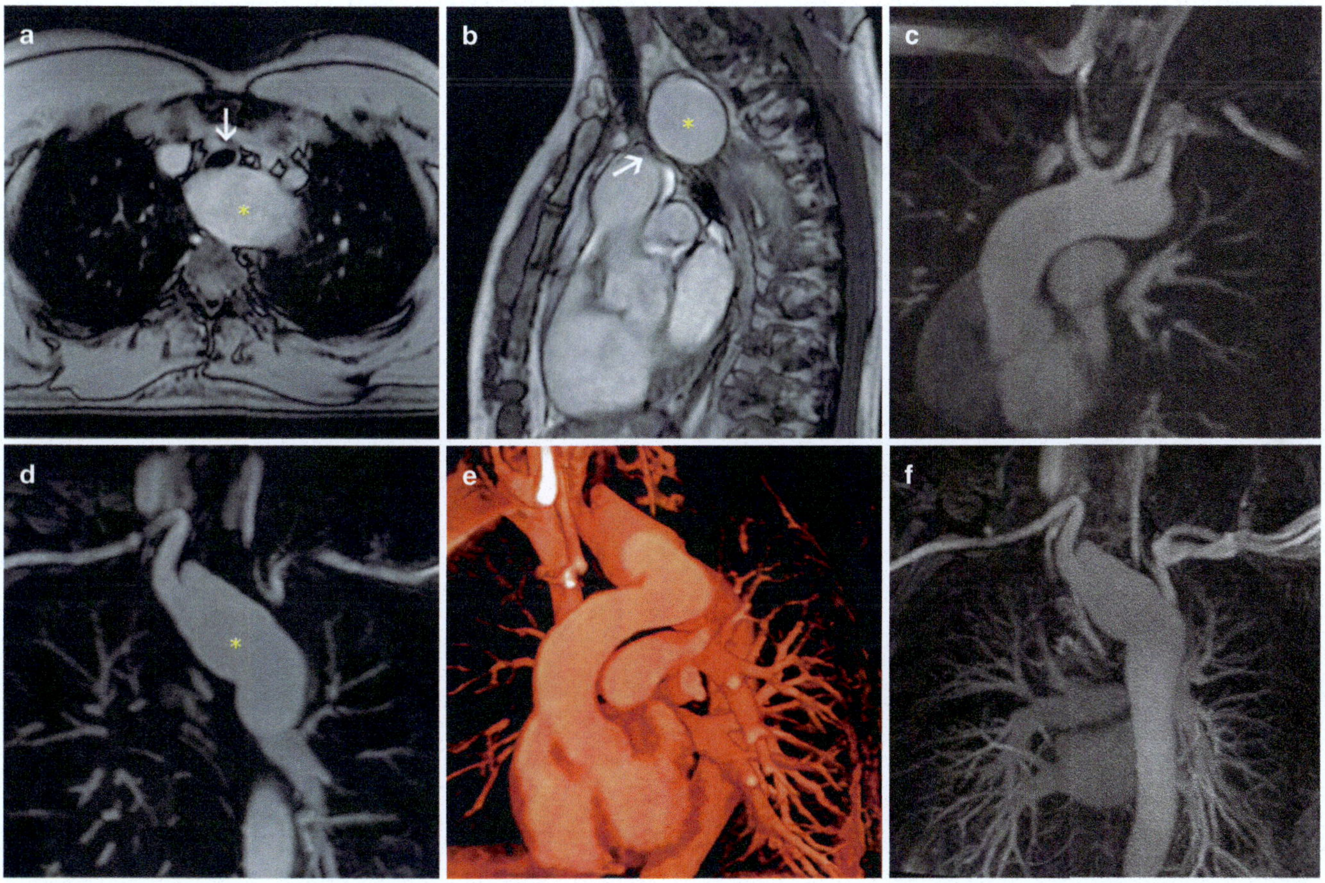

Findings and Interpretation

- Magnetic resonance imaging examination demonstrates an aberrant right subclavian artery that arises as the last supra-aortic vessel, with Type 1 Kommerell diverticulum (KD).
- Axial LAVA post-gadolinium and sagittal FIESTA images (panels A, B) show the aberrant right subclavian artery with KD (maximum diameter of 42 mm), crossing the midline with a retro-esophageal tract (asterisk). It causes anterior displacement and mild tracheoesophageal compression.
- Thin slab coronal MIP images at the level of the aortic arch (panels C, D) illustrate a bovine arch and the aberrant right subclavian artery that emanates most distally from the dorsal side of the aortic arch with an outpouching at the origin (asterisk).
- Volume rending and MIP images (panels E, F) show the left-sided aortic arch with the incomplete vascular ring and KD.
- Aberrant right subclavian artery constitutes the most common of the vascular rings, with an incidence of 1–2%. Its association with KD has been reported in the literature

to be present in 20–60% of individuals with an aberrant subclavian artery.

- KD is considered to be a remnant of the distal portion of the embryonic right aortic arch. In general, it is asymptomatic, but it can cause associated symptoms secondary to tracheal and esophageal compression.
- Current recommendations include elective treatment of diverticula measuring more than 3 cm, due to its highest risk of rupture.
- Salomonowitz et al. classified aortic diverticula into three types:
  - Type 1: Diverticulum associated with left aortic arch with aberrant right subclavian artery
  - Type 2: Diverticulum associated with right aortic arch with aberrant left subclavian artery
  - Type 3: Diverticulum arising from the isthmus of the thoracic aorta not associated with the subclavian artery (non-Kommerell diverticulum)

Further Reading

Fisher RG, Whigham CJ, Trinh C. Diverticula of Kommerell and aberrant subclavian arteries complicated by aneurysms. Cardiovasc Intervent Radiol. 2005;28:553–60.

Kanabuchi K, Noguchi N, Kondo T. Vascular tracheobronchial compression syndrome in adults: a review. Tokai J Exp Clin Med. 2011;36:106–11.

Lv P, Lin J, Zhang W, Hu J. Computed tomography findings of Kommerell diverticulum. Can Assoc Radiol J. 2014;65:321–6.

Salomonowitz E, Edwards JE, Hunter DW, Castaneda-Zuniga WR, Lund G, Cragg AH, et al. The three types of aortic diverticula. AJR Am J Roentgenol. 1984;142:673–9.

Tanaka A, Milner R, Ota T. Kommerell's diverticulum in the current era: a comprehensive review. Gen Thorac Cardiovasc Surg. 2015;63:245–59.

Case 181

Aberrant Right Subclavian Artery

Clinical History

- Eighty-seven-year-old female.
- History of recent loss of appetite and some weight loss. An ultrasound scan showed a 4.2 cm abdominal aortic aneurysm. No other significant abdominal abnormalities were found.
- Past medical history included controlled hypertension, diabetes, and mixed dyslipidemia.
- No respiratory or other gastrointestinal symptoms were present.
- The patient was referred for thoracic computed tomography (CT) angiography to exclude thoracic aortic aneurysm.

Images

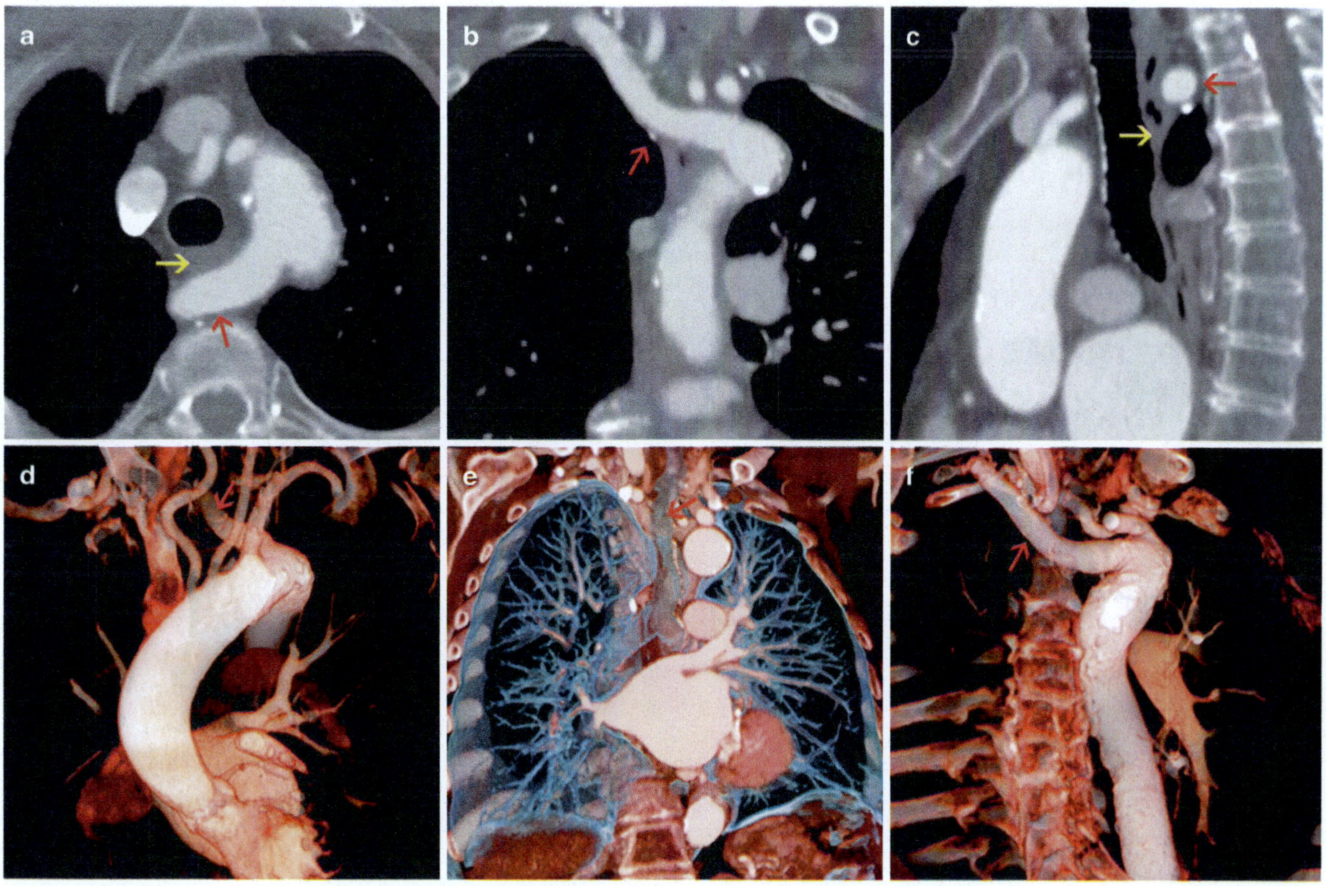

Findings and Interpretation

- CT angiography of the aorta shows a congenital anomaly of the aortic arch that constitutes an incomplete vascular ring.
- Axial, coronal, and sagittal multiplanar reconstructions (panels A–C) and 3D volume rendering images (panels D–F) show an independent origin for both common carotid arteries (first and second arch branches) from a left-sided aorta. The third arch branch is the left subclavian artery. This is followed by a fourth branch that corresponds to an aberrant right subclavian artery following a retro-esophageal path (arrow). Although imaging shows mild external compression of the esophagus (yellow arrow), the patient was asymptomatic.
- Three-dimensional volume rendering images and anterior (panel E) and posterior view (panel F) clearly demonstrate a left-sided aortic arch and the presence of a fourth branch that corresponds to an aberrant right subclavian artery (red arrow). Note in panel E that the aberrant artery is crossing behind the trachea.
- Vascular rings are rare congenital malformations of the aortic arch due to developmental failure of the embryological

aortic arches, representing less than 1% of all cardiovascular congenital malformations. Diagnosis usually occurs in early life, but when compression of the esophagus and/or the trachea is absent or nonsignificant, they can be asymptomatic and incidentally found on unrelated screening exams.

- The most common of the vascular rings is the left aortic arch with an aberrant right subclavian, with an incidence of 1–2%. This anomaly results from interruption of the dorsal segment of the right arch between the right carotid artery and right subclavian artery with regression of the right ductus arteriosus in the developing double aortic arch. The aberrant right subclavian artery arises from the descending aorta as a last branch and crosses the mediastinum from left to right. In 20–60% of cases, an aortic diverticulum (Kommerell diverticulum) may be present at the origin of this vessel.
- CT angiography gives excellent image and accurate preoperative evaluation of the vascular anatomy and its relationship to the trachea and esophagus.

Further Reading

Bonnard A, et al. Vascular ring abnormalities: a retrospective study of 62 cases. J Pediatr Surg. 2003;38:539–43.

Fenández-Tena A, Martínez-González C. Double aortic arch diagnosed in a 44-year-old woman with recurring respiratory infections. Respir Med Case Rep. 2017;20:176–8.

Kanabuchi K, Noguchi N, Kondo T. Vascular tracheobronchial compression syndrome in adults: a review. Tokai J Exp Clin Med. 2011;36:106–11.

Case 182

Aberrant Right Subclavian Artery

Clinical History

- Sixty-four-year-old male.
- Coronary risk factor: hypertension.
- During a routine echocardiogram, a dilated ascending aorta was identified (aortic root, 51 mm; tubular portion, 46 mm). No evidence of aortic regurgitation was detected.
- Referred for aortic computed tomography (CT) angiography for further assessment.

Images

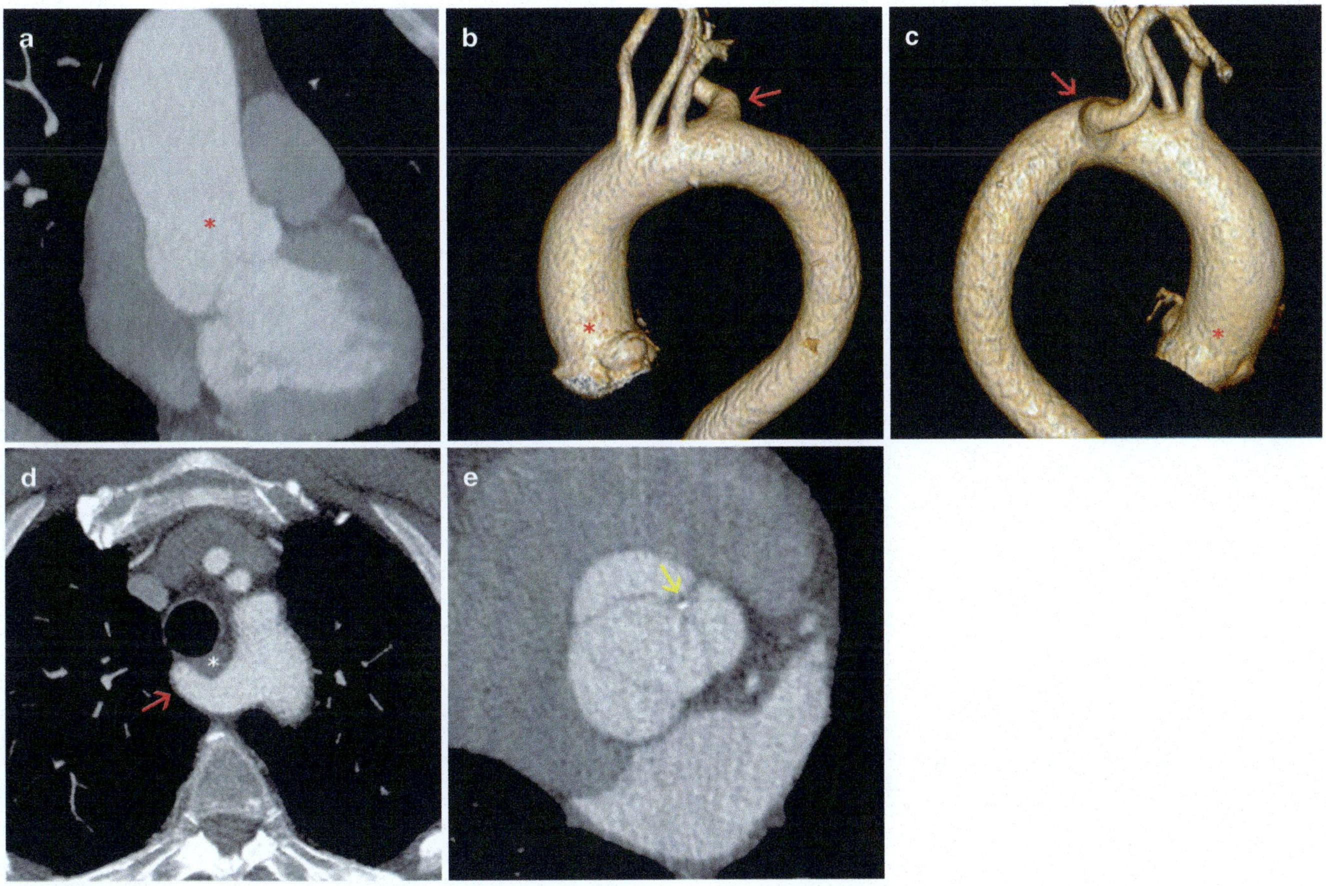

Findings and Interpretation

- Gated CT angiography of the thoracic aorta confirmed a diffusely dilated ascending aorta, comprising the aortic root (50 mm), sinotubular junction (44 mm), and tubular portion (45 mm).
- This is shown using coronal maximum intensity projections (panel A) and volume rendering reconstructions (panels B and C). Red asterisks indicate the dilated aortic root.
- No evidence or aortic atherosclerosis was found.
- An aberrant right subclavian artery was also identified (red arrows in panels B, C, and D). A high, thick-slab axial view is particularly useful in this case to evaluate the relationship between this structure and the esophagus/trachea (asterisk). In this patient, the aberrant right subclavian artery has a retro-esophageal course.
- Using systolic reconstructions (the most accurate for estimating the maximum aortic dimensions), a bicuspid aortic valve is identified, with and minimally calcified raphe between the left and right cusps (panel E). There is no restriction to valve opening, and the non-coronary cusp is the largest, being this the most frequent finding in type 1 form.
- Bicuspid aortic valve is the most common congenital cardiac anomaly (1–2% of the population) and comprises different phenotypes that can have from none or mild to

severe effects over the valve function. The most common classification of bicuspid aortic valve is based on the number of raphes (type 0, purely bicuspid aortic valve without raphe; type 1, valve with 1 raphe; and type 2, valve with 2 raphes).

- Notably, only 7% of patients with bicuspid aortic valve have the type 0 variant, with no raphe.
- A large number of patients with bicuspid aortic valve have dilated ascending aorta and are at increased risk of aortic dissection. Less frequently, aortic coarctation and other pathological findings can be identified in these patients. Given that progressive aortic dilatation commonly occurs, careful surveillance is recommended, until the surgical threshold for asymptomatic patients is reached (generally 55 mm).

Further Reading

Michałowska IM, Kruk M, Kwiatek P, et al. Aortic pathology in patients with bicuspid aortic valve assessed with computed tomography angiography. J Thorac Imaging. 2014;29:113–7.

Nistri S, Sorbo MD, Marin M, et al. Aortic root dilatation in young men with normally functioning bicuspid aortic valves. Heart. 1999;82:19–22.

Sievers HH, Schmidtke C. A classification system for the bicuspid aortic valve from 304 surgical specimens. J Thorac Cardiovasc Surg. 2007;133:1226–33.

Case 183

Annuloaortic Ectasia

Clinical History

- Fifty-seven-year-old male.
- Coronary risk factors: hypertension and obesity.
- During surveillance echocardiogram, a thoracic aorta aneurysm was detected.
- Referred for aortic computed tomography (CT) angiography for further assessment.

Images

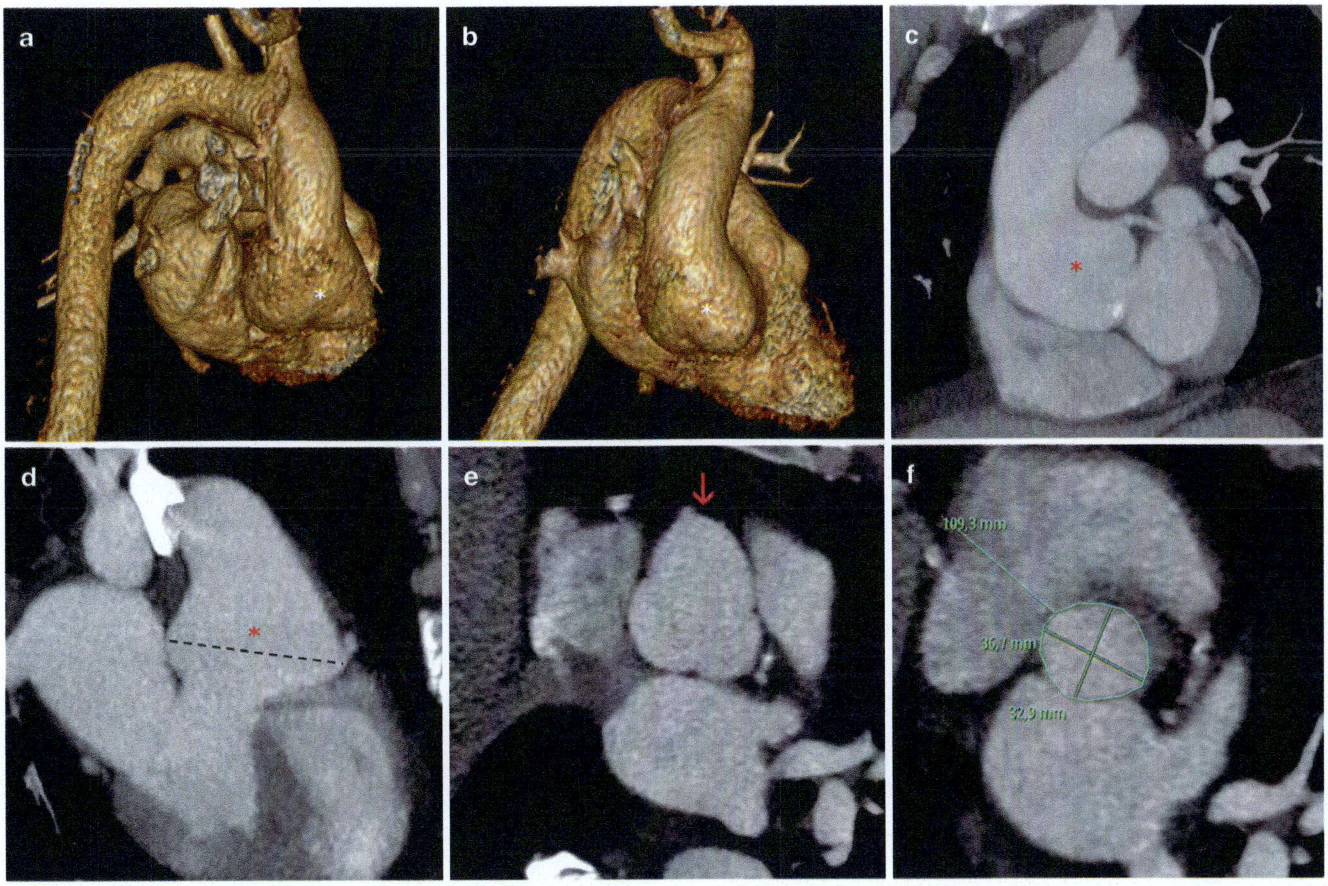

Findings and Interpretation

- Gated CT angiography of the thoracic aorta reveals aortic root aneurysm (asterisk), with a maximum diameter of 63 mm (dashed line). This is clearly depicted using volume rendering images (panels A and B) and thick-slab maximum intensity projections (panel C, oblique coronal view, and panel D, left ventricular outflow tract view).
- Of note, there is an asymmetric dilatation of the right sinus of Valsalva, as depicted using an orthogonal view (red arrow in panel E).
- The aortic annulus is dilated (33 mm × 37 mm, panel F) and has a relatively circular shape (it has lost the physiological oval shape).
- The aortic valve has three cusps, ruling out bicuspid valve as the underlying etiology. No aortic atherosclerosis is detected, and the remaining thoracic and abdominal aorta have a normal size.
- Annuloaortic ectasia is a rare entity, commonly related to connective tissue disorders such as Marfan and Ehlers-Danlos syndrome.
- These patients are at high risk of aortic dissection and rupture.

Further Reading

Evangelista A. Bicuspid aortic valve and aortic root disease. Curr Cardiol Rep. 2011;13:234–41.

Hofmann NP, Abdel-Aty H, Siebert S, et al. Giant dilatation of the right coronary aortic bulb with compression of the right ventricular outflow tract mimicking a ventricular septal defect: diagnostic workup using echocardiography, heart catheterization, and cardiac computed tomography. Case Rep Med. 2012;2012:524526.

Case 184

Saccular Aortic Aneurysm

Clinical History

- Sixty-seven-year-old male.
- Coronary risk factor: diabetes.
- He has a history of papillary thyroid cancer 2 years before.
- During surveillance, an aortic arch aneurysm was identified.
- Referred for aortic computed tomography (CT) angiography for further assessment.

Images

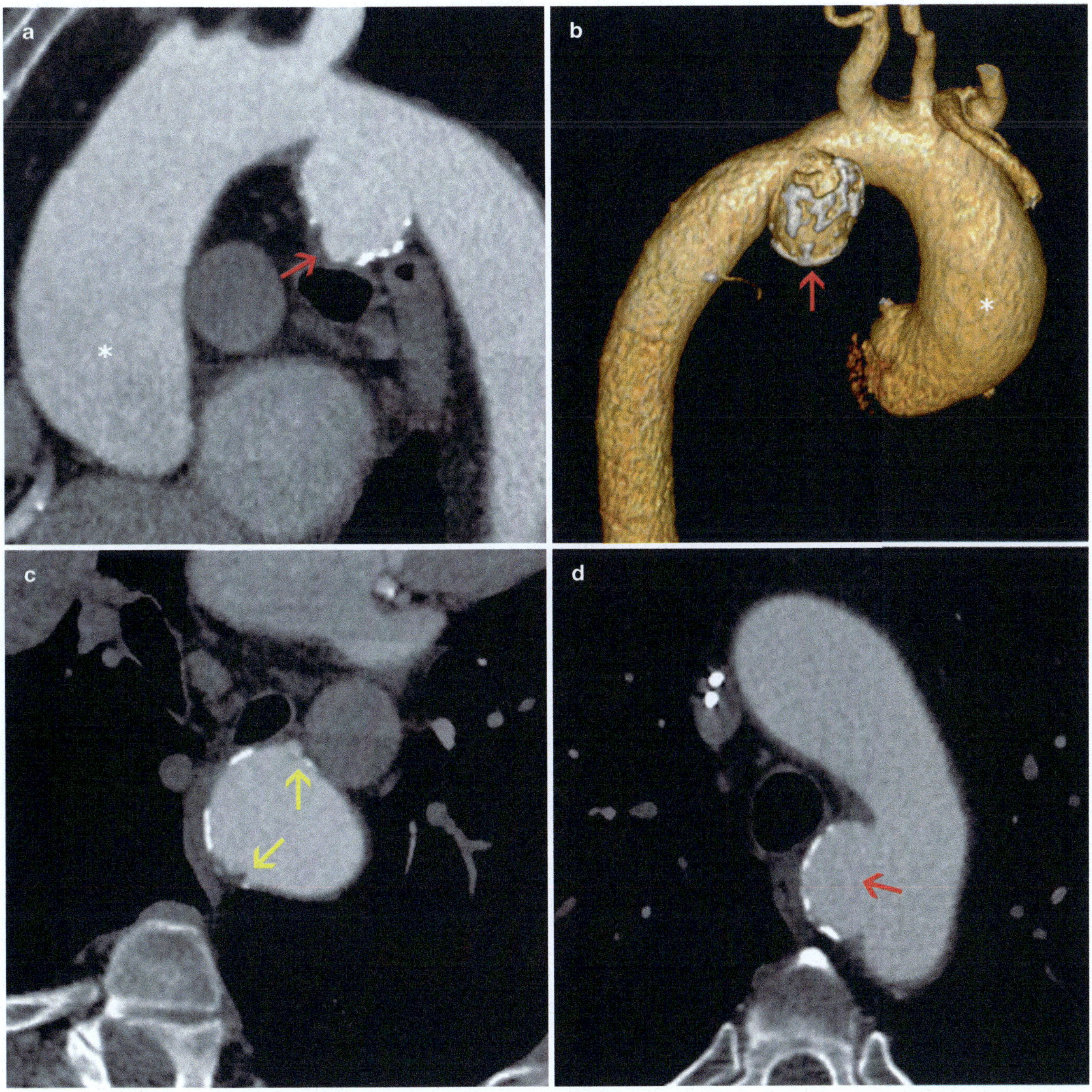

Findings and Interpretation

- Gated CT angiography of the thoracic aorta denotes a dilated ascending aorta (asterisk in panels A and B), with a maximum diameter of 45 mm.
- In addition, a saccular aortic aneurysm is observed at the aortic isthmus (red arrow), with peripheral calcification (yellow arrow) and a maximum diameter of 45 mm (panels A–D).
- Although the discrimination between true and false (pseudoaneurysm) is not easily defined with noninvasive imaging tools, the characteristics of the sac, the presence of normal proximal and distal references, and the identification of focal sites of vessel injury at the saccular neck suggest that this might possibly correspond to an aortic pseudoaneurysm/false aneurysm.

Further Reading

Craviari C, Taggart NW, Cetta F, Hagler DJ, Bower TC, Mauriello DA, Johnson JN. Percutaneous treatment of a complex saccular aortic pseudoaneurysm with covered stenting after subclavian artery translocation. JACC Cardiovasc Interv. 2014;7:e23–4.

Case 185

Descending Aorta Aneurysm

Clinical History

- Seventy-four-year-old male
- Clinical history of controlled arterial hypertension and stable long-standing rheumatoid arthritis
- Incidental diagnosis of a smooth posterior mediastinal lesion with silhouetting of the descending aorta on non-enhanced computed tomography (CT) of the thorax ordered to rule out interstitial lung disease in the clinical setting of shortness of breath and a dry cough.
- Referred for thoracic and abdominal CT angiography to rule out aortic disease

Images

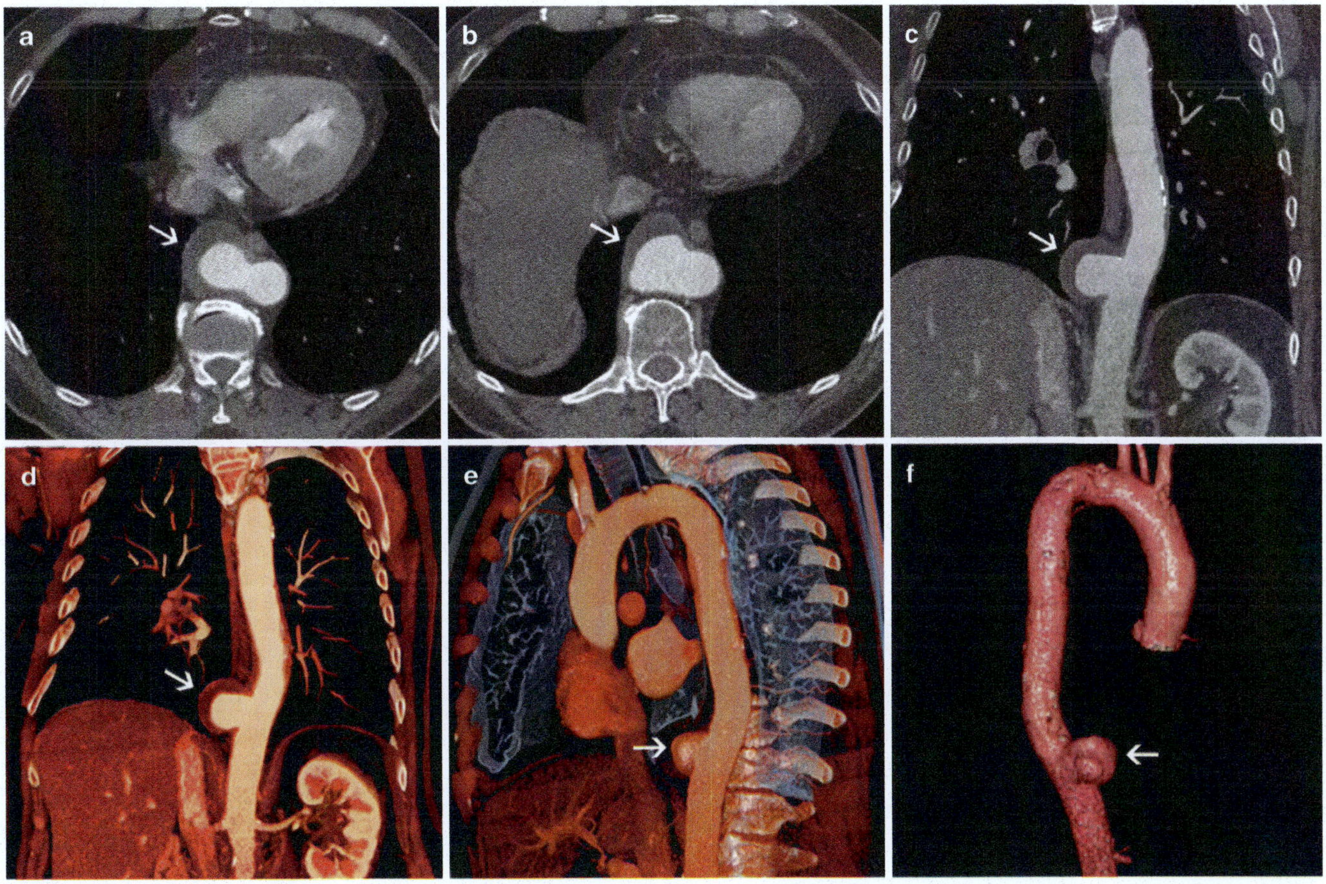

Findings and Interpretation

- CT angiography of the aorta demonstrates mild atherosclerotic aortic disease and the presence of a saccular aneurysm in the distal portion of the descending aorta just above the diaphragm.
- Axial CT images (panels A, B) and coronal multiplanar reconstruction (panel C) show the presence of a saccular aneurysm about 45 mm in diameter with mural thrombus. It determines anterior displacement, without compression, of the adjacent esophagus.
- Coronal slab, left coronal oblique, and right coronal oblique volume rendering views (panels D–F) illustrate a round, localized outpouching of the aortic wall corresponding to a saccular aortic aneurysm.

- Definition of an aortic aneurysm comprises a permanent localized dilatation of the vessel, with at least a 50% increase in the expected normal diameter. The normal diameter of the mid-distal descending aorta in adults varies according to age and sex, and it should not be greater than 3 cm. Descending thoracic aorta aneurysms approximately represent one-third of all aortic aneurysms, being atherosclerosis the most frequent underlying cause. Nevertheless, saccular aneurysms may be secondary to other etiologies including penetrating atherosclerotic ulcer, vasculitis, trauma, and iatrogenic (procedure-related) causes.
- CT angiography allows detailed anatomical assessment, being an excellent imaging test for evaluation of the size and shape of an aortic aneurysm.

Further Reading

Kucukarslan N, Ozal E, Temizkan V, Tatar H. Diagnostic and surgical approach to a descending thoracic aorta saccular aneurysm case. J Card Surg. 2007;22:142–4.

Shang EK, Nathan DP, Boonn WW, Lys-Dobradin IA, Fairman RM, Woo EY, et al. A modern experience with saccular aortic aneurysms. J Vasc Surg. 2013;57:84–8.

Taylor BV, Kalman PG. Saccular aortic aneurysms. Ann Vasc Surg. 1999;13:555–9.

Case 186

Shaggy Aorta

Clinical History

- Sixty-seven-year-old male.
- History of controlled hypertension. No diabetes, dyslipidemia, or obesity.
- Incidental diagnosis of abdominal aortic aneurysm found on abdominal ultrasound indicated for left upper abdominal pain.
- Referred for thoracic and abdominal computed tomography (CT) angiography for a complete pretreatment imaging assessment.

Images

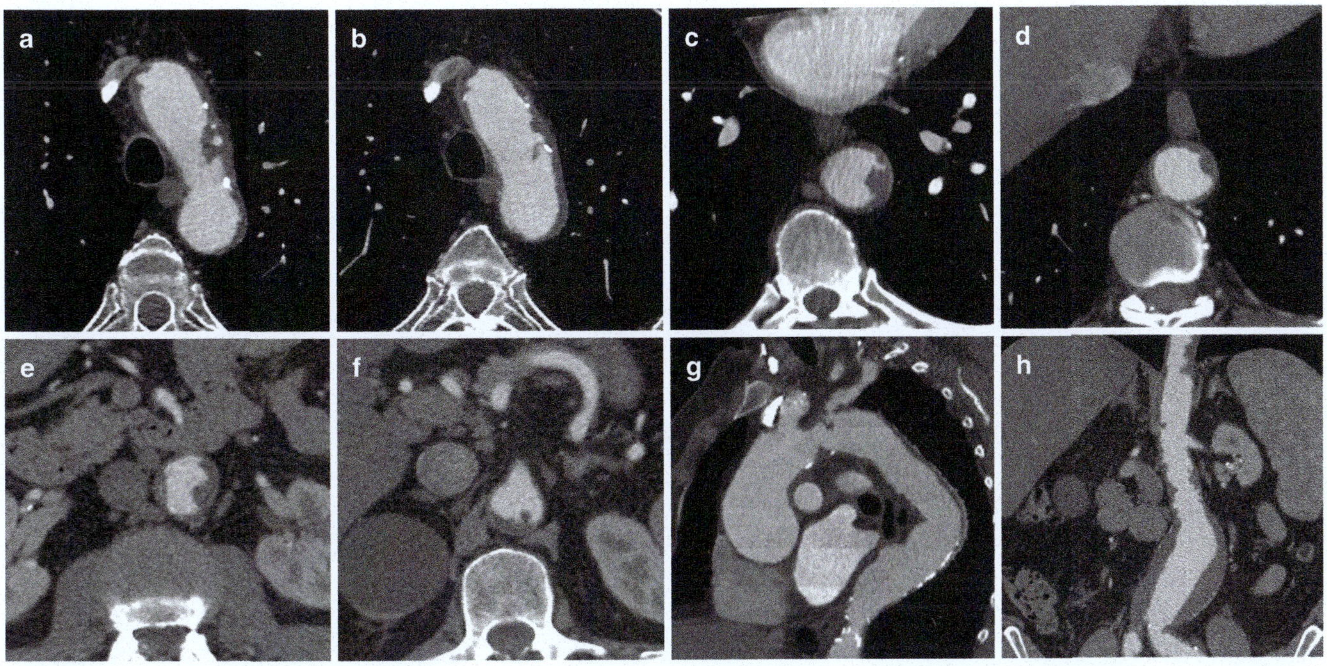

Findings and Interpretation

- CT angiography of the aorta shows extensive, irregular thrombi in the aorta and the presence of a fusiform infrarenal abdominal aortic aneurysm with mural thrombus.
- Axial CT images (panels A–F) and sagittal and coronal multiplanar reconstructions (panels G and H) demonstrate extensive and diffuse, complex aortic plaques in the aortic arch and descending and abdominal aorta. The atheromatous plaque thickness is greater than 4 mm, with presence of (mobile) atherosclerotic aortic debris in the aortic arch lumen.
- The shaggy aorta syndrome is a rare condition. It refers to a severe arterial degeneration of the aorta involving >75% of the length of the aorta, and it is characterized by both, diffuse, irregularly shaped ulcerated atheromatous plaques that can break off, and clinically evident and repeated embolic episodes that can cause cerebral, peripheral, renal, and visceral ischemia.
- CT angiography allows detailed anatomical assessment with excellent spatial and temporal resolution, and it is considered an excellent imaging test for evaluation of the entire aorta, being the modality of choice for preoperative planning as it accurately delineates the size and shape of the abdominal aortic aneurysm and its relationship to branch arteries and the aortic bifurcation.
- In these patients, acknowledgment of the presence of irregular surface of the aortic lumen due to shaggy thrombus prior surgical or endovascular aortic aneurysm treatments helps to prevent undesired complications such as cholesterol and micro- or macro-embolization (shower embolism).

Further Reading

Fukuda I, Daitoku K, Minakawa M, Fukuda W. Shaggy and calcified aorta: surgical implications. Gen Thorac Cardiovasc Surg. 2013;61:301–13.

Kwon H, Han Y, Noh M, Gyo Gwon J, Cho Y-P, Kwon T-W. Impact of shaggy aorta in patients with abdominal aortic aneurysm following open or endovascular aneurysm repair. Eur J Vasc Endovasc Surg. 2016;52:613e9.

Case 187

Subtle-Discrete Dissection of the Ascending Aorta

Clinical History

- Forty-two-year-old male.
- The patient presented to the emergency room with dyspnea and acute anterior chest pain. Electrocardiogram results and troponin levels were normal. Transthoracic echocardiography showed a subtle limited intimal splitting tear at the aortic root. A discrete aortic dissection was suspected.
- Referred for computed tomography (CT) angiography of the aorta to confirm the diagnosis.

Images

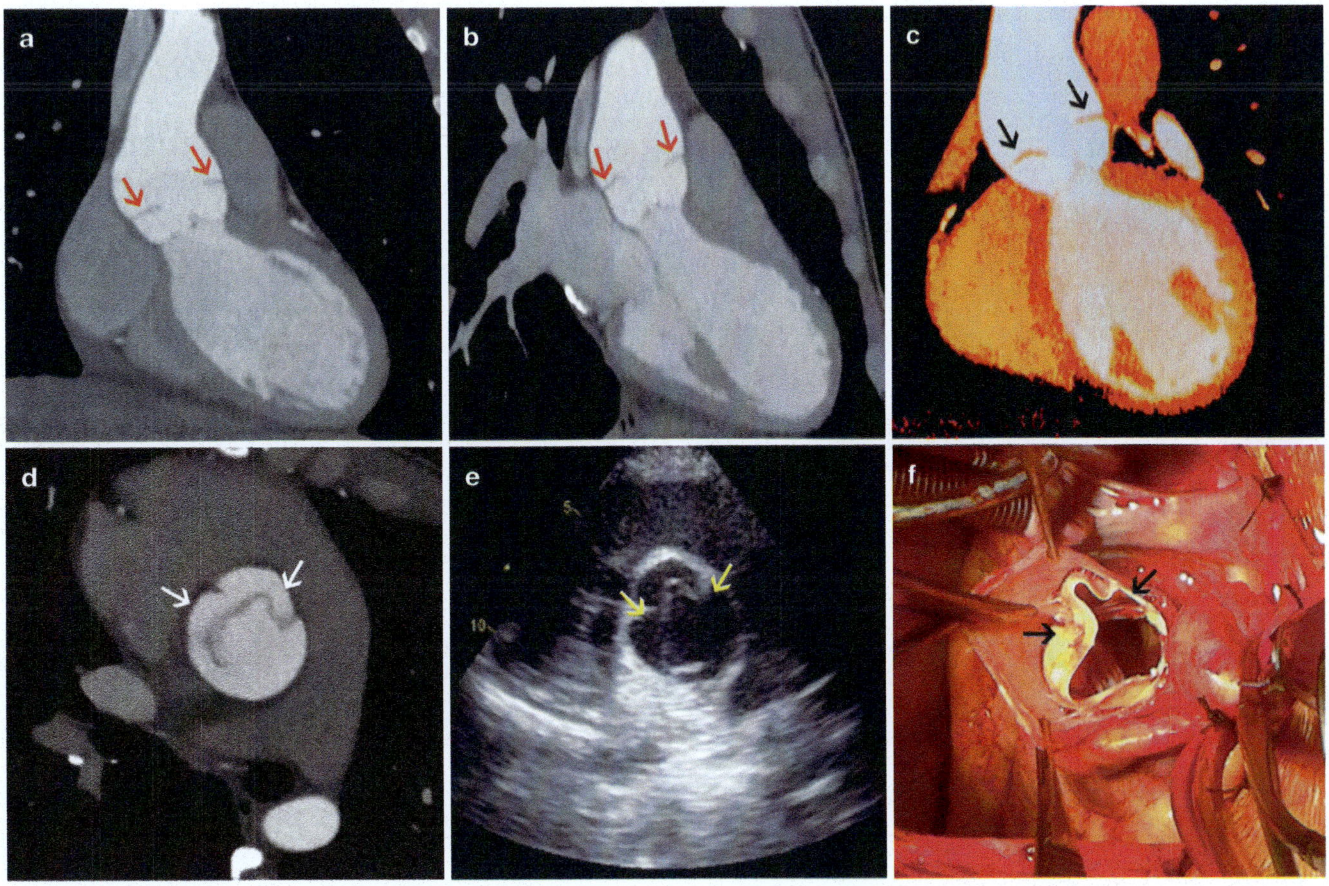

Findings and Interpretation

- A focal, discrete, aortic dissection at few millimeters from the aortic root that mimics a supra-aortic membrane (red arrows) is seen in these coronal and oblique coronal multiplanar reconstructions (panels A and B) and volume rendering coronal view (panel C).
- Correlation findings of the focal aortic dissection (arrows) at the level of the aortic root, seen on orthogonal CT image (panel D), transthoracic echocardiography (panel E), and surgery (panel F).
- A particular Type A aortic dissection that consists in a discrete, subtle aortic dissection (class 3 in the classification of the European Society of Cardiology) is the most neglected variant of aortic dissection; it is very rare and difficult to diagnose.

- It is placed generally at the posterior wall of the ascending aorta at 1–40 mm above the ostium of the main left coronary artery. Its length ranges from 2.8 to 12.3 mm.
- Classification of the European Society of Cardiology (ESC) includes:
  - Class 1: classical aortic dissection
  - Class 2: intramural hematoma
  - Class 3: subtle/discrete aortic dissection
  - Class 4: plaque rupture/ulceration
  - Class 5: iatrogenic/traumatic aortic dissection
- In comparison with typical aortic dissections, the focal dissection is associated with lower intra-surgery mortality, less hospitalization time, and less need of blood transfusion.

Further Reading

Chirillo F, Salvador L, Bacchion F, et al. Clinical and anatomical characteristics of subtle-discrete dissection of the ascending aorta. Am J Cardiol. 2007;100:1314–9.

Erbel R, Aboyans V, Boileau C, et al. 2014 ESC Guidelines on the diagnosis and treatment of aortic diseases: document covering acute and chronic aortic diseases of the thoracic and abdominal aorta of the adult. The Task Force for the Diagnosis and Treatment of Aortic Diseases of the European Society of Cardiology (ESC). Eur Heart J. 2014;35:2873–926.

Case 188

Type A Aortic Dissection

Clinical History

- Sixty-year-old male.
- Breathlessness and transient loss of consciousness. Neither chest nor back pain was present.
- Electrocardiogram demonstrated normal sinus rhythm.
- Posterioranterior chest X-ray showed widening of the mediastinum.
- Cardiovascular risk factor: controlled hypertension.
- Referred for thoracic computed tomography (CT) angiography.

Images

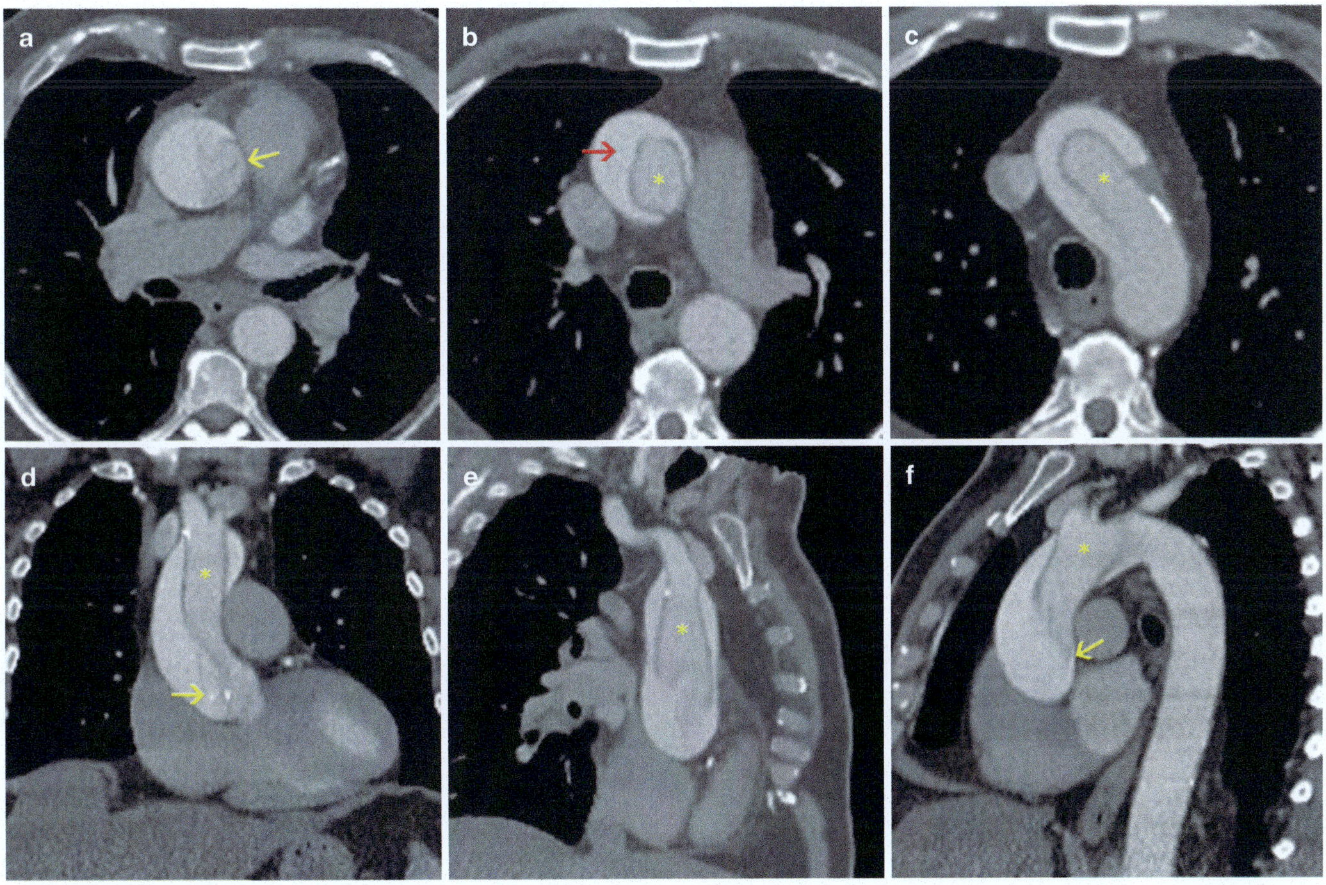

Findings and Interpretation

- CT angiography of atypical appearances of acute Stanford type A aortic dissection.
- Axial (panels A–C), coronal (panel D), sagittal (panel E), and sagittal oblique (panel F) images show atypical appearances of an aortic dissection. There is a circumferential dissection of the intimal layer (red arrow). The intima tears near the coronary orifices (yellow arrows) and an intimo-intimal intussusception between the true and false dissected lumens of the thoracic ascending aorta occur (asterisk).
- The density differences between the dissection lumens which taper distally give rise to a wind sock appearance. In almost all cases, the inner filiform shape lumen corresponds to the true lumen.
- Aortic dissection is the most common form of the acute aortic syndromes. In the majority of cases, it is secondary to spontaneous longitudinal separation of the aortic intima due to circulating blood, splitting the media of the aortic wall. In rare cases, there is a circumferential dissection of the intimal layer, resulting in an intimo-intimal intussusception

between the true and false dissected lumens (wind sock sign).

- Stanford type A aortic dissection involves the ascending thoracic aorta, and it accounts for 60–70% of cases. Type A dissections in almost all cases require urgent surgical intervention to prevent extension into the aortic root, pericardium, or coronary arteries. Non-treated type A dissections have a mortality rate of over 50% within 48 h.
- Early diagnosis is mandatory for improving the prognosis. Multidetector CT angiography allows early detection and classification of aortic dissection as well as recognition of any associated complications. Sensitivity and specificity of nearly 100% have been reported.

Further Reading

Castañer E, Andreu M, Gallardo X, Mata JM, Cabezuelo MA, Pallardó Y. CT in nontraumatic acute thoracic aortic disease: typical and atypical features and complications. Radiographics. 2003;23 Spec No:S93–110.

Karabulut N, Goodman LR, Olinger GN. CT diagnosis of an unusual aortic dissection with intimointimal intussusception: the wind sock sign. J Comput Assist Tomogr. 1998;22(5):692–3.

McMahon MA, Squirrell CA. Multidetector CT of aortic dissection: a pictorial review. Radiographics. 2010;30(2):445–60.

Case 189

Chronic Type B Aortic Dissection

Clinical History

- Fifty-six-year-old male.
- Mild upper back pain and symptoms of lower respiratory tract infection.
- Posteroanterior and lateral chest X-rays showed a prominent aortic knob and an enlarged, elongated thoracic descending aorta.
- Cardiovascular risk factors: hypertension, diabetes, and dyslipidemia.
- Past medical history indicates an abrupt, severe interscapular pain 9 months ago that disappeared shortly after 2 weeks. The patient did not attend the medical consultation.
- Referred for thoracic computed tomography (CT) angiography.

Images

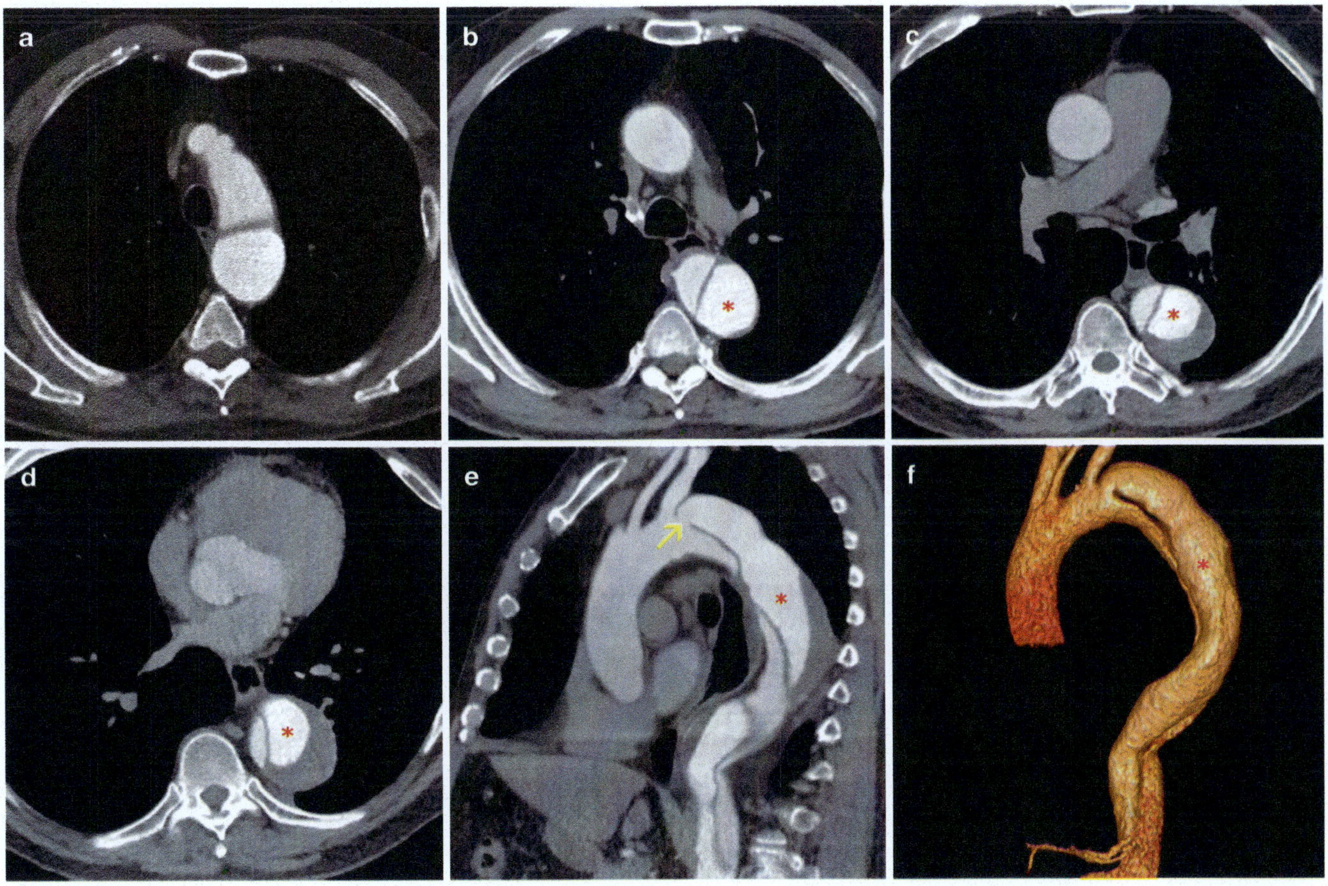

Findings and Interpretation

- CT angiography of the aorta shows chronic Stanford type B aortic dissection, associated with descending aortic aneurysm.
- Axial CT images obtained at different levels (panels A–D) show a Stanford type B aortic dissection that involves the descending thoracic aorta distal to the left subclavian artery. Sagittal multiplanar reconstruction (panel E) and three-dimensional sagittal view (panel F) demonstrate that the dissection flap arises just distal to the left subclavian artery (arrow). The descending thoracic aorta is dilated. The false lumen (asterisk) is larger than the true lumen, and it is partially thrombosed.
- Aortic dissection is the most common form of the acute aortic syndromes. It results from a spontaneous longitudinal separation of the aortic intima due to circulating blood, splitting the media of the aortic wall. The intimal tear permits blood to enter into the media from the vessel lumen, creating the false lumen.

- The type of dissection is determined by the site of origin of the intimal tear according to the Stanford classification system. Type A aortic dissection involves the ascending thoracic aorta and requires urgent surgical intervention, whereas in a type B dissection, the intimal tear is located distal to the left subclavian artery and can often be treated medically.
- CT angiography provides excellent image detail. It enables the diagnosis and classification of the aortic dissection and also the evaluation of its possible complications. Sensitivity and specificity of nearly 100% have been reported.
- The true lumen often is compressed by the false lumen and has a smaller size. The false lumen often has higher luminal pressures than the true lumen, a lower contrast density due to delayed opacification, and it may be partial or totally thrombosed in chronic stages.

Further Reading

Castañer E, Andreu M, Gallardo X, Mata JM, Cabezuelo MA, Pallardó Y. CT in nontraumatic acute thoracic aortic disease: typical and atypical features and complications. Radiographics. 2003;23 Spec No:S93–110.

Fattori R, Cao P, De Rango P, Czerny M, Evangelista A, Nienaber C, et al. Interdisciplinary expert consensus document on management of type B aortic dissection. J Am Coll Cardiol. 2013;61(16):1661–78.

McMahon MA, Squirrell CA. Multidetector CT of aortic dissection: a pictorial review. Radiographics. 2010;30(2):445–60.

Case 190

Intramural Hematoma

Clinical History

- Seventy-nine-year-old female.
- History of controlled hypertension and glucose intolerance.
- Moderate atypical "pleuritic-like" left interscapular back pain and symptoms of lower respiratory tract infection.
- Non-enhanced chest CT showed absence of lung parenchymal abnormalities, demonstrating mild left pleural effusion and the presence of aortic wall hyperattenuation in both the ascending and descending thoracic aorta.
- Referred for thoracic computed tomography (CT) angiography.

Images

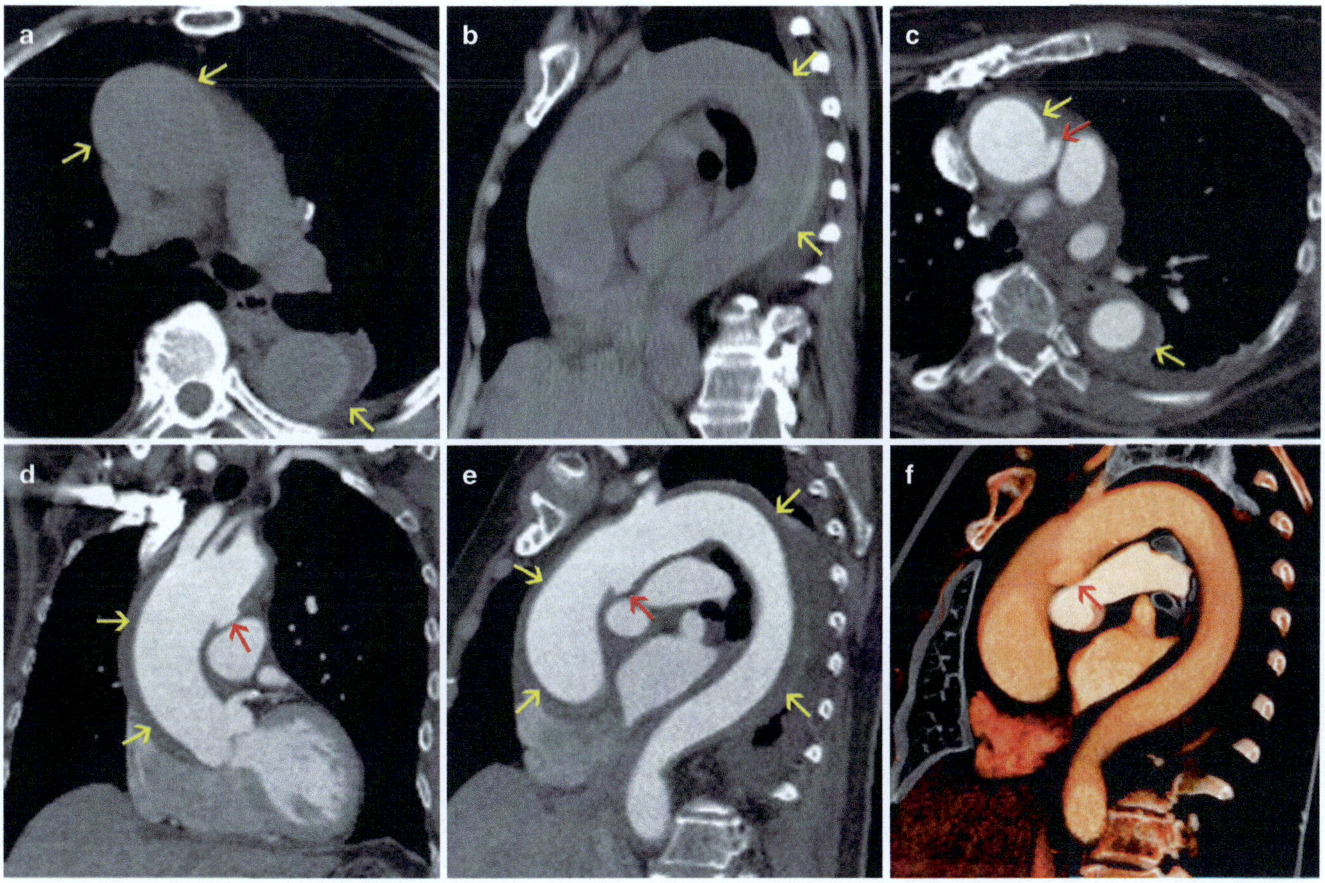

Findings and Interpretation

- Non-enhanced axial CT image (panel A) and sagittal multiplanar reconstruction (panel B) with mediastinal window show an area of hyperattenuating circular and crescentic thickening in both the ascending and descending thoracic aortic wall (arrows).
- CT angiography of the aorta shows Stanford type A aortic intramural hematoma (IMH), complicated by an ulcer-like projection (red arrow). Also a mild left pleural effusion is present (panel C).
- Contrast-enhanced axial CT image (panel C), coronal and sagittal multiplanar reconstructions (panels D and E), and sagittal 3D volume rendering image (panel F) show the presence of an ulcer-like projection (red arrow) at the level of the distal part of the ascending aorta, near its concavity. It is manifest as a localized contrast enhancement extending from the aortic lumen into the IMH with a visible communication. The aortic IMH (yellow arrows) is seen as a non-enhancing, smooth, region of aortic wall thickening. A decreased diameter of the aortic lumen is also observed.
- IMH is included in the spectrum of acute aortic syndromes, representing 6–20% of all cases. Classically considered as the result of ruptured vasa vasorum in the aortic

media, currently there is evidence of the presence of small intimo-medial tears ("microintimal tears") not visible at preoperative imaging that were found at surgery.

- As in aortic dissection, the type of IMH is determined by the location and extension of the thickening of the aortic wall, according to the Stanford classification system. Type A IMH involves the ascending thoracic aorta, whereas in a type B dissection, the IMH is located distal to the left subclavian artery.
- Natural history of IMH may vary between complete resorption of the hematoma to progression to classic aortic dissection due to intimal disruption, aortic aneurysm, or aortic rupture. The presence of ulcer-like projection is a poor prognostic indicator with increased risk for complications.
- On non-enhanced CT images, the crescentic hyperattenuation is better visualized using 5 mm reformatted images and narrow window (width, 200 HU; level, 40 HU). The density of the IMH varies according to the evolution time, being isoattenuating relative to the blood pool in subacute stages.
- CT angiography gives excellent image detail, being able to diagnose and classify the IMH and document the maximal aortic diameter, the thickness of the IMH, the transverse diameters of the aortic lumen, and the presence of ulcer-like projections, pericardial effusion, and periaortic hematoma.

Further Reading

Castañer E, Andreu M, Gallardo X, Mata JM, Cabezuelo MA, Pallardó Y. CT in nontraumatic acute thoracic aortic disease: typical and atypical features and complications. Radiographics. 2003;23 Spec No:S93–110.

Gutschow SE, Walker CM, Martínez-Jiménez S, Rosado-de-Christenson ML, Stowell J, Kunin JR. Emerging concepts in intramural hematoma imaging. Radiographics. 2016;36(3):660–74.

Lee YK, Seo JB, Jang YM, Do KH, Kim SS, Lee JS, et al. Acute and chronic complications of aortic intramural hematoma on follow-up computed tomography: incidence and predictor analysis. J Comput Assist Tomogr. 2007;31(3):435–40.

Case 191

Takayasu Arteritis

Clinical History

- Thirty-three-year-old woman.
- Past medical history of hospitalization for subarachnoid hemorrhage, secondary to posterior communicating artery aneurysm, with subsequent endovascular treatment.
- Currently with malaise, weakness, fatigue, and fever, presenting occasionally since she was 25 years old. At physical examination, a remarkable blood pressure discrepancy between the right and left arms was observed, as well as between radial and brachial pulses, being the left ones impalpable. Signs and symptoms of bilateral subclavian steal syndrome were present.
- In this clinical scenario of multiple vessels involvement, an autoimmune vascular syndrome was suspected.
- Referred for thoracoabdominal computed tomography (CT) angiography.

Images

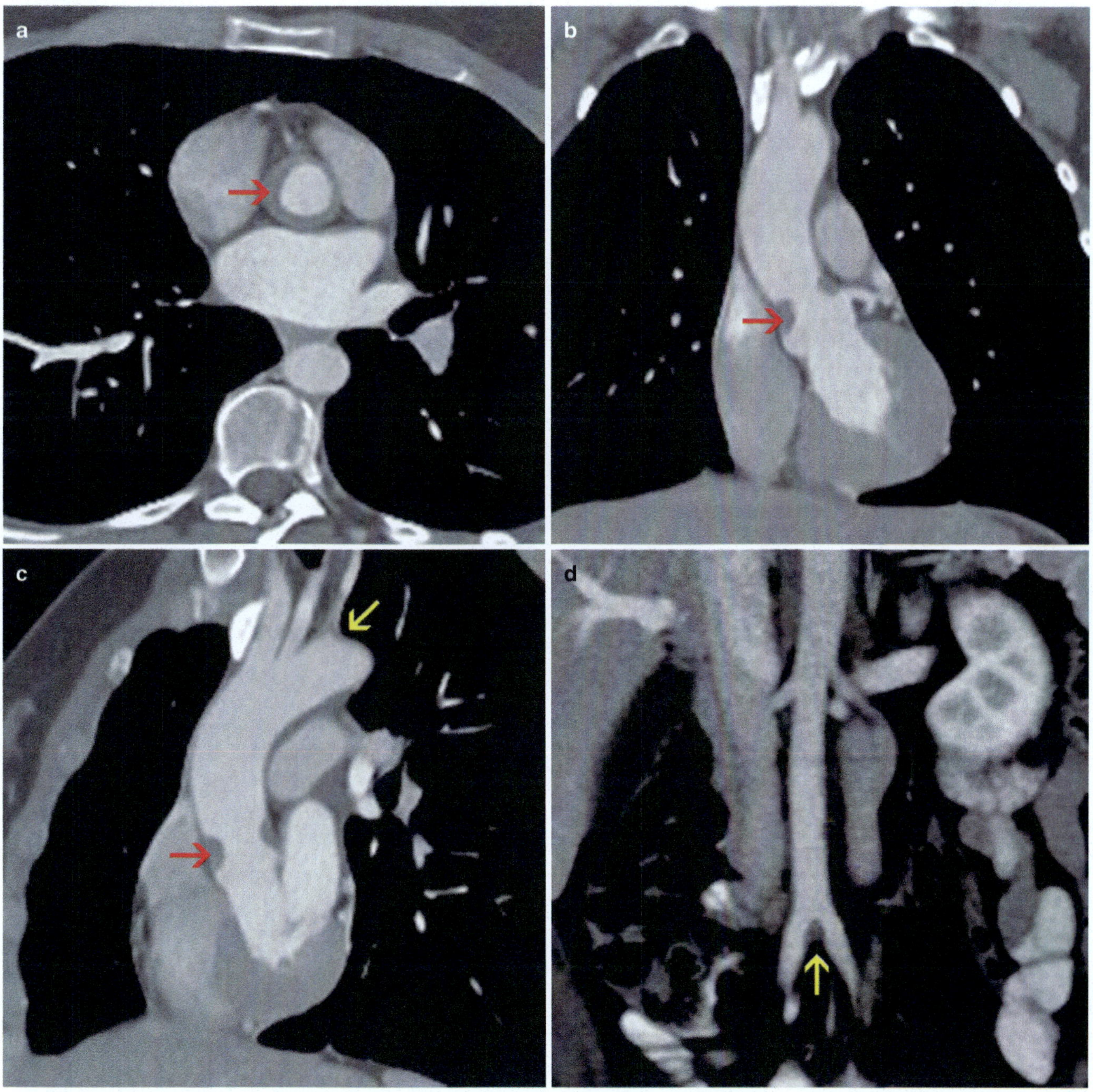

Findings and Interpretation

- Axial CT image (panel A), coronal (panel B), and left oblique (panel C) multiplanar reconstructions show a segmental concentric mural thickening in the ascending aorta at the sinotubular junction. It is located just above the origin of the coronary arteries, which are not compromised, generating mild aortic stenosis. In turn, severe obstruction at the level of the origin of the left subclavian artery secondary to circumferential mural thickening was also documented (yellow arrow in panel C).
- Coronal multiplanar reconstruction at the level of the abdominal aorta (panel D) depicts an asymmetric mural thickening of the infrarenal aorta and the aortoiliac bifurcation (arrow).
- CT angiographic findings show typical manifestations of type V Takayasu arteritis (TA).
- TA is a large vessel systemic granulomatous vasculitis primarily involving the aorta and its major branches. According to vessel involvement, proposed angiographic classification divides TA into five types:
  - Type I: only branches of the aortic arch
  - Type II: (a) ascending aorta and aortic arch and its branches and (b) plus thoracic descending aorta
  - Type III: thoracic descending aorta, abdominal aorta, and/or renal arteries
  - Type IV: only abdominal aorta and/or renal arteries
  - Type V: combined features of Types IIb and IV
- Central nervous system involvement as a clinical manifestation of the disease is seen in 20% of TA patients, being the intracranial aneurysms rare.
- Typical imaging finding for TA on CT images is a concentric mural thickening of the involved arteries; transmural calcification is seen in one of four cases. Such mural thickening may account for several millimeters and is associated with vascular stenosis in almost 90% of the cases. Less common, occlusion or aneurysm of the vessels can be found.
- On non-enhanced axial CT images, mural thickening is highly attenuated compared with the lumen, while on the venous phase CT images, it shows a double ring enhancement pattern, with a low attenuated inside ring (swollen intima) and a highly enhanced outside ring (active inflammation in the medial and adventitial layers).

Further Reading

Brunner, J, Feldman BM, Tyrrell PN, Kuemmerle-Deschner JB, Zimmerhackl LB, Gassner I, et al. Takayasu arteritis in children and adolescents. Rheumatology. 2010;49:1806–14.

Canyigit M, Peynircioglu B, Hazirolan T, Dagoglu MG, Cil BE, Haliloglu M, et al. Imaging characteristics of Takayasu arteritis. Cardiovasc Intervent Radiol. 2007;30:711–8.

Nastri MV, Baptista LP, Baroni RH, Blasbalg R, de Avila LF, Leite CC, et al. Gadolinium-enhanced three-dimensional MR angiography of Takayasu arteritis. Radiographics. 2004;24:773–86.

Zhu FP, Luo S, Wang ZJ, Jin ZY, Zhang LJ, Lu GM. Takayasu arteritis: imaging spectrum at multidetector CT angiography. Br J Radiol. 2012;85:e1282–92.

Case 192

Endovascular Treatment of Postcoarctation Repair Aneurysm Associated with Double Superior Vena Cava and Atrial Septal Aneurysm

Clinical History

- Seventy-year-old female.
- Asymptomatic.
- Past medical history indicates previous surgical repair of aortic coarctation (Dacron patch aortoplasty) at age of 25, without complications. Last cardiology follow-up was 8 years ago.
- A late postcoarctation repair aneurysm after surgical correction was diagnosed on follow-up computed tomography (CT) angiography.
- One month after endovascular repair of the postcoarctation repair aneurysm, the patient was referred to CT angiography for evaluating the endovascular device.

Images

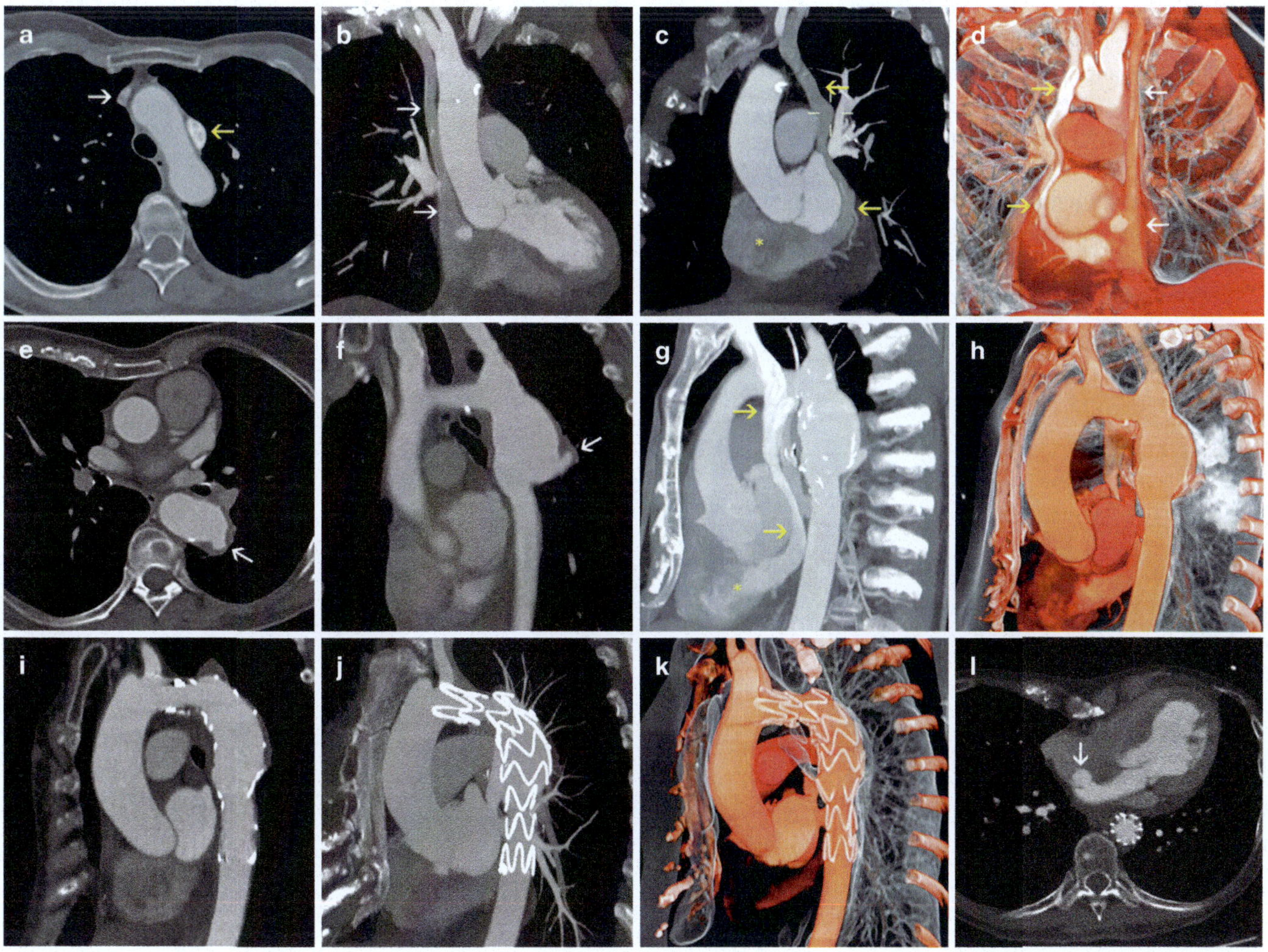

Findings and Interpretation

- Axial CT image (panel A), coronal oblique MPRs (panels B, C) and volume rendering image at posterior view (panel D) show the presence of double superior vena cava (SVC). Right SVC (white arrows) drains into the right atria. Persistent left SVC (yellow arrows) drains to a dilated coronary sinus (asterisk).
- Axial CT image (panel E) and sagittal MPR (panel F) show a postcoarctation repair aneurysm, with the presence of a focal outpouching of contrast into the atheroma in the inferior margin of the aneurism, typical of a penetrating atherosclerotic ulcer (arrow). Sagittal MIP (panel G) and volume rendering image (panel H) demonstrate the postcoarctation repair aneurysm and the persistent left SVC (arrows).

- Sagittal MPR (panel I), sagittal MIP (panel J), and sagittal volume rendering image (panel K) show endovascular repair of the postcoarctation repair aneurysm, without evidence of complications. Axial CT image (panel L) also shows an atrial septal aneurysm (arrow) and the presence of pectus excavatum.
- Coarctation of the aorta is a congenital cardiovascular malformation (CVM) that consists in a congenital narrowing of the thoracic aorta.
- All surgical repair options can be associated with postcoarctation repair aneurysms, being more common after Dacron patch aortoplasty, with reported incidences up to 90% during a follow-up period of more than 20 years. These secondary aneurysms are secondary to suture line disruption between a prosthetic patch and the aortic tissue. As the risk of rupture is increased in these cases, most patients require intervention.
- CVMs are exceptionally common, with an incidence of 0.5–0.7% of all live-born infants. Nearly 20% of infants born with a CVM have other noncardiac malformations or neurodevelopmental disorders. Coarctation of the aorta has been associated with other types of anomalies such as bicuspid aortic valve, tubular hypoplasia of aortic arch, atrial or ventricular septal defects, patent ductus arteriosus, left ventricular inflow/outflow obstruction, and transposition of the great arteries.
- It is common that more than one anomaly is present in these patients, as seen in this case. Duplication of superior vena cava is the most common thoracic venous congenital anomaly.
- Atrial septal aneurysm is a well-delimitated saccular deformity that protrudes to the right or the left atrium.

Further Reading

Abbruzzese PA, Aidala E. Aortic coarctation: an overview. J Cardiovasc Med (Hagerstown). 2007;8:123–8.

Pemberton J, Sahn DJ. Imaging of the aorta. Int J Cardiol. 2004;97 Suppl 1:53–60.

Szkutnik M, Sulik S, Fiszer R, Chodor B, Głowacki J, Bialkowski J. Native aortic coarctation stenting in patients ≥ 46 years old. Postepy Kardiol Interwencyjnej. 2017;13:302–6.

Walhout RJ, Braam RL, Schepens MA, Mulder BJ, Plokker HW. Aortic aneurysm formation following coarctation repair by Dacron patch aortoplasty. Neth Heart J. 2010;18:376–7.

Index

P. M. Carrascosa et al. (eds.), *Clinical Atlas of Cardiac and Aortic CT and MRI*, https://doi.org/10.1007/978-3-030-03682-9

D

E

The manufacturer's authorised representative in the EU is Springer Nature Customer Service Centre GmbH, Europaplatz 3, 69115 Heidelberg, Germany. If you have any concerns regarding our products, please contact ProductSafety@springernature.com

Printed and bound by CPI Group (UK) Ltd, Croydon, CR0 4YY
30/09/2026
02225269-0005